Dr Ante Bilić
liječnik - stomatolog

Ante Bilić

18.12.81

ORTHODONTICS

PRINCIPLES
AND PRACTICE

T. M. GRABER, D.D.S., M.S.D., Ph.D.

Director, Kenilworth Dental Research Foundation
Chairman, Orthodontics, University of Chicago

Third Edition

illustrated with 2150 figures

W. B. SAUNDERS COMPANY
Philadelphia · London · Toronto

W. B. Saunders Company: West Washington Square
Philadelphia, PA 19105

1 St. Anne's Road
Eastbourne, East Sussex BN21 3UN, England

1 Goldthorne Avenue
Toronto, Ontario M8Z 5T9, Canada

Listed here is the latest translated edition of this book together with
the language of the translation and the publisher.

Spanish (3rd Edition) — NEISA, Mexico 4, D.F., Mexico

Orthodontics — Principles and Practice   ISBN 0-7216-4182-2

Print No.:   18   17   16   15   14   13   12   11   10

Dedication

TO MY WIFE, DORIS

Whose example in thought and action
provides a continuing inspiration

Read not to contradict and confute,
nor to believe and take for granted
but to weigh and consider.

Francis Bacon

PREFACE

There are many indications that the orthodontic specialty per se cannot keep up with the need and demand for orthodontic services in this country. It is estimated that by 1975 there will be 40,000,000 children under 18 years of age, out of a total population of 225,000,000 in the United States. This represents a net increase each year of between 1.5 and 1.78 per cent of children generally considered to be of orthodontic age. If this population explosion is coupled with effective public health and patient education programs designed to extend dental services generally to a greater number of our citizens, it is obvious that it will be difficult to satisfy the demand made upon a relatively small number of orthodontists. At least part of the answer to this problem is the training of the *dental student* and *general dentist* in the recognition, prevention and interception of dental malocclusions.

Considerable confusion still exists over just what should be the scope of the dentist's activities in orthodontics. The Council on Orthodontic Education* of the American Association of Orthodontics recommends the following objectives as desirable and important in the training of the dentist so that he may better cope with the orthodontic problems that confront him. Specifically he should be able to:

1. anticipate and detect incipient malocclusion
2. provide preventive measures, where possible
3. recognize conditions which require advanced orthodontic diagnosis
4. understand the possibilities of comprehensive orthodontic treatment
5. use orthodontic principles as an adjunct to treatment procedures in all other phases of dental practice.

This book is intended to serve as a text for the dental student and a guide for the general practitioner of dentistry in managing those orthodontic problems and techniques with which the dentist must be prepared to deal. For the orthodontist this volume will be of value as a reference work. In particular, Chapter 2, Growth and Development, Chapter 3, Physiology of the Stomatognathic System,

---

*Orthodontics: Principles and Policies, Educational Requirements, Organizational Structure. St. Louis, American Association of Orthodontists, 1971.

and Chapter 10, Biomechanical Principles of Orthodontic Tooth Movement, contain collections of material not heretofore available in one place. The two-volume text, "Current Orthodontic Concepts and Techniques," published in 1969, relies strongly on the reader's having a thorough understanding of the background provided by this book, before attempting to comprehend and apply the various mechanotherapies described therein.

If the dental student studies this text thoroughly, he will surely recognize that the specialty of orthodontics demands training far beyond that possible in undergraduate courses. If he heeds the admonitions that are given again and again in conjunction with interceptive and limited corrective orthodontic procedures, he will avoid the pitfall of undertaking orthodontic correction beyond the scope of his training and experience. "Orthodontic sense" requires not only a broad background in general dentistry but also specialized orthodontic indoctrination and ample clinical experience. The general practitioner in medicine does not hesitate to obtain a consultation when a problem arises which a specialist might treat with greater competence. If we in dentistry will emulate this practice more, both the patient and the profession will benefit. There are undoubtedly problems that can be handled by general practitioner and specialist together, with periodic specialist guidance to augment routine therapeutic measures by the general dentist.

This book is written to give the reader an understanding of craniofacial growth and development, the physiology of the stomatognathic system, the incidence, recognition, etiology and unfavorable sequelae of malocclusion and the biomechanical principles of orthodontic tooth movement.

By knowing how to take diagnostic records and understanding their importance, by being familiar with orthodontic appliances in general and by being able to handle cases that are under the guidance of an orthodontist, the dentist can render a higher level of dental service than would otherwise be possible. He can apply orthodontic principles to the broad spectrum of associated problems and render preventive, interceptive and limited corrective assistance. By first educating the patient and parents to the fact that dental service is not a one-shot affair, that it is a long-term and continuing sequence, and then by applying his knowledge, dedicated to the goal of the maintenance of a normal occlusion, the dentist is truly practicing preventive dentistry as an applied biologist.

Twenty-five years of teaching orthodontics to undergraduate and graduate dental students played a significant role in the development of subject matter and in the presentation of the material. More than 1400 student course appraisal questionnaires have been evaluated and suggestions and criticisms heeded wherever possible. Each preventive, interceptive and limited corrective technique described has been student-tested and modified to produce the best possible results with a minimum of teaching difficulty. The book is profusely illustrated because my teaching and lecturing experiences before dental and medical groups indicate that words cannot create the accurate mental picture that a visual impression imparts.

No textbook is a one-man job and this book is no exception. While most of the photographs were selected from my personally taken collection of over 45,000 illustrations, I have been privileged to draw also from the rich collections made by a number of outstanding men in the field. Credit is given under each illustration; I wish to express my gratitude for their significant contribution.

Photographs are important, but there are a number of them in this book that have been re-touched to better bring out their meaning and credit goes to

Sid Piel for his expert touch and re-touch. As far as the drawings are concerned, the majority were done by my associate, Tsuneo James Aoba. His great skill in drawing and the countless hours spent in reproducing technical material in intimate detail earn him a large share of the credit for the favorable reception the first two editions of this book have had. Kenji Shimizu was my fine research associate for the third edition, and an excellent artist. My son, Lee Graber, in between dental school and graduate orthodontics, spent a summer of intense reading and criticism, from the student's viewpoint. His help was invaluable, and the third edition should redound to his credit, if it is as improved as I think it is.

I particularly want to thank the many friends and colleagues for their sound advice and counsel, especially Warren Mayne. And I am deeply indebted to Coenraad Moorrees, and to Joe Jarabak, Don Woodside, Kaare Reitan, George Andreason, Harry Dougherty, Gene West, Bob Isaacson, and to many others for their perceptive critiques. I am grateful to my associates, Donn Chung and Santo Signorino, and to my research assistants, for invaluable help. My "office family" and "home family" had to tolerate me and my absenteeism during the arduous, yet provocative and most stimulating process of producing and revising this text. I thank them for the obvious sacrifices they have made.

T. M. GRABER

CONTENTS

chapter 1

DEVELOPMENT OF A CONCEPT

Christophe Francois Delabarre 1819

Orthodontics as a specialty dates back to the turn of the century. The year 1900 is arbitrarily selected as a date for the beginning of the oldest specialty of dentistry, because it was in that year that the Angle School of Orthodontia was founded in St. Louis and in the following year that the American Society of Orthodontists was formed. Angle's comprehensive textbook, *The Angle System of Regulation and Retention of the Teeth and Treatment of the Fractures of the Maxilla,* was in its fifth edition and in demand at this time.[1] A number of men who were to make significant contributions to the development of the science and art of orthodontics were starting to limit their practices to that specialty.

Weinberger[2] points out that there had been an awareness of unsightly appearance of "crooked teeth" many centuries before. It is mentioned in the writings of Hippocrates (460–377 B.C.), Aristotle (384–322 B.C.), and Celsus and Pliny, contemporaries of Christ. Celsus noted in 25 B.C. that teeth could be moved by finger pressure. The name of the specialty, "orthodontics," comes from two Greek words: "orthos," meaning right or correct, and "dons," meaning tooth. The term "orthodontia" was apparently used first by the Frenchman LeFoulon in 1839. Another Frenchman, Pierre Fauchard, often called the father of modern dentistry, is generally given the credit for the first comprehensive discussion of "regulating teeth." In his *Treatise on Dentistry,* published in 1728, Fauchard discusses the "bandelette," now called the expansion arch. Since Fauchard, many men have written about irregularities of the teeth. Such names as Hurlock, Hunter, Fox, Delabarre, Harris, Kingsley, Brown, Mortimer, Farrar and Talbot are associated with the development of orthodontics in the United States during the nineteenth century.[3] The publication of Angle's first edition in 1887 capped these contributions.[4] More than any other work at the time, Angle's text served to organize the existing knowledge of orthodontics. For the next 30 years he had a profound influence on the growth of what was to become dentistry's first recognized specialty. Almost as important were Calvin Case and Martin Dewey. The constant battles among Angle, Case and Dewey, in the contemporary literature and in and out of society meetings, only served to enhance interest in orthodontics and increase the dedication and devotion of their disciples. The Case-Dewey debates have

(Text continued on p. 5)

1

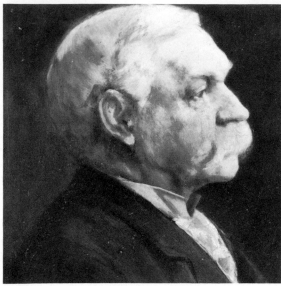

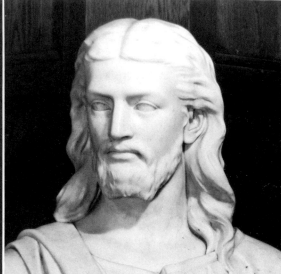

Norman Williams Kingsley
(self-portrait)
1829–1913

Bust of Christ (Kingsley)

"I regard him as orthodontia's greatest genius (Angle)."

Stockholm, New York, was the home of one of dentistry's greatest leaders. On October 2, 1829, Norman W. Kingsley was born. Until he was 19 years old he worked on his father's farm. When the family moved to Pennsylvania he entered the office of his uncle, Dr. A. W. Kingsley of Elizabeth, New Jersey (1849). In 1852 he opened his first office in Oswego, New York. Shortly afterward he moved to New York City.

Very early in his professional career Kingsley became interested in cleft palate rehabilitation. It was in this field that he was to make one of his greatest contributions. In 1859 he made his first obturator. For the rest of his professional career he devoted much of his time to helping the unfortunate victims of this congenital deformity. Through his great skill, Kingsley was able to restore normal speech for many of his cleft palate patients and to improve facial appearance with prosthetic restorations.

In 1865 Kingsley was one of the founders and served as the first dean of New York University College of Dentistry. He also helped organize several dental societies and held the highest offices in them. He received an honorary degree from the Baltimore College of Dental Surgery in 1871.

Kingsley was a prolific writer. Over 100 articles on cleft palate rehabilitation, the inadequacies of cleft palate surgery, obturators, orthodontic diagnosis and orthodontic appliances bear his name. His first book, *A Treatise on Oral Deformities As a Branch of Mechanical Surgery,* was published in 1880. A large number of the 350 illustrations were made by Kingsley himself, His chapters on cleft palate prostheses, the artificial replacement of missing parts and the external immobilization of fractures serve as a foundation for present-day knowledge. (Kingsley was no less skillful as sculptor. His bust of Christ is an example of his superb artistry.)

When Dr. Kingsley died in 1913 in Patterson, New Jersey, on the birthday of George Washington, the father of our country, many of his contemporaries felt that the father of modern orthodontics had passed away. Calvin S. Case wrote: "The longer orthodontia is practiced, the more respect the author has for the general teachings enunciated forty years ago and published in his inestimable text by that most ingenious man of his day, Dr. Norman W. Kingsley."

"Lover of art and nature, intimate friend of trees and flowers, but pre-eminently founder of the science of orthodontia, to which best thought of a life has been given in experiments and in tests."

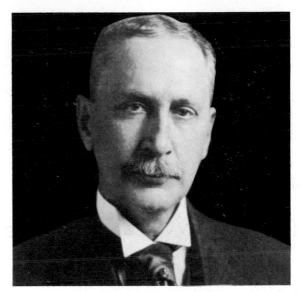

Edward H. Angle
1855–1930

This accolade made at the presentation of an honorary degree to Edward Hartley Angle at the Thomas W. Evans Institute in 1915 is a fitting tribute to a man who has done more than any other single person to organize and systematize our knowledge and to bring orthodontics to the high level it occupies as dentistry's first specialty.

Angle was born on June 1, 1855, in Herrick, Pennsylvania. After spending his childhood on the farm, he attended the Pennsylvania College of Dentistry and graduated in 1878. It was then that he started his first orthodontic case – on his preceptor's son. The problems that arose stimulated him to devote the rest of his life to orthodontics.[9]

Angle had to go west for his health, but later he returned to Minneapolis to teach and practice. He presented his first scientific paper in 1887, before the Ninth International Medical Congress. The first paperbound edition of his book on orthodontics was published the same year, and the last fully revised seventh edition appeared in 1907. This book has served as a reference source to more orthodontists for a longer time than any other volume. In 1892 Angle became Professor of Orthodontics at Northwestern University School of Dentistry and in 1895 he moved to St. Louis, assuming the same post first at Marion Sims Dental College and shortly afterward at Washington University Dental School.

It was in St. Louis in 1900 that Angle started his first school of orthodontics, independent from any university. From 1900 to 1928 Angle was active head of his school, first in St. Louis, later in New London, Connecticut, and finally in Pasadena, California. Over 150 men graduated from the Angle School of Orthodontia, beneficiaries of Angle's rich experience, unorthodox teaching methods and rigid and exacting discipline. From them came many of dentistry's greatest leaders. Under Angle's aegis, the American Society of Orthodontists was founded in 1901.

In addition to introducing the most universally used classification of malocclusion, Angle developed a number of appliances: the "E" arch, the pin and the tube appliance, the ribbon arch appliance and the edgewise appliance. His edgewise appliance is probably used more than any other fixed attachment today. The ribbon arch bracket has been refurbished and re-vamped, and now it is an integral part of the Begg technique. Thus, an overwhelming number of patients today wear appliances that were initially developed by Angle.

Though Angle died August 11, 1930, his influence is still felt very strongly in orthodontics. The entire orthodontic world now uses his classification of types of malocclusion. His excellent description of occlusion is hardly less important than his classification of malocclusion. His strong feelings against extraction of teeth as part of orthodontic therapy have served as a balance wheel against promiscuous tooth removal. His mechanical genius provided some of the most efficient appliances in use at present.

Even his enemies – and he made many of them in a lifetime of zealous endeavor to upgrade his specialty and to establish orthodontics as a separate specialty of medicine – recognized the many contributions made by Edward Hartley Angle. Characteristic of the man was a remark made shortly before he died: "I have finished my work. It is as perfect as I can make it."[8, 9]

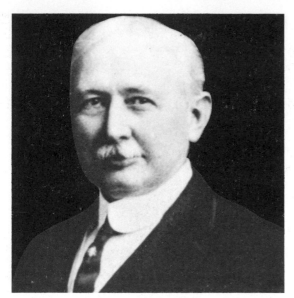

Calvin S. Case
1847–1923

"He waved the magic wand of hope across the deformed faces of little children, and wrought a miracle of symmetry and grace."

One of the great pioneers in orthodontics, Calvin Case, was born in Jackson, Michigan, on April 24, 1847. Following military service in the Civil War, he studied dentistry with Dr. John Stone of Jonesville, Michigan, and then went to the Ohio Dental College, where he graduated in 1871. After private practice in Jackson, he joined the faculty of the dental school of the University of Michigan. He studied medicine at the same time, graduating from the University of Michigan Medical School in 1884.

In 1890 Case moved to Kenilworth, Illinois, and became Professor of Prosthetics and Orthodontics at Chicago College of Dental Surgery. In 1896 he dropped his professorship of prosthetics, continuing in orthodontics only. He taught for the rest of his life. A prolific writer, Case wrote 123 articles in dental literature alone on orthodontic diagnosis, orthodontic appliances, problems of tooth movement, cleft palate and associated speech problems, and prosthetic restoration of normal speech and function. His textbook, *The Techniques and Principles of Dental Orthopedia,* published in 1908, was second only to Angle's text in popularity and influence in the dental profession. He, like Dewey, fought those who would fit all orthodontic procedures into the mold of a single appliance and an empiric philosophy. His most bitter battles were with Angle over the question of extraction of teeth. Case[6] wrote, "A careful study of the question of extraction which is so largely dependent upon causes, and which lies at the very foundation of the advanced dento-facial orthopedia, must convince every receptive truth-seeking mind of the delusiveness of a teaching which asserts the *universal applicability* of the 'normal occlusion theory'—which is: 'every tooth or its artificial substitute is necessary for the perfect correction of dental or dento-facial malocclusions' (Anglè)." Perhaps Case's major contribution, over and above his cephalometrics with plaster facial casts, was his attack on the dogma of Angle's concepts and the regimentation of therapy by the narrow use of the Angle classification of malocclusion.

Case was also a pioneer in orthodontic mechanotherapy. He was one of the first to stress the importance of root movement (1892); one of the first to use rubber elastics in treatment (1892); one of the first to use small gauge, light, resilient wires for tooth alignment (1917); and he pioneered the use of retainers to stabilize orthodontic results. Almost as great a contribution was his work in the field of cleft lip and cleft palate rehabilitation. He is regarded as the outstanding man of his time in the prosthetic aspect of rehabilitation of cleft palate deformities. The Case type of obturator still finds application in the treatment of certain types of clefts.

On his death, Dr. C. N. Johnson said, "Nature was kind to Calvin Case. She endowed him with a wondrous wealth of skill and art which made him the genius he was. He waved the magic wand of hope across the deformed faces of little children, and wrought a miracle of symmetry and grace. He reached down into the nethermost depths of disfigurement and despair, and raised the hopeless one into the dawning of a better day."[15]

been republished in the *American Journal of Orthodontics,* illustrating the fact that many of the problems facing the orthodontic pioneers are still very much with us, and still engender considerable controversy.[5-7]

ORTHODONTIC TRAINING

We would like to think that orthodontics has made tremendous strides as a part of dental education, and that, since it is the first *bona fide* dental specialty, with the second oldest qualifying board in all of medicine and dentistry, similar advances have been made in the dental curriculum. Because of the increasing emphasis on the biologic aspects of dentistry and because orthodontics is a foremost proponent of applied biology, it would be natural to assume that the subject occupies an important place in the dental curriculum. Unfortunately, this is not true. Frank Casto, in looking back over the development of orthodontics since the beginning of the twentieth century, analyzed the status of orthodontics at that time. A few of his observations are listed here.

1. The biologic problems were relegated to a place of secondary importance.
2. The study of occlusion was given but meager attention.
3. The extraction of teeth was generally recommended.
4. Prevention was largely ignored.
5. Treatment was seldom begun until after the full complement of teeth had erupted (except the third molars).
6. Esthetics was the primary object of treatment.
7. The mechanical phase was the most important and was given by far the greatest consideration.
8. Systems of treatment devised by individual men were being strongly promoted and recommended, usually to the exclusion of all other methods.
9. Orthodontia was given a small place in the curricula of schools of dentistry, and its teaching was considered of minor importance.
10. Many persons were attempting to correct malocclusions without having the least conception of the principles involved.[8]

This indictment is largely correct. Indeed, some observers would find most items embarrassingly contemporary in their application. Orthodontics then was considered part of the regular prosthetics course and accorded secondary consideration. This academic affiliation still exists in some areas of the world (Russia, for example) and indicates a primarily mechanical orientation of orthodontic philosophy and treatment procedures. In many of our own dental schools, prosthetics still maintains its stranglehold on hundreds of hours in the dental curriculum, while orthodontics is allotted a few hours here and there, among the "giants"—prosthetics, operative dentistry, crown and bridge, and so forth. Twenty to fifty hours of lecture in the entire undergraduate program are hardly adequate to qualify the budding dentist to perform even the bare minimum of orthodontic procedures. Many orthodontic departments meet a stone wall when trying to increase their allotted time.[11]

Unless dental school curriculum committees are prepared to provide adequate time and space for proper orthodontic training by reapportioning that which is allotted for prosthetics and operative dentistry, then Casto's last observation of many ill-trained and ill-qualified men performing orthodontic services will still be valid—70 years later! Currently, it seems that the setting up of so-called orthodontic societies, made up of general practitioners with inadequate dental school training in orthodontics, the creation of international

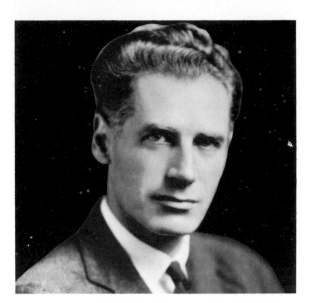

"Science knows no friendship."

Martin Dewey
1881–1933

Martin Dewey was born in 1881 near Kingman, Kansas, where his family had moved from Michigan after the Civil War. Graduating from Keokuk Dental College in 1902, Dewey attended one of the first classes of the Angle School of Orthodontia and joined the faculty of the school as a teacher until he and Dr. Angle came to a parting of the ways. During his time in St. Louis, Dr. Dewey earned his M.D. degree.

He then moved to Kansas City and conducted a private practice. He also taught at the Kansas City Dental School, wrote widely about the problems of orthodontics and earned quite a reputation as an outstanding lecturer. These were turbulent times in orthodontics, and Dewey's speaking ability and debating talent stood him in good stead. Angle's unalterable opposition to any form of extraction in orthodontic procedures and the antagonisms engendered over claims of superiority for various appliances frequently resulted in bitter wrangling in dental society meetings.

In 1915, with the help of Dr. C. V. Mosby, Dewey founded and became editor of the *International Journal of Orthodontia* (now the *American Journal of Orthodontics*), which has become the most complete record of orthodontic literature in existence.

The first session of the Dewey School of Orthodontia, a postgraduate school similar to that formed by Angle in 1900, was held in Kansas City in 1911. Dewey moved the school to Chicago and stayed there two years. When he moved again to New York in 1919, he re-established his orthodontic school there. Classes continued under Dewey's personal supervision until his death in 1933. When the American Board of Orthodontics was set up in 1929 (the second oldest specialty Board in Medicine and Dentistry, the first specialty Board in Dentistry), Dewey was one of the seven men chosen to serve.

Practical Orthodontics, a textbook on orthodontic philosophy and mechanical procedures, was first published by Dewey in 1914. Like the texts of Angle and Case, Dewey's book had wide acceptance both at the teaching level and in private practice. He also wrote a book on dental anatomy and collaborated with Alton Howard Thompson on a comparative anatomy volume. He published some 105 articles in dental and medical journals, covering a broad range of basic scientific and clinical orthodontic subjects. Through his lectures and writings, Dewey stressed the importance of a blend of the biologic and mechanical aspects of orthodontics. He was merciless in fighting for truth and against the empiricism of the day. Like Angle, Dewey stepped on many toes in his fight to elevate his chosen profession, but, as he once said, "science knows no friendship."

boards of orthodontics by general practitioners to "qualify" general practitioners, and the giving of courses in orthodontics by these same self-designated authorities are dubious signs of progress and poor substitutes for formal and comprehensive undergraduate training.[12, 13]

Fortunately, the development of orthodontics as a specialty has been more successful. Angle, recognizing the resistance to more orthodontics courses within the dental school curriculum, turned away from the dental school. He had written in 1899, "If orthodontia is to make any material progress, a separate school, entirely independent of dental schools, must be formed which would amply provide opportunity for those with aptitude and liking for the subject to study in a broad, thorough and comprehensive manner and where it would be relieved from all the blighting, handicapping influences which are necessarily thrown around it in dental colleges."[14]

Angle's school started in 1900 with an 8-week course. That he was successful in training and inspiring his students is shown by the fact that they included such men as Dewey, Noyes, Hellman, Ketcham, Mershon, Pollock, Casto, Weinberger, Hahn and Tweed, among others, who were to make great contributions in their own right during the next 30 years. Martin Dewey also set up a proprietary school outside the confines of the dental college, and graduates from the Dewey School of Orthodontia did much to bring the profession to its present status.

It was not until after World War I that orthodontics turned to the dental colleges for the training of specialists. At the time, the colleges themselves were affiliating with universities and only a few could accommodate the graduate and postgraduate demands for such training. Facilities were limited, faculty was scarce, and the number of students was relatively small. Before the start of World War II there were less than a dozen schools where students could receive bona fide graduate training culminating in an advanced degree. The type and caliber of instruction varied widely. Course length ranged from four months to two years and the number of students was quite limited. Coincident with public dental education and an increased public awareness of the scope and value of such service has been a rapid enlargement of university orthodontic training facilities since World War II. There is greater uniformity of course content, length and instruction. Some 400 orthodontists now complete their training each year. The number of orthodontists has more than doubled in less than 12 years. Orthodontic techniques have assumed integral roles in other phases of dentistry (pedodontics, periodontics, prosthetics, etc.). Interest in orthodontics among members of the general dental profession is at its highest level. The number of graduate students in orthodontics exceeds 10 per cent of the total number of dental students graduating each year. Thus, orthodontics is dentistry's oldest and largest specialty at present.

NEED FOR ORTHODONTIC SERVICES

Despite a decline in the precipitate rate of population increase since World War II, the number of prospective orthodontic patients has increased tremendously. According to the United States Census Bureau statistics of 1970, there are 25,000,000 children under five years of age, with a projected increase to 37,000,000 by 1985. In the 5- to 13-year age group, there are 37,000,000 children in 1972, with a similar rate of projected increase by 1985. In the 14- to 17-year age group, there are over 15,000,000 now, and it is estimated that there may be as many as 20,000,000 by 1985. Even with a conservative estimate of 20 per cent of all these children who could benefit from orthodontic guidance, the number of potential patients in the 5- to 13-year age group alone far exceeds the facilities and personnel available. If we combine the sobering figures of the total population with Medicare, Medicaid, child health legislation, dental insurance programs, and more effective public health and patient education programs, the

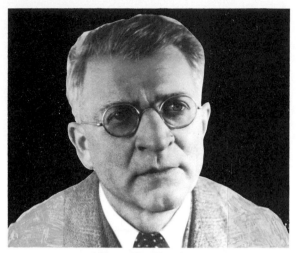

Albert H. Ketcham
1870–1935

"Above all, a feeling of biologic sense."

No list of orthodontics' great pioneers is complete without the name of Albert H. Ketcham. He was born on August 3, 1870, in Whiting, Vermont, and grew up in New England. He graduated from the Boston Dental School in 1892. Then he moved to Colorado because of ill health. When he had overcome the limitations imposed on him by tuberculosis he started a part-time practice in Meeker.

Inspired by the challenge of the young profession of orthodontics and aware of the tremendous potential of a health service whose benefits lasted for a lifetime, he entered the Angle School of Orthondontia in 1902. Thereafter he became one of orthodontics' most dedicated leaders. An inveterate reader and deep thinker with an inquiring mind, Ketcham explored many of the philosophical and mechanical problems and controversies that beset the profession in his day. Though he was a disciple of Angle at first, he questioned some of Angle's arbitrary pronouncements, causing Angle to attack him vehemently as a deviationist. Thereafter Ketcham was to travel the same road as Angle, but in his own inimitable way.

To raise professional standards, Ketcham worked diligently in the American Society of Orthodontists and served as its president in 1929. He was instrumental in founding the American Board of Orthodontics, which was incorporated in the State of Illinois in 1930, and served as its first president.

Completely objective, Ketcham reported his treatment results—both favorable and unfavorable—as they came. Because he was concerned over the possibly damaging consequences of mechanotherapy, he investigated the problem of root resorption. His study did much to alert the profession to the pathologic results of improperly guided treatment and to awaken a feeling of "biologic sense."

Always a teacher, he guided many men in the same meticulous manner as they sought training with him. From this grew the Ketcham Seminar (now the Denver Seminar), which is one of the profession's highlights each year. Orthodontics lost a great leader when Albert Ketcham passed away on December 5, 1935.

In recognition of his services to orthodontics, and in his honor, the American Board of Orthodontics established what is now considered the specialty's most coveted prize—the Albert H. Ketcham Memorial. This award is made annually in recognition of valuable contributions to the science and art of orthodontics. The award not only perpetuates the memory of a great leader in orthodontics, but also inspires those who follow to serve orthodontics with the same devotion and high purpose, the same adherence to objectivity and truth and the same love of service to mankind as were exemplified by Dr. Ketcham.

demand for orthodontic care certainly cannot be met by the approximately 7000 orthodontic specialists in the United States. Undoubtedly, the development of comprehensive auxiliary programs and the delegation of many of the professional responsibilities to the dental and orthodontic nurse will help, but part of the answer to this problem is the better training of general dentists in recognition, prevention and interception of dental malocclusions. Considerable con-

"Gentlemen, we are not arguing whether you or I am right, but what we wish to ascertain is the truth of the question before us."

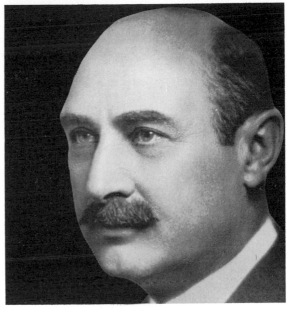

Milo Hellman
1872–1947

The above paraphrase of Socrates appeared in an editorial by Milo Hellman in 1911. Although he was a man of many sides— a talented musician, an esthete, a progressive and learned scholar—this short precept probably characterizes Milo Hellman's career better than any other.

Hellman was born on March 26, 1872, in Jassy, Rumania, and was an accomplished musician before emigrating to the United States in 1888. Because he was a superb flutist, Victor Herbert asked him to join the Pittsburgh Symphony Orchestra, even though he was only 16 years of age. By 1900, however, Hellman decided that he wanted a professional career and graduated *cum laude* from the University of Pennsylvania in 1905.

In 1908 Hellman was one of 12 men to take Angle's course in orthodontics. In this class were three others, Harry E. Kelsey, John Mershon and Frederick B. Noyes, who were to make their own marks in this specialty. The friendship of these men stimulated Hellman in his most formative and productive years. He joined the faculty as an instructor and helped Angle experiment with the new pin and tube appliance. Although he was to become a prolific contributor to orthodontic literature, the first paper did not appear until 1912 and was entitled "Bone tissue: its growth and development: a résumé." This article actually had been an assignment given by Dr. Angle, but Hellman recognized the need for a biologic and anthropologic orientation and took further training at Columbia University under Thomas Morgan and William K. Gregory. First at the Museum of Natural History in the department of anthropology under Professors Boas and Wissler and later under Hrdlicka at the National Museum in Washington, D.C., Hellman studied the development of the human denture and face with precise anthropometric techniques. In 1919 he demonstrated the occlusal relationship of the upper and lower molars in man and indicated the evolutionary trend of the cuspal interdigitation. In 1920 he made his first paleontologic analysis of the Angle classification of malocclusion. Angle had emphasized the first molar as the "key to occlusion." Hellman demonstrated the high percentage of upper first molar rotation and warned against categorizing malocclusion without first checking this rotational tendency and mentally replacing the tooth. With Paul Simon of Germany, Hellman emphasized the broad biologic range and the early use of statistical tools for this purpose. He wrote, "We must use Johnson's newly proposed 'individual normal' reservedly . . . I would prefer the phrase, individual variation.'"

Emphasizing facial growth and dental development, Hellman established his seven stages. Studies on prehistoric American Indians in Arizona in 1929 allowed him to present a diagrammatic profile of facial size, proportions and position in each of the seven stages. His cogent observations on the height, breadth and depth dimensions serve as the basis for our present knowledge that has been gleaned by much more sophisticated techniques on living material. (See Chap. 4.) Hellman also pioneered in the use of wrist and hand x-rays to determine the growth age and status for patients.

Despite the fact that he maintained a practice and conducted independent research, Hellman was professor of orthodontics at New York University from 1927 to 1929 and in his long career he was also a professor at Columbia University.

In 1933 his alma mater awarded him the honorary degree of Doctor of Science. In 1937 Western Reserve University gave him an honorary citation and in 1938 the University of Witwatersrand in Johannesburg, South Africa, awarded him an honorary doctorate. Hellman was the recipient of the Albert H. Ketcham Memorial Award of the American Association of Orthodontists in 1939, in recognition of his contribution to the science of orthodontics.

At a memorial meeting held shortly after Hellman's death in 1947, another eminent anthropologist, Dr. Wilton Marion Krogman, paid tribute: "He took a technique that was dead and static and vitalized it into one that was alive and dynamic . . . and brought to orthodontia a rigorous uncompromising attitude of scientific objectivity. Classification, diagnosis and procedure were all subservient to a thorough study and analysis of each case under observation and/or treatment. If Dr. Hellman's attitude may be reduced to a single phrase, it would be: Know your patient — which really means know the growth pattern of your patient."

fusion exists over just what the dentist should do — and not do — when it comes to orthodontics. It is hoped that this text will serve as a logical outline for a division of labor, the end-result being better service for more patients.

Although demands for orthodontics are greater, the problems are not greatly different from those in 1912 when Lischer[16] wrote:

Now the treatment of dental anomalies involves us in countless difficulties, hence "we seek truth not merely for the pleasure of knowing, but in order to have a lamp for our feet. We toil at building sound theory *that we may know what to do and what to avoid.*" Thus the *process of dentition*, its mechanism, causes and various developmental stages, as exemplified by comparative studies, is not without meaning, but furnishes a field of compelling interest to every intelligent dentist. It is further apparent that a comprehensive knowledge of the *development of the jaws,* and of the nasal passages and accessory sinuses (which are so intimately related to them), is also desirable. A frequent attribute of malocclusion of the teeth is a marked *inharmony of the facial lines.* The true basis of a differential classification of such deformities is a wide familiarity with *ethnic variations of the head form.* A valuable aid in the study of the various forms of malocclusion of the teeth is an inquiry into the classification of all anomalies, the relations of anomalies to disease, and the foundations of teratology in general. Again, a consideration of *the causative factors* opens a large field of inquiry to the student of orthodontics, owing to their intimate connection with *the theories of inheritance, the transmission of acquired characters,* and other allied Darwinian factors and biological problems. Another essential to a scientific comprehension of treatment is a careful consideration of the *tissues of attachment,* i.e., the alveolus and pericementum, and the changes they undergo during and after tooth movement.

All these are questions . . . to investigate and if possible to explain; he (the dentist) must search for the laws underlying them, tell why they are so, and indicate the place they occupy in the scheme of things. Finally, to render our studies less difficult, and to perfect the *nomenclature* of orthodontics, we must strive to develop a greater accuracy of expression and uniformity of usage of the terms we employ in our speech.

DEFINITIONS

If Lischer's final observation is taken first, a definition of terms is in order. In 1907 Angle[17] stated that the objective of the science of orthodontics is "the correction of the malocclusions of the teeth." In 1911 Noyes[18] defined orthodontics as "the study of the relation of the teeth to the development of the face, and the correction of arrested and perverted development." In 1922 the British Society of Orthodontists proposed the following definition: "Orthodontics includes the study of growth and development of the jaws and face particularly, and the body generally, as influencing the position of the teeth; the study of action and reaction of internal and external influences on the development, and the prevention and correction of arrested and perverted development."[19]

For the dental student, a further definition of terms is essential. Such terms as preventive orthodontics, prophylactic orthodontics, interceptive orthodontics, limited orthodontics and pedodontic orthodontics are encountered frequently in the literature. Confusion arises because of the lack of any uniformity in interpretation of the various terms used. Some orderly differentiation should be made.[20] For our purposes, the general field of orthodontics can be divided into three categories—preventive orthodontics, interceptive orthodontics and corrective orthodontics.

Preventive orthodontics, as the name implies, is action taken to preserve the integrity of what appears to be the normal occlusion at a specific time (Chap. 13). Under the heading of preventive orthodontics are any procedures that attempt to ward off untoward environmental attacks or anything that would change the normal course of events. The early correction of carious lesions (particularly in proximal areas) that might change the arch length (Fig. 1–1); proper restoration of mesiodistal dimensions of the teeth; early recognition and elimination of oral habits that might interfere with the normal development of the teeth and jaws; the placing of a space maintainer that is designed to maintain proper positions of contiguous teeth—all these are examples of preventive orthodontics. The dentition is normal to start with, and it is the goal of the dentist to see that it stays that way.

Interceptive orthodontics implies that an abnormal situation exists (Chaps. 14, 15). The definition given in the brochure on orthodontics by the American Association of Orthodontists, Council on Orthodontic Education, is "that phase of the science and art of orthodontics employed to recognize and eliminate potential irregularities and malpositions in the developing dentofacial com-

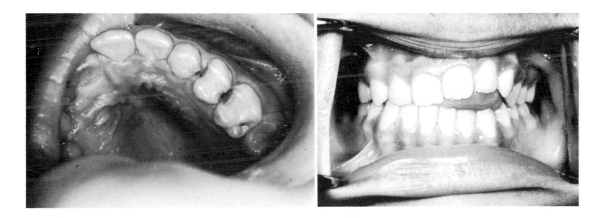

Figure 1–1 A preventive orthodontic problem. Loss of arch length due to proximal carious lesions. (Courtesy W. R. Mayne.)

Figure 1–2 An interceptive orthodontic problem. An anterior open bite is developing as a result of a finger sucking habit coupled with abnormal lip and tongue activity.

plex."[21] When there is a manifest malocclusion developing because of hereditary pattern or extrinsic or intrinsic factors, certain procedures may be taken to lessen the severity of the malformation and, in some instances, to eliminate its cause (Fig. 1–2). A good example here would be a planned program of serial extraction. Recognizing the discrepancy between amount of tooth material and the space available for teeth in the dental arches, the properly timed removal of deciduous

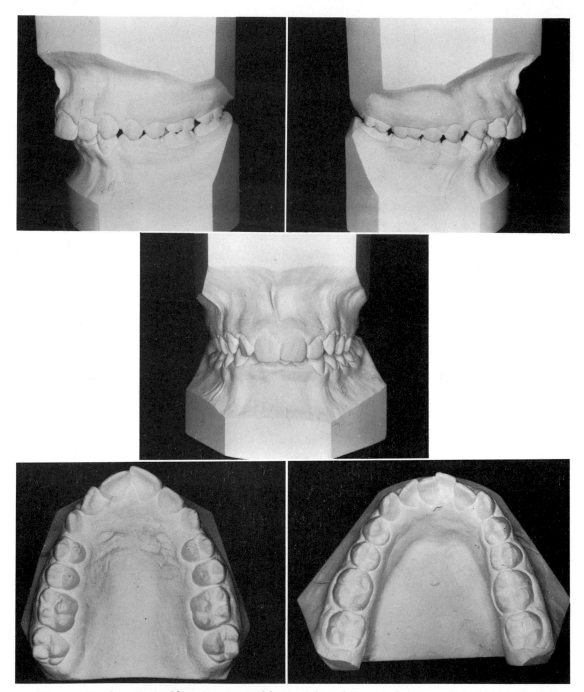

Figure 1–3   Case S. J., Class II type problem, with arch length deficiency. Study models before treatment. (Courtesy W. R. Mayne.)

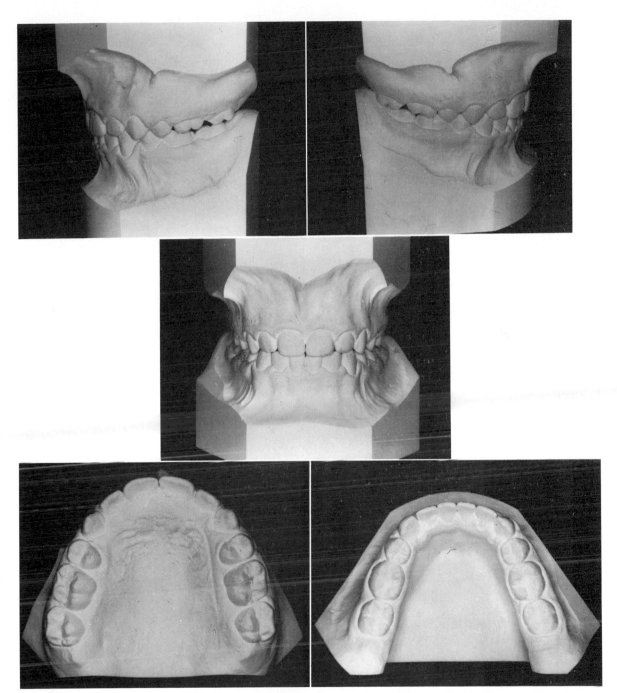

Figure 1-4   Study models after removal of four premolars and orthodontic therapy. (Courtesy W. R. Mayne.)

teeth (and ultimately the first premolar teeth) can allow considerable autonomous adjustment.

Corrective orthodontics, like interceptive orthodontics, recognizes the existence of a malocclusion and the need for employing certain technical procedures to reduce or eliminate the problem and the attendant sequelae (Chaps. 16, 17, 18). These procedures are usually mechanical and of broader

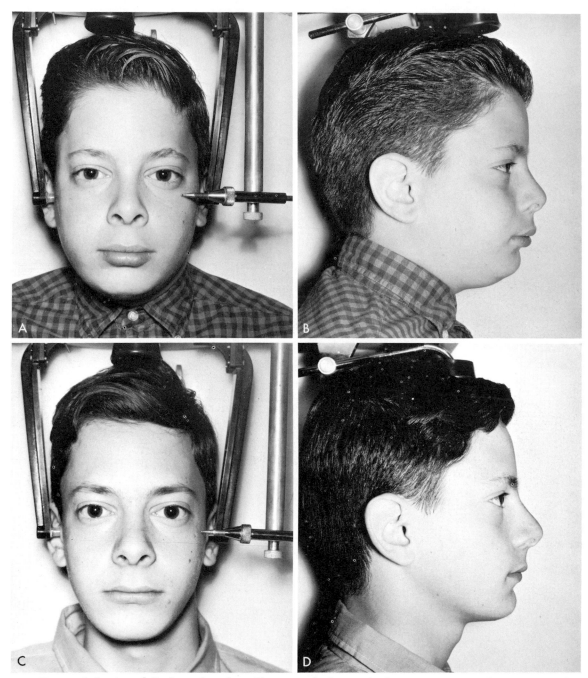

Figure 1–5 A and B, frontal and profile views before orthodontic treatment, showing muscle imbalance and lack of facial harmony; C and D, frontal and profile views after mechanotherapy, illustrating the establishment of a normal facial contour and pleasing esthetics. (Courtesy W. R. Mayne.)

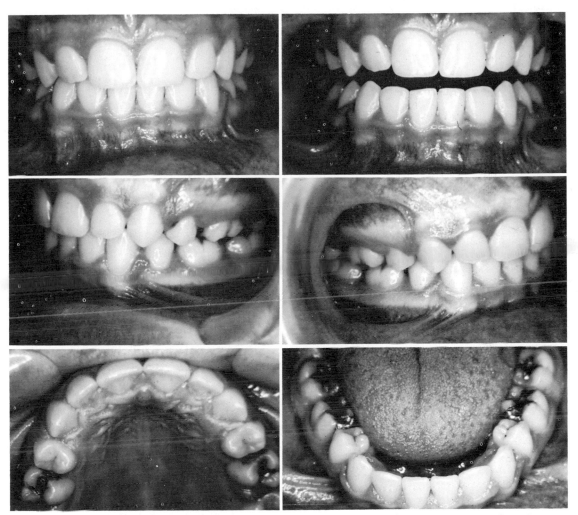

Figure 1-6 Intraoral views out of retention to show continued improvement and settling in of occlusion. (Courtesy W. R. Mayne.)

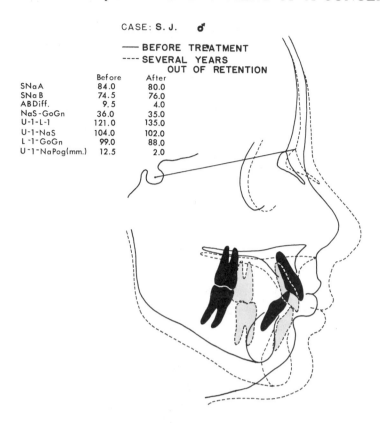

CASE: S. J. ♂

— BEFORE TREATMENT
---- SEVERAL YEARS
         OUT OF RETENTION

	Before	After
SNaA	84.0	80.0
SNaB	74.5	76.0
ABDiff.	9.5	4.0
NaS-GoGn	36.0	35.0
U-1-L-1	121.0	135.0
U-1-NaS	104.0	102.0
L-1-GoGn	99.0	88.0
U-1-NaPog(mm.)	12.5	2.0

Figure 1-7 Case S. J., tracings before and after therapy to demonstrate elimination of excessive apical base difference, excessive overjet. (Courtesy W. R. Mayne.)

scope than techniques used in interceptive orthodontics. It is in this type of problem that demands for special training are greatest (Figs. 1–3 to 1–8).

A CONCEPT AND DIAGNOSTIC DISCIPLINE

Any arbitrary division of orthodontic services, necessary as it is, implies that each entity is separate unto itself. This is not true in many instances. Much depends on the nature of the deviation from normal occlusion and at what time the problem is first seen and recognized. As Mayne has pointed out, the important thing is to be able to analyze the dentofacial complex early and by a differential diagnosis to know whether preventive, interceptive or corrective measures are to be employed. Even properly timed preventive measures alone are not always the whole answer. In many instances the patient may require a combination of preventive and interceptive procedures, or of interceptive and corrective measures. Based on the knowledge, training and experience of the dentist, corrective orthodontics should be divided into *limited* corrective procedures that can be administered by the general practitioner and pedodontist (see Chaps. 16, 17, 18) and *extensive* corrective procedures requiring the guidance and services of a qualified orthodontic specialist. Periodic observation and the timing of all services are vitally important. Orthodontics is no "one shot" remedy. Continuing guidance throughout the formative years is essential. Mayne[22] writes:

Such a program requires considerable specialized knowledge, but such knowledge is not beyond the scope of the dental curriculum. Most preventive efforts must be

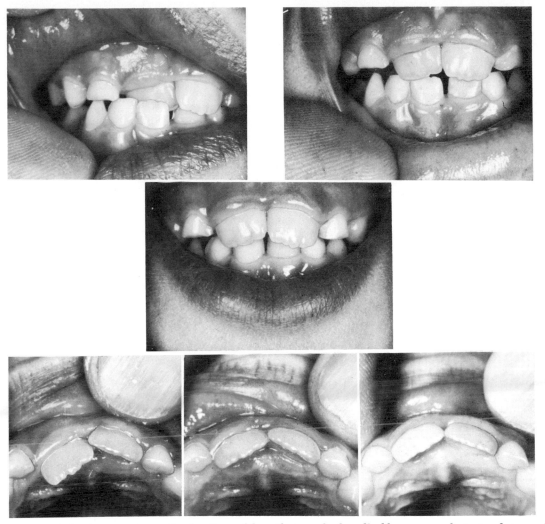

Figure 1–8 A corrective orthodontic problem that can be handled by a properly trained general dentist. Cross-bite has been corrected by an acrylic guide plane. (See Chap. 17.)

handled by the general practitioner. Interceptive measures, on the other hand, are generally more complex and it is questionable whether certain or all of these should be employed by the general practitioner. Corrective procedures fall more within the realm of the specialist than the general practitioner. Training, experience, interest, geography plus standards of perfection desired will determine which cases are to be treated by the family dentist. In any event, study and considered judgment are required of the general practitioner in analyzing the dentofacial complex, in order to direct most constructively the total dental health care of the child.

From the orthodontic standpoint, directing the total dental health care means more than asking the patient to close his teeth together to "check the bite." While the interdigitation of the teeth is important, it is only part of the total knowledge needed. Additional dental and occlusal aspects are essential in a dentofacial analysis (Chap. 8). Since occlusion is so important the dentist must have a biometric concept of the *normal*. Such a concept must encompass a dynamic appreciation of growth and developmental contributions (Chap. 2) and of the functional mechanics, demands and possibilities of the stomatognathic system (Chap. 3). Only then can he recognize the normal (Chap. 4), categorize a malocclusion (Chap. 5) and search for etiologic factors (Chaps. 6, 7). Such concepts are not reserved for orthodontics alone. They are an integral part of dentistry. The dental student must learn them and apply them constantly. Indeed, the dentist must be an applied biologist.

There are four *tissue systems* recognized in dentofacial development: the bone system, the muscle system, the nerve system, and the tooth system. Only the laboratory technician deals with the tooth system. It is essential that the dentist recognize at the outset that the tissue system orientation requires a thorough knowledge of the bone system (two-thirds of malocclusions treated by orthodontists involve basal bone abnormalities) and of the vital and dynamic role of the nerve and muscle systems. Equally important is an appreciation of facial esthetics—the relationship of the parts of the face to each other and to the face as a whole. The position the dentition assumes in the face and its effect on the total profile become vital considerations. Facial balance, both at postural resting position and with the teeth in occlusion, is important. Is the dentition complementary to facial appearance? Is it contributing harmony and balance to the face (Figs. 1–9, 1–10), or is the reverse true? Do the lips close effortlessly or with obvious strain when the teeth are placed in centric occlusion (Fig. 1–11)? Would a change in the anteroposterior position of the dentition contribute greater harmony and balance to the face? And what of the relationship of the maxilla and mandible to each other and to the cranial base (Figs. 1–12 to 1–15)?

The family dentist may readily acquire sufficient knowledge to answer many of these questions. Trained observation requires a sense of facial artistry and an appreciation of balance and harmony of parts. The development of a concept such as this cannot be reduced to simple rules and formulas; however, certain diagnostic criteria can be used to make this information more readily available (Chap. 8).

If the dentist detects a defect or abnormality, he should discuss this with the parents (Chap. 9). The parents should be informed of future needs and possible management of their child's problem. Such a discussion would serve to convince the parents that there is considerably more to the total dental care of the child than finding and filling cavities. The dentist's interest in orthodontic problems cannot help but create keener and more constant interest in the dental health of the growing child. The need for public education is paramount. It has been estimated that one third of the total population of the United States has never seen a dentist and that less than one third is getting regular dental care.[23] A recent survey estimates that only 5 per cent of the dentists make routine orthodontic referrals. How does this compare with medical referrals? Not very favorably. Relatively little improvement in the public's unsatisfactory attitude toward adequate dental health can be expected until there is a more concerted intraprofessional interchange, with cross-referral of patients becoming the usual and commonly accepted procedure.

Mayne lists four major conditions which must prevail before interceptive orthodontics can be practiced with wide success: (1) The dentist must have adequate knowledge of the subject as well as sustaining interest in its application. (2) He must have a patient who is under continual care so that such knowledge may be applied. (Preventive or interceptive orthodontics is not a one-operation procedure but generally a long-term program of care. The all-too-frequent indiscriminate change of dentists mitigates against a successful program of preventive or interceptive orthodontics.) (3) The patient's parents must recognize that a defect or deformity is developing or exists, and appreciate

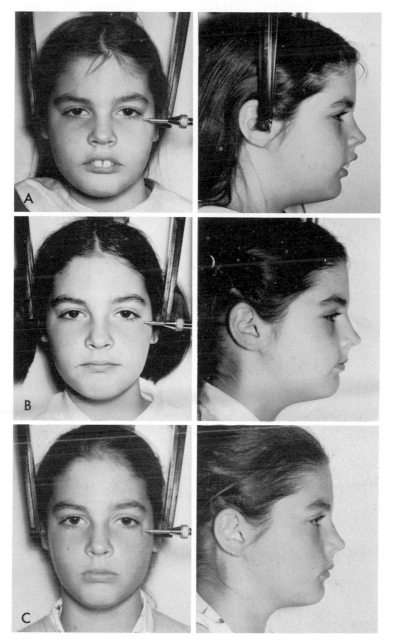

Figure 1–9 Facial changes that can be achieved in a relatively short time by properly guided orthodontic procedures. A, At beginning of treatment. B and C, After orthodontic treatment. (Courtesy W. R. Mayne.)

the need for correction. More concentrated patient education is essential. (4) Finally, the parents of the patient must have sufficient confidence in the dentist to carry out his recommended program (either through his own efforts or in conjunction with an orthodontist) and be willing to assume the financial obligation involved.

Thus, as the guardian of occlusion, the general practitioner assumes special responsibilities concerning the young patient. It is his duty to direct the destiny of the developing dentition. To do so, he must at all times have an in-

(*Text continued on page 24*)

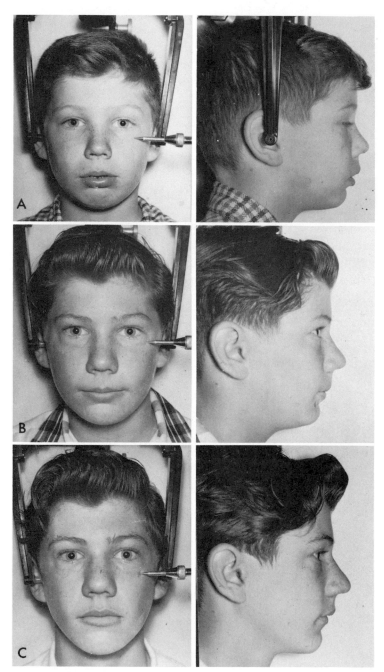

Figure 1–10   Perverted perioral muscle function. A hypotonic upper lip and a redundant lower lip require a plan of mechanotherapy that utilizes growth increments, maximum control of individual teeth and possible tooth sacrifice, to achieve the desired result. A, Before treatment. B, Immediately after treatment. C, Two years out of all appliances. (Courtesy W. R. Mayne.)

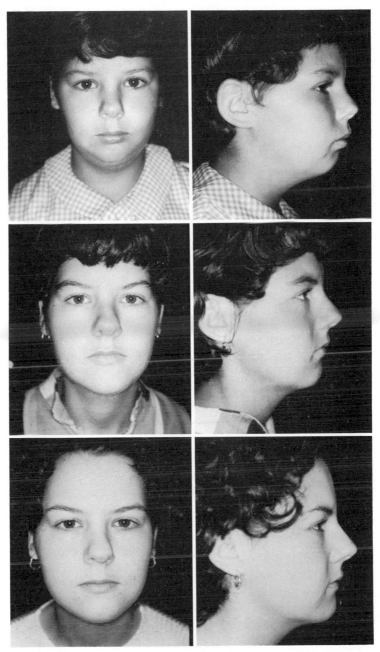

Figure 1–11 Facial views of patient at 8, 15, and 20 years, demonstrating gratifying facial changes associated with proper orthodontic guidance. Significant increments of favorable facial growth and a reduction of the excessive apical base dysplasia contribute to the profile improvement (see Figs. 1–12 to 1–14).

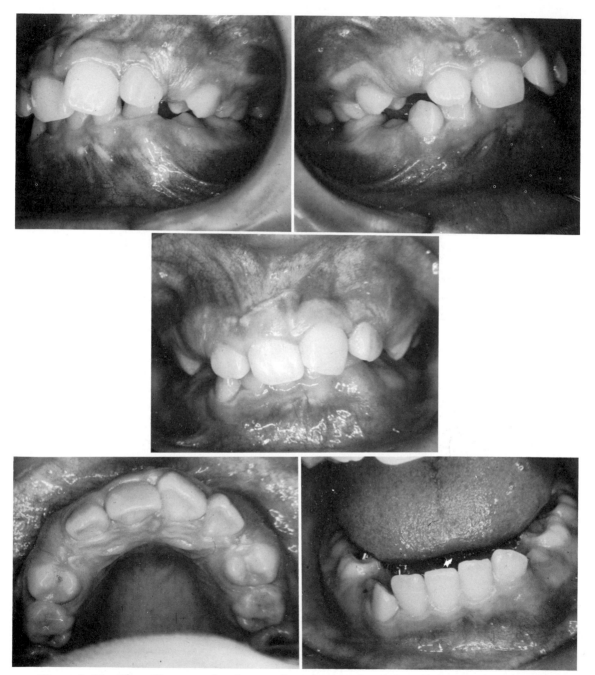

Figure 1–12   Class II type malocclusion, deep bite, and arch length deficiency go with facial photos of top row, Figure 1–11. This is a difficult case to treat because of need for tooth sacrifice, despite deep bite and steep mandibular plane.

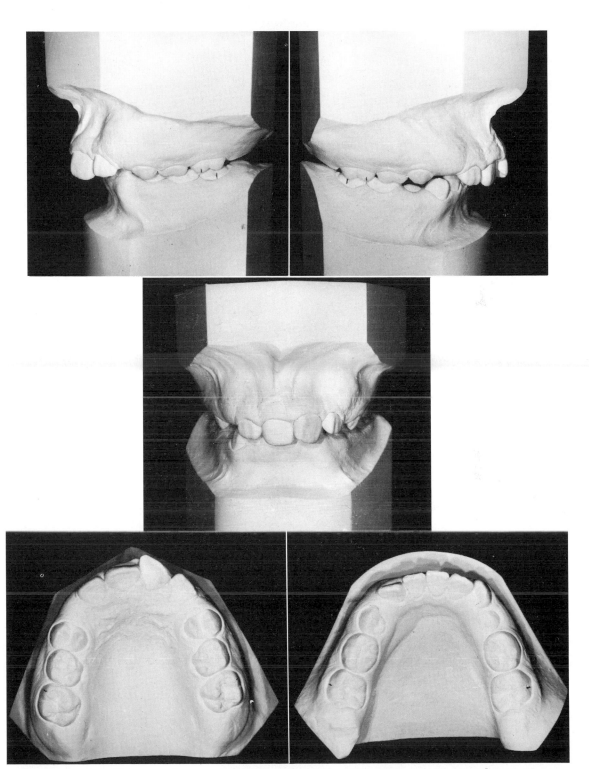

Figure 1–13 Plaster study casts before treatment of patient in Figures 1–11 and 1–12. Torque demands with overbite control provide a major challenge in treatment.

timate appreciation of the dentofacial complex of the patient. This is acquired from a dentofacial analysis, which must be completed as early as possible, and from continuing observations on subsequent visits. Although this requires specialized knowledge, it is knowledge he must have or know where to acquire.

The occlusal aspects of the dentofacial analysis may be readily learned in the classroom. The esthetic aspects, which are of increasing importance, are less easily subjected to rules or measurements. They depend largely on the development of a concept of facial harmony or balance (Fig. 1–11). Yet this concept must also be developed in the dental school.[23, 25, 26] The social and psychological implications of malocclusions and dentofacial deformities are becoming more

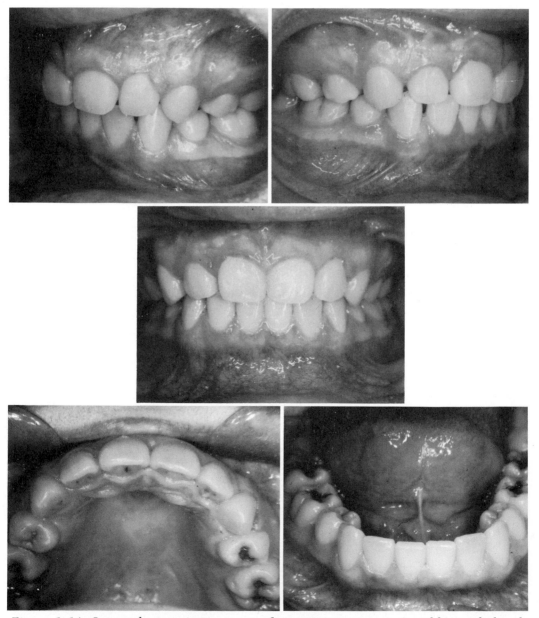

Figure 1–14 Intraoral views, nine years after active treatment. A stable result has been achieved, with elimination of excessive overbite and arch length deficiency.

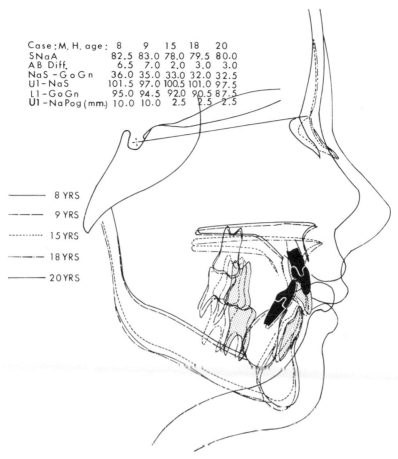

Case:M. H. age:	8	9	15	18	20
SNaA	82.5	83.0	78.0	79.5	80.0
AB Diff.	6.5	7.0	2.0	3.0	3.0
NaS – GoGn	36.0	35.0	33.0	32.0	32.5
U1 – NaS	101.5	97.0	100.5	101.0	97.5
L1 – GoGn	95.0	94.5	92.0	90.5	87.5
U1 – NaPog (mm.)	10.0	10.0	2.5	2.5	2.5

——— 8 YRS

— — — 9 YRS

·········· 15 YRS

—·—·— 18 YRS

——— 20 YRS

Figure 1–15 Cephalometric tracings of lateral cephalograms of patient in Figure 1–11. Despite excessive apical base difference, steep mandibular plane, and need to remove four first premolars, overbite and overjet are completely normal and well out of retention. Significant growth increments with counter-clockwise mandibular rotation contributed to the excellent orthodontic result. (Figures 1–11 through 1–15, courtesy Warren Mayne.)

important all the time.[27, 28] These aspects, as well as those of dental health and esthetics, should be recognized and evaluated.

As you have the rare opportunity of serving children, as you guide them past those roadblocks standing in the way of optimum dental health, never forget for a moment that you play a significant role in the *total* development of each child under your care. The psychologic implications of a severe malocclusion can be enormous. Many an adult neurosis or impotent or misdirected motivational drive can be traced to childhood attitudes begot by the cruel intolerance of a face-conscious society. The shy, sensitive and self-conscious child is like a fragile flower during the formative years of orthodontic guidance. Do not crush it in your eagerness to fulfill the mechanical requirements of being the "guardian of occlusion." Kindness, patience, understanding, empathy and good humor go hand-in-hand with digital dexterity. It is well to heed the admonitions of Edmund H. Wuerpel,[30] a great artist and friend of Edward H. Angle:

The mind of a child is as tender and as lovely as the petals of a full-blown rose. Beware how you touch it! Meet it with all the reverence of your being. Use it with gentle respect and fill it with the honey of love, the perfume of faith and the tenderness of tolerance. Thus shall you fulfill the mission of your life.

REFERENCES

1. Angle, E. H.: The Angle System of Regulation and Retention of the Teeth and Treatment of Fractures of the Maxilla. 5th ed. Philadelphia, S. S. White Manufacturing Co., 1897.
2. Weinberger, B. W.: Orthodontics: An Historical Review of Its Origin and Evolution. St. Louis, C. V. Mosby Co., 1926.
3. Shankland, W. M.: The Biography of a Specialty Organization. St. Louis, The American Association of Orthodontists, 1971.
4. Angle, E. H.: The Angle System of Regulation and Retention of the Teeth. 1st ed. Philadelphia, S. S. White Manufacturing Company, 1887.
5. Pollock, H. C.: The extraction debate of 1911 by Case, Dewey and Cryer. Am. J. Orthodont., 50:656–657, 1964.
6. Case, C. S.: The question of extraction in orthodontia (1911 debate). Am. J. Orthodont., 50:658–691; 751–768; 843–851; 900–912, 1964.
7. Dewel, B. F.: The Case-Dewey-Cryer extraction debate: A Commentary (Ed.) Am. J. Orthodont., 50:862–865, 1964.
8. Casto, F. M.: The trend of orthodontic treatment. Internat. J. Orthodont. Oral Surg. Radiol., 16:1078–1092, 1930.
9. Hahn, G. W.: Edward Hartley Angle (1855–1930). Am. J. Orthodont., 51:529–535, 1965.
10. Moyers, R. E., and Jay, P.: Orthodontics in Mid-Century. St. Louis, C. V. Mosby Co., 1959.
11. Graber, T. M.: The countdown in orthodontic education. J. Dent. Educ., 31:128–137, 1967.
12. Baker, R. W.: Contemporary orthodontic education. Angle. Orthodont., 40:249–259, Discussion by Weinstein, S., 260–261, 1970.
13. Graber, T. M.: Foreword to symposium on interceptive orthodontics. D. Clin. North America, July, 1959, pp. 279–280.
14. Noyes, F. B.: The teaching of orthodontia as Dr. Angle viewed it. D. Cosmos, 73:802–808, 1931.
15. Baker, C. R.: Calvin Suveril case. Am. J. Orthodont., 43:210–218, 1957.
16. Lischer, B. E.: Principles and Methods of Orthodontics. Philadelphia, Lea & Febiger, 1912.
17. Angle, E. H.: Treatment of Malocclusion of the Teeth. 7th ed. Philadelphia, S. S. White Manufacturing Company, 1907.
18. Noyes, F. B.: What should be the relation of the orthodontist and the dentist? D. Cosmos, 13:69–70, 1911.
19. White, T. C., Gardiner, J. H., and Leighton, B. C.: Orthodontics for Dental Students. London, Staples Press, Ltd., 1954.
20. Moore, A. W.: A critique on orthodontic dogma. Angle Orthodont., 39:69–82, 1969.
21. Orthodontics: Principles and Policies; Educational Requirements; Organizational Structure. Council on Orthodontic Education. St. Louis, American Association of Orthodontists, 1971.
22. Mayne, W. R.: A concept, a diagnosis and a discipline. D. Clin. North America, July, 1959, pp. 281–288.
23. Graber, T. M.: More Undergraduate Orthodontics: A Necessity. Kellogg Orthodontic Seminar, Ann Arbor, 1965.
24. Graber, T. M.: The case for orthodontic specialty training. Schweiz. Mschr. Zahnheilk., 80: 471–479, 1970.
25. Weber, F. N.: Orthodontic Education for the nonorthodontist: why, where, and how. Am. J. Orthodont., 48:436–443, 1962.
26. Pollock, H. C.: Iatrogenic orthodontics. Am. J. Orthodont., 48:770–773, 1962.
27. Horowitz, H. S., Thorburn, B. R., and Summers, C. J.: Occlusal relations in children born and reared in an optimally fluoridated community. Angle Orthodont., 40:59–67, 1970.
28. Horowitz, H. S., and Cohen, L. K.: Occlusal relations in an optimally fluoridated community. IV. Clinical and social-psychological findings. Angle Orthodont., 41:189–201, 1971.
29. Björk, A., and Helm, S.: Need for orthodontic treatment as reflected in the prevalence of malocclusion in various ethnic groups. Sartryck Ur. Acta socio-med. Scand., Suppl. 1, 1969.
30. Wuerpel, E. H.: Ideals and idealism in orthodontia. Angle Orthodont., 1:14–31, 1931.

chapter 2

GROWTH AND DEVELOPMENT

Growth was conceived by an anatomist, born to a biologist, delivered by a physician, left on a chemist's doorstep, and adopted by a physiologist. At an early age she eloped with a statistician, divorced him for a psychologist, and is now being wooed, alternately and concurrently, by an endocrinologist, a pediatrician, a physical anthropologist, an educationalist, a biochemist, a physicist, a mathematician, an orthodontist, a eugenicist and the Children's Bureau!

This facetious formulation by Krogman[1] illustrates the complex nature of the biologic process we are to discuss in this chapter. Ten years ago, it was not difficult to compile and present the existing information on craniofacial growth and development. Since then, however, the truly dynamic nature of the concepts, i.e., functional matrix, is evident in the intensive research and writings of a number of men in the field. Since much of our knowledge is still on the level of the working hypothesis, our synthesis of concepts is really a current "state of affairs" report and undoubtedly will be altered with ongoing research in the field. An extensive reading list at the end of the chapter should stimulate the serious student of growth and development to make a firsthand appraisal of the multiple efforts that are being made to solve the complexities of craniofacial development.

Like two Siamese twins joined at the head, growth and development are practically inseparable. According to Todd, "Growth is an increase in size; development is progress toward maturity."[2] But each process relies on the other and, under the influence of the morphogenetic pattern, "the three-fold process works its miracles: self-multiplication, differentiation, organization—'each according to its own kind.'"[1] A fourth dimension is time. Growth increments and developmental progress rates vary considerably during the two major periods of the human being.

During the prenatal period, the height increase is 5000 fold as opposed to only a threefold increase during the entire postnatal period. The weight increase, according to Krogman,[1] is 6.5 billion fold from ovum to birth and only 20 fold from birth to adulthood. But in the postnatal period this growth rate differential is also operating. By the end of the fourth month of life, birth weight has doubled. If growth continued at this rate, human size would be astronomical. Even if we project only the absolute increase of 7 pounds during the four postnatal months, a man would weigh 1000 pounds and would be 50 feet tall at 50 years of age. But the accomplishment of normal human proportions is not due merely to a general slowing down. Different tissues grow at different rates, and at different times. As will be pointed out in detail in this chapter, brain case growth, but not gonadal growth, is completed quite early. Although growth is an orderly process, there are times when "spurts" occur. As more information is available on growth processes and as this information is fed into the computer, there is a certain amount of predictability with respect to growth and developmental phenomena. With the increasing importance of orthopedic concepts and growth guidance, the clinical application of this information is quite apparent. A thorough knowledge of postnatal growth particularly is essential for the dentist, pediatrician, endocrinologist, psychologist, teacher or whoever works with the growing child, if he is to make significant clinical application of this information.

PRENATAL DEVELOPMENT OF CRANIAL, FACIAL AND ORAL STRUCTURES

Prenatal life may be arbitrarily divided into three periods:

1. The period of the ovum (from fertilization to the end of the fourteenth day).
2. The period of the embryo (from the fourteenth day to about the fifty-sixth day).
3. The period of the fetus (from about the fifty-sixth day until the two hundred and seventieth day—birth).

PERIOD OF THE OVUM

This period of about two weeks consists primarily of cleavage of the ovum and its attachment to the uterine wall. At the end of this period the ovum is only 1.5 mm. in length, and cephalad differentiation has not begun.

EMBRYONAL PERIOD

As early as 21 days after conception, when the human embryo is little more than 3 mm. in length, the head begins to take shape.[3] At that time, just before the connection exists between the oral cavity and the foregut, the head is primarily made up of the prosencephalon (Fig. 2–1). The most inferior portion of the prosencephalon is to become the frontal prominence, which overhangs the developing oral groove. Bounding the oral groove laterally are the rudimentary maxillary processes.[4] There is little indication at this time that these processes will migrate toward the midline and ultimately join with the medial and lateral nasal components of the frontal process (Fig. 2–2). Below the oral groove is the broad mandibular arch. The primitive oral cavity (bounded by the frontal process), the two maxillary processes and the mandibular arch are together called the *stomodeum.*

Between the third and eighth weeks of intrauterine life a major part of the development of the face takes place. The primitive oral cavity deepens, and the *oral plate,* which is made up of two layers (the entodermal lining of the foregut and the ectodermal floor of the stomodeum), ruptures. During the fourth week,

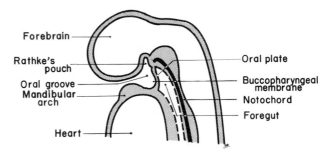

Figure 2–1 Midsagittal section of 3 mm. embryo. Oral groove and foregut still separated.

when the embryo is only 5 mm. long, it is easy to see the ectodermal proliferations on either side of the frontal prominence. These nasal placodes or thickenings will ultimately form the lining of the nasal pits and the olfactory epithelium.

The maxillary processes grow forward and unite with the frontonasal process to form the maxillary jaw. Since the medial nasal processes grow downward more rapidly than the lateral nasal processes, the latter do not contribute to the structures which ultimately form the upper lip. The depression that forms in the midline of the upper lip is called the *philtrum* and indicates the line of fusion of the medial nasal and maxillary processes.

Those primordia responsible for facial development are readily observed by the fifth week of life. Inferior or caudal to the stomodeum and the maxillary processes, which are growing toward the midline to form the lateral parts of the upper jaw, are the four pharyngeal pouches (and possibly a transitory fifth pharyngeal pouch), which form the branchial arches and furrows. The lateral walls of the pharynx are divided both inside and outside into branchial arches. Only the first two arches are named; these are the mandibular and the hyoid. The arches are divided by grooves which are usually identified by number. Special visceral efferent nuclei of the central nervous system supply the branchial arches and activate the visceral muscles. The embryonal development actually begins relatively late, after the primordia of other cranial structures (brain, cerebral nerves, eyes, muscles, and so forth) have already

MEDIAL NASAL PROCESS
MAXILLARY PROCESS
MANDIBULAR ARCH

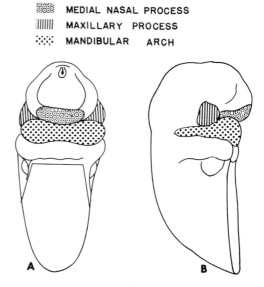

Figure 2–2 Drawing of 3 mm. embryo. A, Frontal and B, lateral views, before formation of nasal pits. (After Sicher, from Orban, B. J.: Oral Histology and Embryology. 7th ed. C. V. Mosby Co., 1972.)

developed. At this time, between and around these structures, mesenchymal tissue condensations appear, providing a shape that we recognize as the skull. Mesenchyme also appears in the branchial arch area. By the fifth week of life of the human embryo, the mandibular arch is quite distinct, bounding the caudal aspect of the oral cavity. Over the next two to three weeks of embryonal life, the medial notch that signifies the area of the union of the paired primordia gradually disappears so that by the eighth week, there is little to indicate the region of merging and fusion.

The medial nasal process and the maxillary processes grow toward each other and are almost in contact. The fusion of the maxillary processes occurs in the 14.5 mm. embryo during the seventh week. The eyes are migrating medially.

Condensed mesenchyme in the area of the cranial base, and also in the branchial arches, differentiates into cartilage. The cartilaginous skull primordium, the chondrocranium, thus develops (Fig. 2–3). As Limborgh points out, the condensed mesenchyme reduces to a thin layer, the perichondrium, which covers the cartilage.[5] The base of the skull is part of the chondrocranium, joining the nasal capsule in front and otic capsules laterally. The first centers of endochondral ossification appear, with cartilage being replaced by bone, leaving only the synchondroses, or cartilaginous growth areas.

About the same time, the mesenchymal condensations of the calvarium and facial areas appear and intramembranous bone formation takes place. As with cartilage, there is a condensation of mesenchyme to form the periosteum. In addition, the sutures with proliferating mesenchyme remain between the bone.

At the beginning of the eighth week the nasal septum has narrowed further, the nose is more prominent, and the external ear may be seen forming (Fig. 2–4). The embryo has quadrupled in length by the end of the eighth week. The nasal pits have broken through into the upper part of the oral cavity and may now be

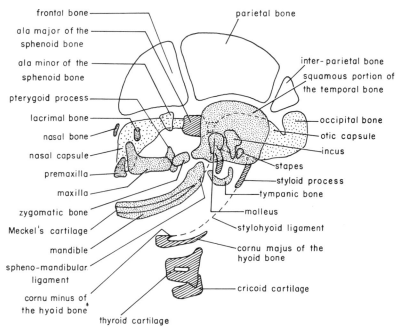

Figure 2–3 Schematic drawing of the skull of a 12-week-old embryo. Dotted white and shaded: chondrocranium; white and dotted gray: desmocranium. (From Limborgh, J. van: A new view on the control of the morphogenesis of the skull. Acta Morphol. Neerl. Scand., 8:143–160, 1970.)

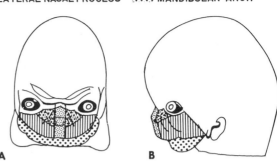

Figure 2–4 Drawing of 18 mm. embryo, eighth week. Nasal septum narrowed down, nose more prominent; external ear may be seen forming. (After Sicher, from Orban, B. J.: Oral Histology and Embryology. 7th ed. C. V. Mosby Co., 1972.)

called the nostrils. At this time also, the cartilaginous septum is being constructed from the mesenchymal cells of the frontal prominence and the medial nasal process. Simultaneously, it will be noted that there is a sharp demarcation between the lateral nasal and the maxillary processes (the nasolacrimal groove). As this closes over, it is converted into the nasolacrimal duct.

The primary palate has formed and actual communication exists between the nasal and oral cavities through the primary choanae. The primary palate develops into the premaxilla and the alveolar process underlying it, and part of the inside of the upper lip.

The lidless eyes start migrating toward the midsagittal plane. Even though the lateral halves of the mandible have fused by the time that the embryo is 18 mm. long, the mandible is still relatively short. It is recognizable in shape by the end of the eighth week of intrauterine life. At this time the head starts to assume human proportions.

FETAL PERIOD

Between the eighth and twelfth weeks the fetus triples in length from 20 to 60 mm.; the eyelids and nostrils form and close. There is relatively greater increase in mandibular size, and the anteroposterior maxillomandibular relationship approaches that of the newborn infant. Great changes have taken place in the facial structures (Fig. 2–5). But the changes seen during these last two trimesters of intrauterine life, arbitrarily labeled the fetal period, are largely an increase in size and a change in proportions. Tremendous acceleration is the theme. During prenatal life the body weight increases several billion times,

Figure 2–5 Drawing of 60 mm. embryo, twelfth week. Embryo has tripled in length in 4 weeks. Maxillomandibular relationship more nearly normal, nostrils closed, eyelids formed and closed. Face approaches human proportions. Adult face has approximately same division as embryonal precursor. (After Sicher, from Orban, B. J.: Oral Histology and Embryology. 7th ed. C. V. Mosby Co., 1972.)

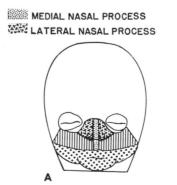

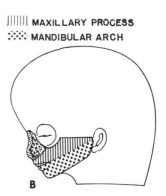

but from birth to maturity rate of increase is only 20 fold. The rate slows down appreciably before birth, as is shown in the following table, which indicates the ratios of weight increase within each of the ten lunar months (28 days), arrived at by taking the weight at the end of each month as compared with the weight at the beginning of the same lunar month.[3]

first lunar month	8000
second lunar month	499
third lunar month	11.0
fourth lunar month	4.0
fifth lunar month	1.75
sixth lunar month	0.82
seventh lunar month	0.67
eighth lunar month	0.60
ninth lunar month	0.50
tenth lunar month	0.33

More specifically in the area of the developing dentition, the maxilla and mandible are of concern.

Dixon[6] divides the maxilla, arising as it does from a single center of ossification, into two areas, based on the relationship to the infraorbital nerve: (1) neural and alveolar areas and (2) frontal, zygomatic and palatal processes. The "unloaded nerve" and neurotrophic influences are discussed later on in the chapter under mandibular growth.

With the exception of the paranasal processes of the nasal capsule and the cartilaginous areas at the alveolar border of the zygomatic process, the maxilla is essentially a membranous bone. This is important clinically, because of the apparent difference in responses of membranous and endochondral bones to pressure. In the last half of the fetal period the maxilla increases in height through bone growth between the orbital and the alveolar regions.[7]

Freiband[8] has described the pattern of fetal growth of the palate. In numerous measurements taken to establish indices, he showed that the form of the palate is quite narrow in the first trimester of fetal life, of moderate width in the second trimester of pregnancy, and wide in the last fetal trimester. Palatal breadth increases more rapidly than length, which accounts for the morphologic change. Palatal height changes are less dramatic.

For the mandible the changes are summarized by Ingham.[9]

1. The alveolar plate (ridge) lengthens more rapidly than does the ramus.
2. The ratio of alveolar plate length to total mandibular length is reasonably constant.
3. The width of the alveolar plate shows a more rapid increase than does total width.
4. The ratio of the width between the mandibular angle to the total width is relatively constant during fetal life.

Table 2–1 shows a comparison of the maxilla with the mandible, which was made by Dixon.[7]

TABLE 2–1

STRUCTURES RELATED TO DEVELOPING JAWS		DEVELOPMENTAL ELEMENTS	
Mandible	*Maxilla*	*Mandible*	*Maxilla*
1. Inferior dental nerve	1. Infraorbital nerve	1. Neural	1. Neural
2. Meckel's cartilage	2. Nasal capsule	2. Alveolar	2. Alveolar
3. Tooth germs	3. Tooth germs	3. Ramal	3. Zygomatic
		4. Muscular	4. Palatal
		5. Cartilaginous	5. Cartilaginous

GROWTH OF THE PALATE

The main part of the palate arises from that part of the upper jaw which originates from the maxillary processes. Also contributing to the formation of the palate is the medial nasal process whose deeper aspects give rise to a small triangular medial portion of the palate, identified as the premaxillary segment. The lateral segments arise from shelf-like projections of the maxillary processes, which grow toward the midline by differential proliferations (Fig. 2–6). As the nasal septum proliferates downward and backward, the shelf-like palatal ridges take advantage of the rapid mandibular growth which allows the tongue to drop caudally. With the tongue mass no longer interposed between the palatine processes, the oronasal communication is narrowed down (Figs. 2–7, 2–8, 2–9). The palatine processes continue to grow toward each other

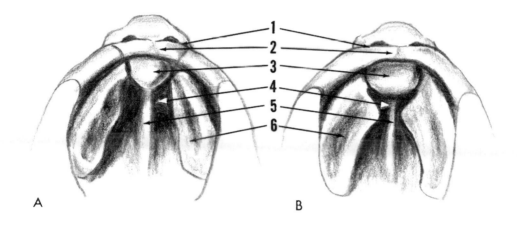

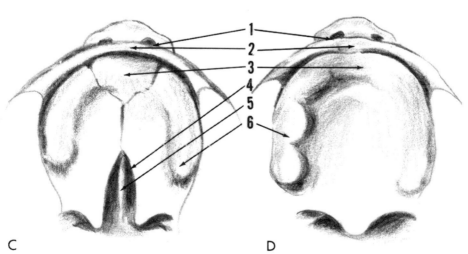

Figure 2–6 Drawings of four successive stages of palatal development. (1) External nares; (2) median nasal process; (3) median palatal process; (4) nasal cavity; (5) nasal septum; (6) lateral palatal processes. (From Avery, J. K., Happle, J. D., and French, W. C.: Development of the nasal capsule in normal and cleft palate formation. Cleft Palate Bull., 7:8–14, 1957.)

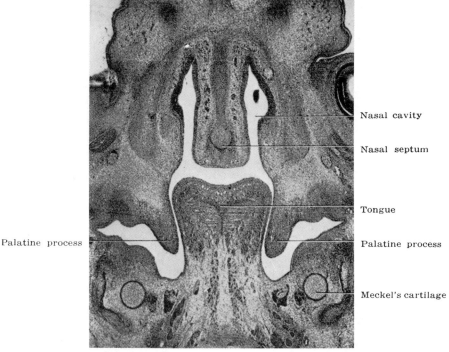

Nasal cavity

Nasal septum

Tongue

Palatine process

Palatine process

Meckel's cartilage

Figure 2–7 Frontal section, 24 mm. embryo, eighth week. Tongue interposed between vertical palatine processes. (From Orban, B. J.: Oral Histology and Embryology. 7th ed. C. V. Mosby Co., 1972.)

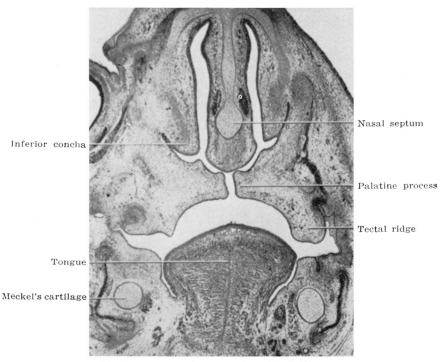

Inferior concha

Nasal septum

Palatine process

Tectal ridge

Tongue

Meckel's cartilage

Figure 2–8 Frontal section, 30 mm. embryo, eleventh week. Through differential growth, palatine processes have become horizontal and approach each other and the nasal septum. Large mandibular growth increments have allowed the tongue to drop below the level of the palate. (From Orban, B. J.: Oral Histology and Embryology. 7th ed. C. V. Mosby Co., 1972.)

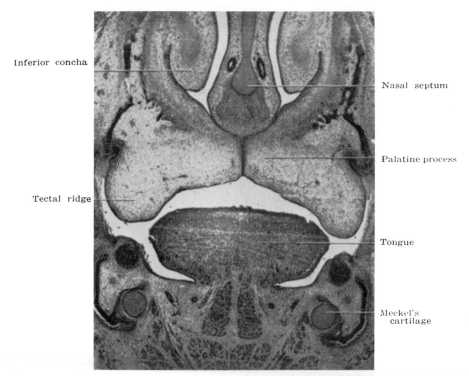

Inferior concha

Nasal septum

Palatine process

Tectal ridge

Tongue

Meckel's cartilage

Figure 2-9 Frontal section, slightly older than Fig. 2-8. Fusion taking place between palatine processes and nasal septum. (From Orban, B. J.: Oral Histology and Embryology. 7th ed. C. V. Mosby Co., 1972.)

anteriorly and unite with the downward proliferating nasal septum to form the hard palate. This fusion progresses from anterior to posterior and reaches the soft palate. Failure of fusion of the palatine processes with each other and the nasal septum gives rise to one of the most frequent congenital defects known — cleft palate. It would appear that perforation of the epithelial covering of the processes is essential. There is some evidence to substantiate the thesis that failure of mesodermal perforation of the resistant epithelial covering and the retention of epithelial bridges can cause cleft palate.[10-14]

GROWTH OF THE TONGUE

Because of the importance of the tongue in the functional matrix and its role in the epigenetic and environmental influences on the osseous skeleton, as well as its possible role in dental malocclusion, the development of the tongue is of considerable interest. Patten refers to the tongue initially as a sack of mucous membrane which becomes filled with a mass of growing muscle.[10] The surface of the tongue and the lingual muscles are from different embryonal origins and undergo changes which make it desirable to consider them separately. During the fifth week of embryonal life, rapidly proliferating mesenchymal swellings, covered with a layer of epithelium, appear on the internal aspect of the mandibular arch. These are referred to as the lateral lingual swellings. A small medial projection rises between them, the *tuberculum impar*. Caudal to this is the *copula* which unites the second and third branchial arches to form a midcentral elevation extending backward to the epiglottis. Mesodermal tissue from the second, third and fourth arches grows on either side of the copula and contributes to the tongue structure. The point at which the first and second branchial arches merge is marked by the foramen caecum just behind the *sulcus terminalis.* This serves as a boundary line between the base or root of the tongue and its active portion. Since the mucosal sac or covering of the body of the tongue originates from the first lateral lingual swellings of the mandibular arch, part of its innervation comes from the mandibular branch of the fifth cranial nerve. The hyoid or second arch contributes the taste bud innervation, or the seventh nerve. The largest part of the tongue is covered with tissue that originated from the stomodeal ectoderm. The papillae of the tongue are seen as early as 11 weeks of fetal age. By 14 weeks the taste buds can be observed in the fungiform papillae, and they appear in the circumvallate papillae at about 12 weeks.

Beneath the ectodermal covering is a kinetic mass of specialized and well-developed muscle fibers, admirably prepared well before birth to cope with the manifold functional demands being made on it by deglutition and suckling. In no other area of the body is precise muscle activity as far advanced.

GROWTH OF THE MANDIBLE

There is a marked acceleration of mandibular growth between the eighth and twelfth weeks of fetal life. As a result of the mandibular length increase, the external auditory meatus appears to move posteriorly. The development of a slender cartilage rod (Meckel's cartilage) during the second month serves as a precursor of mandibular mesenchyme which forms around it and is responsible for mandibular growth activity. At its proximal aspect, nearest to the chondro-cranium, it is actually possible to discern the incus, the malleus and the stapes of the ear. The form of the incus, malleus and stapes at the end of three months is essentially complete.

Bone begins to develop lateral to Meckel's cartilage during the seventh week and continues until the posterior aspect is covered with bone. Ossification stops at the point which will later become the mandibular lingula, and the remaining part of Meckel's cartilage continues on its own to form the spheno-mandibular ligament and the spinous process of the sphenoid. The part of Meckel's cartilage that has been encapsulated with bone appears to have served its purpose as a splint for the intramembranous ossification, and it largely deteriorates. The early development and ossification of the bones of the stoma-tognathic system are quite evident in a lateral radiogram of a 69 mm. fetus taken at 14 weeks (Fig. 2–10). Ossification in the downward proliferating condylar cartilage does not appear until the fourth or fifth month of life. There is good evidence that final ossification in this center does not occur until the twentieth year of life.

GROWTH OF THE CRANIUM

Early cranial base growth is due to proliferation of cartilage and its replace-ment by bone, primarily at the synchondroses. In the cranial vault, or desmo-

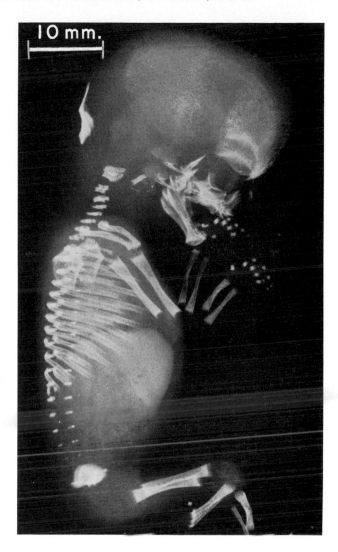

Figure 2–10 Lateral radiogram, 69 mm. fetus, 14 weeks. Radiopacity has been increased by use of silver. Portions of occipital, parietal, frontal, nasal, maxillary, zygomatic, sphenoid, temporal and mandibular bones, together with the arches of the cervical vertebrae, can be identified. Early development of the bony skeleton of the stomatognathic system is evident. (From Gardner, Gray and O'Rahilly: Anatomy.)

cranium, growth is accomplished by proliferation of connective tissue between the sutures and its replacement by bone. The periosteum also grows but it is a limiting membrane, of course, determining the size and shape changes. Despite the rapid ossification of the cranial vault in the terminal stages of fetal life, the bones of the desmocranium are separated from each other by the fontanels when the child is born (Fig. 2–11).

The changes that occur during the first three months in utero are the most important. Those that continue for the balance of intrauterine life are largely growth in size and change in position. What we have reported thus far has been largely a "bird's eye view" of surface changes. Patten points out the importance of the underlying developmental mechanisms that few anatomists discuss.[10] As important as the surface configurations are known to be, beneath the ectodermal covering lie masses of developing mesenchymal cells which arise from mesoderm and migrate, aggregate, and differentiate to form structures. The fantastic ability of this versatile tissue to form muscle, bone, connective tissue, cartilage and vessels, depending on the type of aggregation and the differentiation, is a thing to behold!

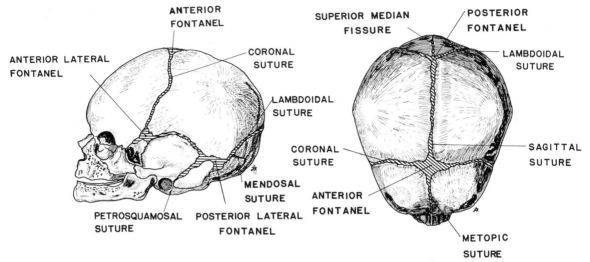

Figure 2–11   Fontanels, fissures and sutures in the newborn skull.

GROWTH OF THE PHARYNX

The pharynx develops early from the lateral wall of entodermal tissue and from the underlying mesenchyme. As has been pointed out already, there are four main pairs of branchial arches and furrows. These differentiate into a number of structures, with the mandibular and hyoid arches forming the mandible, malleus, incus, stapes, styloid process, and so forth. The proximal ends of the first and second branchial arches provide the articulation for the mandible. The temporomandibular joint may be seen in an embryo of seven to eight weeks, with the condyloid process being formed shortly thereafter, and is situated between the superior end of Meckel's cartilage and the developing zygomatic bone.[14] By the end of the eleventh week, the two joint cavities are formed. The articular disk and the external pterygoid muscle are seen in the second trimester. Pterygoid muscle fibers have actually been traced to the retrodiskal portion of the joint. Cartilaginous concentrations appear in the head of the mandible and are first seen during the tenth week. They may also be observed in the articular portion of the temporal bone. The fibrous tissue covering of the articular surfaces is already present at birth.

As the embryo grows, the pouches and branchial arches differentiate into a number of organs. The tympanic cavity of the middle ear and the eustachian tube come from the first pouch. The palatine tonsil rises, in part, from the second pouch. The thymus and parathyroids arise from the third and fourth pouches. It is of interest to note that neither the pharyngeal nor the lingual tonsils are of pharyngeal pouch origin.

POSTNATAL DEVELOPMENT OF CRANIAL, FACIAL AND ORAL STRUCTURES

Growth of the face and skull in the immediate postnatal period is a direct continuation of embryonal and fetal processes. Most of the synchondroses, still present at the time of birth, close fairly early, although the experimental information is not conclusive. Limborgh estimates closure between the second and fourth year of life for all except the spheno-occipital synchondrosis, which closes around the seventeenth year.[5] Growth of the calvarium and facial skeleton, which is largely intramembranous, continues until about the twentieth year of life, largely through the medium of sutural and periosteal growth. As Noyes points out, the fact that man's face is his most recent phylogenetic factor may be the reason that it is so unstable.[15] It does seem that there are more disharmonious relations in the face than in any other part of the body. The changes that occur do not appear to be uniform and do not occur simultaneously. The complex processes of transformation (bone deposition and resorption) and translation differ from site to site and from time to time. The disharmonious relations that do occur are not due solely to aberrations of growth and development. The broader controlling processes must be analyzed and evaluated. They are the intrinsic genetic, local, and general epigenetic factors and the local and general environmental factors. While we cannot completely resolve the continuing conflict between the geneticists and environmentalists concerning the development of the craniofacial complex during the postnatal period, we can construct a fairly logical picture that attributes significant roles to each of the controlling factors in various parts of the complex at different times.

BONE GROWTH

Before we study the growth of the various parts of the craniofacial complex, it is important to have a full appreciation of how bone grows. The forerunner of all bone is always connective tissue.[14] The terms cartilaginous or endochondral and membranous or intramembranous identify the type of connective tissue. Bone is composed of two entities—bone cells, or osteocytes, and intercellular substance. Osteocytes are of two kinds: (1) bone-forming cells, or osteoblasts, and (2) bone-resorbing cells, or osteoclasts (see Chap. 10).

In endochondral bone formation chondrocytes (cartilage cells) differentiate from the original mesenchymal cells and form a rough model, enclosed by perichondrial cells, of the future bone. While the cartilage mass grows rapidly, both by interstitial and appositional increments, a primary bone-forming center becomes apparent. At this point the mature cartilage cells hypertrophy and the matrix between the chondrocytes begins to calcify. Simultaneously from the perichondrium there is a proliferation of blood vessels into the changing cartilage mass. These proliferating vessels carry with them undifferentiated mesenchymal cells which eventually form osteoblasts. The new osteoblasts deposit bone on the surface of the degenerating calcified cartilage matrix, forming bone spicules. During the time the osteoblasts are forming a medullary type of bone inside the former cartilage mold, the perichondrium differentiates to become the periosteum which in turn begins to form bone "around the mold" in an intramembranous fashion.

In membranous or intramembranous bone formation, the osteoblasts arise from a concentration of undifferentiated mesenchymal cells. Osteoid matrix is formed by the newly differentiated osteoblasts and then calcifies to form bone. As the osteoblasts continue to form osteoid they become "entrapped" in their own matrix and become osteocytes. The blood vessels that originally nourished the undifferentiated mesenchyme are now found passing through the remaining connective tissue, interlaced between the bony trabeculae. The final bone's vascularity depends on the speed with which it was formed. The faster the bone forms, the more vascular channels one will see. As the osteoid matrix in the surrounding trabeculae calcifies, there occur certain organic changes, as yet only partly understood. A major factor in the initiation of calcification, however, appears to be the enzymatic activity of the osteocytes themselves.

Bone growth, per se, is additive or appositional. Unlike cartilage, bone cannot grow by interstitial or expansive activity. Connective tissue cells next to the bone already formed differentiate into osteoblasts to deposit new bone on the old. Bone can, however, reorganize its type by a complex combination of osteoclastic and osteoblastic activity. For example, osteoclasts can remove the coarse, less mineralized, spongy and immature bone so that osteoblasts might replace it with lamellae of evenly distributed and relatively uniform trabeculae of mature bone. Bone may be either spongy (i.e., cancellous) or compact (i.e., cortical), depending upon the density and arrangement of the trabeculae. Reorganizational activity does not stop here. Bone is a highly metabolized tissue; it is biologically plastic. Throughout life bone is responsive to the demands of function by changes in its structure. Resorption and deposition can be observed continuously (see Chap. 10, Biomechanical Principles of Orthodontic Tooth Movement). During the growth period, deposition outstrips resorption. The two processes are in balance in the adult but may reverse as old age approaches.

As previously indicated, bones grow toward each other, and in the cranium, the osteogenic region between them is composed of connective tissue. This zone is called a *suture*. As bone replaces the sutural connective tissue, each bone grows larger. One cannot ignore, however, the role of the periosteum in growth of bone. Its sac-like guiding effect is only partly understood, but when periosteal growth stops, bone growth seems to stop. In a discussion of bone growth, environmental modification should be recognized. *Bone grows in the direction of least resistance and soft tissue dominates bone growth.*

GROWTH OF THE SKULL

The human head has a complex growth pattern. A study of anatomy, of the ontogenetic and phylogenetic origins, and of the multiple functions of the skull makes it apparent why this is so. Growth of the brain case or calvarium is tied to the growth of the brain itself, while growth of the facial and masticatory bones is relatively independent of brain growth, even though these bones are in actual contact with the cranial superstructure. Growth of the endochondral cranial base seems to be under less influence from brain growth than the calvarium.[5] At birth the infant skull consists of about 45 bony elements separated by cartilage, or connective tissue. This number is reduced to 22 bones in the adult after the completion of ossification. Fourteen of these bones are in the face, and the remaining eight form the cranium. In the newborn the cranium is eight to nine times larger than the facial portion. The face makes up one fourth of the entire skeletal height at this time (Fig. 2–12). Through accomplishment of the inherited pattern and differential growth rates, this discrepancy is reduced to the point that in the adult the face makes up half the size of the cranium, and head height is reduced to one eighth of total body height.

Obviously, in nature's plan, growth of any part of the skull is coordinated with that of the other parts. The original pattern of the skeleton is maintained, with the stationary biologic center lying in the body of the sphenoid bone. Despite the shift from neurocranial dominance after the fifth year of life to orofacial dominance thereafter, with the emergence of the lower face from beneath the cranium, cephalometric analyses show that certain angular relations between various parts of the skull remain rather constant. The correlation of

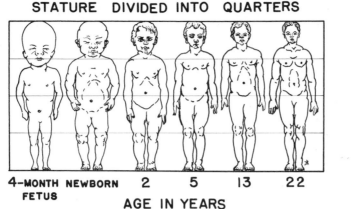

STATURE DIVIDED INTO QUARTERS

4-MONTH NEWBORN 2   5   13   22
FETUS

AGE IN YEARS

Figure 2–12 Changing proportionality of face height to total body height. (After Krogman.)

orofacial growth with the gradual growth and increasing use of the muscles of mastication is emphasized by Moss,[100] and will be discussed in detail later on in this chapter.

Limborgh poses the three main questions concerning the control of morphogenesis of the skull[5]:

1. Are there, in the embryonic phase, any causal relationships between the development of the skull on the one hand, and the presence of the primordia of the other head structures on the other?
2. How is coordination between the endochondral and intramembranous bone growth brought about within the skull once it is formed?
3. In which way is coordination between the skull growth and that of the other structures realized?

To answer these questions, analysis must be made of the more obvious controlling and modifying factors. These are, first, the intrinsic genetic factors, or those inherent in the skull tissues themselves. Second are the epigenetic factors, which are genetically determined but which manifest their influence in an indirect way by intermediary action on associated structures (i.e., eye, brain, and so forth). Structural or functional modifications of these associated structures would exert a modifying effect on the primary craniofacial complex. Third, local and general environmental factors are also controlling entities and require a value judgment in the overall picture. Just how these controlling factors work, separately and together, is not known. The role of RNA (ribonucleic acid) and DNA (deoxyribonucleic acid) at the cellular level, the establishment and maintenance of electric fields and the piezo-electric effect provide fertile fields for research activity at the genetic and epigenetic level. More readily interpretable are the local and general environmental factors.[16, 17]

With regard to the specific application to craniofacial development, the classic idea that cranial differentiation is largely genetically determined (Fig. 2–13) seems now to be challenged by the high degree of individuality of certain parts of the cranium. Spontaneous and experimental malformations prove the very close relationships between the primordia of the other head structures and the development of the skull. Apparently, if there is no eye primordium there will be no orbit. If there is only a single eye primordium, only one orbit will develop.[18] If, as in cleft palate, the eye primordia are abnormally spaced, the

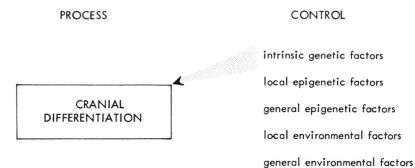

Figure 2–13   Diagram showing the hitherto generally accepted view on the control of embryonic skull differentiation. (From Limborgh, J. V.: A new view on the control of the morphogenesis of the skull. Acta Morphol. Neer-Scand., 8:143–160, 1970.)

orbits will also be laterally displaced. If there are three eye primordia, three orbits will develop. Yet, in a rare case of cebocephalia, congenital absence of eye primordia had relatively little effect on orbit size. Orbits at birth were 55 per cent of adult size (as opposed to approximately 80 per cent normally); they grew 15 per cent in eight years, with no globe and no orbital contents. Explanation of how the orbits attained their size is difficult.[66] What the primary stimulus for existence and growth was cannot be explained under current working hypotheses. This will be discussed in more detail under maxillary growth, later in this chapter. Clearly, these epigenetic factors must be considered. There are other examples of powerful morphogenetic influences of adjacent structures on the development of the skull. As Limborgh says, "The role of local epigenetic factors is quite strong, despite the experiments of Benoit which indicate the presence of the intrinsic factors in the condensed skull mesenchyme."[5, 19] The new view of embryonic skull differentiation is shown in Figure 2–14.

SUTURAL VERSUS CARTILAGINOUS VERSUS FUNCTIONAL MATRIX GROWTH

There are three major working hypotheses that have been advanced for skull growth which we should analyze. These are associated primarily with such investigators as Sicher,[14] Scott[20] and Moss,[21] or, based on tissue dominance concepts, sutural growth versus cartilaginous growth versus functional matrix growth.

The traditional theory of skull growth is shown in Figure 2–15, which indicates that intrinsic genetic factors are the major concern, with only modeling

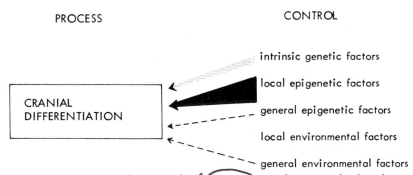

Figure 2–14   Diagram showing the new view on the control of embryonic skull differentiation. (From Limborgh, J. V.: A new view on the control of the morphogenesis of the skull. Acta Morph. Neer-Scand., 8:143–160, 1970.)

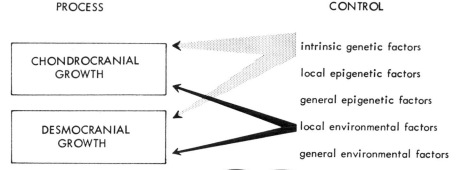

Figure 2–15   Diagram showing the classic view on the control of skull growth. (From Limborgh, J. V.: A new view on the control of the morphogenesis of the skull. Acta Morph. Neer-Scand., 8:143–160, 1970.)

resorptive and depository changes under the influence of muscles and other environmental factors.[5] In this classic explanation, skull growth is largely independent of adjacent structure growth, or both are under the same genetic stimulus. Sicher ascribes equal value to all osteogenic tissues, cartilage, sutures and periosteum. However, his theory is generally referred to as the sutural dominance theory, with proliferation of connective tissue and its replacement by bone in the sutures being a primary consideration.[14]

Figure 2–16 shows the Scott hypothesis, which emphasizes that the intrinsic growth-controlling factors are present in the cartilage and in the periosteum, with the sutures being only secondary and dependent on extrasutural influence. Scott feels that the cartilaginous parts of the skull must be recognized as primary centers of growth, with the nasal septum being a major contributor in maxillary growth, per se.[20] Sutural growth is responsive to synchondrosis proliferation and local environmental factors.

Figure 2–17 shows the most popular current working hypothesis of Moss, which emphasizes that osseous growth of the skull is entirely secondary. Based on the functional cranial component theory of van der Klaauw, Moss supports

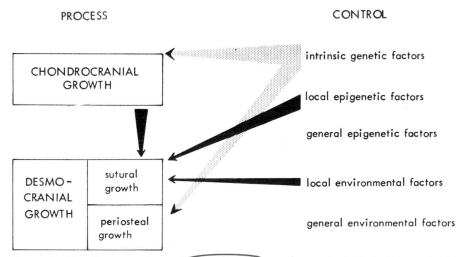

Figure 2–16   Diagram showing Scott's view on the control of skull growth. (From Limborgh, J. V.: A new view on the control of the morphogenesis of the skull. Acta Morph. Neer-Scand., 8:143–160, 1970.)

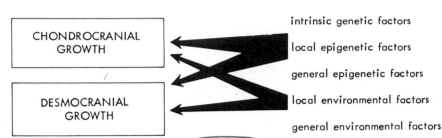

Figure 2–17   Diagram showing Moss' view on the control of skull growth. (From Limborgh, J. V.: A new view on the control of the morphogenesis of the skull. Acta Morph. Neer-Scand., 8:143–160, 1970.)

the concept of the role of the "functional matrix."[21–25] He stresses the dominance of nonosseous structures of the craniofacial complex over the bony parts. Moss claims that the growth of the skeletal components, whether endochondral or intramembranous in origin, is largely dependent on the growth of the functional matrices. This is analogous to Limborgh's designation of local epigenetic factors. Moss recognizes no intrinsic regulatory mechanism in the growing skull tissues.

Before the discussion of the growth of the individual parts of the craniofacial complex, a discussion of the three relevant hypotheses should be made. Genetic factor control ascribed by Sicher to skull tissues themselves could just as well be operating indirectly through the local epigenetic factors. Abnormalities like microcephaly and hydrocephaly cast grave doubt on the dominance of intrinsic genetic stimulus. Overgrowth or undergrowth of associated structures brings about a corresponding response in the contiguous osseous skeleton.[26]

Histologic research validates much of the Scott hypothesis. Both pressure and tension have little effect on cartilaginous growth. On the contrary, intramembranous bone is immediately responsive[27] (Fig. 2–18). Thus, there is support for the contention that sutural growth is secondary to synchondral growth and occurs at the same time. Hunter and Enlow, in their growth equivalents theory analyzing the effect of cranial base growth on facial growth, emphasize both the timing of endochondral and intramembranous growth and the correlation of vectors and increments.[28] Thus, early midface horizontal growth is tied to endochondrally induced anterior cranial base increase. As Figure 2–19 shows, the orientation of the cranial base synchondroses is favorable for this development. The relatively lesser response of the endochondral cranial base to brain growth, as opposed to the immediate response of the intramembranous cranial vault, again points to the possibility of a different reaction to environmental and even to epigenetic factors. The viewpoint that synchondroses are primary centers of growth is supported by research of Sarnat, Burdi, Baume, Petrovic, and others.[29–36]

Supporting the Scott hypothesis is the research by Ohyama on rats.[37] With experimental resection of the septum, using the most delicate and atraumatic procedures, significant interference with growth is still produced. The strong impression is gained in this research that the nasal septum is a primary growth center for nasal, frontal, premaxillary and maxillary bones. In cleft palate cases, where maxillary growth has been retarded by scarified tissue, the nasal septum continues to grow and even bends on itself into the characteristic "S" shape.

The inhibition of sutural growth is considered a concomitant of lack of

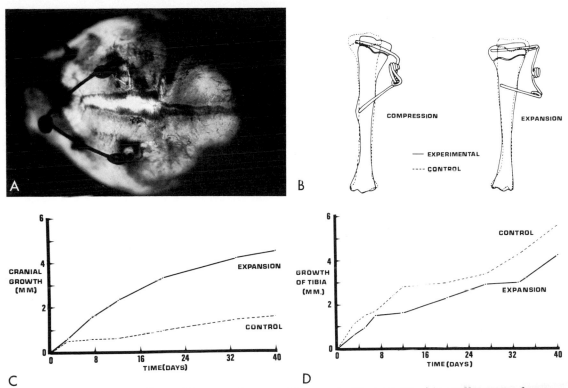

Figure 2–18   The effect of force on bone and bones. A, Photograph of transilluminated guinea pig cranium with helical torsion spring applying tension (expansion) to parietal bones after 40 days. The interparietal suture is widened and new bone trabeculae oriented in the direction of the movement are seen on either side of the translucent sutural connective tissue. The interfrontal suture (right) is also slightly widened. B, Drawing of the changes in the tibia following both tension (expansion) and compression helical torsion springs. In both cases, growth was *decreased* and perverted. This contrasts endochondral response to the previous membranous bone reaction in A. C, Graph showing the rate of lateral movement of parietal bones during normal growth and under increased lateral force. Rapid expansion occurs initially. D, Graph showing that the rate of the control bone growth is greater than that of the endochondral bone site that is under high tensile (expansive) stress. (Courtesy Hinrichsen, G. J., and Storey, E.: The effect of force on bone and bones. Angle Orthodont., 38:155–165, 1968.)

cartilage growth—no cartilage growth, no sutural growth, no proliferation of connective tissue. Scott has attributed an epiphysial platelike effect to the nasal septum.[38–44] Recent research indicates that the nasal septum seems to be more important in anteroposterior than in vertical growth.[66, 158] Mandibular growth is considered more of an adaptive shift.[37] One might question Scott's hypothesis that periosteal growth is controlled by intrinsic factors or ask why the periosteal membrane should be different in its action than sutural growth. Further, what causes the adaptive, developmental response—cartilage growth, soft tissue growth, growth of the functioning spaces, neurotrophism and so forth?

Moss considers periosteal growth entirely secondary just as he does sutural growth.[21, 45–47] The role of muscle forces and environmental factors must be recognized. The dominance of the functional matrix is apparent even in the case of children with craniostenosis.[48] When there is a local discontinuation of intramembranous sutural growth of the calvaria, with the brain still growing, pressure is exerted on other areas, causing the eye to bulge, and producing other effects.

The lumping together of both endochondral and intramembranous bone

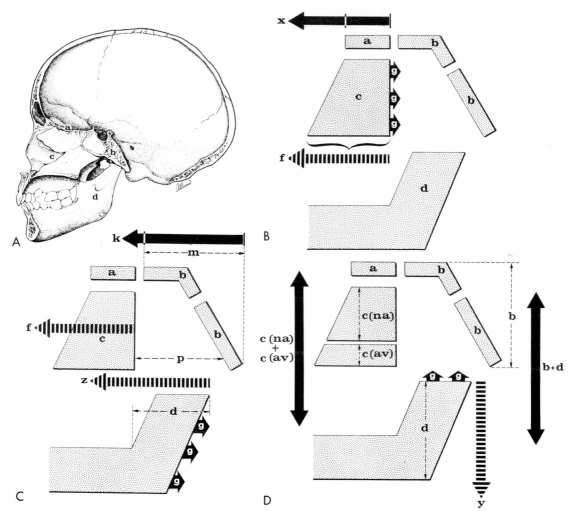

Figure 2–19 Hunter-Enlow growth equivalents concept. A, Component regions of skull (a = anterior cranial base; b = spheno-occipital complex; c = nasomaxillary complex; d = mandible). Diagram in B shows that the elongation of the anterior cranial fossa (a) is related to corresponding enlargement of nasomaxillary complex (c). Arrows show that maxillary growth is dominantly posterior, but resultant displacement is anterior. Diagram C illustrates that lengthening of spheno-occipital region (m) is a growth equivalent to corresponding enlargement of the underlying pharyngeal region (p) and the increasing length of the ramus distance (d). These growth equivalents are associated with normal positioning of the mandibular arch relative to the forward-moving displacement of the nasomaxillary complex (c). Note approximate alignment of maxillary tuberosity growth area with spheno-ethmoidal synchondrosis. In Diagram D, the composite vertical lengthening of the clivus and the mandibular ramus (b and d) is a growth equivalent to the total vertical elongation of the nasomaxillary region (c). The latter is a growth composite of the nasal (na) and the maxillary alveolar (av) regions. Again, although the ramus grows in a predominantly cephaloposterior direction (g), it becomes displaced in the opposite direction (y). (From Enlow, D. H., and Hunter, W. S.: The growth of the face in relation to the cranial base. Trans. Europ. Soc. Orth., 321–335, 1968.)

formation and response by Moss is questioned by others.[26, 30–44] To these observers, hydrocephaly, anencephaly and microcephaly point out the differential response of the endochondral base. There is no doubt that the desmocranium (membranous calvarium) responds directly to pressure but the chondrocranium (endochondral base) which would seem to be under the same pressures or lack of pressures, remains practically normal. As Enlow has shown, the desmocranium shows a much greater incremental change than the chondrocranium during the normal growth process.[49-50] Yet, the brain rests on the chondrocranium and theoretically exerts the same amount of force downward as it would upward and outward. This apparent high degree of independence of endochondral bone growth is further substantiated by the fact that it is very difficult to distort the chondrocranium in contrast with the relative ease of deforming the desmocranium. Thus, there is apparent support for at least part of the Scott hypothesis while much research supports to a large measure the Moss functional matrix explanation.

Limborgh lists the essential elements of the three hypotheses that seem to bear up under current research.

1. Growth of the synchondroses and the ensuing endochondral ossification is almost exclusively controlled by intrinsic genetic factors.
2. The intrinsic factors controlling intramembranous bone growth, i.e., the growth of the sutures and the periosteum, are small in number and of a general nature.
3. The cartilaginous skull parts must be seen as growth centers.
4. Extent of sutural growth is controlled by both the cartilaginous growth and the growth of the other head structures.
5. The extent of periosteal bone growth largely depends on the growth of adjacent structures.
6. The intramembranous processes of bone formation can be additionally influenced by local environmental factors, muscle forces inclusive.[26]

Taking these six observations and constructing a diagram on the basis of their likely validity, Figure 2–20 shows the interrelationship of genetic, epigenetic and environmental controls with chondrocranium and desmocranium growth processes. Note also the influence of the chondrocranium on the membranous bone structures. Yet, the chondrocranium is primarily under the influence of intrinsic genetic factors with some lesser influence from general epigenetic factors and, perhaps from general environmental factors.

This synthesis of parts from the three basic theories of craniofacial growth, while representing a logical interpretation, does not answer all the questions. The growth of the mandible, for example, is not explained completely. An added question of the possible difference between control of appositional cartilaginous growth and interstitial cartilaginous growth can be raised.[26] Also,

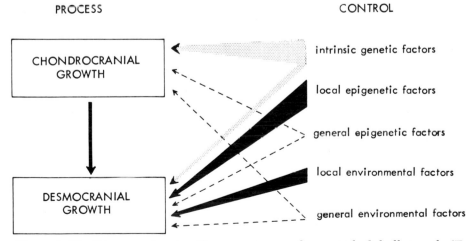

Figure 2–20 Diagram showing the new view on the control of skull growth. (From Limborgh, J. V.: A new view on the control of the morphogenesis of the skull. Acta Morph. Neer-Scand., 8:143–160, 1970.)

since the neurocranium is completed quite early and thus provides a stable base for continued membranous growth in other areas, a question is asked concerning the influence of these membranous bones on other membranous bones which are still growing. Thus, differential growth gradients are also a conditioning factor.

GROWTH OF THE CRANIUM

With the previous discussion serving as a basis, let us now analyze growth of the various parts of the craniofacial complex. Growth of the cranium may be divided into that of the brain case proper, or the brain capsule which primarily concerns the bones that make up the calvarium; and growth of the cranial base, which divides the craniofacial skeleton.

GROWTH OF THE CRANIAL BASE

The cranial base grows primarily by cartilage growth in the sphenoethmoidal, intersphenoidal, spheno-occipital and intraoccipital synchondroses, mostly following the neural growth curve, but partially the general growth curve (Figs. 2–19, 2–21, 2–22). Activity at the intersphenoidal synchondrosis disappears at birth.[51] The intraoccipital synchondrosis closes in the third to the fifth year of life. The spheno-occipital synchondrosis is a major contributor; endochondral ossification does not stop here until the twentieth year of life.[36]

It is quite possible that the spheno-occipital synchondrosis has been overstressed as a growth center. Koski indicated that this suture existed primarily as a means of adjusting the cranial base to the needs of the growing brain and the upper respiratory area.[52] Subsequent research by Koski, transplanting pieces of cranial base from different sutures, showed little growth of the transplant. Since subcutaneously transplanted synchondroses showed little or no growth, a repeat experiment was done on 166 specimens, this time transplanting into brain

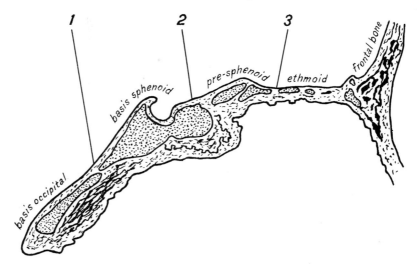

Figure 2–21 Growth sites of the base of the skull. 1, Spheno-occipital synchondrosis. 2, Intersphenoid synchondrosis. 3, Sphenoethmoidal synchondrosis. (After Maronneaud.)

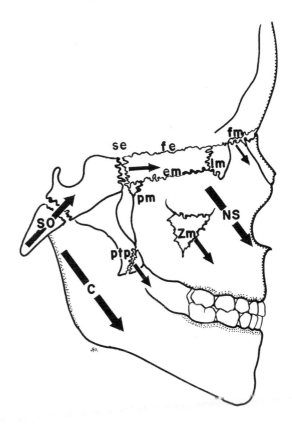

Figure 2–22 Growth directions of cranial base and facial sutures, with resultant "expanding V" accomplishment as the cranial portion moves upward and forward and the facial portion downward and forward. SO, Spheno-occipital synchondrosis; C, reflection of condylar mandibular growth; NS, nasal septum; se, sphenoethmoid suture; ptp, pterygopalatine suture; pm, palatomaxillary suture; fe, frontoethmoidal suture; em, ethmoidal-maxillary suture; lm, lacrimal-maxillary suture; fm, frontomaxillary suture; zm, zygomaticomaxillary suture. Surface apposition and resorption are shown by stippled area. (From Coben, S. E.: Growth and Class II Treatment. Am. J. Orthodont., 52:5–26, 1966.)

tissue. Most of the transplants did not increase in size.[54] However, summarizing the work that Koski and Rönning have done together, "Cartilaginous epiphyses transplanted into brain tissue differentiate into normal, growing long bones, whereas condylar cartilages of the mandible, similarly transplanted, rapidly lose their structure and evidently do not continue to promote bone growth."[55–59] Cranial base synchondroses thus seem to represent an intermediate form of so-called growth cartilage between those two just mentioned, in that they appear to possess an inherent bone growth promoting potential which is greater than that of condylar cartilage but not as great as that of epiphyseal cartilages of long bones.[54] The functional matrix theory is thus strongly supported.

According to some authors, the sphenomesethmoidal synchondrosis and the cartilage between the mesethmoidal and frontal bones are equally important. In addition, there is the growth of the frontal bone itself, increasing in thickness through pneumatization and creation of the frontal sinus. All except the frontal bone portion develop in the chondrocranium. Just when the sphenoethmoidal synchondrosis closes is not definitely known.[60] Claims range from 5 to 25 years of age. It is likely, however, that its major contribution has been made by the time the first permanent molar erupts. Recent research indicates that growth or lack of growth at the sphenoethmoidal synchondrosis may have important ramifications in cleft palate rehabilitation[29, 38–44] (see Chap. 6).

The influence of the cranial base on growth of the maxilla and mandible is discussed in the Enlow-Hunter Growth-Equivalents Theory[50] (Fig. 2–19). The location of synchondroses and maxillary sutures and the dominance of endochondral over intramembranous bone seem to explain some of the changes that occur in the maxilla. These will be discussed later. The possible influence of the cranial base on the growth of the brain case itself must also be recognized.

GROWTH OF THE BRAIN CASE

The cranium grows because the brain grows (Fig. 2–23). This growth is accelerated during infancy. By the end of the fifth year of life, over 90 per cent of the growth of the brain capsule, or brain vault, has been achieved. This increase in size under the influence of an expanding brain is accomplished primarily by proliferation and ossification of sutural connective tissue and by appositional growth of the individual bones that make up the cranial vault. Some selective resorption occurs early in postnatal life on the inner surfaces of the cranial bones to help flatten them out as they expand. Apposition can be seen on both the internal and external tables of the cranial bones as they become thicker. This increase in thickness which permits the development of the diploë is not uniform. Sicher attributes this to the fact that the inner cranial table is primarily under the influence of the growth of the brain—the brain capsule—while the outer plate has certain mechanical influences operating upon it.[14] These mechanical influences contribute to the growth of the cranial superstructures. Of particular significance are the supraorbital, otic and mastoid regions. These structures are usually more marked in the male than in the female.

The newborn not only has his frontal bone separated by the soon-to-close metopic suture, but also has no frontal sinuses. Both outer and inner surfaces are parallel and quite close together. With the general growth and thickening of the cranial vault there is an increase in the distance between the external and internal plates in the supraorbital region. This may be seen on the external surface as the formation of a ridge. The spongy bone between the external plates is gradually replaced by the developing frontal sinus. Benninghoff and others attribute the pneumatization of the skull and the development of ridges and eminences to postural and functional stresses.[61] (This concept is discussed in greater detail in Chapter 3, Physiology of the Stomatognathic System.) The cranial vault increases in width primarily through "fill-in" ossification of pro-

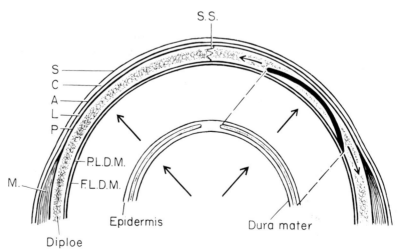

Figure 2–23 The calvarial bones (desmocranium) are embedded within a neurocranial capsule. This capsule expands in response to a volumetric increase of the capsular neural matrix. The embedded bones are passively carried outward, by processes of translative growth. Periosteal transformative processes add bone at sutural margins but these are secondary and compensatory, rather than primary. (From Moss, M. L., Salentijn, L.: The primary role of functional matrices in facial growth. Am. J. Orthodont., 55:571, 1969.)

liferating connective tissue in the coronal, lambdoidal, interparietal, parieto-sphenoidal and parietotemporal sutures. It should be recognized that there is actual translation as well as remodeling of the individual bones, with the structures being moved outward by the growing brain. Despite early accomplishment of pattern and almost adult size, the midsagittal suture between the parietal bones does not close until the middle of the third decade of life.

Increase in the length of the brain case may be primarily due to the growth of the cranial base with active response at the coronal suture.

The brain case grows in height largely owing to the activity of the parietal sutures along with the occipital, temporal and sphenoidal contiguous osseous structures. Davenport lists the following percentages for growth in length of the brain case at different ages[62]:

Brain Case Growth

Birth	63%
6 months	76%
1 year	82%
2 years	87%
3 years	89%
5 years	91%
10 years	95%
15 years	98%

Emphasizing the early and heavy growth contributions, Davenport also gives a table for the number of millimeters per year that the head grows in width: for the first 9 months before birth it is 100 mm.; at the end of 6 months an additional 50 mm.; from 6 to 12 months the head grows 20 mm.; from 1 to 2 years it grows 9 mm.; 2 to 3 years 1.5 mm.; and from 3 to 14 years it grows approximately 0.5 mm. per year.[63]

GROWTH OF THE FACIAL SKELETON

It has already been pointed out that the brain case and the facial skeleton grow at different rates. Scammon and his co-workers diagram the differential growth rate for different body tissues (Figs. 2–24, 2–25) and show that the neurocranium follows the neural timetable of growth.[51] The lower face, or splanchnocranium, more nearly approximates the general or bodily growth curve. The cranial base, unlike the calvarium, is not completely dependent on brain growth and may have some intrinsic genetic guidance and a pattern that is similar, in some dimensions, to that of the facial skeleton.[64] By differential growth, however, the face literally emerges from beneath the cranium (Fig. 2–22). The dentition is translated forward spatially by craniofacial growth, moving it away from the vertebral column. The upper face, under cranial base inclination influence, moves upward and forward; the lower face moves downward and forward on an "expanding V." The divergent pattern permits vertical growth of the dentition through tooth eruption and alveolar bone proliferation.[65] To better understand the growth of the face itself, a detailed analysis of the developmental pattern of the maxilla and its associated structures and of the mandible is essential. Moss points out that the growth of the sinuses, the nasal capsule and the spaces of the facial skeleton must also be recognized for their role in increased size of the skeletal components. The role of the capsule and functional matrices in orofacial growth is discussed in the analysis of maxillary and mandibular growth[67] (Fig. 2–26).

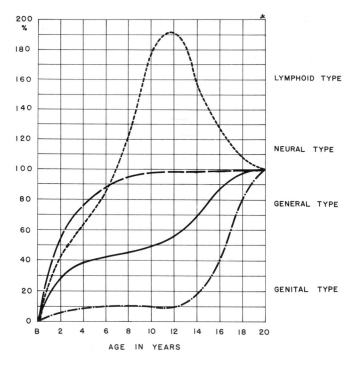

Figure 2–24 Differential growth rate for different body tissues. The neurocranium follows the neural type of growth. The lower face most nearly approximates the general or bodily growth curve. Thus, for a particular age there is a differential in the total growth accomplished (i.e., 10 years of age, neurocranium 96 per cent complete; lower face growth 50 per cent complete). (After Scammon, R. E., et al.: The Measurement of Man. Minneapolis, University of Minnesota Press.)

GROWTH INCREMENTS

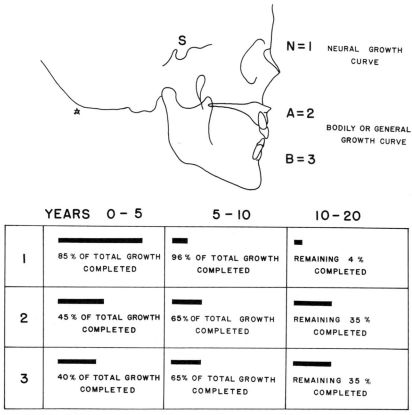

YEARS	0 – 5	5 – 10	10 – 20
1	85 % OF TOTAL GROWTH COMPLETED	96 % OF TOTAL GROWTH COMPLETED	REMAINING 4 % COMPLETED
2	45 % OF TOTAL GROWTH COMPLETED	65% OF TOTAL GROWTH COMPLETED	REMAINING 35 % COMPLETED
3	40% OF TOTAL GROWTH COMPLETED	65% OF TOTAL GROWTH COMPLETED	REMAINING 35 % COMPLETED

Figure 2–25 Differential growth rate of cranial and facial profile components. Cranial structures follow neural growth curve; facial structures parallel bodily or general growth curve.

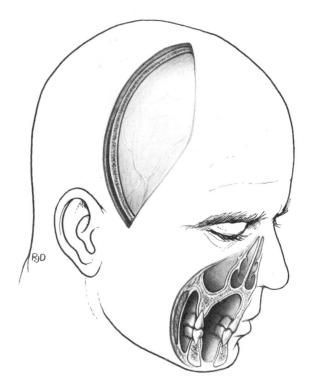

Figure 2–26 Even as the calvarial bones are embedded in a neurocranial capsule and are translated thereby, so are the oronasomaxillary bones embedded in the orofacial capsule (i.e., a capsular matrix). The primary expansion of the functioning oronasopharyngeal spaces on a morphogenetic stimulus brings about secondary compensatory expansion of the orofacial capsule. (From Moss, M. L., and Salentijn, L.: Functional matrices in facial growth. Am. J. Orthodont., 55:569, 1969.)

MAXILLA

We must remember as we study the growth of the maxillary complex that it is joined to the cranial base. Hence, as indicated previously, the cranial base naturally influences the development of this region. There is no sharp line of demarcation between the cranial and maxillary growth gradients. Undoubtedly, the position of the maxilla is dependent on the growth at the spheno-occipital and sphenoethmoidal synchondroses. We are dealing then with two problems: (1) the shift in position of the maxillary complex and (2) the enlargement of the complex itself. Both are intimately related and are separated only for the sake of describing the details that lead to the accomplishment of the adult pattern. Enlow and Bang apply the principle of "area relocation" to the complex and multidirectional growth movements.[68] As the dynamic process continues, "specific local areas come to occupy new actual positions in succession, as the entire bone enlarges. These growth shifts and changes involve corresponding and sequential remodeling adjustments in order to maintain the same shape, relative positions and constant proportions of each individual area in the maxilla as a whole" (Figs. 2–27, 2–30). *Translation* and *transposition* are the words used by Moss to describe the same phenomenon.[69] While growth of the cranial base is largely due to endochondral ossification, with bone replacing the proliferating cartilage, the growth of the maxilla is intramembranous and similar to that of the cranial vault. Sutural connective tissue proliferations, ossification, surface apposition, resorption and translation are the mechanisms for maxillary growth.

The maxilla is hafted to the cranium at least partly by the frontomaxillary suture, the zygomaticomaxillary suture, zygomaticotemporal suture and the pterygopalatine suture. Weinmann and Sicher have pointed out that these sutures are all oblique and more or less parallel with each other.[14] Thus, growth

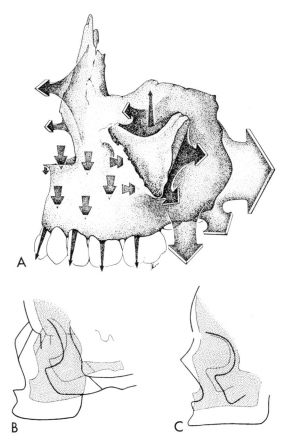

Figure 2–27   The growth and remodeling of the maxilla are represented in A. This involves a complex pattern of deposition and resorption. The classic cephalometric superimposition of cephalometric tracings using sella as a registration point is shown in B. In C, the tracings are oriented according to the actual directions of growth, rather than the composite of growth and displacement seen in B. (From Enlow, D. H., and Hunter W. S.: The growth of the face in relation to the cranial base. Trans. Europ. Soc. Orth., 321–335, 1968.)

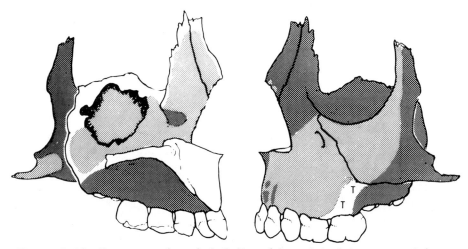

Figure 2–28   Diagrams of medial (left) and lateral (right) aspects of the maxilla, summarizing the distribution of various periosteal (dark crosshatch) and endosteal (light crosshatch) bone deposits. Note zone of variable endosteal-periosteal transition (T) on the lateral cortex in the molar area. (From Enlow, D. H., and Bang, S.: Growth and remodeling of the human maxilla. Am. J. Orthodont., 51:446–464, 1965.)

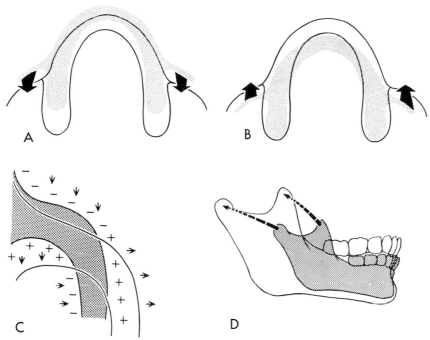

Figure 2–29 A, Schematic interpretation of posterior growth of the maxillary arch and the zygomatic processes. Bone growth proceeds along the entire inner (lingual) side of the arch as well as along its posterior margin (maxillary tuberosity) and the posterior face of the zygomatic process. Resorptive removal occurs from the outer cortex of the premaxillary area and from the anterior surface of the zygomatic process. B schematizes the *apparent* direction of growth which results from the anterior thrust of the maxillary body accompanying its actual growth in a posterior direction. C, Schematic diagram illustrating the mechanism of posterior and lateral movement of the combined zygomatic process of the maxilla and the adjacent zygomatic bone. Bone deposition (+) proceeds in lateral and posterior directions (arrows), together with complementary resorption (−) from anterior and medial surfaces. D, The generalized mode of maxillary growth and remodeling parallels that of the human mandible, shown here for comparison. During posterior growth of the condyle and ramus, the coronoid process is continuously relocated in a posterior direction (arrows). Similarly, the zygomatic process of the maxilla also receives proportionate posterior relocation as the maxillary body grows in this direction. (From Enlow, D. H., and Bang, S.: Growth and remodeling of the human maxilla. Am. Orthodont., 51:446–464, 1965.)

in these areas would serve to move the maxilla downward and forward (or the cranium upward and backward). There is increasing evidence, however, that the sutural growth activity is secondary to primary stimuli from epigenetic factors. First, it is quite possible that the endochondral growth of the cranial base and the growth of the nasal septum may dominate membranous bone response and stimulate the downward and forward growth of the maxillary complex. Our studies of cleft palate growth patterns show the difficulty of retarding nasal septum growth, even with traumatic surgery.[70] If endochondral bone does dominate intramembranous bone and if the synchondroses of the cranial base can influence maxillary translative changes, then there is at least the possibility that the septum may have some influence on the surrounding membranous bone structures. But when one asks, "What is the primary growth center or pacemaker for the maxilla?" he must turn to the extensive research on the functional matrix.

The technique of mapping the localized distribution of various kinds of endosteal and periosteal bone deposits as done by Enlow tells us *what* is

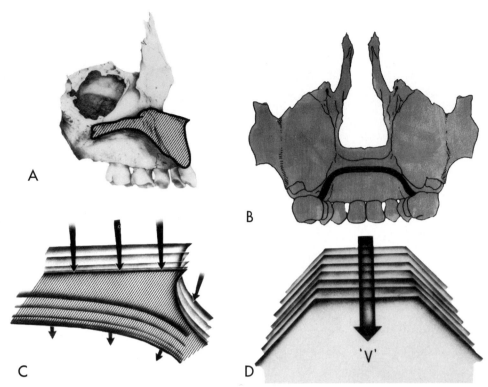

Figure 2-30   A and B, The oral plate and floor of the nasal cavity as well as the nasal spine move in a downward direction as a result of bone deposition on the various inferior surfaces, in conjunction with resorption from contralateral superior surfaces. The premaxillary area moves simultaneously downward and somewhat posterior by a similar process. C and D illustrate the "expanding V" principle, as the palate grows in an inferior direction by subperiosteal bone deposition on its entire oral surface, with corresponding resorptive removal on the opposite surfaces. The entire V-shaped structure thereby moves in a direction toward the wide end of the V and increases in overall size at the same time. (From Enlow, D. H., and Bang, S.: Growth and remodeling of the human maxilla. Am. J. Orthodont., 51:446–464, 1965.)

happening but not *why* it is happening. With the complex changes, as illustrated in Figures 2–27 – 2–30, we can no longer oversimplify and attribute maxillary growth solely to sutural location and activity. We must turn to functional cranial analysis: as Moss says, "The head is a composite structure, operationally consisting of a number of relatively independent functions: olfaction, respiration, vision, digestion, speech, audition, equilibration and neural integration. Each function is carried out by a group of soft tissues which are supported and/or protected by related skeletal elements. Taken together, the soft tissues and skeletal elements related to a single function are termed a functional cranial component. The totality of all the skeletal elements associated with the single function is termed a skeletal unit. The totality of the soft tissues associated with a single function is termed the functional matrix. It may be further demonstrated that the origin, growth and maintenance of the skeletal unit depend almost exclusively upon its related functional matrix."[67] Moss and Greenberg point out that the basic maxillary skeletal unit is the infraorbital neurovascular triad.[71] As in the mandible, where the basal bone largely protects the mandibular nerve canal, the maxilla basal bone serves as a protection mechanism for the trigeminal nerve. It is this neurotrophic influence which maintains the spatial constancy for the infraorbital canal with respect to the anterior cranial base. Thus, indirectly it produces a similar constancy of the basal maxillary skeletal unit relative to the same base.

The possibility that the capillary distribution, which parallels that of the innervation, is a factor should also be explored. But the spatial stability of the infraorbital canal relative to the cranial base and, in addition, the stability of the infraorbital neurovascular triad relative to the other maxillary components seems to indicate neurotrophic dominance.

If we are to analyze the growth of the maxilla, we must turn to the concept of the functional matrices (Fig. 2–26). It was noted previously that the growth of the eyeball seems essential for the development of the orbital cavity. Some experimental research suggests that if there is no primordium for the eye, there is no orbit.[18] It is clear that this functional matrix has a direct effect on the contiguous osseous structures. Also, just as the neurocranial bones are enclosed within a neurocranial capsule, as Moss points out, the facial bones are enclosed within an orofacial capsule. Just as the calvarial bones are passively carried outward by the expansion of the enclosed capsule in direct response to the growth of the neurocranial matrices (the neural mass), so the facial bones are passively carried outward (downward, forward and laterally) by the primary expansion of the enclosed orofacial matrices (orbital, nasal, oral matrices).[69] In addition, there is the essential growth of the sinuses and spaces themselves, which perform important functions. The resultant maxillary changes in the skeletal elements would thus be secondary, compensatory and mechanically obligatory. The actual growth observed in the orbital floor, for example, is secondary and compensatory so that the orbital cavity is not unduly enlarged. In the anteroposterior vector, the forward, passive motion of the maxilla is constantly being compensated for by accretions at the maxillary tuberosity and at the palatal processes of both the maxillary and palatine bones.

Moss cites three types of bone growth change to be observed in the maxilla. First, there are those changes associated with compensation for the passive motions of the bone brought about by the primary expansion of the orofacial capsule. Second, there are changes in bone morphology associated with alterations in the absolute volume, size, shape or spatial position of any or all of the several relatively independent maxillary functional matrices, such as the orbital mass. Thirdly, there are bone changes associated with the maintenance of the form of the bone itself, as diagrammed by Enlow in the accompanying illustrations. It must be emphasized that these three processes do not necessarily occur simultaneously. Judging from recent research, differential or sequential expression is likely.[72]

Turning to the specific workings of maxillary change, a major factor in the increase of height of the maxillary complex is the continued apposition of alveolar bone on the free borders of the alveolar process as the teeth erupt. As the maxilla descends, continued bony apposition occurs on the orbital floor, with concomitant resorption on the nasal floor and apposition of bone on the inferior palatal surface. By the alternate process of bone deposition and modeling resorption, the orbital and nasal floors and the palatine vault move downward in a parallel fashion.

As Figure 2–30 shows, the palatal growth follows the principle of "the expanding V."[68] Thus, additive growth on the free ends increases the distance between them. The buccal segments move downward and outward, as the maxilla itself is moving downward and forward. This, of course, increases the width of the maxillary dental arch.

It is not easy to demonstrate the particulars of maxillary width completion. The functional matrix concepts of Moss largely explain the stimulus, with compensatory changes at the midpalatal suture. However, the suture closes quite early. Some orthodontic techniques employ rapid expansion of the lateral and palatal segments or "splitting the palate" for maxillary deficiency cases, and these cases demonstrate connective tissue fill-in and replacement by bone at the midline.[73, 74] It is highly questionable that midpalatal growth is a primary motivating force. Rather, the likelihood of its adjustive or adaptive response to functional matrix stimulus is evident. The research of Hinrichsen and palate-splitting experiences demonstrate the largely adjustive and compensatory reaction of sutural connective tissue and the immediate and sensitive response of membranous bone to tensional forces[27] (Fig. 2–18).

In an attempt to analyze possible areas for change in accomplishing the ultimate width dimension of the maxilla, the junction of the maxilla with the outward divergent pterygoid processes provides an area for "fill-in activity." Other sutures with similar potential are the ethmoid, zygomatic, lacrimal and nasal bone sutures. Of course, as Enlow shows, appositional growth on the lateral walls of the maxilla itself, on the palatal process of the premaxilla and on the palatal process of the palatine bones all play a role in the accomplishment of final form.[49]

One cannot get away from the observation that the maxilla completes its width quite early in life. Because of its intimate association with the cranial base and because of the possibility of endochondral dominance over membranous bone changes, there are a number of observers who feel that the maxillary width more nearly follows the neural growth curve, which is differentially complete quite early. This is in contrast with the downward and forward maxillary growth which follows the general growth curve and continues to parallel pubertal changes elsewhere.

Lebret confirmed the minimal change in the shape of the top of the palatal vault, with only the alveolar process increasing in height and breadth continuously.[75] Her work substantiated studies by Korkhaus, who pointed out the constancy of the midsagittal curvature from a few millimeters posterior to the incisive foramen to the region of the first permanent molars.[76-78, 83]

Our current knowledge of maxillary growth and development is well summarized by Enlow and Bang.[68]

As the maxilla increases in size, its various parts and regions come to occupy, in sequential order, new positions in the bone. This requires a mechanism of structural adjustment which brings about actual shifts in the location of specific parts in order to maintain constant shape and relative positions.

The postnatal growth of the human maxilla parallels that of the mandible in that forward and downward movement of the growing bone as a whole is a result of growth which takes place in a posterior direction with corresponding repositioning of the entire bone in a forward course. This growth pattern is one of several adaptations to the presence of teeth in the maxilla and mandible, and it makes possible elongation of the dental arch at its free (distal) ends. Such growth permits a progressive increase in the number of teeth which can take place only at the posterior ends of the dental arch. It also involves a complex series of corresponding remodeling changes in all of the various parts of both the maxilla and the mandible.

The generalization that the maxilla is thrust downward and forward by growth in posterior and superior parts of the bone is an oversimplification and, if not qualified, can lead to inaccurate assumptions. Growth does occur in this manner in certain specific areas, but it also proceeds in a complex variety of other directions in different major regions of the maxilla. The over-all size of the face increases by a series of specific growth movements in several individual areas which proceed away from each other, thereby drawing out the dimensions of the maxilla in several different directions.

Bone deposits are added along the posterior margin of the maxillary tuberosity. This functions to lengthen the dental arch and to enlarge the anterior-posterior dimensions of the entire maxillary body. Coordinated with this increase is the progressive movement of the entire zygomatic process in a corresponding posterior direction. This sequence serves to maintain continuously the constant position of the zygomatic process relative to the remainder of the maxilla. The separate zygomatic bone also moves in a posterior course by a combination of resorption from its anterior surfaces and deposition along its posterior side. The face simultaneously enlarges in breadth by proportionate bone apposition on the lateral surface of the zygomatic arch with corresponding resorption from its medial surface.

The floor of the orbit faces superiorly, laterally, and slightly anteriorly. Surface deposition results in growth proceeding in all three corresponding directions. Resorption from the lateral surface of the orbital rim functions to make way for the laterally-moving orbital surface of the maxilla in the floor of the orbital cavity. The nasal area of the maxilla, together with its separate nasal bones, also faces in similar lateral, anterior, and superior directions. Growth proceeds in these same directions by surface bone deposition, thereby increasing the internal size of the nasal cavity by an elongation and expansion of its vertical and horizontal dimensions. The bony cortex lining the inner surface of the nasal cavity undergoes periosteal surface removal of bone as its endosteal side receives simultaneous deposits of new bone.

The palatine processes of the maxilla grow in a generally downward direction by a combination of surface deposition on the entire oral side of the palatal cortex with resorptive removal from the opposite nasal side, as well as from periosteal labial surfaces of the anterior maxillary arch.

The premaxillary part of the maxilla grows in a downward direction. The surface orientation of this area is such that downward movement is brought about by resorptive removal from the periosteal surface of the labial cortex which faces away from the direction of growth. The endosteal side of its cortex and the periosteal surface of the lingual cortex receive new bone deposits. This growth pattern also produces a slight "recession" of the incisor area in a posterior direction, a situation also present in the human mandible.

It is suggested that the various remodeling movements of the growing maxillary bone contribute to a functional basis for the drifting of teeth. Adjustments in the position of erupted as well as unerupted teeth appear to be required as a result of growth and remodeling movements of tooth-bearing bone.

It is also suggested that the variety of specific remodeling processes associated with maxillary (and mandibular) growth contributes to the characteristic age changes in the gross appearance of the human face.

It should be emphasized that the actual changes that occur in the maxilla are very probably under the influence of epigenetic factors such as neurotrophic stimulus, development of the functional matrices, growth of the functioning spaces, and so forth. Although Moss is quite willing to discount cartilaginous growth as a primary stimulus, despite Scott's support, this author could well add it to the list just given above.

Clinical evidence, as well as the experimental research already cited, seems to support Scott's thesis.[33] In achondroplastic dwarfs, the midface shows marked concavity and retardation, owing to deficient cartilage growth. In the cebocephalia case reported by Ackerman et al., the severe midface deficiency is obvious, owing to congenital lack of the cartilaginous nasal septum. The insult here is primarily horizontal, indicating that the septum may be most involved in this vector of growth.[66] Since the orbits were present, despite the absence of the eye mass, and since there was apparently some orbital growth in the child with cebocephalia (albeit less than normal), the only possible explanation is that the shiny pink lining, which was deduced as Tenon's capsule and conjunctiva, could have performed as a periosteal or capsular matrix, as outlined by Moss. It is quite probable that fluid was present in the orbital cavities, at least during the period in utero. But this is surmise and it illustrates the limitations of making interpretation about the normal from the pathologic. Even the role of nasal septum is open to some question (Fig. 2–31). Babula, Smiley and Dixon were not able to substantiate its dominance in their study of A/Jax rats.[81]

It is quite easy to construct a hypothesis whereby the early growth of the anterior cranial base with its synchondrosis dominance over membranous bone would be a time-linked factor in the forward movement of the maxilla itself. When the cranial base ceases to be a major area of change, the continued downward and forward growth of the nasal septum could well "take over" as the vertical growth becomes dominant and, as Enlow shows, the palate descends with significant increases in nasomaxillary height (Fig. 2–31).[80, 82]

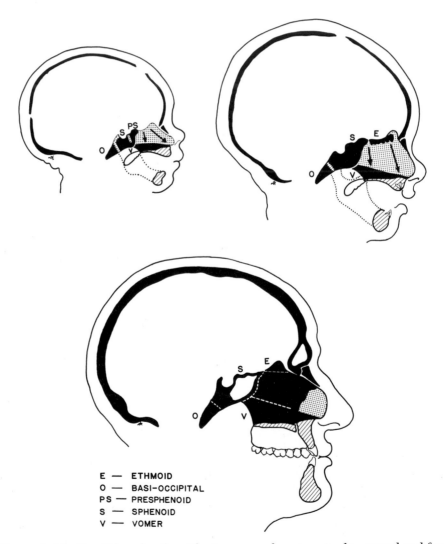

E — ETHMOID
O — BASI-OCCIPITAL
PS — PRESPHENOID
S — SPHENOID
V — VOMER

Figure 2–31 Possible role of cartilaginous nasal septum in downward and forward growth of the maxillary complex (bone is black or crosshatched; cartilage, stippled). (Adapted from Ford, E. H. R.: Growth of the human cranial base. Am. J. Orthodont., 44:498–506, 1958.)

Savara and Singh confirm the greatest increase in maxillary height, next in depth and least in width in their study of children from 3 to 16 years of age.[79] The width is complete relatively early with no sex difference. But the downward and forward growth is sex-linked at puberty, with boys' growth one to three years later than girls' growth. Cephalometric studies of late changes by the author show a dominance of vertical growth over horizontal maxillary growth in the late stages, in both boys and girls, somewhat in contrast with mandibular directional changes, as is pointed out in the section on the mandible.

MANDIBLE

At birth the two rami of the mandible are quite short. Condylar development is minimal and there is practically no articular eminence in the glenoid fossa. A thin line of fibrocartilage and connective tissue exists at the midline of the symphysis to separate right and left mandibular bodies. Between four months of age and the end of the first year, the symphysial cartilage is replaced by bone. Although growth is quite general during the first year of life, with all surfaces showing bone apposition, there is apparently no significant growth between the two halves before they unite. During the first year of life, appositional growth is especially active at the alveolar border, at the distal and superior surfaces of the ramus, at the condyle, along the lower border of the mandible and on its lateral surfaces (Fig. 2–32).

CONDYLAR GROWTH.   Endochondral growth does occur during the accomplishment of the full morphogenetic pattern of the mandible. Weinmann and Sicher have strongly supported their contention that the condyle is the major growth center of the mandible and is endowed with an intrinsic genetic potential.[14] However, this concept is overly simplified. In many circles, the condyle is no longer considered the dominant primary growth factor for the mandible.[84, 85] The explanation has been that differentiation and proliferation of hyaline cartilage and its replacement by bone in the deepest layer is quite similar to changes that occur at the epiphysial plate and in the articular cartilage of the long bone. Indeed there is a similarity of these areas histologically[30] (Fig. 2–33).

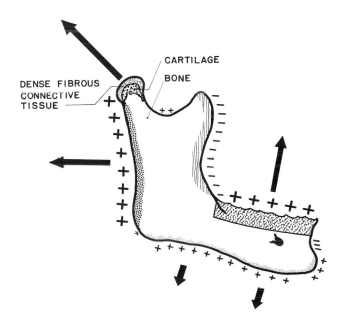

Figure 2–32   The unique growth mechanism of the mandibular condylar region employs both interstitial and appositional proliferation. Appositional growth at the posterior border of the ramus, alveolar margin, inferior margin of the mandibular body, and on the lateral surfaces (to a lesser degree) accounts for the increase in size. Concomitant resorption occurs on the anterior ramus margin, in effect increasing the dental arch length.

CARTILAGE

BONE

DENSE FIBROUS CONNECTIVE TISSUE

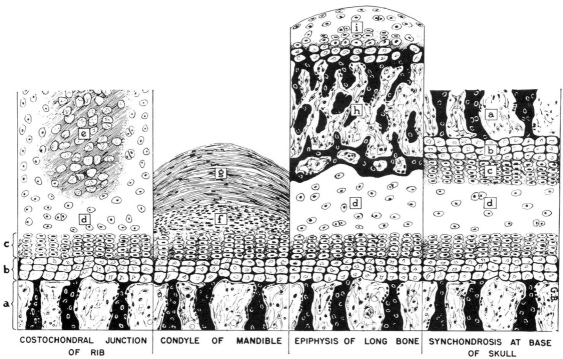

Figure 2–33 Diagrammatic representation of the variation in tissue arrangement adjacent to endochondral bone formation at the costochondral junction of a rib, condyle of the mandible, epiphysis of a long bone, and cranial base synchondrosis. Note that the zones of endochondral bone formation (a, b, c) are the same. Also note the variation in tissue arrangement adjacent to the four separate areas of endochondral bone formation. Letters designate different tissues: a, bone; b, prechondroblasts; c, chondroblasts or proliferating cartilage; d, zone of resting cartilage; e, mature cartilage with a calcified core; f, transitional zone of cartilage; g, dense fibrous connective tissue; h, bone and marrow of epiphysis; i, articular cartilage. (From Sarnat, B. G.: Growth of bones as revealed by implant markers in animals. Am. J. Phys. Anthrop., 29:255–286, 1968.)

There is, however, a unique difference which is observed in no other articular cartilage of the body. The hyaline cartilage of the condyle is covered by a dense and thick fibrous connective tissue layer. Thus, the cartilage of the condyle not only increases by interstitial growth, as the long bones of the body, but is able also to increase in thickness by appositional growth beneath connective tissue covering.[86]

Sicher's explanation of the role of this tough condylar covering seems to be logical. Since pressure mitigates against apposition of bone—and the condyle is under constant pressure during function as the articulating element of the mandible—the fibrous condylar covering allows a thickening of the hyaline cartilage in the transitional zone directly beneath it. It further protects the prechondroblastic zone in the neck of the condyle. It is here that pressures might find a more sensitive response as Charlier and Petrovic have shown with the reduction of prechondroblastic activity under excessive pressures, resulting in the diminution of production of chondroblasts later.[87] If the Sicher-Weinmann theory is correct, then the mandibular condyle would grow by two mechanisms: by the usual epiphysial plate-like interstitial proliferation of cartilage and its replacement by bone and by appositional growth of cartilage beneath a unique fibrous covering.

Intensive research on the functional matrix growth theory questions the primacy of this area and also whether it is analogous to an epiphysial plate at all. Moss does not deny the cellular changes but he feels that this is under the influence of the growth of the orofacial capsular matrices. As these matrices grow, as the vital spaces and airway remain in patent form and as the mandible itself is translated by growth of other structures, the cellular changes take place. Thus, the concept of the dominance of epigenetic and environmental factors is supported. Bone yields to soft tissue pressure, as Sicher himself has stressed. Condylar growth is regarded as a secondary or "fill-in" response.[88-90]

To test the functional matrix thesis and to explain some of the observations of Björk[91-93] which did not agree with the Sicher-Weinmann hypothesis, Koski and Makinen did an extensive study on transplanted components of the mandibular ramus of the rat.[94, 95] One hundred and seventeen hosts received a total of 222 transplants. One hundred and forty-nine transplants were recovered after periods of 30, 45, 60 and 90 days. Transplants were well tolerated but the shape of the recovered tissue was largely that of the original transplant. Only when the condyles were transplanted with a part of the ramus or with bone tissue was there measurable growth. Koski writes, "It appears as if the presence of the ossified portion of the ramus would be necessary for the condylar cartilage to function as a growth center in a limited sense."[94] In addition, Koski did another series of transplants, using different tissues: condylar cartilage with primary spongiosa and pieces of ramus with primary spongiosa.[58] The placement of a 1 mm. thick radial epiphysial cartilage, inserted into the subcutis, produced a well-organized epiphysiometaphysial unit; after this was transplanted into the brain, Koski secured pieces up to 9 mm. long with complete epiphysis and diaphysial bony tail. For transplanted condylar cartilages, however, there was no bony growth. These experiments again seemingly refute the Sicher-Weinmann concept of similarity of condylar cartilage to epiphysial cartilage.

Further supporting evidence comes from the experimental work of Sarnat, and Muchnic, Irving and Rönning, Gianelly and Moorrees[96-99] (Figs. 2–34, 2–35). Strongly supportive is the Rankow-Moss study of a young female who had been subjected to condylectomy, following ankylosis.[100] The immediate resumption of downward and forward mandibular growth, basal mandibular translation and

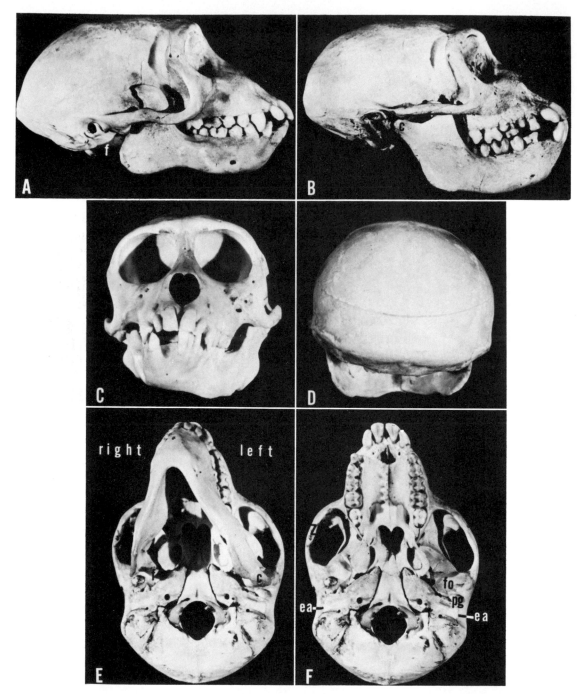

Figure 2-34 Skulls of growing rhesus monkeys. Right mandibular condyle was resected at about 8 months of age (A, C, D, E, and F). A and C, Lateral and anterior views. Postoperative survival was 29 months. Note that facial height is less in A than in B (unoperated on animal No. 2–2). No true condyle, fossa, or articular eminence is visible. Note also considerably wider and heavier coronoid process directed more posteriorly and above zygomatic arch; shorter, wide, anteriorly positioned ramus; relation of posterior border of ramus to where true fossa should be; mandibular angle, which is less than 90 degrees; accentuation of antegonial notch; and lesser height of mandibular body. In C, note lesser amount of total facial height on operated right side as compared with unoperated left side, relatively lower level of zygomatic arch, and lesser height of ramus. D, posterior view of animal, with postoperative survival of 14 months. Note higher level of mandible on operated right side. E and F, Ventral views of animal, with and without mandible in occlusion.

the increase in vertical height indicate that the condyle certainly is not the controlling factor of mandibular development.[101] Obviously, we reach the frontiers of our knowledge pretty quickly. Until we learn the growth timing and incremental changes for the muscles associated with the mandible, as well as the growth gradients for other elements of the functional matrix, including the tongue, our knowledge remains at the convenient working hypothesis level. It is difficult to analyze the growth of vital spaces and more difficult to measure the primacy of orofacial matrices. If there is, indeed, a dominant neurotrophic influence, more must be done to demonstrate this experimentally.[102] At present, we are in a better position to demonstrate what mandibular growth is not, than what it is. A more detailed description of the functional matrix concepts is given later in ths section.

A study of the effects of orthopedic appliances gives every indication that they can guide mandibular growth, redirecting it and interfering specifically with alveolar bone growth.[103] (See Chaps. 11, 14). Of course, more than clinical substantiation is necessary. Longitudinal cephalometric studies of a large number of cases under orthopedic guidance by the author provide confirmatory evidence that growth can, indeed, be influenced or redirected.

MANDIBULAR GROWTH AFTER THE FIRST YEAR OF LIFE. The fact that we cannot tell precisely *why* the mandible grows does not prevent us from giving an accurate description of *how* it grows and changes. After the first year of extrauterine life, mandibular growth becomes more selective. The condyle does show considerable activity as the mandible moves and grows downward and forward. Heavy appositional growth occurs on the posterior border of the ramus and on the alveolar border. Significant increments of growth are still observed at the tip of the coronoid process. Resorption occurs along the anterior border of the ramus lengthening the alveolar border and maintaining the anteroposterior dimension of the ramus (Fig. 2–32). Cephalometric studies indicate that the body of the mandible maintains a relatively constant angular relationship to the ramus throughout life. The gonial angle changes little after muscle function has become well defined. With approaching senescence and a marked reduction of muscle activity, there is evidence that the gonial angle tends to become more acute.

Although growth at the condyle, together with apposition of bone on the posterior border of the ramus, contributes to the length of the mandible, and the condyle, together with significant alveolar growth, contributes to the height of the mandible, the third dimension—width—shows a more subtle change. Actually, after the first year of life, during which there is appositional growth on all surfaces, the major width contribution of the mandible is growth at the

---

Figure 2–34 Continued.
Right condyle was resected 25 months before death. Note, on right side in E, increased distance of articulating surface of mandible from temporal bone and position of left unoperated-on condyle in fossa. Also note, on operated right side, that postglenoid process is less prominent, mandible articulates with temporal bone anterior to fossa, and body is shorter than the unoperated left side, so that entire mandible is directed toward operated side. Left zygomatic arch extends more posteriorly and is longer, thinner, and straighter than one on right. There is no semblance of articular fossa in right temporal bone, and remaining right postglenoid process is not as far posterior as left one. External auditory canal is more posterior than unoperated left side. c, Condyle; ea, external auditory canal; f, false articulation; fo, articular fossa; pg, postglenoid; z, zygomatic arch. (From Sarnat, B. G., and Muchnic, H.: Facial skeletal changes after mandibular condylectomy in growing and adult monkeys. Am. J. Orthodont., 60:33–45, 1971.)

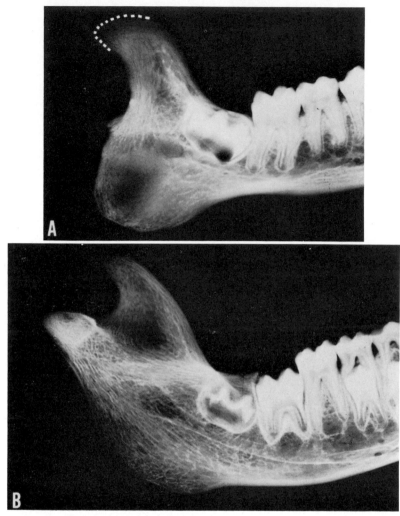

Figure 2–35 Postmortem lateral roentgenograms of disarticulated, dissected mandibles of two growing rhesus monkeys. A, Mandibular condyle was resected 29 months before death. Note deficiency of posterior ramus and relatively prominent coronoid process, with some accentuation of antegonial notch. Also note trabecular pattern along posterior border of ramus and coronoid process and increased radiopacity of bone at new articular area. Entrance to mandibular canal is close to articular area. Contrast with B, unoperated side of mandible. Principal trabecular masses appear to be directed in form of "N" along the following axes: (1) condylar-angular, from condyloid process to angle and lower border of mandible; (2) condylar-retromolar, from condyloid process to retromolar area; and (3) coronoid-retromolar, from coronoid process to retromolar area. Last molars are not fully calcified and erupted. (Sarnat and Muchnic.)

posterior border. Literally, the mandible is an "expanding V". Additive growth at the ends of this "V" naturally increases the distance between the terminal points. The two rami also diverge outward from below to above so that additive growth at the coronoid notch, coronoid process and condyle also increases the superior inter-ramus dimension.[49, 104] Patterns of cortical structure based on the growth of 25 young human mandibles are recorded in Figure 2–36. Growth patterns in condyle, coronoid process, ramus and body are recorded in Figures 2–37 to 2–39.

Alveolar growth is another factor. Continued growth of alveolar bone with the developing dentition increases the height of the mandibular body. But we are again dealing with a three-dimensional object. The alveolar process of the mandible grows upward *and* outward on an expanding arc. This permits the dental arch to accommodate the larger permanent teeth. Relatively little increase in mandibular body width is noted after the cessation of lateral surface appositional growth. Modeling deposition at the canine eminence and along the lateral inferior border is seen. Measurements between the right and left mental foramina,

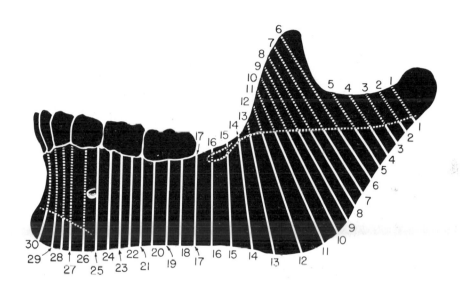

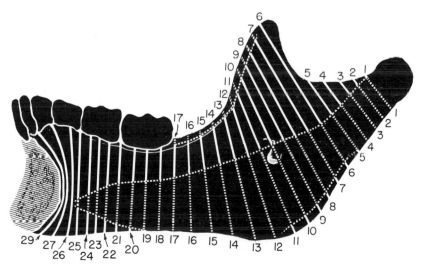

Figure 2–36 A composite figure based on 25 young human mandibles. The most frequently observed patterns of cortical structure in various areas are summarized. The numbered lines indicate the serial locations of entire transverse sections. Solid white lines represent cortical surfaces which have received periosteal deposits and which have grown in an outward or periosteal direction. Broken lines indicate resorptive surfaces with an underlying cortex composed of endosteal bone. (Top) Buccal aspect. (Bottom) Lingual aspect. (From Enlow, D. H., and Harris, D. B.: A study of the postnatal growth of the human mandible. Am. J. Orthodont., 50:25–50, 1964.)

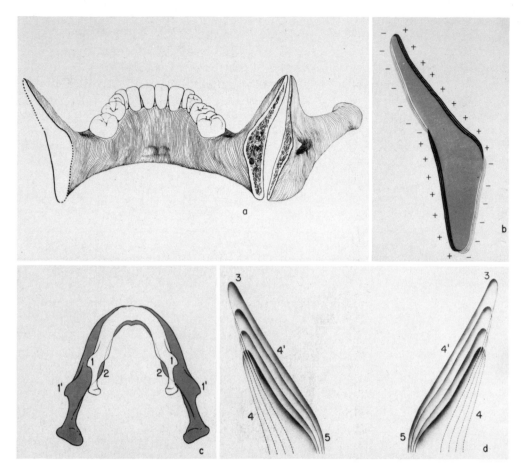

Figure 2–37 A vertical section through the ramus and coronoid process (a) shows a characteristic growth pattern (b) which involves periosteal deposition (+) on the lingual surface of the coronoid process together with removal (−) from the buccal surface. The basal part of the ramus receives periosteal deposits on the buccal side with contralateral resorption from the lingual surface. In (c) the coronoid process moves laterally from 1 to 1'. Note that the coronoid process of the younger mandible occupies the same level as the lingual tuberosity in the older growth stage. The remodeling mechanism involved in this relocation is shown partly by (d) which illustrates the "expanding V" principle. As the coronoid processes become higher, their termini grow farther apart at their apices (3) by additions on the *lingual* surface (4') with contralateral removal from the buccal side (4). Note also that this same mechanism of lingual deposition brings their bases toward each other (5). This combination of growth movements serves to move and enlarge the coronoid process from 1 to 1' in (c) and to bring about simultaneously the lingual direction of movement seen at 2 in diagram (c), as the mandibular body becomes lengthened. (From Enlow, D. H., and Harris, D. B.: A study of the postnatal growth of the human mandible. Am. J. Orthodont., 50:25–50, 1964.)

for example, show that this dimension changes relatively little after the sixth year of life.

Some observers attribute a great role to the musculature in the development of the characteristics mandibular morphology and size. Scott divides the mandible into three basic types of bone—basal, muscular and alveolar, or tooth-supporting.[39] The basal portion is a tube-like central foundation running from the condyle to the symphysis (Fig. 2–40). The muscular portion (the gonial angle and coronoid process) is under the influence of the masseter, internal pterygoid and temporal muscles. Muscle function determines the ultimate form of the mandible in these areas. The third portion, alveolar bone, exists to hold the teeth. When the teeth are lost there is no further use for alveolar bone and it is gradually resorbed. Reduced muscle activity would account for the flattening of the gonial angle and reduction of the coronoid process. This functional matrix concept is supported by those who regard the visceral growth as dominant and the bone growth as adjustive.[45-48, 58] Moss speaks of the mandible as a group of microskeletal units.[89] Thus, the coronoid process is one skeletal unit, under the influence of the temporalis muscle. The gonial angle is another skeletal unit under the influence of masseter and internal pterygoid muscles. The alveolar bone is under the influence of the teeth. Biggerstaff shows in his research that when a tooth is transplanted, it actually grows its own alveolar supporting bone around it.[105] The basal tubular portion of the mandible serves as protection for the mandibular canal ("unloaded nerve" concept) and apparently follows a logarithmic spiral in its downward and forward movement from beneath the cranium. It would certainly appear that the most constant portion of the mandible is the arc from foramen ovale to mandibular foramen to mental foramen.[90]

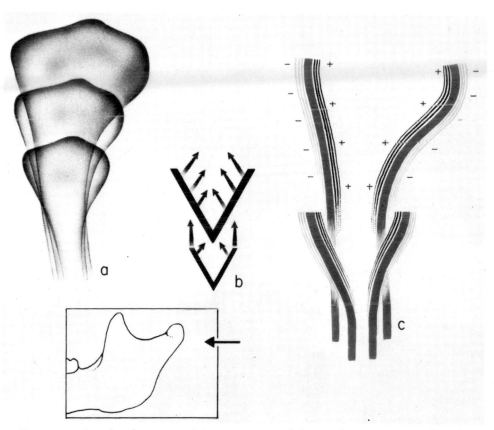

Figure 2–38   The diameter of the narrow condylar neck is progressively reduced from the wider dimensions of the posterior-moving condyle. Inward growth of the buccal and lingual cortices (c) is accomplished by a combination process of periosteal resorption (−) and endosteal deposition (+). This is also an example of the "expanding V" principle (b) and as seen in Figure 2–37 (d). (From Enlow, D. H., and Harris, D. B.: A study of the postnatal growth of the human mandible. Am. J. Orthodont., 50:25–50, 1964.)

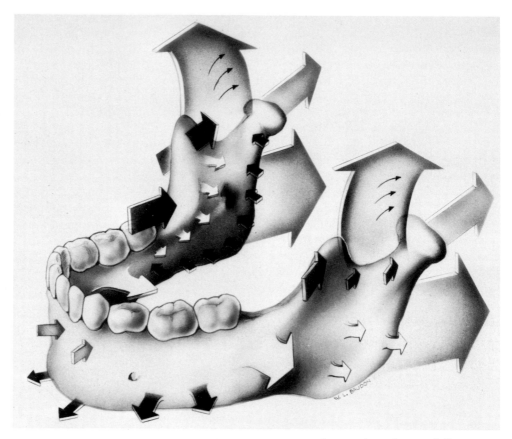

Figure 2–39 Composite of all the various regional growth and remodeling movements of the mandible as shown in Figures 2–36 to 2–38. (From Enlow, D. H., and Harris, D. B.: A study of the postnatal growth of the human mandible. Am. J. Orthodont., 50:25–50, 1964.)

In a discussion of the role of muscles and functional matrices, it might be well to point out that Moss delineates two basic types of functional matrices. These are the periosteal and the capsular matrices.[85] The periosteal matrix is exemplified by the functional component consisting of the temporalis muscle and the coronoid process. This process first arises within the earlier form of anlage of the temporalis muscle whose contractile abilities are well developed in prenatal stages. Its subsequent growth also occurs within this muscular matrix. The fibrous noncontractile portion of the temporalis muscle is attached to the coronoid process in a variable manner: indirectly to the outer fibrous layer of the periosteum for the most part, and to a slight degree by insertion into the skeletal tissue itself, chiefly at a relatively late postnatal stage. The experimental removal of the temporalis muscle or its denervation invariably results in the actual diminution of the size and shape of the coronoid process or even its total disappearance.[89] Thus, Moss feels that the total growth changes of the coronoid process are at all times a direct compensatory response to morphogenetic and functional demands of the temporalis muscle function. "All responses of the osseous portions of skeletal units to periosteal matrices are brought about by the complementary and interrelated process of osseous deposition and resorption. The resultant effect of all such skeletal unit responses to periosteal matrices

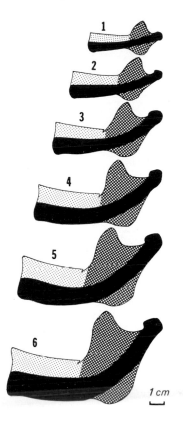

Figure 2–40 Protected nerve concept with central core straight at first, but following logarithmic curve, with progressing mandibular growth and development. "Unloaded nerve" concept also accounts for stress trajectory alignment and trabecular structure from condyle to symphysis.

is to alter their size and/or their shape."[89] Although muscles are excellent examples of periosteal functional matrices, they do not comprise this entire category. Blood vessels, nerves and glands produce morphologic changes in their related skeletal units in a completely homologous manner. The same analysis can be made of the alteration of relative proportions of the contiguous microskeletal units, for example, in the mandible. Analyzing the net backward displacement of the microskeletal units of the ramus during growth points to more than mere deposition and resorption (Figs. 2–41 – 2–44). Any definition

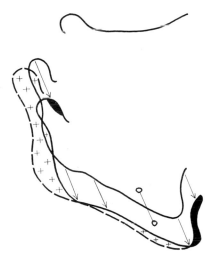

Figure 2–41 An overlay of the tracings produces this picture, which shows both transformation and translation. In effect, the two positions of the younger mandible show what would occur if the mandible were only translated (passively moved within the expanding orofacial capsule), without transformation occurring simultaneously. The magnitude and direction of this translation are shown by the arrows. However, transformation occurs also and is shown as areas of resorption (black) and deposition (plus signs). This figure is an approximate mean and clearly shows that the downward and forward motion of the mandible primarily is passive translation, whereas active transformation produces minor changes anteriorly and inferiorly while being entirely responsible for the posterior and upward compensatory growth of the ramus. (From Moss, M. L., and Salentijn, L., Am. J. Orthodontics; 56:474, 1969.)

—— 7 yrs.

—— 15 yrs.

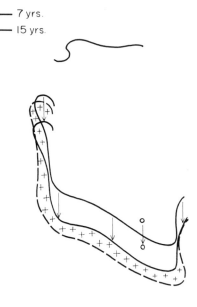

Figure 2–42 In this and in Figures 2–43 and 2–44, mandibles are superimposed as in Figure 2–41, to show translative and transformative changes. In this patient, the net result is a vertical vector of growth. (From Moss, M. L., and Salentijn, L., Am. J. Orthod. 56:474, 1969.)

—— 6 yrs., 11 mo.

– – 15 yrs., 5 mo.

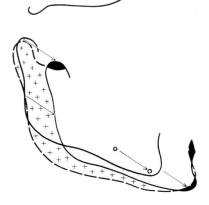

Figure 2–43 Superimposed tracings which indicate transformative and translative aspects of mandibular growth. Here the net result is a strongly horizontal component. (From Moss, M. L., and Salentijn, L.: The capsular matrix. Am. J. Orthodont., 56:474–490, 1969.)

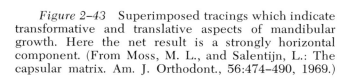

—— 9 yrs., 6 mo.

– – 14 yrs., 5 mo.

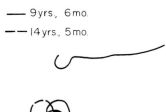

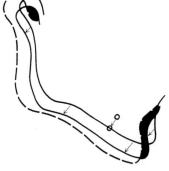

Figure 2–44 Despite additive growth at the posterior border of the ramus, the net effect, because of translative or transpositional aspects of growth, is a downward and backward vector. The resorption shown here at the symphysis seems to be independent of the direction of translative growth. (From Moss, M. L., and Salentijn, L.: The capsular matrix. Am. J. Orthodont., 56:474–490, 1969.)

of growth must include spatial translation of bones in addition to the size and shape changes which can often occur simultaneously.

Capsular matrices are a bit harder to describe.[67, 69] All skeletal units, and so all bones in the formal sense, arise, exist, grow and are maintained and respond morphologically while totally embedded within their functional periosteal matrices. At the same time these functional cranial components (functional matrices together with skeletal units) organize in the form of cranial capsules. Each of these capsules is an envelope which contains a series of functional cranial components which are sandwiched between two covering layers. In the neurocranial capsule, for example, the covers consist of skin and the dura mater. In the orofacial capsule, the skin and mucosa form the limiting layers. Spaces intervening between the functional components themselves and between them and the capsule are filled with undifferentiated loose connective tissue. Each capsule surrounds and protects a capsular functional matrix: in one case the neural mass which consists of the brain, and leptomeninges and, most important, cerebral-spinal fluid; in the other case the oronasopharyngeal functioning spaces. The common fact in both cases is that the capsular matrices exist as volumes. In the case of the neural skull, it is quite easy to visualize the calvarial bones lying within a neural cranial capsule. For the orofacial matrices, all functional cranial components of the facial skull arise, grow and are maintained within an orofacial capsule. Moss indicates that the volumetric growth of the spaces is the primary morphogenetic event in the facial skull growth. The three functioning spaces (oral, nasal and pharyngeal) are not simply leftover areas. The functional reality of the respiratory and digestive systems is the patency of these spaces. The volume of the patency is related to the general metabolic demands of the body as a whole. The concept of the morphologic and functional primacy of the oronasopharyngeal spaces receives strong support from the independently developed work of Bosma.[106] The patency of the airway, maintained by the dynamic musculoskeletal postural balance, has been demonstrated for some time.

Mandibular growth demonstrates the integrated activity of periosteal and capsular matrices in facial growth. Since the condyles are not primary sites of mandibular growth but loci with secondary, compensatory growth potential, condylar removal does not inhibit the spatial translation of contiguous mandibular functional components. Nor does condylectomy inhibit the changes in the form of their microskeletal units as their individual matrices alter functional demands.[100] If there are no condylar processes how does the mandible alter its spatial position? No combination of periosteal growth changes of microskeletal unit form (size and shape) is capable of explaining this. It is only by considering that the orofacial capsule expands in response to the morphogenetically previous volumetric expansion of the orofacial functioning spaces that we can comprehend the observed translation in space. Mandibular growth is seen now to be a combination of the morphologic effects of both capsular and periosteal matrices. The capsular matrix growth causes an expansion of the capsule as a whole. The enclosed and embedded microskeletal unit (the mandible) is passively and secondarily translated in space to successively new positions. Under normal conditions then the periosteal matrices related to the constituent mandibular microskeletal unit also respond to this volumetric expansion. Such alteration in spatial position inevitably causes them to grow. This now calls for direct alteration in the size and shape of the microskeletal units. The sum of *translation* plus changes in *form* comprises the totality of mandibular growth.

If the functional cranial analysis of Moss and his co-workers is correct, it is important to know how functional stimuli are translated at the skeletal unit interface and how functional matrices are regulated and controlled. This involves neurotrophic processes. Neurotrophism "is a non-impulse transmittive neurofunction, involving axoplasmic transport, providing for the long term interactions between neurons and innervated tissues which homeostatically regulate the morphological, compositional and functional integrity of those tissues. The nature of neurotrophic substances and the process of their introduction into the target tissue are unknown at present."[102] Moss does indicate that there are three general categories: neuro-epithelial, neurovisceral and neuromuscular.

As an example of neuroepithelial trophism, amphibian limb regeneration is initiated only after intimate neuroepithelial contact. Also, the mitotic activity necessary for normal epithelial turnover of taste buds, the maintenance in being, the expression of their genomic potential in such processes as DNA, and enzymatic synthesis are all under the direct and continuous afferent gustatory neurotrophic control. From such examples, it is tempting to ask whether the growth of the epithelially lined and covered orofacial capsule which reflects the growth of the naso-oral functioning space (as the capsular matrix) similarly is trophically regulated. Certainly, some patients with facial hypoplasia or anatomic and physiologic abnormalities of hard and soft palate exhibit a concurrent cluster of sensory deficits, as do many other patients with cleft palate (Chap. 6) or with disordered articulation.[107]

NEUROVISCERAL TROPHISM. "Considering only the orofacial region, it is clear that the salivary glands, among other splanchnocranial viscera, are trophically regulated, at least partially." Experimental data have shown increase and decrease of mature salivary glands under trophic influence. More recently, these techniques have extended to glandular ontogenesis. There is a consensus developing that the normal rate of growth, expressed in part as regulation of cell number and size, is under neurotrophic control.[102]

NEUROMUSCULAR TROPHISM. Moss indicates that skeletal muscle ontogenesis normally requires motoneuron innervation to proceed past the stage of myotubes. Neurotrophic rather than conductive influences are involved. Cross-innervation experiments are provocative. They show that significant morphologic biomechanical and functional parameters of re-innervated muscle come to more closely resemble those of the muscle formerly innervated by the now ectopically implanted nerve.[108] In other words, these parameters of skeletal muscle are nerve-specific not muscle-specific. Diculescu *et al.* state, "The complex chain of events leading to particular expression of the genetic-embryonic potential is not wholly within the cell, but also includes informational elements contributed by the nerve."[109] Samaha, Guth and Albers write, "A new species of protein has been synthesized, and we therefore suggest that the nerve influences gene expression of the cell."[110] Moss feels that if this is true, that periosteal (muscular) functional matrices actually regulate the size and shape of specifically related skeletal units, it is apparent that the genetic control of the structural, chemical and functional attributes of the same matrices cannot reside solely in the matrices themselves. They reflect constant neurotrophically regulated, homeostatic control of the genome. Carrying this one step further, similar trophic controls probably exist for the capsular functional matrices which passively regulate the position of both the skeletal units and the periosteal matrices. If some degree of visceral neurotrophic control is probable, then we are close to knowing the ultimate stimulus for growth.

THE CHIN.   The last word has yet to be stated on growth of the chin.[159] Enlow and Harris feel that the chin is "associated with a generalized process of cortical recession in the flattened regions positioned between the canine teeth. The process involves a mechanism of endosteal cortical growth."[104] On the lingual surface behind the chin, heavy periosteal growth occurs, with the dense lamellar bone merging and overlapping on the labial side of the chin. The point of periosteal to endosteal contact is variable but usually occurs at a level just superior to the projecting apex of the chin. Most studies have been made before the chin assumes its final morphology.[111] Particularly in the male, the apposition of bone at the symphysis seems to be about the last change in shape during the growing period. This means that some time between 16 and 23 years of age, modeling apposition fashions a new shape to the symphysis in the male. This change is much less apparent in the female. Since the chin is missing in anthropoids, we can only conjecture reasons for this evolutionary change in man. We do not know whether the chin is due to the expansion of the brain case and reduction of the facial and dental skeleton, as claimed by Weidenreich,[112] or the result of muscle activity and the function of mastication, deglutition, respiration and speech or a reduction and retrusion of the jaws and ventral migration of the foramen magnum and change of the angle of the cranial base, as claimed by DuBrul.[111] It is quite possible, however, that the change of means of locomotion and the assumption of a vertical posture may be contributory. Certainly, if we make a functional analysis of osseous changes, a change in posture and locomotion should produce a corresponding change in bony morphology.

THE DYNAMICS OF FACIAL GROWTH

The growth and development of the human face provides a fascinating interplay of form and function. The mosaic of the morphogenetic pattern, as it is influenced by epigenetic and environmental forces, requires an understanding of many factors if we are to fully appreciate the phenomenon. This has more than artistic value as far as the orthodontist is concerned. Surveys have shown that two thirds of the cases seen for orthodontic therapy involve types of malocclusion in which growth and development play a significant role in the success or failure of mechanotherapy.

DIFFERENTIAL GROWTH.   Even before the advent of cephalometrics (longitudinal study of the head by oriented lateral and frontal x-ray images), Hellman had outlined the general growth picture as a result of his anthropologic studies.[113-114] He had pointed out that of the three dimensions—height, width and depth—the vertical growth, or height, and the anteroposterior length, or depth, increased most. Width showed the least change. He indicated that facial growth was more than a mere increase in size. Different organs grew at different rates (this is termed *differential growth*).

It has already been pointed out that the cranium grows quite rapidly and approaches adult size considerably before the face. But even in this instance, not all cranial dimensions show the same percentage of growth pattern at the same time. Growth in cranial depth is most rapid, with growth in width and height following in that order. In the face, height shows the greatest incremental change, followed by depth and width. In the differential growth of the various parts of the face, the height of the cranium and the width of the face are closest to adult size at birth. Then, "Growth is generally completed first in the head, then in the width of the face, and last in length or depth of face."[114]

Thus, it is apparent from any study of growth that we must take into consideration a fourth dimension—time. This is of vital importance to the orthodontist who must schedule his therapy so that it coincides with the most favorable growth period. Differential growth is time-linked. Those who study growth of the human head would like to know how much growth *per unit of time* occurs in the various structures that make up the craniofacial complex. Despite much that has been written on the constancy of facial growth and on its uniform rate (this has been deduced largely from longitudinal studies of cephalometric radiographs) a considerable body of evidence points to growth "spurts." Longitudinal studies have been made by the author on normal children and those with cleft palate from birth to six years of age. Significant and marked differences in the *rate* of growth within the same individual are uniformly evident[70] (Fig. 2–45). Not only is the rate of growth for both normal and cleft palate children highly variable, but the *direction* of growth at a particular time is occasionally unpredictable.

Similar studies made on orthodontic patients between the ages of 11 and 19 years also show varying rates of growth accomplishment and directional change.[115] A number of investigators point out the sex-linked nature of growth, with female pubertal spurt occurring ahead of that of the male[115, 116] (Figs. 2–46 to 2–48).

Mandibular downward and forward growth rate follows the general growth curve, i.e., precipitate growth early, leveling off in the deciduous dentition period, picking up somewhat in intensity during the mixed dentition period, and then showing significant growth spurts in the prepubertal and pubertal period as shown by Woodside. Mandibular growth in width, which is accomplished relatively early in the child, shows less total change than the vertical and anteroposterior dimensions in which change is significant. This is fortunate for the orthodontist, who must change anteroposterior and vertical jaw relationships in over half of the patients he treats. Timing treatment with mandibular growth particularly is most important, reducing the demands made on tooth position changes and the potential iatrogenic damage of prolonged appliance wear. This is discussed in greater detail under the Clinical Application of Growth and Development Data.

Woodside, in his study of the Burlington group, points out that growth spurts are really possible.[116] They seem to be sex-linked. The greatest increments of growth, as shown in the chart (Figs. 2–47, 2–48), are actually at the 3-year age level. The second peak is from 6 to 7 years in girls and 7 to 9 years in boys. The third peak is 11 to 12 years in girls and 14 to 15 years in boys. The tendency is for more boys to have two or three peaks, while the largest number of girls show only two peaks. The following chart shows the distribution.

	Male (114)	Female (104)
One peak	7	35
Two peaks	73	64
Three peaks	34	5

The clinical implications are obvious for orthopedic correction of maxillomandibular malrelationships. Very few girls seem to show the mixed dentition growth spurt; all show the pubertal growth spurt. This would seem to indicate that mixed dentition jaw change objectives are more likely to be successful in the boy. Pubertal increments still offer the best time for a large number of cases, as far as predictability, growth direction, patient management and total treatment time are concerned.

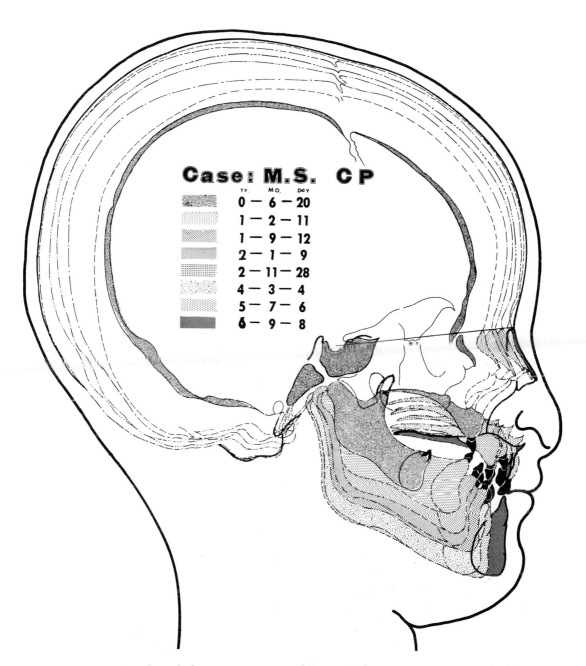

Figure 2–45 Serial cephalometric tracings of Pierre Robin patient. Note marked horizontal vector (catch-up growth) for first two years, with vertical dominance for the next two years, followed by a horizontal mandibular change. Although changes are more dramatic in this case, they demonstrate a normal phenomenon—variability in both direction and amount of growth, even before puberty and the classic growth spurt.

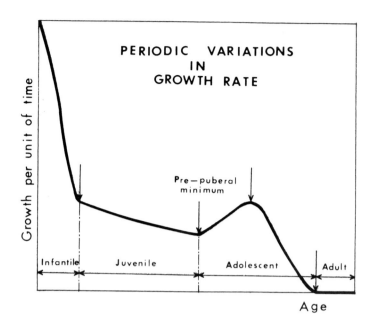

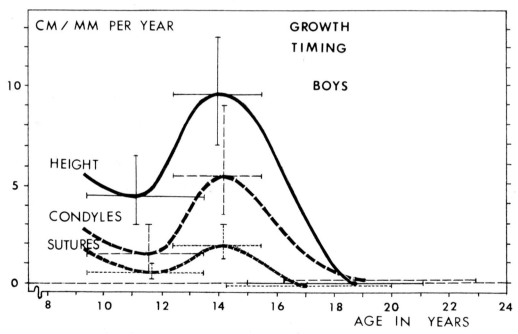

Figure 2–46 Growth gradients are age-linked, as the chart of this time-linked phenomenon shows. Note the high level of change in the infantile era, showing a decline to prepubertal minimum and then an acceleration during adolescence. For boys, maximum condylar change occurs concurrently with sutural and skeletal height peaks. This is one and a half years later than for girls, on the average. (From Björk, A., and Helm, S.: Prediction of the age of maximum puberal growth in body height. Angle Orthodont., 37:134–143, 1967.)

PEAK VELOCITY CURVES FOR FEMALES

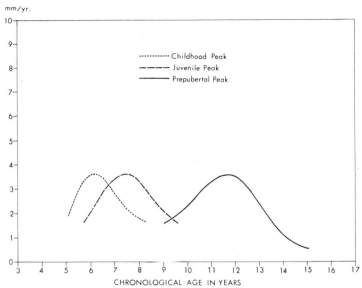

Figure 2–47 These peak velocity curves, taken from the Burlington study, show three possible periods of accelerated growth that are of interest clinically, if growth amounts are to be optimal. All three peaks for the female are ahead of comparable spurts for males (see Fig. 2–48). (From Woodside, D. G.: Distance, velocity and relative growth rate standards for mandibular growth for Canadian males and females age three to twenty years. Unpublished manuscript, 1969.)

PEAK VELOCITY CURVES FOR MALES

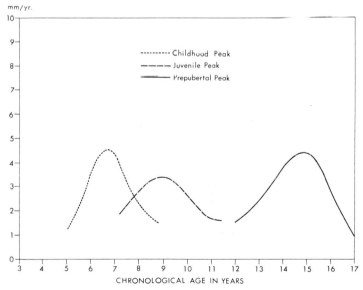

Figure 2–48 Male peak growth increments also show three possible age-linked associations, but with less overlap than females, and with later spread, particularly of prepubertal and pubertal spurt. Predictability of just when each individual will have a particular spurt is still not accurate enough. And this does not take into account the direction of growth, even though the increments may be large (see Figs. 2–41 to 2–44). (From Woodside, D. G.: Distance, velocity and relative growth rate standards for mandibular growth for Canadian males and females age three to twenty years. Unpublished manuscript, 1969.)

Savara and associates at the University of Oregon Child Study Clinic have developed a method of obtaining three-dimensionally corrected distances from cephalograms and have applied it on a longitudinal basis to 103 boys and girls between 3 and 16 years of age.[117-119] In their study of growth changes in the cranium, maxilla and mandible, they have corroborated the observations of Nanda, Meredith, Harris, Björk, Woodside and others concerning the adolescent growth acceleration.[92, 120-123] Distances measured on the mandible are shown in Figure 2–49. Figures 2–50 and 2–52 show Woodside's graphs of the velocity curves of mandibular dimensions and the mean annual increments for boys and girls from 3 to 17 years of age. Norms developed from the 50th to the 97th percentile should provide valuable data over an age range of considerable interest to the pedodontist and orthodontist.

In a discussion of the dynamics of facial growth, one other thought should be introduced. The accommodating and adjustive changes that occur within the structure that is growing and changing its spatial relationship may be unpredictable, but they are of significant importance. Specifically with respect to the maxilla and mandible, the teeth themselves are juggling, vying or competing for space as growth occurs. For the dentist, the "space age" surely is during the period of mixed dentition. There is no set "path of eruption" that follows a straight line. Summarizing graphs of various studies sometimes give this oversimplified impression. Rather there is a nonpredictable migration of teeth through bone per unit of time, intimately linked to the gross changes in the bony environment of these teeth. This is partly adaptive to changing bone relations, partly a physiologic response to functional pressures, partly attributable to that nebulous entity referred to as "pattern."

CLINICAL IMPLICATIONS.   It is obvious that certain growth factors are of vital importance to the pedodontist and orthodontist. If he is looking for growth in

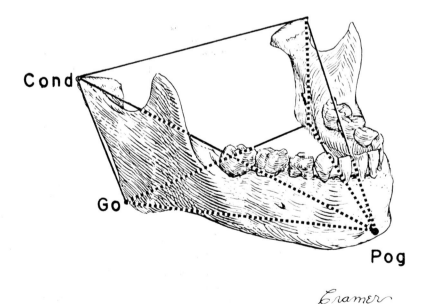

Figure 2–49   Distances measured on mandible in three-dimensional study by Savara and associates at University of Oregon Child Study Clinic. (From Savara, B. S., Tracy, W. E., and Brant, J. W. A.: Relation of height, width and depth of the mandible. Angle Orthodont., 35:270, 1965.)

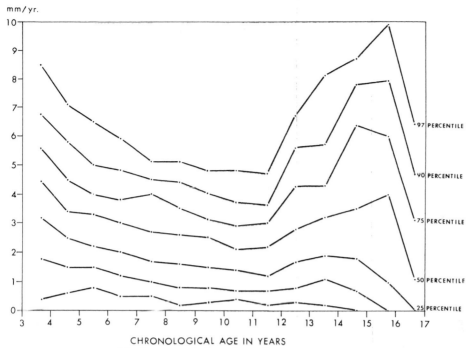

Figure 2–50 Mandibular growth for selected percentiles is shown for boys. Curves roughly approximate those shown by Björk in his study (see Fig. 2–46). Late teen-age spurt important clinically, both for therapy and for effect on stability of finished result. (From Woodside, D. G.: Distance, velocity and relative growth rate standards for Canadian males and females age three to twenty years. Unpublished manuscript, 1969.)

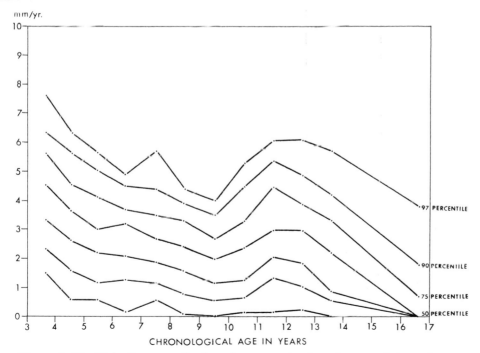

Figure 2–51 Velocity curve for females seems to show less precipitate change and a broader spread. Comparing percentile with percentile, the actual incremental change is less for girls than for boys. (From Woodside, D. G.: Distance, velocity and relative growth rate standards for mandibular growth for Canadian males and females age three to twenty years. Unpublished manuscript, 1969.)

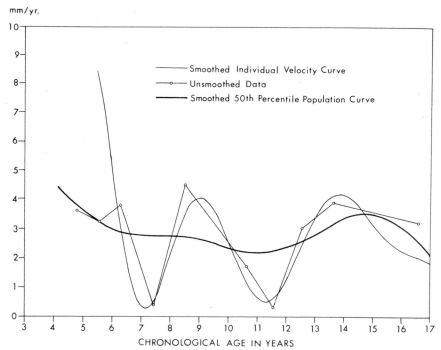

Figure 2-52   The effect of "smoothing" a velocity curve from a given sample, in this case the Burlington study, is shown here. Compare the smoothed curve with the unsmoothed data. Smoothing out irregularities at the 50th percentile masks the potential highs and lows, and reduces clinical interpretative value. (From Woodside, D. G.: Distance, velocity and relative growth rate standards for mandibular growth for Canadian males and females age three to twenty years. Unpublished manuscript, 1969.)

width in the denture area, he is likely to be disappointed after the fifth or sixth year of life since then there is little change in the width of the dental arch anterior to the first permanent molars. In the mandibular dentition, mandibular intercanine width is relatively complete by nine to ten years of age in both boys and girls.[126, 128] In the maxilla, intercanine width is essentially complete by 12 years of age in girls but continues to grow until 18 years of age in boys. The clinical implications here are quite obvious. The final horizontal growth increments in the mandible, particularly in the male, cause a forward movement of the mandibular base with its teeth. This basal change eliminates any flush terminal plane tendencies that have persisted beyond the mixed dentition. However, the bodily mandibular thrust forward is unmatched by comparable maxillary horizontal growth changes. Hence, the maxillary intercanine dimension serves as a "safety valve" for this basal discrepancy.

As already indicated, many of the problems confronting the orthodontist involve disturbance of the anteroposterior relationship of the teeth and jaws. What growth factors will help him here? Since both mandible and maxilla grow downward and forward at a more rapid rate with reference to the cranium after the fifth or sixth year of life, can something be done to adjust maxillary and mandibular growth and thus eliminate the dental malrelationship? Can the orthodontist, for example, stimulate deficient maxillary or mandibular growth by means of mechanical appliances? Can he make one jaw "catch up" with the other? Can he retard growth of one jaw or the other, in the hope of gaining adjustment of the teeth in the jaws? Or, at least, can he change the direction of growth?

For centuries the Chinese bound the feet of their women and kept them from increasing beyond four and a half inches in length; some South American Indian tribes have greatly changed the shape of the cranium by means of selective binding techniques. It does appear that channeling or redirection of growth offers the greatest hope to the orthodontist at present.[103] Evidence already mentioned, the research of Hinrichsen and Storey on the susceptibility of membranous bone to pressures, has therapeutic implications.[27] The guiding of maxillary and mandibular growth (or, more accurately, the redirection of specific growth vectors and spatial changes of the maxillary and mandibular dentition and alveolar bone support by means of mechanical appliances), has been utilized with uniformly successful results. This is an orthopedic concept since the orthodontist is literally an "orthopedic surgeon" of the craniofacial complex. (See Chaps. 14 and 18.) A large percentage of cases involve anteroposterior basal dysplasia with abnormal or adaptive muscle activity and tooth positions which reflect a multisystemic involvement. Since the cranial and facial structures grow at different times and at different rates, the question arises: Which is the best time to influence growth, to exert a retarding influence or growth directional change? Logically, the greatest success would be likely at the time of the greatest change. This means that the period just before and during puberty offers the best possibility. However, changes can and should be wrought at other times, depending on the severity of the malocclusion and basal bone and muscle involvement. Interceptive orthodontics is more than a noble concept; it is an established fact. Growth guidance in the deciduous dentition as well in the mixed dentition may be called upon frequently prior to therapy in the permanent dentition, so that the ultimate stability and the optimum level of accomplishment are ensured. Treatment timing must be based on the individual's own pattern of growth and accomplishment per unit time. As growth prediction becomes more practicable, the technique of ulna sesomoid interpretation introduced by Björk and other wrist and hand x-ray clues (used by Graves, together with Björk's technique) will provide the orthodontist with even better indications for timing of therapy with growth.[115] (Table 2–2). (See Chapter 8.)

Another variable to be considered is the *direction* of growth. While the face as a whole grows downward and forward, there are times when growth is predominantly in one direction or the other. Growth direction can change autonomously or can be changed by means of mechanical orthodontic appliances. Studies of hundreds of longitudinal records bear out this observation.[129, 130] As a generalization based on the fundamental concept of predominance of the morphogenetic pattern, the growth direction in mandibular retrusion cases is more vertical than in normal cases, while it is more nearly horizontal where there is a tendency toward a mandibular prognathism or protrusion. But even this is not always true Figs. 2–53, 2–54). The student of anatomy soon learns that there is no "always" or "never" for most phenomena occuring in the human body. Björk points out the late changes that occur in the mandible and shows that there is a significant "rotational vector of mandibular growth, with the mandible itself following an arc which tends to bring the chin point forward and reduce the mandibular plane steepness."[92] Moss refers to a logarithmic spiral which accomplishes the same thing, as the mandible follows the curve from foramen ovale, mandibular foramen and mental foramen. This is the concept of an "unloaded" nerve and exemplifies the neurotrophic dominance and stimulus for growth amounts and direction.[90]

TABLE 2–2   MAJOR PHYSICAL GROWTH TRAITS FROM BIRTH TO ADULTHOOD*

AGE PERIOD	GROWTH				DENTITION		OSSIFICATION		ENDOCRINES	
	Brain case	Face	H & W	Trunk, limbs	Decid.	Perm.	Appear.	Union	Gonads	Sex traits
1. Infancy (B–1 yr)	Rapid	Slow	Rapid (H 50%, W 300%)	Trunk fast; limbs slow	Calcif. rapid; begin eruption	Calcif. begins	Rapid	...	...	...
2. Early childhood (1–6 yrs)	Rapid; 95% finished	Faster esp. in depth	Slower (rate 25–100%)	Both slower	Decid. completed	Calcif. complete but for M3; eruption begins	Rapid; most are present by 6 yrs.	...	...	...
3. Mid-childhood (6–10 yrs)	None	Moderate	In slow phase (rate 5–10%)	Slow; adult proports. attained	Replacement of decid. by perm.	Perm. in rapid eruptive phase; all calcif.	Slow; inc. in size is chief factor	...	Trace of sex hormones	...
4. Late childhood (10–14 yrs)	Final 5%(?)	Faster, espec. hts. & depths	Faster, prepubertal accel.	Faster, esp. trunk trans. & sag.	All decid. are replaced	All erupted except M3	Growth of epith. about complete	Begins in hands and feet	Sex hormones inc. in amount	Early maturers ♀ ca. 11:0 ♂ ca. 12:0
5. Puberty (♀ 12–13 yrs) (♂ 13–14 yrs)	None	Slow: resting phase	Both decel. in rate, H more than W	Trunk bulk increases	...	...	Little change	Proc. of union moving into rapid phase	Sex hormones up to ad. values	Average maturers ♀ ca. 12:6 ♂ ca. 13:6
6. Postpubertal (13–20 yrs)	None	Sl. final increase in ht.	Slow decel. to final adult value	Slow inc. in trunk vol; limb proports. adult.	...	M3 erupts, if early	...	Very rapid union in long bones	Continue as above	Late maturers ♀ ca. 13:0+ ♂ ca. 14:0+ adult patterns achieved

*From Krogman, W. M.: Principles of human growth. Ciba Sympos., 5:1458–1466, 1943.

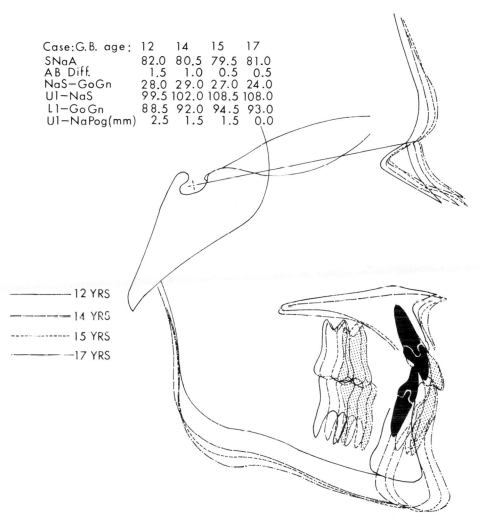

Case:G.B. age:	12	14	15	17
SNaA	82.0	80.5	79.5	81.0
A B Diff.	1.5	1.0	0.5	0.5
NaS−GoGn	28.0	29.0	27.0	24.0
U1−NaS	99.5	102.0	108.5	108.0
L1−GoGn	88.5	92.0	94.5	93.0
U1−NaPog(mm)	2.5	1.5	1.5	0.0

——————— 12 YRS

— —— — —— 14 YRS

----- ------- 15 YRS

— ·—— · —— 17 YRS

Figure 2–53 Directional change of mandibular growth after orthodontic therapy usually has some effect on incisor inclination, if overjet is minimal. Here, maxillary incisors have tipped labially to accommodate the basal change. This counterclockwise pattern reduces mandibular plane angle, but not at the expense of deepening the overbite for this patient.

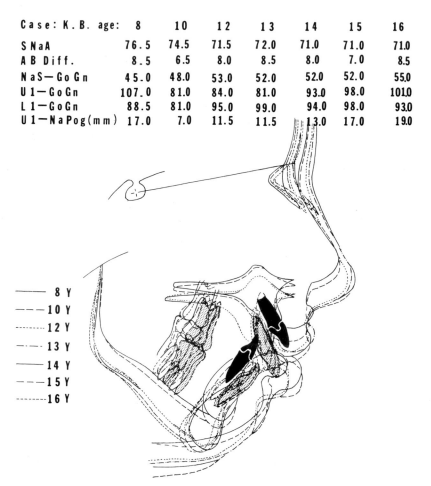

Case: K. B. age:	8	10	12	13	14	15	16
S N a A	76.5	74.5	71.5	72.0	71.0	71.0	71.0
A B Diff.	8.5	6.5	8.0	8.5	8.0	7.0	8.5
N a S — Go Gn	45.0	48.0	53.0	52.0	52.0	52.0	55.0
U 1 — Go Gn	107.0	81.0	84.0	81.0	93.0	98.0	101.0
L 1 — Go Gn	88.5	81.0	95.0	99.0	94.0	98.0	93.0
U 1 — Na Pog (mm)	17.0	7.0	11.5	11.5	13.0	17.0	19.0

——— 8 Y
— — — 10 Y
········· 12 Y
— · — 13 Y
——— 14 Y
— — — 15 Y
········· 16 Y

Figure 2–54   Unfavorable growth direction in a birth injury case. Despite stringent orthopedic procedures, restricting maxillary horizontal growth, as evidenced by reduction of SNaA by 5 degrees, and lingual positioning of maxillary incisors, the apical base dysplasia remains at 8.5 degrees. Clockwise growth changes opened up mandibular plane from 45 degrees to 55 degrees. No hoped for directional changes occurred. Geneoplasty or mandibular resection offers greatest profile help at this stage.

THE DEVELOPMENT OF THE DENTITION

BIRTH TO TWO YEARS

Since most histology texts cover the initial stages of dental development and the processes of tooth formation, it is not necessary to go into detail about the changes that occur during the first two years of life. Figure 2–55 shows an interesting roentgenogram of an infant at birth and points out the long road that must be traveled before the permanent teeth achieve their ultimate developmental and positional status. The student is urged to refresh his knowledge of dental development and of the eruption sequences for the first two years of life since aberrations may occur and interceptive procedures may occassionally be necessary.[152]

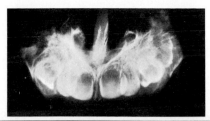

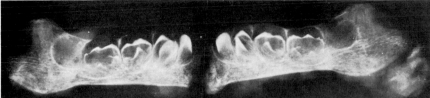

Figure 2–55   Roentgenogram of infant at birth (wet specimen; actual size). In the mandible, the central incisors show calcification of about half the crown, with the lateral incisors nearly as advanced. The cusps of the canines and deciduous molars are shown, but with little calcification of their crowns. In the maxilla, calcification corresponds to that of the mandible but is a little less advanced. (From McCall, S., and Wald, J.: Clinical Dental Roentgenology. 4th ed. W. B. Saunders Co., 1957.)

TWO YEARS TO SIX YEARS

At two years of age, a large number of children have 20 teeth that are clinically present and functioning. Hence, this is a good place to begin a more detailed analysis of the age-linked status of the dentition. This is important because preventive and interceptive measures are possible, when the orthodontist knows the normal range and timing of developmental phenomena. Certainly, by two years of age the deciduous second molars are usually in the process of erupting or will erupt within the next several months (Fig. 2–56). Deciduous incisor root formation is finished and root formation of the deciduous canines and first molars is approaching completion. The permanent first molars continue to develop with a shift in their position within their respective bones toward the occlusal plane. Calcification is also proceeding in the developing permanent teeth, anterior to the first permanent molars. In some children the developing crypts of the second permanent molars may be seen distal to the first permanent molars.

By two and a half years of age the deciduous dentition is usually complete and in full function.

By three years of age the roots of all the deciduous teeth are complete. First permanent molar crowns are fully developed and the roots are starting to form. The crypts of the developing permanent second molars are now definite and can be seen in the space formerly occupied by the developing first permanent molars. Although calcification is proceeding in the developing permanent successors, little shift can be noted in the position of these teeth at this time with the exception of the first permanent molars. At three years of age there is some indication of the future status of the occlusion. Normally there may be what would later be called an excessive overbite, with the upper incisors almost hiding the lower incisors when the teeth are brought into occlusion. Frequently there is a retrognathic tendency in the mandible. With differential growth and the emergence of the splanchnocranium from beneath the neurocranium, both the vertical and the horizontal discrepancy will be diminished or eliminated.

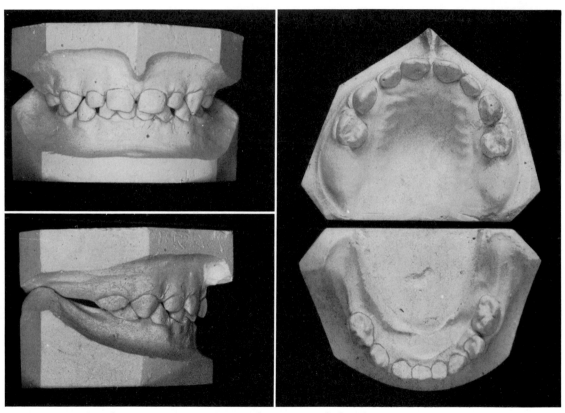

Figure 2-56   Case D. M., 2 years, 11 days. Second deciduous molars have not yet erupted. Overbite appears excessive, but such is normal at this age. (Courtesy J. H. Sillman.)

At this time, a precise long cone technique radiographic examination should determine the approximate width of the crowns of the permanent incisor teeth.

A clinical examination of the deciduous dentition and measurement of available arch length will show whether these teeth have enough room to erupt later (Chaps. 8, 13). Spacing in the upper and lower anterior segments is usual and desirable to accommodate the larger permanent teeth. It was formerly thought that "developmental spacing" appeared spontaneously between the baby teeth between three and six years of age, but recent research contradicts this. Relatively little change occurs in the width dimensions of the deciduous dentition from the time it is completed at two and a half years of age until the permanent successors erupt. There is, as has been indicated before, increase in width posterior to the deciduous dentition. But a perimeter of circumferential measurement from the distal of the second deciduous molar on one side to the distal of the second deciduous molar on the opposite side will show relatively little change until the permanent incisors erupt (Fig. 2–57).

Between three and six years of age the development of the permanent teeth continues, with the maxillary and mandibular incisor teeth most advanced (Fig. 2–58). From five to six years of age, just before the shedding of the deciduous incisors, there are more teeth in the jaws than at any other time. Space is quite critical within both the alveolar process and the deciduous dental arches themselves.[131] Early, average and later eruption times for girls and boys are shown in Figure 2–59 and demonstrate a broad range of "normalcy." Developing permanent teeth are shifting closer to the alveolar border; the apices of the deciduous incisors are being resorbed; the permanent first molars are about ready to erupt. Very little bone exists between the permanent teeth and their crypts and the "front line" of deciduous teeth. A cross-section of the maxilla and mandible illustrates this remarkable phenomenon (Figs. 2–60, 2–61). It seems impossible that the permanent teeth would have enough room to assume their normal place in the dental arches; but the juggling for vital space continues, as if according to some grand master plan, and somehow the teeth erupt properly at the last moment. The complex interplay of forces makes it imperative that the integrity of the dental arch be maintained at this time. Loss of arch length through caries may make the difference between normal occlusion and malocclusion. It does not take very much to upset the delicate timetable of tooth formation, eruption and resorption within a viable osseous medium. As Owen points out, space loss is most likely in the maxillary second deciduous molar area.[128]

Between three and six years of age, the broad variation in individual accomplishment of pattern becomes quite apparent. Chronologic or calendric age conveys only a rough approximation of the developmental timetable. As Moorrees says, "Physiologic (biologic or developmental age) is based on maturation of one or more tissue systems."[132] In the Forsyth Infirmary, Harvard School of Dental Medicine Laboratories, four systems are delineated: the dentition, as well as bone age, height and weight, and secondary sex characteristics. Tooth formation is a more reliable measure of dental age than tooth eruption and is less susceptible to the environment. Except during the circumpubertal period, there is a fair degree of correlation among the maturity indicators. Figures 2–62 and 2–63 illustrate the age variation in the formation of maxillary and mandibular incisors in boys and girls. Figure 2–64 graphs the crown and root development in a similar manner for permanent mandibular canines, premolars and molars for girls. Boys may be charted similarly.[132]

(*Text continued on page 100*)

DECIDUOUS DENTITION

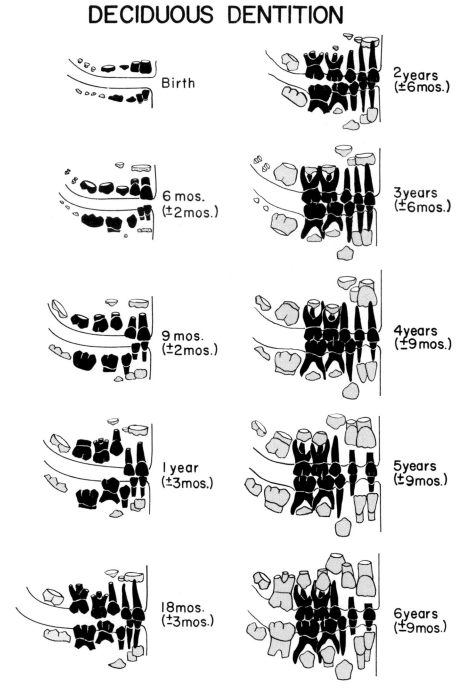

Figure 2–57   Development of human dentition. (Modified from Schour and Massler.)

MIXED DENTITION   PERMANENT DENTITION

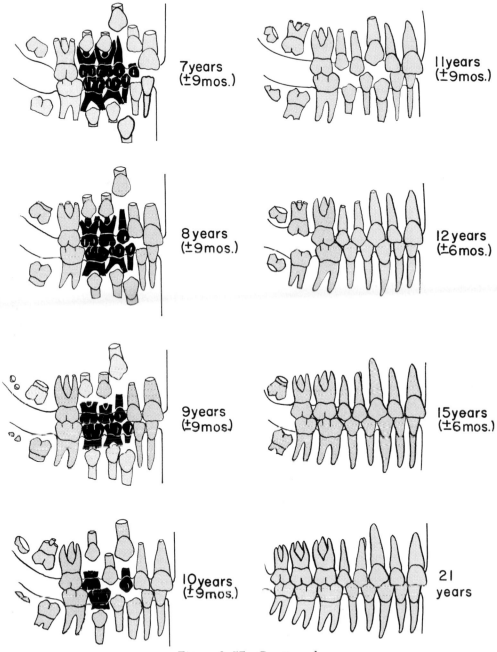

7 years (±9 mos.)

8 years (±9 mos.)

9 years (±9 mos.)

10 years (±9 mos.)

11 years (±9 mos.)

12 years (±6 mos.)

15 years (±6 mos.)

21 years

Figure 2–57   Continued.

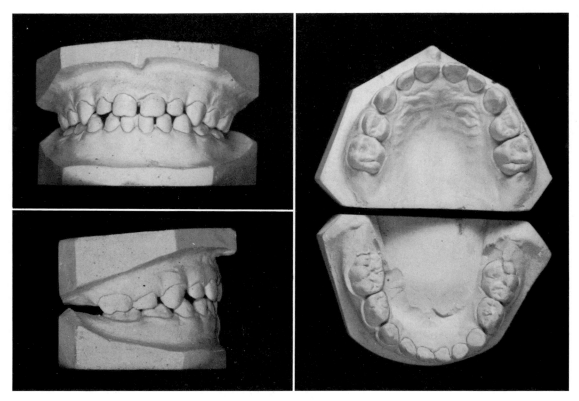

Figure 2–58   Case D. M., 4 years, 1 month, 20 days. There has been some reduction in over-bite. Note spacing present between incisor teeth.

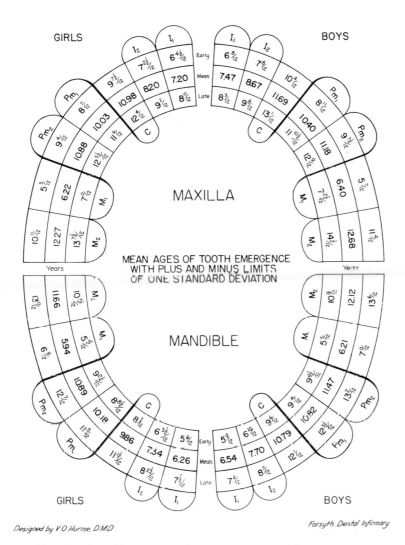

Figure 2–59 Graphic illustration of early, mean and late eruption ages for girls (left) and boys (right). Such an age range as depicted would include two thirds of any sample. (Courtesy V. O. Hurme.)

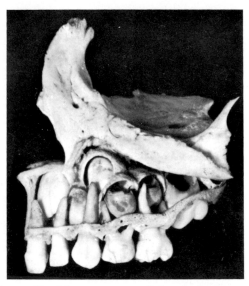

Figure 2–60   Left maxilla. Note position of developing premolars and first permanent molar. (From Wheeler, R. C.: Textbook of Dental Anatomy and Physiology. 4th ed. W. B. Saunders Co., 1965.)

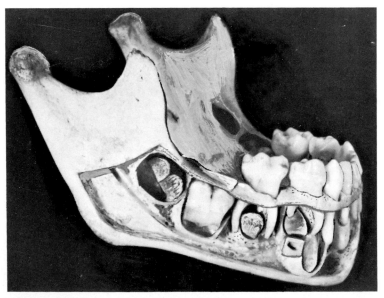

Figure 2–61   Right lateral view of dissected mandible, same patient as Figure 2–60. Position of developing permanent teeth should be noted. The second molar is still actually behind the anterior margin of the ramus. (From Wheeler, R. C.: Textbook of Dental Anatomy and Physiology. 4th ed. W. B. Saunders Co., 1965.)

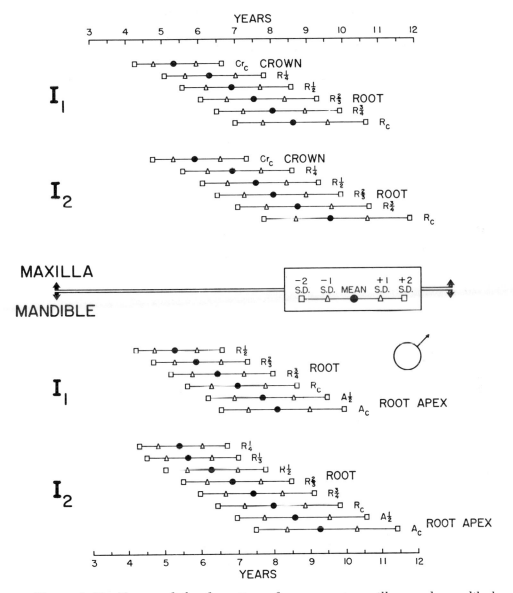

Figure 2-62 Norms of the formation of permanent maxillary and mandibular incisor roots of males, including the crown-complete stage of the maxillary incisors. (From Moorrees, C. F. A., Fanning, E. A., and Hunt, E. E., Jr.: Age variation of formation stages for ten permanent teeth. J. Dent. Res., 42:1490–1502, 1963.)

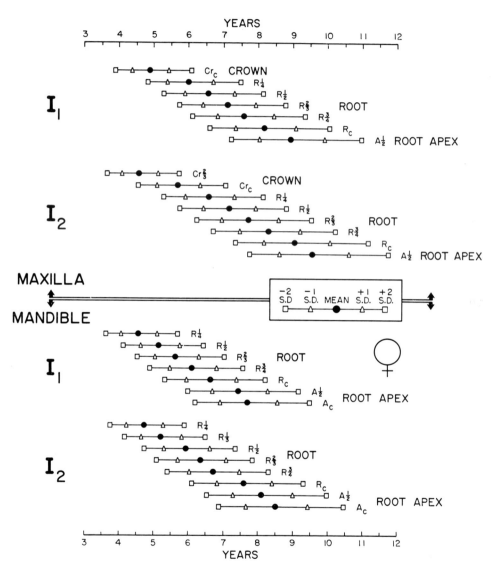

Figure 2-63 Norms of the formation of permanent maxillary and mandibular incisor roots of females, including terminal stages of crown formation of the maxillary incisors. (From Moorrees, C. F. A., Fanning, E. A., and Hunt, E. E., Jr.: Age variation of formation stages for ten permanent teeth. J. Dent. Res., 42:1490–1502, 1963.)

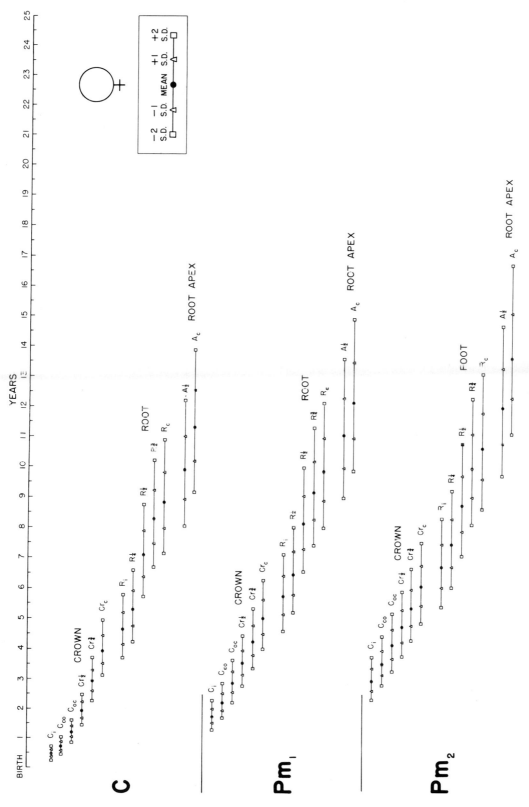

Figure 2-64 Norms of tooth formation of permanent mandibular canines, premolars and molars of females. (From Moorrees, C. F. A., Fanning, E. A., and Hunt, E. E., Jr.: Age variation of formation stages for ten permanent teeth. J. Dent. Res., 42:1490–1502, 1963.)

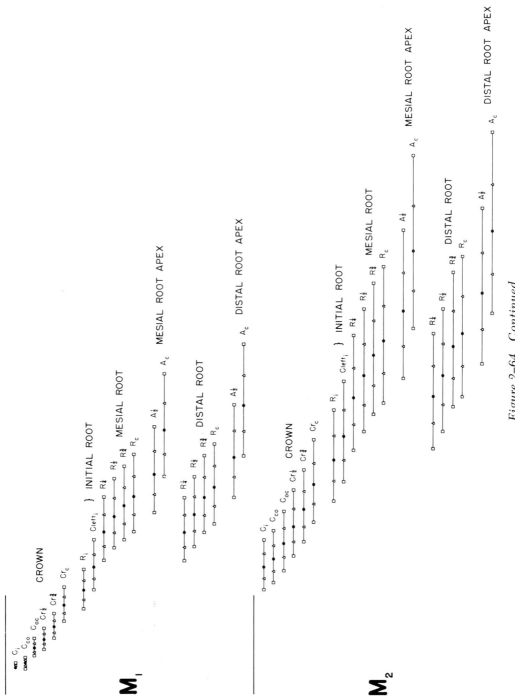

Figure 2-64 Continued.

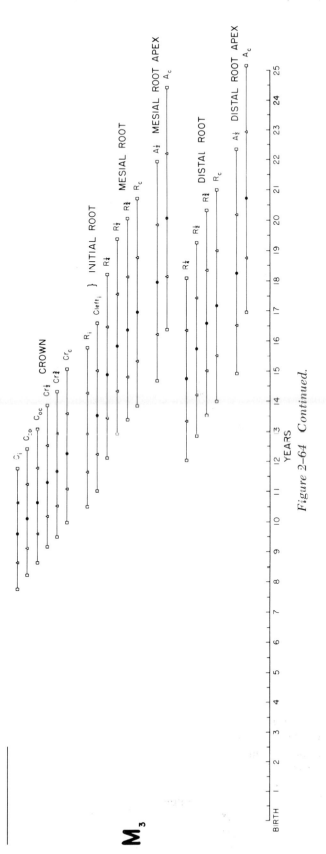

Figure 2-64 Continued.

SIX YEARS TO TEN YEARS

Between six and seven years of age the first permanent molars erupt into the mouth. It is at this time that the first of three assaults on the excessive overbite occurs. As Schwarz says, "There are three periods of physiologic raising of the bite, with the eruption of the first permanent molars at six with the eruption of the second permanent molars at twelve and with the eruption of the third molars at around 18."[133] As the upper and lower first permanent molars erupt, the pad of tissue overlying them creates a premature contact. Proprioceptive response conditions the patient against biting on this natural "bite opener," and thus the deciduous teeth anterior to the first permanent molar area erupt, reducing the overbite. About this time, the deciduous central incisors are lost and their permanent successors start their eruptive path toward contact with the incisors of the opposing arch. Usually the mandibular central incisors erupt first, followed by the maxillary permanent central incisors. These teeth frequently erupt lingual to the deciduous counterparts and move forward under the influence of tongue pressure as they erupt. The maxillary central incisors appear as large bulges in the mucobuccal vestibule above the deciduous incisors before they erupt. A significant factor in normal or abnormal eruption of succedaneous teeth is the space available as provided by the deciduous teeth plus "developmental spacing," compared with the width of the permanent successors.

Moorrees, in his study of 184 North American white children from 12 to 15 years of age, made careful measurements of tooth widths and subjected the results to a biometric analysis. Tables 2–3 to 2–6 show the mesiodistal crown diameters of the deciduous and permanent teeth, the mesiodistal crown diameters of tooth groups and the mesiodistal crown diameters of the deciduous teeth expressed as a percentage of those of their permanent successors.[124] These tables should prove to be of considerable value to the orthodontist as he carefully measures the width of the deciduous and succedaneous teeth before embarking on a planned program of serial extraction, before placing a space maintainer, etc. (see Chap. 15).

The time between seven and eight years of age is critical for the developing dentition (Fig. 2–65). Will there be enough space or not? Frequent observation by the dentist is essential at this time. Sometimes radiographic examination discloses abnormal resorption of the deciduous roots. Congenitally missing or supernumerary teeth may be discovered. A mucosal barrier may be preventing the permanent incisors from erupting. (These, and many other factors, will be discussed in more detail in Chapters 6 through 9). It is apparent that constant vigilance is essential. If there is obviously inadequate space, for example, the patient should be referred for an orthodontic consultation. Complete diagnostic records taken at this time may indicate the advisability of guided extraction procedures, i.e., removing deciduous teeth ahead of schedule to allow autonomous adjustment of permanent teeth already in the mouth and reducing the orthodontic challenge later on (Chap. 15).

Calendric age is even less reliable as a basis for projection of eruption of maxillary and mandibular incisors. More sophisticated research and the accumulation of precise developmental data from several "growth centers" has indicated that physiologic age provides a better yardstick. Those neat and simplified "tooth eruption charts," based on specific ages, posted in schools, physicians' offices, etc., with no indication of range, standard deviation or standard error, provide little useful information. By themselves these charts are often misleading and can delude an inquiring parent into a sense of false security.

TABLE 2–3 MESIODISTAL CROWN DIAMETERS OF DECIDUOUS TEETH

TOOTH	SEX	MEAN (mm)		S.E._M (mm)	S.D. (mm)	C.V. (per cent)	RANGE (mm)	NUMBER
			Maxilla					
di_1	♂	6.55		0.05	0.36	5.53	5.8–7.2	64
	♀		6.44	0.05	0.43	6.65	5.4–7.5	69
di_2	♂	5.32		0.05	0.39	7.39	4.5–6.6	64
	♀		5.23	0.04	0.33	6.37	4.5–6.2	69
dc	♂	6.88		0.04	0.36	5.16	6.1–7.9	65
	♀		6.67	0.04	0.35	5.29	5.9–7.6	69
dm_1	♂	7.12		0.05	0.38	5.33	6.3–8.3	64
	♀		6.95	0.04	0.36	5.14	6.3–7.9	68
dm_2	♂	9.08		0.06	0.46	5.07	8.0–10.4	63
	♀		8.84	0.07	0.55	6.21	7.5–10.0	68
			Mandible					
di_1	♂	4.08		0.04	0.30	7.23	3.0–4.7	64
	♀		3.98	0.04	0.30	7.42	3.2–4.7	68
di_2	♂	4.74		0.04	0.35	7.43	4.1–6.0	65
	♀		4.63	0.05	0.39	8.48	3.9–5.7	69
dc	♂	5.92		0.04	0.32	5.39	5.1–6.7	65
	♀		5.74	0.04	0.35	6.06	5.0–6.6	68
dm_1	♂	7.80		0.05	0.42	5.38	7.0–8.9	65
	♀		7.65	0.04	0.35	4.55	6.7–8.5	69
dm_2	♂	9.83		0.07	0.52	5.32	8.5–11.0	63
	♀		9.64	0.06	0.49	5.07	8.6–10.9	69

[a]Moorrees, C. F. A.: The Dentition of the Growing Child: A Longitudinal Study of Dental Development Between 3 and 18 Years of Age. Harvard University Press, 1959.

Since the question of adequate space seems to be particularly critical in the incisor segments, where there is no leeway space to help, a study on available space for incisors during dental development based on physiologic age is of significant value.[125]

In a longitudinal study of over 200 children with excellent tooth alignment, casts were carefully measured for available space. Figure 2–66 charts average amounts of spacing or crowding. The sudden change during the eruption of the central and lateral incisors is illustrated by over 1.5 mm. crowding in both boys and girls. The study showed that the average female recovers slightly better than the average male. Recovery is tied to significant increases in arch length and breadth during the actual eruption. Moorrees and Chadha note that, after full eruption, a plateau is reached in arch dimension increases. Only a slight width increase is noted in maxillary intercanine width with the later eruption of the maxillary canines. The clinical implication is that "no great relief of crowding in the incisor segment can be expected after the complete eruption of lateral incisors."[125]

Figure 2–67 is a scale drawing of the deciduous maxillary and mandibular dentitions of the average male, showing available space in the incisor, canine and premolar segments. Figures 2–68, 2–69 and 2–70 are drawings of the

TABLE 2-4   MESIODISTAL CROWN DIAMETERS OF PERMANENT TEETH

TOOTH	SEX	MEAN (mm)		S.E.$_M$ (mm)	S.D. (mm)	C.V. (per cent)	RANGE (mm)	NUMBER
			Maxilla					
I_1	♂	8.78		0.05	0.46	5.29	7.9–10.0	87
	♀		8.40	0.06	0.53	6.30	7.1–9.8	87
I_2	♂	6.64		0.07	0.63	9.42	4.5–8.2	84
	♀		6.47	0.07	0.62	9.60	4.5–8.5	86
C	♂	7.95		0.05	0.42	5.24	6.6–9.0	87
	♀		7.53	0.04	0.37	4.94	6.9–8.5	85
Pm_1	♂	7.01		0.04	0.38	5.24	6.1–8.2	87
	♀		6.85	0.05	0.42	6.12	5.8–7.8	84
Pm_2	♂	6.82		0.04	0.37	5.43	5.9–7.6	86
	♀		6.62	0.05	0.43	6.49	5.2–7.8	81
M_1	♂	10.81		0.06	0.56	5.18	9.9–12.4	83
	♀		10.52	0.06	0.51	4.86	9.4–11.9	85
M_2	♂	10.35		0.08	0.63	6.11	8.5–11.7	65
	♀		9.81	0.07	0.49	4.96	8.3–11.8	50
			Mandible					
I_1	♂	5.42		0.03	0.31	5.75	4.5–6.1	85
	♀		5.25	0.04	0.36	6.86	4.3–6.1	87
I_2	♂	5.95		0.04	0.38	6.32	5.2–6.9	85
	♀		5.78	0.04	0.38	6.60	4.7–6.8	87
C	♂	6.96		0.04	0.36	5.22	6.2–8.1	84
	♀		6.47	0.04	0.32	5.00	5.8–7.4	87
Pm_1	♂	7.07		0.04	0.35	4.94	6.4–8.1	85
	♀		6.87	0.04	0.38	5.59	5.9–7.9	87
Pm_2	♂	7.29		0.06	0.52	7.11	6.3–9.6	82
	♀		7.02	0.04	0.40	5.67	6.2–7.9	83
M_1	♂	11.8		0.05	0.47	4.22	10.0–12.7	76
	♀		10.74	0.06	0.56	5.24	9.4–12.2	84
M_2	♂	10.76		0.10	0.71	6.62	9.3–12.5	53
	♀		10.34	0.08	0.62	5.96	9.2–11.7	53

*Moorrees, C. F. A.: The Dentition of the Growing Child: A Longitudinal Study of Dental Development Between 3 and 18 Years of Age. Harvard University Press, 1959.

TABLE 2–5   MESIODISTAL CROWN DIAMETERS OF TOOTH GROUPS*

TOOTH GROUP	SEX	MEAN (mm)	S.E.$_M$ (mm)	S.D. (mm)	C.V. (per cent)	RANGE (mm)	NUMBER
				Maxilla			
Deciduous incisors	♂	37.31	0.24	1.79	4.80	33.2–44.0	57
and canines	♀	36.44	0.22	1.78	4.88	33.4–41.1	63
Permanent incisors	♂	47.00	0.33	2.53	5.38	41.0–55.3	57
and canines	♀	45.07	0.29	2.31	5.13	40.3–50.5	63
Deciduous molars	♂	32.29	0.19	1.51	4.68	28.8–35.8	61
	♀	31.60	0.24	1.85	5.85	28.6–35.1	59
Premolars	♂	27.86	0.16	1.24	4.45	22.6–30.5	61
	♀	26.85	0.20	1.51	5.62	21.9–30.0	59
				Mandible			
Deciduous incisors	♂	29.35	0.19	1.49	5.08	25.9–32.3	60
and canines	♀	28.68	0.22	1.75	6.10	25.8–33.1	64
Permanent incisors	♂	36.70	0.22	1.69	4.60	33.0–40.3	60
and canines	♀	35.12	0.24	1.93	5.50	29.9–39.0	64
Deciduous molars	♂	35.09	0.22	1.63	4.65	32.1–38.9	56
	♀	34.53	0.19	1.52	4.40	32.4–38.0	64
Premolars	♂	28.77	0.20	1.46	5.07	25.6–32.4	56
	♀	27.89	0.20	1.58	5.67	24.6–31.4	64

*Moorrees, C. F. A.: The Dentition of the Growing Child: A Longitudinal Study of Dental Development Between 3 and 18 Years of Age. Harvard University Press, 1959.

TABLE 2–6   MESIODISTAL CROWN DIAMETERS OF THE DECIDUOUS TEETH EXPRESSED AS A PERCENTAGE OF THOSE OF THEIR PERMANENT SUCCESSORS

TEETH	SEX	MEAN (per cent)	S.E.$_M$ (per cent)	S.D. (per cent)	C.V. (per cent)	RANGE (per cent)	NUMBER
		Incisors and canines					
Maxillary	♂	79.51	0.60	4.56	5.74	72.65–86.32	57
	♀	80.98	0.43	3.41	4.21	73.20–88.79	63
Mandibular	♂	80.06	0.53	4.09	5.11	70.77–91.89	60
	♀	81.74	0.73	5.82	7.12	69.23–95.76	64
		Deciduous molars (premolars)					
Maxillary	♂	116.03	0.73	5.67	4.89	101.35–133.20	61
	♀	117.32	0.88	6.72	5.73	100.68–138.36	59
Mandibular	♂	122.13	0.81	6.08	4.98	106.29–135.13	56
	♀	124.03	0.74	5.94	4.79	114.56–143.57	64

*Moorrees, C. F. A.: The Dentition of the Growing Child: A Longitudinal Study of Dental Development Between 3 and 18 Years of Age. Harvard University Press, 1959.

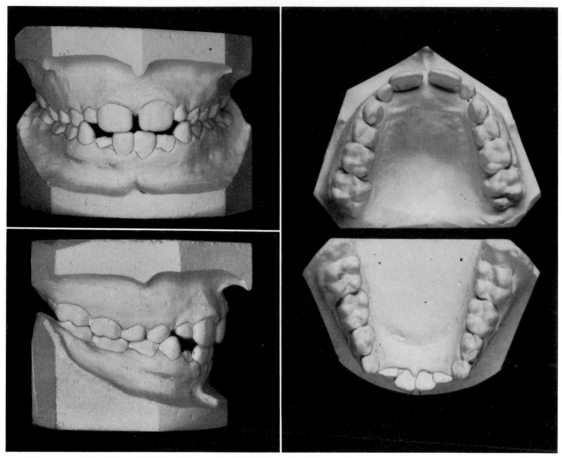

Figure 2–65   Case D. M., 7 years, 4 months, 8 days. Observe the irregularity of the erupting mandibular incisors. (Courtesy J. H. Sillman.)

transitional dentition of the average male child. Arch length changes are illustrated, with actual shortening and elimination of leeway space mesial to the first permanent molars.[124–127]

As with the mandibular central incisors, the mandibular lateral incisors frequently erupt lingually and are brought labially into the correct position by a combination of the direction of the path of eruption and the functional forces. The maxillary central incisors seem to erupt from the labial. Seldom can bulges be seen on the labial gingival tissue before the eruption of the maxillary lateral incisors. If there is inadequate space, the eruption time is delayed for these teeth, or they erupt markedly to the lingual or are rotated. A decision may have to be made, on the basis of a careful radiographic examination, on the removal of the deciduous cuspids ahead of the time at which they would normally be shed. Orthodontic consultation is desirable before making a decision. If removal is postponed, the lateral incisors may erupt palatally and in lingual cross-bite with the lower incisors. In that case, considering the constant struggle of the erupting teeth for space in the jaws, the permanent canine and its crypt will probably move mesially toward the midline and encroach on the space that would normally be occupied by the lateral incisor (Chap. 15). Eruption of the incisors is usually completed by eight and a half years of age. Maxillary inter-canine width in the girl will show relatively little increase, except with the eruption of the permanent canines, and is complete by twelve years. While permanent canine eruption causes a similar time-linked increase in the boy, there still remains a significant intercanine incremental increase between 12 and 18 years. This latter developmental change is tied to basal horizontal mandibular growth increments, as has been indicated already. After the eruption of the incisors, mandibular intercanine width increase is minimal, again coinciding with permanent canine eruption. In both the boy and the girl, it is essentially complete by ten years of age. Clinically, then, mandibular intercanine growth is relatively complete in the latter stages of the mixed dentition.

Arch length is influenced by morphogenetic pattern, however. In Class III malocclusion (mandibular prognathism) cases, the mandibular incisors tend to erupt more vertically and are lingually tipped, often reducing the perimeter measurement. In Class II malocclusion, the mandibular incisors are flared more labially by tongue action and freedom from incisal contact.[123] This has the effect of increasing incisor arch length, unless there is a confirmed mentalis muscle hyperactivity, with the lower lip cushioning between upper and lower incisors during function. In such cases, mandibular incisor arch length is reduced by a flattening and retrusion of the anterior segment, concomitantly with an increase in overjet. Overbite may also influence the space availability in the mandibular incisor region with excessive overbite having a constricting and crowding effect on lower incisors in Class I and Class II, Division 2 malocclusions (see Chap. 5).

Even though the central and lateral incisors erupt into the normal position,

AVAILABLE SPACE - INCISOR SEGMENT

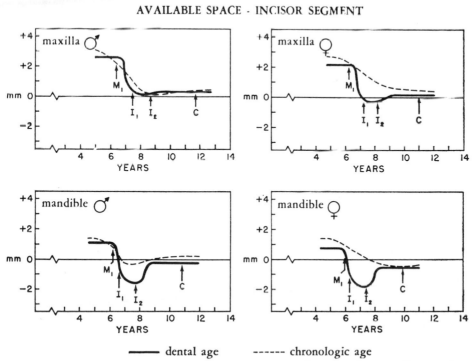

——— dental age   ------ chronologic age

Figure 2–66 Average amounts of spacing or crowding for the maxillary and mandibular incisor segments of males and females obtained with reference to dental age. The arrows refer to the mean ages of emergence of the permanent teeth. (From Hurme *in* Moorrees, C. F. A., and Chadha, J. M.: Available space for the incisors during dental development. Angle Orthodont., 35:12–22, 1965.)

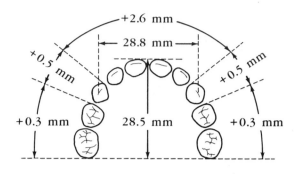

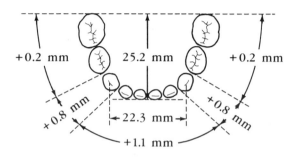

Figure 2-67 The deciduous maxillary and mandibular dentitions of the average male child, drawn to scale for all measurements of available space in the incisor, canine and premolar segments; arch lengths, the intercanine distances as well as mesiodistal crown diameters of the teeth. (From Moorrees, C. F. A., and Chadha, J. M.: Available space for the incisors during dental development. Angle Orthodont., 35:12–22, 1965.)

Figure 2-68 The transitional dentition of the average male child after eruption of the permanent maxillary and mandibular central incisors and first molars (note closing of spaces between deciduous molars). (From Moorrees, C. F. A., and Chadha, J. M.: Available space for the incisors during dental development. Angle Orthodont., 35:12–22, 1965.)

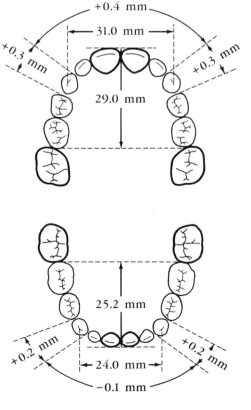

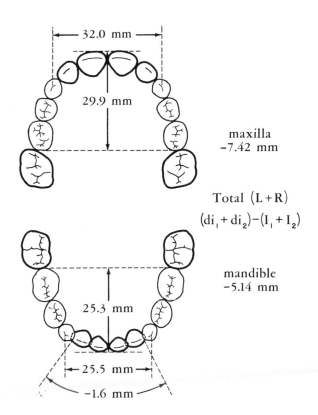

maxilla
−7.42 mm

Total (L+R)

$(di_1 + di_2) - (I_1 + I_2)$

mandible
−5.14 mm

Figure 2–69 The transitional dentition of the average male child after eruption of all permanent incisors (note differences in size of permanent and deciduous incisors, crowding of mandibular incisors, increments in the maxillary and mandibular intercanine distances and increase only in the maxillary arch length). (From Moorrees, C. F. A., and Chadha, J. M.: Available space for the incisors during dental development. Angle Orthodont., 35:12–22, 1965.)

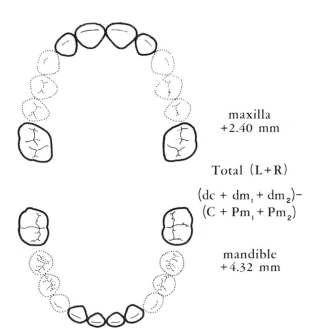

maxilla
+2.40 mm

Total (L+R)

$(dc + dm_1 + dm_2) - (C + Pm_1 + Pm_2)$

mandible
+4.32 mm

Figure 2–70 The transitional dentition of the average male child at an imaginary phase where all deciduous posterior teeth (dc, dm_1, dm_2,) are shed, just prior to the emergence of their permanent successors (note so-called leeway space). (From Moorrees, C. F. A., and Chadha, J. M.: Available space for the incisors during dental development. Angle Orthodont., 35:12–22, 1965.)

root formation is not complete. The apices are wide open and do not close for at least another year. At this time, nine to ten years of age, all the permanent teeth except the third molars have completed crown formation and enamel deposition. Even the third molar is in the process of forming. Its crypt appears as an oval-shaped radioparency well behind the margin of the ramus. Extensive laminagraphic study of the developing dentition shows that there is a high degree of variability in the time of onset of third molar development. In some instances, third molars have not started to form until as late as 14 years of age. There seems to be relatively little correlation between chronologic age, dental age and third molar formation.

Between nine and ten years of age, the apices in the deciduous canines and molars begin to resorb. Individual variation is also great here. Girls are usually a year to a year and a half ahead of boys (Fig. 2–59). A full mouth radiographic examination, made by the long cone technique, provides interesting information. At this time, in the mandible the combined width of the deciduous cuspid, the first deciduous molar and the second deciduous molar is approximately 1.7 mm. greater on the average than the combined width of the canine and first and second premolar teeth. In the maxilla the combined width difference averages only 0.9 mm. (Fig. 2–71). This space differential for each maxillary and mandibular buccal segment is called the "leeway space" by Nance.[134, 135] It is this temporary increase in arch length, particularly due to the relatively large size of the mandibular second deciduous molar, that often prevents the normal interdigitation of the permanent first molars. They maintain an end-to-end relationship until the first and second deciduous molars are lost. This is a normal

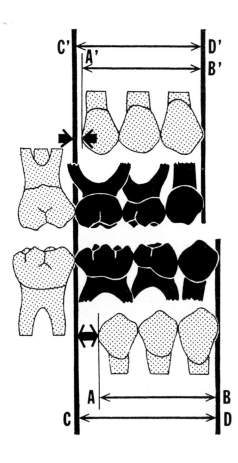

Figure 2–71 "Leeway space" in maxillary and mandibular arches, as described by Nance. On the average, the combined width of the mandibular deciduous canine and first and second deciduous molars is 1.7 mm. greater than the permanent successors. The deciduous versus permanent tooth dimension for the comparable maxillary arch segment is only 0.9 mm. Mesial drift is consequently greater in the mandibular arch, often adjusting for a flush terminal plane. Arrows indicate segmental space differential.

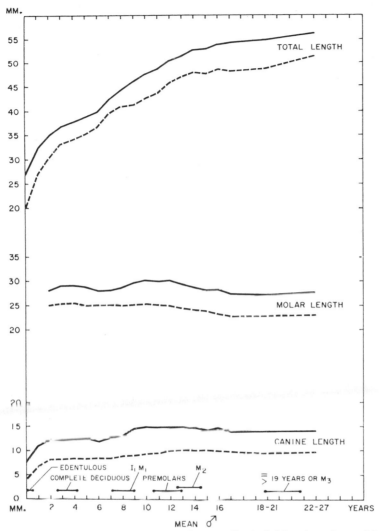

Figure 2–72   Mean arch lengths of male maxilla (solid line) and mandible (broken line). Time span of each stage (mean ± 1 S.D.) of groups of erupted teeth is also indicated. (From Sillman, J. H.: Dimensional changes of dental arches: longitudinal studies from birth to 25 years. Am. J. Orthodont., 50:824–842, 1964.)

phenomenon and need cause no concern. The flush terminal plane relationship, as it is called, is seen in at least 50 per cent of the youngsters in the normal development of the dentition[136] (Fig. 15–2). The flush terminal plane is eliminated and the correct cusp and fossa interdigitation occurs only after the exchange of the deciduous molars and canines for permanent successors. The mesial drift of the lower molars takes up the greater leeway space that is present in the lower arch. This accounts for the reducing distance from molar to molar as seen in various studies (Fig. 2–72). If there is a distal step instead of a flush terminal plane, then a developing Class II malocclusion may be likely. A mesial step, of course, may mean a developing Class III malocclusion or a mandibular prognathism.[137] In any event, a careful measurement should be made of the leeway space to see if there is adequate space to effect the necessary changes in the arch without any appliance intervention.

Another important clue to the question of adequacy of space in the dental arches at this time is the mandibular deciduous canine. Where there is inadequate space, the mandibular deciduous canine root resorbs ahead of schedule and is lost prematurely. In acute space deficiency problems the crown of the permanent lateral incisor may contact the mesial surface of the first deciduous molar after the loss of the deciduous canine (see Chap. 15). Normally, however, the mandibular canine root resorbs more slowly than that of the first deciduous molar in the maxilla and a trifle ahead of the first deciduous molar in the mandible.

Availability of space is not the only factor which influences the eruption of permanent teeth and the resorption of the deciduous teeth. Endocrine disturbances can markedly change this pattern. Thyroid abnormalities, for example, are not at all uncommon and their effect is noticed in the developing occlusion (see Chap. 6). Febrile disease may also upset the timetable, as may local environmental disturbances. Sometimes it is possible for a blow to cause a variation in the sequence of eruption of the permanent teeth. Abnormal muscle pressures, induced either by malrelationship of the dental arches and inherent morphologic variations or by finger, lip or tongue sucking habits, may influence the mixed dentition development. (see Chap. 6).

AFTER TEN YEARS

Between 10 and 12 years of age there is considerable variability in the sequence eruption of the canines and premolars. The most common sequence is shown in Figure 2–73. In about half the cases, the mandibular canine erupts ahead of the mandibular first and second premolars.[131] In the maxilla, the first premolar usually erupts before the canine. The maxillary second premolar and the maxillary canine erupt at about the same time. Not too much significance should be attached to a variation in this order if there appears to be adequate space. At times, deciduous teeth are retained beyond the time that they should normally be shed. A good rule of thumb is to try to maintain the left and right sides on approximately the same schedule. If the upper left deciduous molar is lost naturally and the upper right first deciduous molar is still firm, radiographic evidence may show that the mesial or distal root has not resorbed properly. It is then advisable to assist with the removal of the tooth.

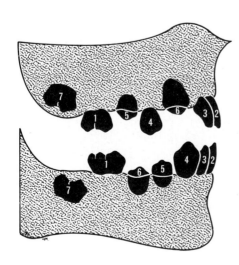

Figure 2–73 Most common sequence of eruption of permanent teeth. (Adapted from Moyers, R. E.: Handbook of Orthodontics. 3rd ed. Year Book Medical Publishers, 1972.)

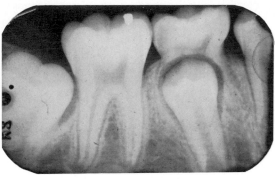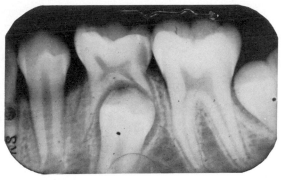

Figure 2-74   Normal resorption pattern, mandibular second deciduous molars.

Following the loss of the second deciduous molars, there is an adjustment in the occlusion of the first molar teeth. The mesiobuccal cusp of the maxillary first molar moves forward to occlude with the mesiobuccal groove of the mandibular first molar, as the flush terminal plane is eliminated. The Class II tendency which has been present throughout the deciduous and mixed dentition no longer exists. It cannot be stressed enough that it is important to keep the patient under careful surveillance during this critical period of interchange (Figs. 2–74, 2–75). Frequently preventive or interceptive orthodontic procedures can prevent the development of a full-fledged malocclusion or the establishment of occlusal aberrations which will cause considerable periodontal disturbance in later life. Certainly the philosophy here is to preclude an occasion when "for want of a tooth the battle was lost." There is no exaggeration to say that it is possible to prevent a deep bite and a functional retrusion and Class II malocclusion in some cases by interceptive guidance at the right time. A more complete discussion of this all-important period and the means of control in the hands of the dentist is given in Chapters 13 to 17.

Eruption of the second molar teeth usually occurs shortly after the appearance of the second premolars (Fig. 2–76). Since the second premolar and second molar teeth show the greatest variability in order of eruption of any of the teeth (third molars excepted), the second molar teeth may be expected to erupt before the second premolar teeth in about 17 per cent of the cases in Caucasians.[137]

Both maxillary and mandibular second molars ordinarily erupt at about the

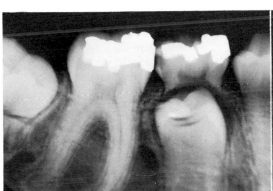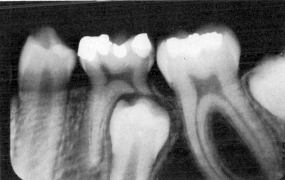

Figure 2-75   Abnormal resorption pattern, lower left second deciduous molar. Molar on right side is resorbing normally.

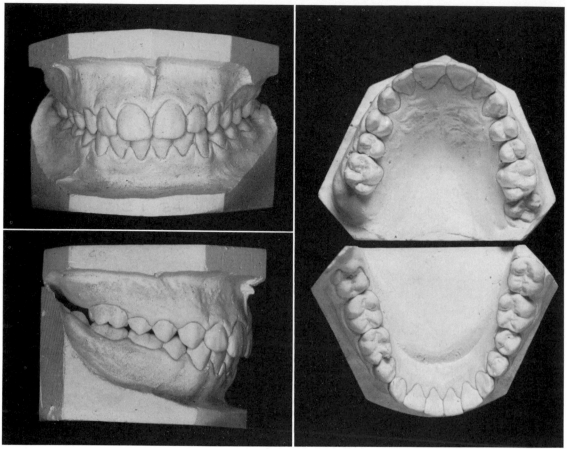

Figure 2-76   Case D. M., 12 years, 1 month, 24 days. The maxillary right second premolar has finally erupted and the second molars are making their appearance. Mandibular incisor irregularity has disappeared. (Courtesy J. H. Sillman.)

same time. Here again, we are confronted with the three stages of physiologic raising of the bite—this being stage 2. The gingival pads overlying the second molars contact prematurely again, blocking open the bite anteriorly, allowing the eruption of teeth anterior to the second molar for a period of a couple of weeks while this situation exists. The reduction in overbite is minimal and variable, being greater in some cases and less in others, but it is a phenomenon that occurs so frequently that it should be watched. This natural bite plate may be augmented with a prosthetic appliance. Before therapy is started, it is a good idea to see how much overbite correction nature produces spontaneously. There is still sufficient vertical growth in the alveolodental complex after the eruption of the second molars to allow a bite plate to work.

If the second permanent molars erupt before the second premolars, occasionally the first permanent molars may tip to the mesial. This is especially true in patients with premature loss of second deciduous molars. If the molars are tipped mesially, the eruption of the second premolar is further delayed. It may erupt belatedly to the lingual, or it may not erupt at all. In a large number of Class II, Division I malocclusions, the maxillary second molar tends to erupt before its mandibular opponent. Reasoning *a posteriori*, this has been explained on the basis of possible mesial drift of the maxillary denture due to perverted perioral muscle function, pressure habits, abnormal swallowing, and so forth. A contributing factor in slower second molar eruption is the apparently more critical space problem that may exist in the mandibular denture. In a contained arch there is less possibility of adjustment in tooth position. Also, deep bite and the retrusive effect of abnormal lip activity may exacerbate the problem.

Radiographs taken shortly after the eruption of the second permanent molars often show an image of the developing third molar teeth that is difficult to interpret. This is especially true of the mandibular third molars. Usually inadequate space exists in the dental arch to accommodate these teeth, which appear to be forming in the ramus. The tooth appears to be facing sideways (Fig. 2–77). In actuality, the long axis of the developing third molar is obliquely

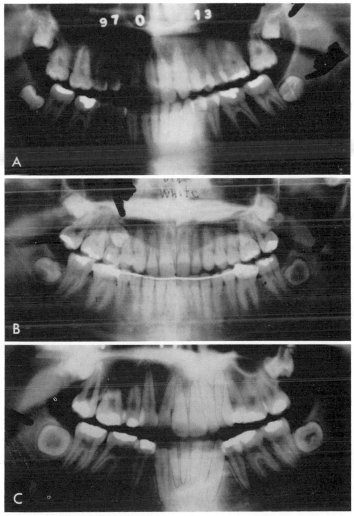

Figure 2–77 Panoral radiographs show the status of third molars early. Lingually inclined mandibular third molars may not become upright autonomously. Despite removal of four premolars, C, mandibular third molars are almost horizontal in their lingual malposition, and will have to be removed. A four tooth extraction thus becomes an eight tooth sacrifice, if a careful diagnostic study is not made with adequate radiographic analysis.

directed toward the tongue in midplane at an angle of from 55 to 70 degrees.[139] This inclination tends to become less obtuse between the ages of 12 and 16 years, but the occlusal surface is still lingually inclined. Since the alveolar process curves lingually at the point of juncture with the anterior border of the ramus the third molar may frequently have enough room to erupt, even though the tooth appears radiographically to be in the ramus itself. It is, of course, lingual to the ramus. Although the maxillary second molars erupt in a downward and forward direction, the maxillary third molars erupt downward and more backward. To this might be added the direction "outward." As Dempster, Adams and Duddles showed (see Chap. 4, Figs. 4–16 to 4–19), the axial inclinations of the maxillary teeth tend to converge, particularly at the end of the arch.[140] The mandibular long axes tend to diverge, following the curve of Spee. (This creates certain problems with serial extraction procedures, as will be discussed in Chapter 15.) Of more immediate concern, however, is the fact that with the maxillary third molars erupting in a posterior and buccal direction, it is no wonder that a cross-bite exists in many cases where the third molars have sufficient room to erupt. It is not possible to state a definite time for the eruption of third molars. Hurme estimates the median time for eruption at 20.5 years.[138] In general, these teeth appear in girls before they do in boys, and eruption is completed more rapidly in girls. In the male, the eruption of third molars is quite erratic and the emergence of these teeth into the oral cavity is much more variable chronologically than in the female. By 20 years of age most females have their third molars, if they are going to get them. This is not true of males.

It is easy to understand that problems arise frequently in the third molar area, considering the initial deficiency in arch length, the tendencies for the maxillary and mandibular third molars to by-pass each other, their varying axial inclinations and the unpredictable timing of the eruption of these teeth. The third molar problem can be not only a painful experience, but it can cause functional disturbances that affect longevity of the dentition and create and aggravate temporomandibular joint pathology.

Many orthodontists feel that when they remove the four first bicuspid teeth and complete orthodontic therapy, the third molars now have a better chance to erupt normally because they have more room. However, panoramic laminagraphic surveys show that in many of these cases the addition of space allows the mandibular third molar to tip forward and to impact under the distal convexity of the second molar.[139] Constant supervision is essential, and surgical uprighting is often a possible interceptive procedure (see Chap. 15).

CLINICAL APPLICATIONS OF GROWTH AND DEVELOPMENT DATA

The preceding pages of this chapter outline the prenatal and postnatal development of the cranial, facial and oral structures. I have described the phenomena of bone tissue growth, bone organ growth and the development of the dentition. Since highly organized and complex procedures are involved here, the discussion has been time-linked, describing the changes occurring in the progress toward maturity at different age levels. Those who wonder at the marvels of nature as they watch the unfolding of a beautiful flower should find an appreciation of craniofacial growth and development no less fascinating. But there is more to be gained than esthetic appreciation. As was pointed out at the beginning of this chapter, the practicing dentist will find that very real, concrete benefits can accrue from a working knowledge of the growth and development processes.

More than ever, a knowledge of the intricacies of dentofacial development is essential. Unsubstantiated claims of appliance success by "expanding" the dental arches to stimulate development are encountered often in the literature. The significant increase in the types and numbers of removable appliances being foisted upon general dental practitioners and being taught privately in "courses" or in "study groups" may be considered an unfavorable development. Use of such appliances should be justified by objective scientific data, not by claims of success for which there have not been sufficient follow-up studies after the patients have discarded their appliances.

Longitudinal studies of dimensional changes in the dental arches from birth to 25 years provides sobering evidence of the futility of expansionist philosophies of orthodontic treatment.[141-143] Arch length and arch width changes are illustrated in Figures 2–72, 2–78. The minimal changes in intermolar and intercanine length and width are dramatically evident. The clinical implications are obvious, particularly for treatment of Class I malocclusions. Arbitrary expansion, the first and foremost objective of most removable appliances, is fraught with failure. Relapse, periodontal involvement and a tarnished dental image are likely sequelae if the biologic and physiologic evidence such as that shown in Figure 2–78 is ignored.

Most crowding seems to occur in the mandibular anterior segment. How much growth occurs between the canines? When is maxillary and mandibular intercanine dimensional change completed? This is obviously important for the man who would increase intercanine distance, waiting for growth to catch up. As shown in Chapter 15 (Fig. 15–1), in the girl the mandibular intercanine dimension is essentially completed at nine; in the boy at ten years of age.[124, 154] In the maxillary arch, intercanine dimension is complete by 12 in the girl; in the boy at 18. In both male and female, the maxillary intercanine dimension serves as a "safety valve" for pubertal growth spurts, where there is a basal horizontal mandibular growth, partly unmatched by the maxilla, as the mandible grows downward and forward. It is during the pubertal growth period that there is often a directional change from vertical to the horizontal, as Figure 2–53 shows. The maxillary intercanine dimension adjusts as the mandibular dentition is brought forward, helping to eliminate the flush terminal plane relationship, or any residual Class II tendencies. The biologist knows that an erupting third molar cannot push the buccal segments forward and crowd the incisors. However, the presence of third molars does interfere with retropositioning of the mandibular dentition on its base, since the incisors tend to upright under the terminal horizontal growth increments. Early removal of third molars may be indicated in some instances. Continued radiographic survey is essential to prevent increasing or relapsing malocclusion.

Entirely too many mechanical procedures which ignore the equally important anatomic and physiologic considerations have been taught in the past. A six-year-old child loses a maxillary deciduous first molar. Since this is a "baby" tooth, do we ignore the loss and wait for the successor? No, for we have been taught that the maintenance of space is vital for the establishment of a normal occlusion. Teeth drift when their neighbors are lost. This is not always true, however, and we must know a good deal more before we rush in and place a space maintainer. Is the occlusion normal? Are there any abnormal finger, tongue or lip muscle habits? What is the size of the succedaneous tooth as compared with the deciduous counterpart? Does the anatomy of the cusps and

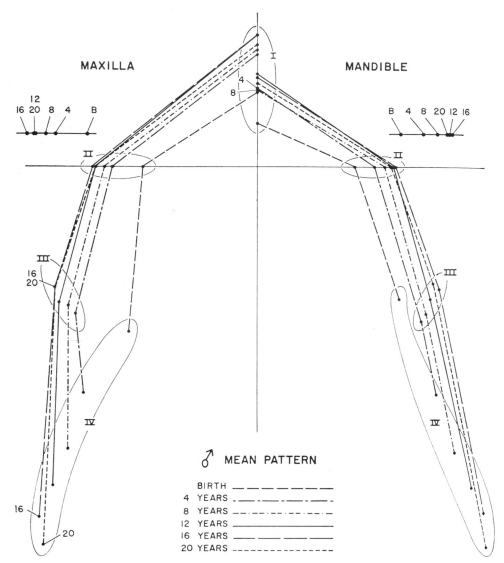

Figure 2–78 Composite mean pattern of male maxilla and mandible from birth to 20 years of age. (From Sillman, J. H.: Dimensional changes of dental arches: longitudinal studies from birth to 25 years. Am. J. Orthodont., 50:824–842, 1964.)

inclined planes "lock" the occlusion so that the loss of a deciduous molar may be ignored? Is the morphogenetic pattern one of generalized deficiency of space to accommodate all the teeth? Is the overbite excessive, creating a restricting influence upon arch length in the mandibular arch? If such is the case, maintaining the space of a prematurely lost tooth may well interfere with the autonomous adjustment of the remaining teeth. Perhaps a planned program of serial extraction is indicated (Chap. 15).

Odontometry provides valuable information for the dentist at this critical stage. What are the correlations among crown diameters of human teeth?[144] "Considerable discordance can occur in the relations of mesiodistal crown diameters among permanent or deciduous, successional, as well as maxillary and mandibular teeth and tooth groups."[126]

This corroborates an earlier study in which it was concluded: "The space demands of the permanent central and lateral incisors relative to the size of their deciduous predecessors differed markedly among children. Similarly, the space that became available during the replacement of the deciduous canines and molars by their permanent successors contributed in varying degrees to the alignment of the teeth in the permanent dentition."[125] The immediate clinical implications are that there is considerable variability in the leeway space of Nance, so that we cannot arbitrarily accept the 1.7 mm. on each side in the lower arch and the 1 mm. space in the upper arch as a rule. It is only a mean and the range is appreciable. Actual measurement of the deciduous teeth on the cast and the permanent successors on properly taken intraoral radiographs offers the best prediction of space adequacy for that particular patient. Various analyses, such as the Moyers Mixed Dentition Analysis, are helpful, but they should serve only as a guide and as corroborative evidence. Obviously, frequent orthodontic consultations should be had where there is any question at all about the need for future orthodontic guidance. It is better that the orthodontist make the decision on the best time for treatment, correlating therapy with the most favorable biologic factors, than to have to "make do" at a less than optimum time.

What contributions can be expected from craniofacial growth and development? *Magnitude* of growth increments is important, and so is *timing* with the best amount of growth per unit time, to keep therapeutic intervention as short as possible. But what about growth *direction*? Is it downward and forward or downward and backward?[153] Treatment time, tooth position changes, decisions on extraction, and ultimate prognosis and stability all depend on growth direction (Fig. 2–79).

Is overeruption of the opposing tooth or teeth a factor? Is the premature loss of the first deciduous molar nature's clue to arch length problems in the near future — problems that growth and development cannot solve — or is the loss of the tooth due to caries or some other pathologic process?[128] Are there any congenitally missing teeth? Any tooth size discrepancies?

Obviously, the answers to these and many other questions transcend the mere mechanical substitution of the missing dental unit. Complete diagnostic records will provide some of the answers (Chap. 8). Many of the answers are found in the foregoing pages on growth and development. If the loss of the deciduous first molar is indeed a sign of lack of space in the dental arch, we know that ordinary growth procedures will not make up that space. While the combined width of the deciduous cuspid, first deciduous and second deciduous molars is on the average 1.7 mm. greater than the permanent successors in the mandibular arch and 0.9 mm. greater in the maxillary arch, adjustive changes following the loss of a tooth can quickly dissipate this advantage (Fig. 2–71).

Histologic studies show that teeth erupt rapidly during the tooth exchange period and continue to erupt even though they are in occlusal contact with their opposing members.[145] (Remember, occlusal contact is only 2 to 6 per cent in any 24-hour period.) Eruption is more rapid, however, with no opposing tooth. Another factor, then, is the elongation of the clinical crown into the edentulous area, beyond the level of the contiguous teeth.

Frequently, the maxillary lateral incisors erupt into the oral cavity with a strong distal inclination of their crowns. What relevant information does knowledge of the growth and development pattern give us? Studies have shown that this may well be part of the "ugly duckling pattern"[146] (Fig. 2–80). As the lateral incisors erupt, the canines higher up in the alveolar process are also erupting but are literally sliding down the developing roots of lateral incisors.

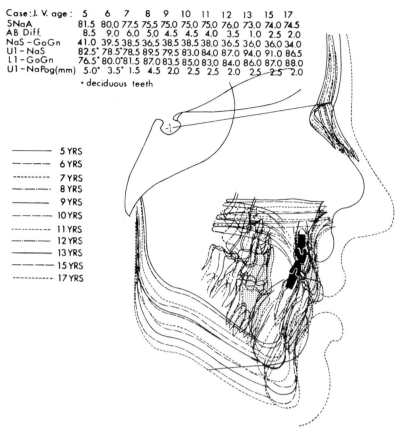

Case: J. V. age:	5	6	7	8	9	10	11	12	13	15	17
SNaA	81.5	80.0	77.5	75.5	75.0	75.0	75.0	76.0	73.0	74.0	74.5
AB Diff.	8.5	9.0	6.0	5.0	4.5	4.5	4.0	3.5	1.0	2.5	2.0
NaS – GoGn	41.0	39.5	38.5	36.5	38.5	38.5	38.0	36.5	36.0	36.0	34.0
U1 – NaS	82.5°	78.5°	78.5	89.5	79.5	83.0	84.0	87.0	94.0	91.0	86.5
L1 – GoGn	76.5°	80.0°	81.5	87.0	83.5	85.0	83.0	84.0	86.0	87.0	88.0
U1 – NaPog (mm)	5.0°	3.5°	1.5	4.5	2.0	2.5	2.5	2.0	2.5	2.5	2.0

• deciduous teeth

————— 5 YRS
– – – – 6 YRS
- - - - - 7 YRS
—·—·— 8 YRS
————— 9 YRS
– – – – 10 YRS
- - - - - 11 YRS
—·—·— 12 YRS
————— 13 YRS
– – – – 15 YRS
- - - - - 17 YRS

Figure 2–79   Changes over a 12-year period in a familial Class III pattern. Chincap therapy from 5 to 10 years of age produced a primarily vertical component. More horizontal growth without cap from 10 to 12 years was followed by further wear from 13 to 15 years. Vertical vector again dominated. The mandibular growth was counterclockwise, reducing inclination of mandibular plane, and apical base difference from 8 degrees to 2 degrees. A tightly restricting repaired cleft lip undoubtedly helped reduce SNaA from 81.5 degrees to 74.5 degrees.

This tends to force the apices of these teeth toward the midline, while the crowns tend to flare laterally (Fig. 2–81). As the canines continue to erupt, however, there is an autonomous straightening up of the lateral incisors. The temporary spacing that often occurs between the central incisors and the lateral incisors is usually closed as the canines erupt into complete occlusion. It would be most hazardous to place appliances at this critical stage. The chances of damage to the apices of the maxillary lateral incisors and the possibility of deflecting the permanent canines from their normal path of eruption are great.

Many deciduous dentitions present themselves with what we would call an excessive overbite.[147] Is this normal? Does this overbite restrict the development of the mandibular incisor segment as is sometimes claimed? Will growth and developmental processes take care of the overbite spontaneously? Should anything be done? Here again, a thorough knowledge of the growth and developmental processes is essential to interpret the situation and answer these questions. Many five- and six-year-olds have what would be considered an excessive overbite at a later stage. Quite frequently there is an end-to-end flush terminal plane type of bite in the buccal segments, with the appearance of a mandibular retrusion. In many instances the eruption of the first molars does

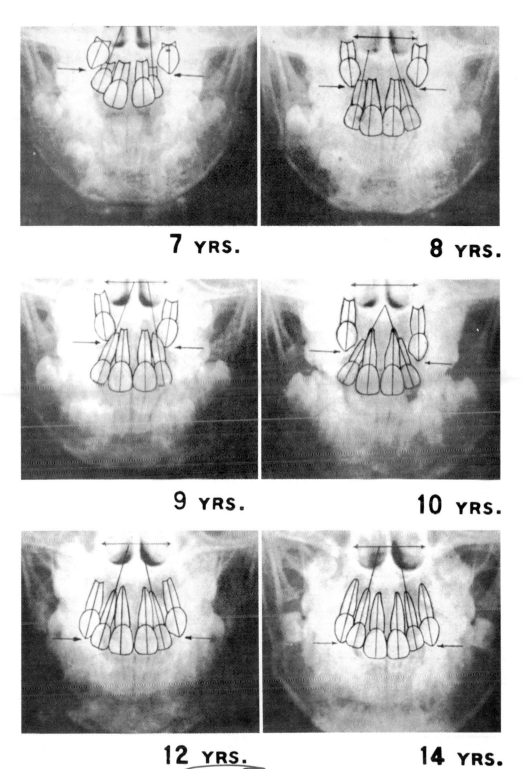

7 YRS.   **8 YRS.**

9 YRS.   **10 YRS.**

12 YRS.   **14 YRS.**

Figure 2–80   So-called "ugly duckling" developing dental patterns. (From Broadbent, B. H.: Ontogenetic Development of Occlusion, Angle Orthodontist, *11*:223–241, 1941.)

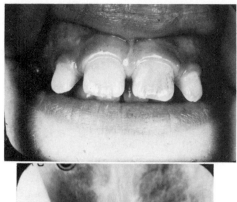

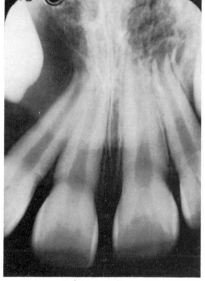

Figure 2–81   Photograph and radiograph showing transient flaring of maxillary incisors as canines migrate through the alveolar bone toward the oral cavity.

not change the end-to-end bite tendency and terminal plane relationship. Not until the deciduous molars are lost and the premolars erupt does the occlusion really settle into proper interdigitation. This transient malocclusion, as was mentioned previously, may be attributed to the fact that the combined width of the deciduous canine and first and second deciduous molars is, on the average, 1.7 mm. greater on each side in the mandibular arch than the combined width of the permanent canine and first and second premolars (Nance's "leeway space"). It can be wrong to hurry and place orthodontic appliances to correct what appears to be a developing Class II malocclusion during the mixed dentition when the exchange of the deciduous for the permanent teeth would correct this tendency spontaneously. The change in growth direction in the terminal stages of pubertal growth, with horizontal increments often appearing, may be all that is necessary to correct the Class II tendency. Carefully examined periodic cephalograms may give us the clue and prevent needless therapy.

With mandibular retrusion there is usually a tendency toward a deeper than normal overbite. With this excessive overbite there is the likelihood of more vertical axial inclination of the lower anterior teeth. In the deciduous dentition, the teeth are more vertical and the angle formed by the intersection of the long axis is greater (Fig. 2–82). In the permanent dentition the long axes of the upper and lower incisors form a more acute angle. It is a well-known fact in dentistry that the more upright the incisors, the greater the likelihood of excessive overbite. This is true in the permanent dentition, as many orthodon-

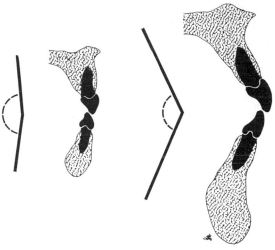

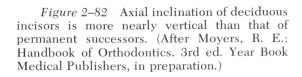

Figure 2–82   Axial inclination of deciduous incisors is more nearly vertical than that of permanent successors. (After Moyers, R. E.: Handbook of Orthodontics. 3rd ed. Year Book Medical Publishers, in preparation.)

tists have found, after the removal of teeth during orthodontic therapy. But the phenomenon is quite natural in the deciduous dentition. A combination of the more acute axial inclination of the permanent incisors as they erupt and simultaneous vertical alveolar growth often reduces the temporarily excessive overbite.

An examination of any series of six-year-old children will show that the lower incisor teeth have quite a struggle to erupt into the dental arch. Space almost always seems to be at a premium. With a deep overbite, the lower incisors are literally crowded lingually, being part of the contained arch. It is possible, with the use of a simple bite plate, to reduce this tendency, to allow the full development of mandibular intercanine width and to enhance the normal eruption of the lower incisors. This procedure will be discussed in greater detail in Chapter 16.

The question has often been asked, "Why are there so many children with severe malocclusions, while there are relatively few adults with the same degree of deformity?" Although this question derives primarily from a clinical impression, it has some basis in fact. Here again a thorough knowledge of cranial and facial growth and development helps provide the answer. It was pointed out in the first part of this chapter that the cranial, facial and dental width increments are completed quite early. Anteroposterior growth continues much longer. Vertical growth, particularly in the lower third of the face, is the last to be completed. It is accomplished through the growth of alveolar bone and eruption of teeth. A mandibular retrusion looks less severe in a long face than a short face. The mandible can be just as far behind the maxilla in the adult as it is in the child, but the angle of convexity of the profile is reduced (Fig. 2–83).

The severity of the malocclusion and the associated profile abnormality is not likely to diminish, if the study of Frölich on 51 untreated Class II malocclusions is to serve as a guide. In the longitudinal appraisal, he observed that both overbite and especially overjet increase in Class II malocclusions. Generally, the sagittal relationship of the dental arches does not improve, but may actually become more severe. Frölich concludes that "since the malrelationship of the dental arches increases, as determined by overjet and by canine and molar relationships, it is of no advantage to postpone therapeutic measures,

Case: S.E. age:	7	12 1/2	14	14 1/2
AB Diff.	8.0	8.0	8.0	8.0
NaS-GoGn	36.0	40.0	38.0	38.0
U1-NaS	107.0	97.0	101.0	101.0
L1-GoGn	101.0	101.0	101.0	101.0
U1-NaPog(mm.)	13.0	13.0	14.0	14.0

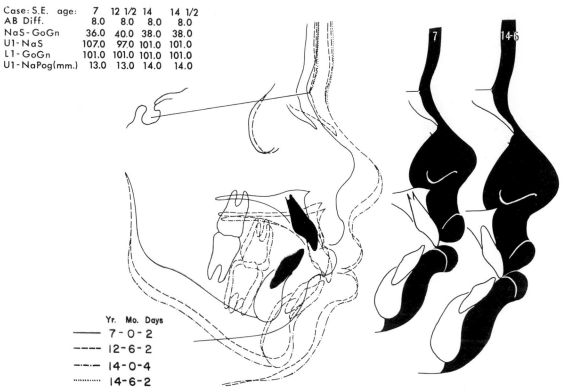

Yr. Mo. Days	
———	7- 0- 2
----	12- 6- 2
-·-·-	14- 0- 4
··········	14- 6- 2

Figure 2-83   Case S. E., showing decreasing angle of facial convexity over an 8-year period, despite the fact that the anteroposterior relationship of the mandible and maxilla remains the same. The decrease may be attributed to a significant increase in facial height, moving the points on the profile farther away from each other.

once the distocclusion is observed."[148] However, in cases where there is a marked horizontal vector and change of direction of mandibular growth, particularly in boys, there may actually be some reduction in anteroposterior dysplasia. This change can be seen on cephalograms, and the patient is entitled to the benefit of orthodontic knowledge on the subject.

Many observers feel that with the maturation and increased tonicity of the perioral soft tissue the role of the musculature is a favorable factor in reducing a maxillary protrusion. This is discussed in greater detail in Chapter 3. We have shown that growth gradients are not uniform.[103] Growth spurts and directional changes are quite demonstrable, as Woodside has shown in the deciduous and mixed dentitions as well as in the permanent dentition[116] (Fig. 2–38). The astute orthodontist recognizes that with the onset of puberty, significant accelerated growth increments can be observed along with frequently favorable change in growth direction. This is of real value in the treatment of Class II malocclusions, where a face that has been largely growing downward will at once show horizontal mandibular growth increments (Fig. 2–53, 2–54). Finally, there are modeling bony changes that occur, particularly at the symphysis of the mandible, with approaching maturation. Excellent longitudinal cephalometric studies illustrate these phenomena (Chap. 8).

Björk's study of 322 12-year-old pupils and 281 Swedish conscripts in the 20-year age group illustrates the role of pubertal and postpubertal mandibular growth.[149] In the 12-year-olds, there were only eight cases of mandibular prognathism (Class III, Angle), or 2.5 per cent. In the 20-year-olds, 26 of the conscripts had mandibular prognathisms, or 9.3 per cent of the sample. Even considering the fact that the conscripts were selected on the basis of physical fitness, the almost 4 to 1 ratio is significant. To the orthodontist treating a Class II malocclusion characterized by a mandibular retrusion, this latent growth spurt, coupled with emphasis on the horizontal vector of growth, may mean the difference between restoration of normal jaw relationship and residual Class II characteristics. Whether it is a Class II or a Class III malocclusion, proper treatment timing, based on a thorough knowledge of growth, is an essential prerequisite for successful therapy.

Although we may not be able to significantly reduce the *amount* of growth during this circumpubertal period, perhaps we can alter the *direction* (Figs. 2–84, 2–85). In patients with scoliosis who wear the orthopedic Milwaukee brace, basal morphologic changes are created.[103] The work of Elgoyhen and co-workers and Joho on the Macaque provides additional substantiating evidence of the ability to make changes in growth direction.[150, 151] Extensive clinical experience by the author using chin caps in Class III malocclusions for the past 15 years, strongly supports these pilot studies (see Chap. 14). Since a large

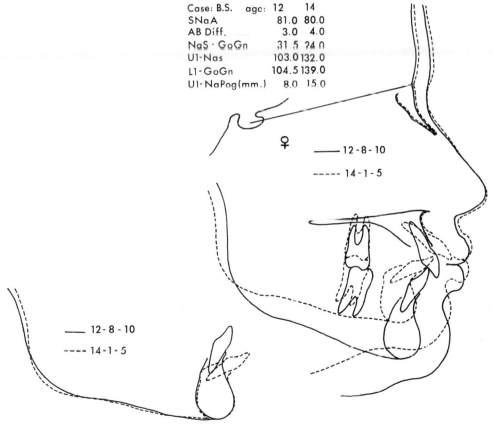

Case: B.S.   age: 12   14
SNaA   81.0 80.0
AB Diff.   3.0   4.0
NaS - GoGn   31.5 24.0
U1-Nas   103.0 132.0
L1-GoGn   104.5 139.0
U1-NaPog(mm.)   8.0 15.0

——— 12-8-10
----- 14-1-5

——— 12-8-10
---- 14-1-5

Figure 2–84   Milwaukee brace effect. Note closing down of bite due to orthopedic effect on mandible, alveolar bone, teeth, and maxilla. Membranous bone response is apparently more sensitive to pressures than endochondral bone response (scoliosis). This adverse effect has favorable therapeutic potential, however, in basal malrelationships, such as Class II, Class III and open bite problems. See Figure 2–85 for lateral cephalograms. (Courtesy S. Weinstein.)

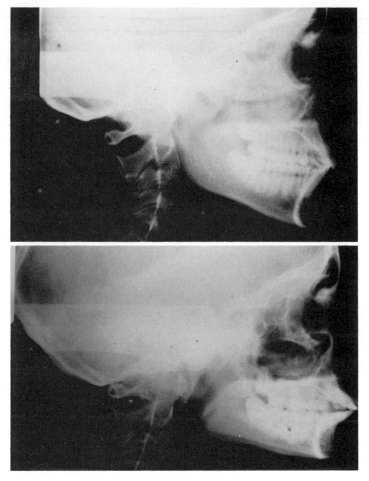

Figure 2–85. Dramatic reduction in lower face height, in less than two years of scoliosis brace (i.e., Milwaukee brace) wear. Orthopedic force has significant effect in a period of peak growth acceleration. (Courtesy of S. Weinstein.)

number of cases treated by the orthodontist are jaw malrelationships, the future emphasis on orthopedic guidance of growth may well be one of the most significant advances in the specialty of orthodontics. It is essential that the dentist be an applied biologist. The traditional overconcern with the alignment of teeth must be subordinated to a broader appreciation of bone system and neuromuscular system involvement.[112, 128]

REFERENCES

1. Krogman, W. M.: Principles of human growth. Ciba Sympos., 5:1458–1466, 1943.
2. Todd, T. W.: Differential skeletal maturation in relation to sex, race variability, and disease. Child Develop., 2:49–65, 1931.
3. Arey, L. B.: Developmental Anatomy. 7th ed. Philadelphia, W. B. Saunders Co., 1965.
4. Orban, B.: Oral Histology and Embryology. 7th ed. St. Louis, C. V. Mosby Co., 1972.
5. Limborgh, J. Van: A new view on the control of the morphogenesis of the skull. Acta Morph. Neerl. Scand., 8:143–160, 1970.
6. Dixon, A. D.: The early development of the maxilla. Dent. Pract., 3:331–356, 1953.
7. Dixon, A. D.: The development of the jaws. Dent. Pract., 9:10–18, 1958.
8. Freiband, B.: Growth of the palate in the human fetus. J. Dent. Res., 16:103–122, 1937.

9. Ingham, T. R.: Study of the human fetal mandible. J. Dent. Res., 12:647–650, 1932.

10. Patten, B. M.: The normal development of the facial region *in* Pruzansky, S. (ed.): Congenital Anomalies of the Face and Associated Structures. Springfield, Ill., Charles C Thomas, 1961.

11. Avery, J. K., Happle, J. D., and French, W. C.: A possible factor in cleft palate etiology. J. Dent. Res., 37:79–81, 1958.

12. Avery, J. K., and Devine, R. K.: The development of the ossification centers in the face and palate of normal and cleft palate human embryos. Cleft Palate Bull., 9:25–26, 1959.

13. Avery, J. K.: The nasal capsule in cleft palate. Anat. Anz. Erganz., 109:722–726, 1960–1961.

14. Weinmann, J. P., and Sicher, H.: Bone and Bones. St. Louis, C. V. Mosby Co., 1955.

15. Noyes, H. J.: The role of growth and development in interceptive orthodontics. D. Clin. North America, July, 1959, pp. 289–298.

16. Yasuda, I.: On the piezoelectric activity of bone. J. Jap. Orthop. Surg. Soc., 28:267–269, 1954.

17. Bassett, C. A. L.: Biologic significance of piezo-electricity. Calcu. Tissue Res., 1:252–272, 1968.

18. Coulombre, A. J., and Crelin, E. S.: The role of the developing eye in the morphogenesis of the avian skull. Am. J. Phys. Anthrop., 16:25–38, 1958.

19. Tonneyk-Müller, I.: Das Wachstum von Augen und Augenhöhlen beim Hühnerembryo. Acta Morphol. Neerl.-Scand. 8:303–319, 1971.

20. Scott, J. H.: The cartilage of the nasal septum. A contribution to the study of facial growth. Brit. Dent. J., 95:37–43, 1953.

21. Moss, M. L.: The functional matrix *in* Kraus, B. S., and Riedel, R. A. (eds.): Vistas in Orthodontics. Philadelphia, Lea & Febiger, 1962.

22. Klaauw, C. J. van der: Cerebral skull and facial skull. A contribution to the knowledge of skull structure. Arch. Neerl. Zool., 9:16–36, 1946.

23. Klaauw, C. J. van der: Size and position of the functional components of the skull. A contribution to the knowledge of the architecture of the skull, based on data in the literature. Arch. Neerl. Zool., 9:1–176, 1948.

24. Klaauw, C. J. van der: Size and position of the functional components of the skull (continuation). Arch. Neerl. Zool., 9:177–368, 1951.

25. Klaauw, C. J. van der: Size and position of the functional components of the skull (conclusion). Arch. Neerl. Zool., 9:369–560, 1952.

26. Limborgh, J. van, and Verwoerd-Verhoef, H. L.: Effects of artificial unilateral facial clefts on growth of the skull in young rabbits. J. Dent. Res., 47:1013, 1968.

27. Hinrichsen, G. J. and Storey, E.: The effect of force on bone and bones. Angle Orthodont., 38:155–165, 1968.

28. Enlow, D. H., and Hunter, W. S.: The growth of the face in relation to the cranial base. Trans. Europ. Soc. Orth., 321–335, 1968.

29. Sarnat, B. G.: Postnatal growth of the nose and face after resection of septal cartilage in the rabbit. Oral Surg., 26:712–727, 1968.

30. Sarnat, B. G.: Growth of bones as revealed by implant markers in animals. Am. J. Phys. Anthrop., 29:255–286, 1968.

31. Burdi, A. R.: Sagittal growth of the nasomaxillary complex during the second trimester of human development. J. Dent. Res., 44:112–125, 1965.

32. Latham, R. A.: The sella point and postnatal growth of the human cranial base. Am. J. Orthodont., 61:156–162, 1972.

33. Baume, L. J.: Patterns of cephalofacial growth and development. Int. Dent. J., 18:489–513, 1968.

34. Petrovic, A., Charlier, J. P., and Hermann, J.: Les Mecanismes de croissance du crane. recherches sur le cartilage de la cloison nasale et sur les sutures craniennes et faciales de jeunes rats en culture d'organes. Bull. Assoc. Anat., Extrait, no. 143, April 7–11, 1968.

35. Petrovic, A., and Charlier, J. P.: La synchondrose spheno-occipitale de jeune rat en culture d'organes: mise en evidence d'un potentiel de croissance independent. C. R. Acad. Soc. (Paris), 265:1511–1513, 1967.

36. Dorenbos, J.: Craniale Synchondroses. Doctoral thesis, Central Drukkerij n.v. Nijmegen, University of Nijmegen. April, 1971.

37. Ohyama, K.: Experimental study on growth and development of dentofacial complex after resection of cartilagenous nasal septum. Bull. Tokyo Med. Dent. Univ., 16:157–176, 1969.

38. Scott, J. H.: The growth of the human face. Proc. Roy. Soc. Med., 47:91–100, 1954.

39. Scott, J. H.: Craniofacial regions; contribution to the study of facial growth. Dent. Pract., 5:208–214, 1955.

40. Scott, J. H.: Growth at facial sutures. Am. J. Orthodont., 42:381–387, 1956.

41. Scott, J. H.: The cranial base. Am. J. Phys. Anthrop., 16:319–348, 1958.

42. Scott, J. H.: The analysis of facial growth. Part 1. The anteroposterior and vertical dimensions. Am. J. Orthodont., 44:507–512, 1958. Part 2. The horizontal and vertical dimensions. Am. J. Orthodont., 44:585–589, 1958.

43. Scott, J. H.: The doctrine of functional matrices. Am. J. Orthodont., 56:38–44, 1969.

44. Ford, E. H. R.: Growth of the human cranial base. Am. J. Orthodont., 44:498–506, 1958.

45. Moss, M. L.: Inhibition and stimulation of suture fusion in the rat calvaria. Anat. Rec., 136:457–468, 1960.

46. Moss, M. L. and Greenberg, S. N.: Postnatal growth of the human skull base. Angle Orthodont., 25:77–84, 1955.

47. Moss, M. L.: The pathogenesis of artificial cranial deformation. Am. J. Phys. Anthrop., 16:269–286, 1958.
48. Moss, M. L.: Fusion of the frontal suture in the rat. Am. J. Anat., 102:141–166, 1958.
49. Enlow, D. H.: The Human Face. Hoeber Medical Division, New York, Harper & Row, 1968.
50. Enlow, D. H., Moyers, R. E., Hunter, W. S., and McNamara, J. A.: A procedure for the analysis of intrinsic form and growth. Am. J. Orthodont., 56:6–23, 1969.
51. Scammon, R. E., Harris, J. A., Jackson, C. M., and Patterson, D. G., The Measurement of Man. Minneapolis, University of Minnesota Press, 1930.
52. Koski, K.: Some aspects of growth of the cranial base and the upper face. Odont. Trans., 68:344–358, 1960.
53. Koski, K., and Ronning, O.: Growth potential of subcutaneously transplanted cranial base synchondroses of the rat. Acta Odont. Scand., 27:343–357, 1969.
54. Koski, K., and Ronning, O.: Growth potential of intracerebrally transplanted cranial base synchondroses in the rat. Arch. Oral Biol., 15:1107–1108, 1970.
55. Koski, K., and Ronning, O.: Pitkän luun rustoisen pään sürrännäisen kasvupotentiallista rotalla. Suom. hammaslääk. toim., 62:165–169, 1966.
56. Koski, K., and Ronning, O.: Growth potential of transplanted components of the mandibular ramus of the rat III. Suom. hammaslääk. toim., 61:292–297, 1965.
57. Ronning, O.: Observations on the intracerebral transplantation of the mandibular condyle. Acta Odont. Scand., 24:443–457, 1966.
58. Koski, K.: Cranial growth centers, facts or fallacies? Am. J. Orthodont., 54:566–583, 1968.
59. Koski, K. and Ronning, O.: Intracerebral isologous transplantation of the condylar cartilage with and without the articular disc. Am. J. Orthodont., 60:86, 1971.
60. Melsen, B.: Time of closure of spheno-occipital synchondrosis determined on dry skulls. Acta Odont. Scand., 27:73–90, 1969.
61. Benninghoff, A.: Form und Bau der Gelenknorpel in ihren Beziehungen zur Funktion. Z. Zellforsch., 2:783–862, 1925.
62. Davenport, C. B.: How We Came By Our Bodies. New York, Henry Holt Co., 1936.
63. Davenport, C. B.: Bodily growth of babies during the first post-natal year. Contributions to Embryology, No. 169, Carnegie Institute, Washington, D.C., 496:271–305, 1938.
64. Baer, M. J., and Harris, J. E.: A Commentary on the growth of the human brain and skull, Am. J. Phys. Anthrop., 30:39–44, 1969.
65. Cannon, J.: Craniofacial height and depth increments in normal children. Angle Orthodont., 40:202–218, 1970.
66. Ackerman, J. L., Takagi, Y., Proffit, W. R., and Baer, M. J.: Craniofacial growth and development in cebocephalia. Oral Surg., 19:543–554, 1965.
67. Moss, M. L.: The primacy of functional matrices in orofacial growth. Dent. Pract., 19:65–73, 1968.
68. Enlow, D. H., and Bang, S.: Growth and remodelling of the human maxilla. Am. J. Orthodont., 51:446–464, 1965.
69. Moss, M. L., and Salentijn, L.: The capsular matrix. Am. J. Orthodont., 56:474–490, 1969.
70. Graber, T. M.: Growth of the cleft palate and normal child from birth to six years of age in Hotz, R. (ed.): Early Treatment of Cleft Lip and Palate. Zurich, Hans Huber, 1964.
71. Moss, M. L., and Greenberg, S. N.: Functional cranial analysis of the human maxillary bone. Angle Orthodont., 37:151–164, 1967.
72. Walker, D. G.: A facial index of oral surgery. Proc. Roy. Soc. Med., 59:71–74, 1966.
73. Isaacson, R. J., Wood, J. L., and Ingram, A. H.: Forces produced by rapid maxillary expansion. Angle Orthodont., 34:256–270, 1964.
74. Wertz, R. A.: Skeletal and dental changes accompanying rapid midpalatal suture opening. Am. J. Orthodont., 58:41–66, 1970.
75. Lebret, L.: Growth changes of the palate. J. Dent. Res., 41:1391–1404, 1962.
76. Korkhaus, G.: Present orthodontic thought in Germany. Am. J. Orthodont., 46:187–206, 1960.
77. Burdi, A. R., and Faist, K.: Morphogenesis of the palate in normal human embryos with special emphasis on the mechanisms involved. Am. J. Anat., 120:149–160, 1967.
78. Joondeph, D. R., and Wragg, L. E.: Facial growth during the secondary palate closure in the rat. Am. J. Orthodont., 6:88–89, 1971.
79. Savara, B. S., and Singh, I. J.: Norms of size and annual increments of seven anatomical measures of maxillae in boys from three to sixteen years of age. Angle Orthodont., 38:104–120, 1968.
80. Scott, J. H.: Development, structure and function of alveolar bone. Dent. Pract. 19:19–22, 1968.
81. Babula, W. J., Smiley, G. R., and Dixon, A. D.: The role of cartilagenous nasal septum in midfacial growth. Am. J. Orthodont., 58:250–263, 1970.
82. Scott, J. H.: Dento-facial Development and Growth. London, Pergamon Press, 65–137, 1967.
83. Shapiro, B.: A twin study of palatal dimensions partitioning genetic and environmental contributions to variability. Angle Orthodont., 39:139–151, 1969.
84. Moss, M. L.: Functional cranial analysis of the mandibular angular cartilage in the rat. Angle Orthodont., 39:209–214, 1969.
85. Moss, M. L.: Functional cranial analysis and the functional matrix. ASHA Reports, no. 6, 5–18, 1971.
86. Sicher, H.: The growth of the mandible. Am. J. Orthodont., 33:30–35, 1947.

87. Charlier, J. P., Petrovic, A., and Stutzmann, J.: Effects of mandibular hyperpropulsion of the prechondroblastic zone of young rat condyle. Am. J. Orthodont., 55:71–74, 1969.

88. Moss, M. L.: Functional cranial analysis of mammalian mandibular ramal morphology. Acta anat., 71:423–447, 1968.

89. Moss, M. L.: Functional cranial analysis of the coronoid process in the rat. Acta anat., 77:11–24, 1970.

90. Moss, M. L., and Salentijn, L.: The logarithmic growth of the human mandible. Acta anat., 77:341–360, 1970.

91. Björk, A.: Variations in the growth pattern of the human mandible: longitudinal radiographic studies by the implant method. J. Dent. Res., 42:400–411, 1963.

92. Björk, A.: Prediction of mandibular growth rotation. Am. J. Orthodont., 55:585–599, 1969.

93. Björk, A.: The use of metallic implants in the study of facial growth in children: method and application. Am. J. Phys. Anthrop., 29:243–254, 1968.

94. Koski, K., and Makinen, L.: Growth potential of transplanted components of the mandibular ramus of the rat. I. Suom. hammaslääk. toim., 59:296–308, 1963.

95. Koski, K., and Mason, K. E.: Growth potential of transplanted components of the mandibular ramus of the rat. II. Suom. hammaslääk. toim., 60:209–217, 1964.

96. Sarnat, B. G., and Muchnic, H.: Facial skeletal changes after mandibular condyllectomy in the adult monkey. J. Anat., 108:323–338, 1971.

97. Sarnat, B. G., and Muchnic, H.: Facial skeletal changes after mandibular condylectomy in growing and adult monkeys. Am. J. Orthodont., 60:33–45, 1971.

98. Irving, J. T., and Rönning, O. V.: The selective action of papain on calcification sites. Arch. Oral Biol., 7:357–363, 1962.

99. Gianelly, A. A., and Moorrees, C. F. A.: Condylectomy in the rat. Arch. Oral Biol., 10:101–106, 1965.

100. Moss, M. L., and Rankow, R. M.: The role of the functional matrix in mandibular growth. Angle Orthodont., 38:95–103, 1968.

101. Castelli, W. A., Ramirez, P. C., and Burdi, A. R.: Effect of experimental surgery on mandibular growth in Syrian hamsters. J. Dent. Res., 50:356–363, 1971.

102. Moss, M. L.: Neurotrophic processess in oro-facial growth. J. Dent. Res., 50:1492–1494, 1971.

103. Graber, T. M., Chung, D. D. B., and Aoba, J. T.: Dentofacial orthopedics versus orthodontics. J. A. D. A., 75:1145–1166, 1967.

104. Enlow, D. H., and Harris, D. B.: A study of postnatal growth of the human mandible. Am. J. Orthodont., 50:25–50, 1964.

105. Biggerstaff, R. H.: The biology of the chin. Am. J. Phys. Anthrop. (in press).

106. Bosma, J. F.: Evaluation of oral function of the orthodontic patient. Am. J. Orthodont., 55:578–584, 1969.

107. Bosma, J. F.: Facial hypoplasia, growth retardation, impairment of oral sensation and perception and hyposmia: a new syndrome in The Second Symposium on Oral Sensation and Perception. Springfield, Ill., Charles C Thomas, 1970.

108. Robbins, N.: Trophic effect of gustatory nerves, in The Second Symposium on Oral Sensation and Perception. Springfield, Ill., Charles C Thomas, 1970.

109. Diculescu, I., Gotinard, L., and Popescu, M.: Les terminaisons nerveuses cholinergiques du tissue conjonctif. Exp. Cell Res., 54:251–253, 1969.

110. Samaha, F. J., Guth, L., and Albers, W.: The neural regulation of gene expression in the muscle cell. Exp. Neurol., 27:276–282, 1970.

111. DuBrul, E. L., and Sicher, H.: The Adaptive Chin. Springfield, Ill., Charles C Thomas, 1954.

112. Droschl, H.: The effect of heavy orthopedic forces on the maxilla in the growing saimiri sciureus (Squirrel monkey). Am. J. Orthodont., 63:449–461, 1973.

113. Hellman, M.: A preliminary study in development as it affects the human face. D. Cosmos, 71:250–269, 1927.

114. Hellman, M.: The face in its developmental career. D. Cosmos, 77:685–699, 1935.

115. Björk, A., and Helm, S.: Prediction of the age of maximum puberal growth in body height. Angle Orthodont., 37:134–143, 1967.

116. Woodside, D. G.: Distance, velocity and relative growth rate standards for mandibular growth for Canadian males and females age three to twenty years. American Board of Orthodontics thesis, Toronto, Canada, 1969.

117. Tracy, W. E., and Savara, B. S.: Norms of size and annual increments of five anatomical measures of the mandible in girls from three to sixteen years of age. Arch. Oral Biol., 11:587–598, 1966.

118. Tracy, W. E., Savara, B. S., and Brant, J. W. A.: Relation of height, width and depth of the mandible. Angle Orthodont., 35:269–277, 1965.

119. Savara, B. S.: A method of measuring facial bone growth in three dimensions. Arch. Hum. Biol., 37:245–255, 1965.

120. Nanda, R. S.: Growth changes in skeletal-facial profile and their significance in orthodontic diagnosis. Am. J. Orthodont., 59:501–513, 1971.

121. Meredith, H. V.: Serial study of change in a mandibular dimension during childhood and adolescence. Growth, 25:229–242, 1961.

122. Marschner, J. J., and Harris, J. E.: Mandibular growth and Class II treatment. Angle Orthodont., 36:89–93, 1966.

123. Rothstein, T. L.: Facial morphology and growth from ten to fourteen years of age in children presenting class II, division 1 malocclusion. Doctoral thesis, University of Pennsylvania, 1971.

124. Moorrees, C. F. A.: The Dentition of the Growing Child. A longitudinal study of dental development between 3 and 18 years of age. Boston, Harvard University Press, 1959.

125. Moorrees, C. F. A., and Chadha, J. M.: Available space for the incisors during dental development. A growth study based on physiologic age. Angle Orthodont., 35:12–22, 1965.

126. Moorrees, C. F. A., and Reed, R. B.: Changes in dental arch dimensions expressed on the basis of tooth eruption as a measure of biologic age. J. Dent. Res., 44:129–141, 1965.

127. Moorrees, C. F. A.: Normal variation in dental development determined with reference to tooth eruption status. J. Dent. Res., 44:161–173, 1965.

128. Linge, L.: Tissue changes in facial sutures incident to mechanical influences. Ph.D. thesis, University of Oslo, 1973.

129. Graber, T. M.: Craniofacial and dentitional development in Falkner, F. (ed.): Human Development. Philadelphia, W. B. Saunders Co., 1966, pp. 510–581.

130. Graber, T. M.: Implementation of the roentgenographic cephalometric technique. Am. J. Orthodont., 44:906–932, 1958.

131. Mills, L. F.: Changes in dimension of the dental arches with age. J. Dent. Res., 45:890–894, 1966.

132. Moorrees, C. F. A., Fanning, E. A., and Hunt, E. E., Jr.: Age variation of formation stages for ten permanent teeth. J. Dent. Res., 42:1490–1502, 1963.

133. Schwarz, A. M.: Lehrgang der Gebissregelung. Vienna, Verlag Urban & Schwarzenberg, 1961.

134. Nance, H. N.; The limitations of orthodontic treatment. Part I. Am. J. Orthodont., 33:177–223, 1947.

135. Nance, H. N.: The limitations of orthodontic treatment. Part II. Am. J. Orthodont., 33:253–301, 1947.

136. Moyers, R. E.: A Handbook of Orthodontics. 3rd ed., Chicago, Yearbook Medical Publishers, Inc., in preparation.

137. Moyers, R. E.: Development of occlusion. D. Clin. North America, 13:523–536, 1969.

138. Hurme, V. O.: The human dentition in forensic medicine. J. Forensic Sci., 2:377–388, 1957.

139. Graber, T. M.: Diagnosis and panoramic radiography. Am. J. Orthodont., 53:799–821, 1967.

140. Dempster, W. T., Adams, W. J., and Duddles, R. A.: Arrangement in the jaws of the roots of the teeth. J.A.D.A., 67:779–797, 1963.

141. Clinch, L. M.: An analysis of serial models between three and eight years of age. Dent. Rec., 42:61–79, 1951.

142. Muzj, E.: Oro-facial anthropometrics. Hempstead, Index Publishers, Inc., 1970.

143. van der Linden, F. P. G.: Interrelated factors in the morphogenesis of teeth, the development of the dentition and craniofacial growth. Schweiz. Mschr. Zahnheilk., 80:518–526, 1970.

144. Hasund, A., and Sivertsen, R.: Dental arch space and facial type. Angle Orthodont., 41:140–145, 1971.

145. Glickman, I., Pameijer, J. H. N., Roeber, F. W., and Brion, M. A. M.: Functional occlusion as revealed by miniaturized radio transmitters. D. Clin. North America, 13:667–679, 1969.

146. Broadbent, B. H.: The face of the normal child. Angle Orthodont., 7:183–208, 1937.

147. Mathews, J. R.: Functional considerations of the temporomandibular articulation and orthodontic implications. Angle Orthodont., 37:81–93, 1967.

148. Frölich, F. J.: Changes in untreated class II malocclusions. Angle Orthodont., 32:167–179, 1962.

149. Björk, A.: The face in profile. Lund, Berlingska Boktrycketiet, 1947.

150. Elgoyhen, J. C., Riolo, M. L., Graber, L. W., Moyers, R. E., and McNamara, J. A.: Craniofacial growth in juvenile Macaca Mulatta. J. Phys. Anthrop. (in press).

151. Joho, J. P.: Die Reaction der Zähne und Kiefer auf Veränderung der Bisslage. University of Zurich, Zurich, Juris Druck Verlag, 1968.

152. Richardson, A. S., and Castaldi, C. R.: Dental development during the first two years of life. J. Canad. Dent. Ass., 33:418–429, 1967.

153. Krogman, W. R.: Biological timing and dentofacial complex. J. Dent. Child., 35:178–185; 228–241; 377–381, 1968.

154. Grewe, J. M.: Intercanine width variability in American Indian children. Angle Orthodont., 40:353–358, 1970.

155. Gates, R. E.: Computation of the median age of eruption of permanent teeth using probit analysis and an electronic computer. J. Dent. Res., 45:1024–1028, 1966.

156. Enlow, D. H., Kuroda, T., and Lewis, A. B.: The morphological and morphogenetic basis for craniofacial form and pattern. Angle Orthodont., 41:161–188, 1971.

157. Enlow, D. H.: The growth and development of the craniofacial complex in Grabb, W. C., Rosenstein, S. W., and Bzoch, K. R. (eds.): Cleft Lip and Palate, Boston, Little, Brown and Co., 1971.

158. Latham, R. A.: Mechanism of maxillary growth in the human cyclops. J. Dent. Res., 50:929–933, 1971.

159. Berger, H.: The chin problem from an orthodontists point of view. Am. J. Orthodont., 56:516–522, 1969.

160. Moss, M. L., and Salentijn, L.: Differences between the functional matrices in anterior openbite and in deep overbite. Am. J. Orthodont., 60:264–280, 1971.

chapter 3

PHYSIOLOGY OF THE STOMATOGNATHIC SYSTEM

The description of the parts that make up the dentofacial complex, their intimate relations with each other and their role in the accomplishment of the overall pattern are only part of the story. When we look at a patient we usually are examining that person in repose or at rest. We say, almost automatically, "hold still." When we want to check the occlusion of the teeth, we have the patient close his mouth and then we open the lips to see how the upper and lower teeth meet. Or, we carefully articulate the plaster casts in fullest contact. This static analysis is important, but equally important is a dynamic appreciation of how these parts function. It is becoming increasingly apparent that function can influence the overall pattern and the relationship of parts, the very foundations of the stomatognathic system. We must do more than analyze the teeth in occlusion. We must know more about function than just how mastication works. Equally important is the full appreciation of deglutition, respiration, speech and even the maintenance of the head in the constant postural position. This chapter will be divided into four parts: (1) functional osteology, (2) myology, (3) the temporomandibular joint and (4) functions of the stomatognathic system.

One might wonder why a discussion of bone should be part of a chapter on physiology. Although bone is one of the hardest materials in the body, it is one of the most plastic and most responsive to functional forces. An orthodontist can establish a perfect occlusal relationship of the teeth, but unless he takes into consideration the effects of the use of these teeth, unless he makes allowances for the manifold environmental functional influences, the delicately responsive bony structures are apt to change, and the tooth positions will change with them.

Form and function are intimately related. The role of the functional matrix has already been discussed in Chapter 2. Historically, the apparent effect of function on bone was noted first in the femur. In 1867 an anatomist named Meyer, with the help of the mathematician Culmann, propounded what was later to be called the trajectorial theory of bone formation.[1] He pointed out that the alignment of the bony trabeculae in the spongiosa followed definite engineering principles. If lines were drawn following discernible columns of oriented bony elements, these lines showed a remarkably similar structure to the trajectories seen in a crane (Fig. 3–1). Many of these trajectories crossed at right angles — an excellent arrangement to resist the manifold stresses on the condyle of the femur. The theory was developed further to show that the design of the femur in its entirety was in harmony with the best engineering principles. Even the fact that the body of the femur is a hollowed tube, instead of a solid bar, was cited to show that, using the same amount of material, it was better able to resist the bending and shearing stresses to which the bone is subjected during function. If the cross section of the femur was solid, but the same cross-sectional area of material, the shaft would be smaller, and consequently weaker.

In the 1870's Julius Wolff carried this theory one step further.[2, 5] He claimed that the trabecular alignment was due primarily to functional forces. A change in the intensity and direction of these forces would produce a demonstrable change in the internal architecture and external form of the bone. He thought that his observation could be expressed by definite mechanical mathematic laws. This concept was referred to as the law of orthogonality. Roux and others introduced functional factors in the development of the so-called law of transformation of bone.[3] In essence, the law stated that the stresses of tension or pressure on bone stimulate bone formation.

Subsequent research has qualified the theories of these early bone physiologists. Endochondral bone may respond differently at its growth centers than membranous bone (see Chap. 2). It has been shown that both tension and pressure can produce a loss of bone tissue, that the trabeculae do not all cross each other at right angles but at varying angles and that they do not form predominantly straight lines. Many of the so-called trajectories are irregular and wavy, varying from bone to bone depending on the stresses encountered. Changes in functional forces produce measurable changes in bony architecture. These changes are, of course, within the limits of inherent morphogenetic pattern. Lack of function leads to reduction of the density of bone tissue, or

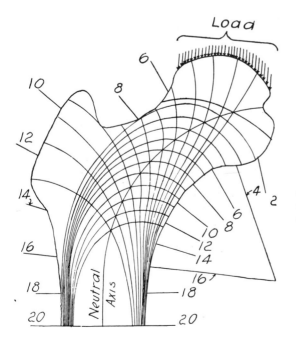

Figure 3–1 Diagrammatic representation of the alignment of bony trabeculae in stress trajectories to better prepare the femur to resist a variety of functional forces. (After J. C. Koch.)

osteoporosis. Increased function produces a greater density of bone in a particular area, or osteosclerosis. An example is a condition called kyphosis, or curvature of the spine, in which some of the vertebrae are stressed unevenly (Fig. 3–2).[4] Frost, the orthopedic surgeon, provides similar evidence in his studies of bone biology and functional response. Electric field effects on cellular activity, piezo-electric effects, nutritional influence, neurotrophism, the roles of RNA and DNA—all offer fertile fields for the investigation of the modus operandi of the physiologic response of bone.[5–7]

Abnormal pressures on bone can cause actual change, as shown in studies of patients with scoliosis who are being treated with the Milwaukee brace. Constant pressure on the mandible produces a marked effect on the vertical dimension, as well as on the teeth (Figs. 2–84, 2–85). Although the reaction to pressure is unfavorable in this type of case, it is most favorable for an open bite problem and can be employed to great advantage in dentofacial orthopedics.[8] (See Chap. 14.)

It is important to note that the stimulating influence of muscles causes bone

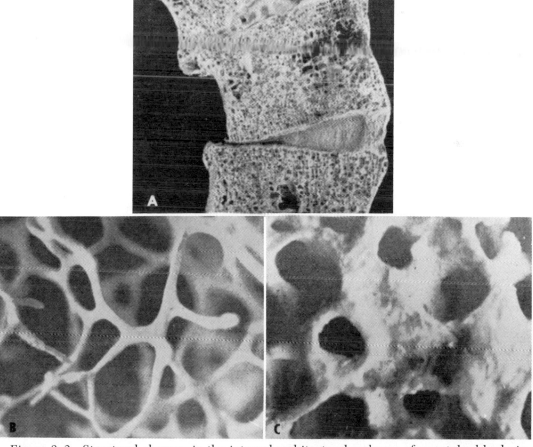

Figure 3–2 Structural changes in the internal architectural make-up of a vertebral body in an acute curvature of the spine. A, General view with osteosclerosis on concave or compressed side, osteoporosis on convex side. B, Osteoporotic region showing thin and widely spaced bony trabeculae. C, Osteosclerotic region illustrating the thick and closely knit trabecular structure. (From Weinmann, J. P., and Sicher, H.: Bone and Bones. 2nd ed. C. V. Mosby Co., 1955.)

to change. Adaptive changes occur in bone.[9] Muscles and soft tissues grow, of course, but once the growth is complete, the muscles cannot lengthen to accommodate an increase in bony bulk. This means that in a pathologic situation like acromegaly there is a morphologic change in the bone as it adapts to the length of the mature muscles which are not as responsive to the same erratic endocrine stimulus (Fig. 3–3).

Closer to our field, the effects of function or lack of function are seen in a study of the alveolar process surrounding teeth that have no opposing dental units. Dental radiographs show a loose trabecular structure resulting in a generalized radiolucency surrounding the nonfunctional teeth. Restoration of function to such teeth by the artificial replacement of opposing teeth brings an increase in the bony trabeculae and a demonstrable increase in radiopacity. This enables the bone to better resist the functional stresses. Benninghoff made an exhaustive study of the architecture of the cranial and facial skeleton, and of the so-called stress trajectories, similar to those seen in the head of the femur.[10] He showed that these trajectories, or lines of stress, involve both the compact and spongy bone. They exist in direct response to epigenetic and local functional influences, not as manifestations of intrinsic genetic potential.

It soon becomes apparent that a remarkable purposefulness of design accounts for the shape of the human head. First of all there is a maximum of strength with a minimum of material. This structural purposefulness alone is a good reason for the presence of the various sinus cavities in the head. While we think of the skull as composed of many bones, functionally it is a single unit or a group of units (see Chap. 2, functional matrix theory). Benninghoff showed that the stress trajectories obeyed no individual bone limits, but rather the demands of the functional forces. Following his reasoning, the head is composed of only two bones—the craniofacial skeletal unit and the mandible, the only movable bone. We can demonstrate the presence of stress trajectories, emanating from above the teeth in the maxillary arch and passing superiorly to the zygomatic or jugal buttress. There are three main vertical pillars of trajectories, all arising from the alveolar process and ending in the base of the skull: the canine pillar, the zygomatic pillar and the pterygoid pillar. These trajectories curve around the sinuses and nasal and orbital cavities (Fig. 3–4).[4] The supraorbital and infraorbital bony eminences and the zygomatic buttresses are horizontal reinforcing members for the vertical stress trajectory columns. Also included with these buttressing structures are the hard palate, the walls of the orbits, and the lesser wings of the sphenoid bone. Actual stress trajectories crossing the palatal structure itself also exist. Sicher emphasizes the importance of the supraorbital rim as a receptor of the forces transmitted to it by the canine and zygomatic pillars.[4] He believes that the development of the supraorbital ridge in lower primates and man is an adaptive response to the strong prognathism and heavy masticatory pressures.

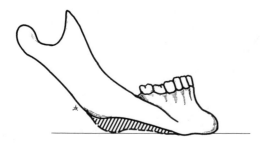

Figure 3–3 Changes in contour of lower border of mandible as a result of acromegaly. Strong increments of bone growth were not matched with a lengthening of the masseter muscle. The shaded portion has thus been lost due to remodeling resorption. (After Sicher, H., and du Brul, E. L.: Oral Anatomy. C. V. Mosby Co., 1970.)

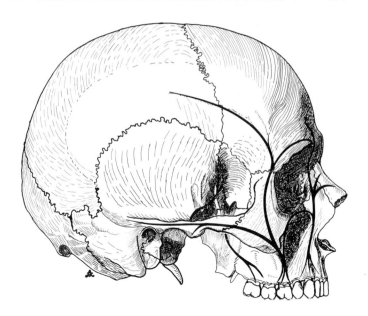

Figure 3-4 Stress trajectories to absorb functional forces in the middle face and cranium. Three main concentrations or pillars of trajectories, the pterygoid, zygomatic and canine elements, are shown with the heavy solid lines. Note the buttressing horizontal supra- and infraorbital components. (From Sicher, H., and du Brul, E. L.: Oral Anatomy. C. V. Mosby Co., 1970.)

The mandible, because it is a unit by itself and a movable bone, has a different trabecular alignment from that of the maxilla (Fig. 3–5). Trabecular columns radiate from beneath the teeth in the alveolar process and join together in a common stress pillar, or trajectory system, that terminates in the mandibular condyle. The mandibular canal and nerve are protected at the same time by this concentration of trabeculae, demonstrating the "unloaded nerve" concept. The thick cortical layer of compact bone along the lower border of the mandible offers the greatest resistance to the bending forces (Fig. 3–6). Other trajectory patterns are seen at the symphysis, at the gonial angle and leading downward from the coronoid process into the ramus and body of the mandible. These accessory stress trajectories probably are due mainly to the direct effect of attachment of the muscles of mastication. The role of the temporomandibular joint in the transmission of functional forces to the base of the cranium and the implementation of its rotary and translatory activity will be discussed in greater detail at the end of this chapter, after the role of the muscles themselves has been described.

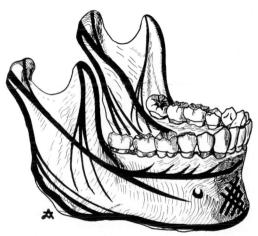

Figure 3–5   Stress trajectories in the mandible. (From Sicher, H., and du Brul, E. L.: Oral Anatomy. C. V. Mosby Co., 1970.)

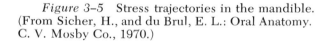

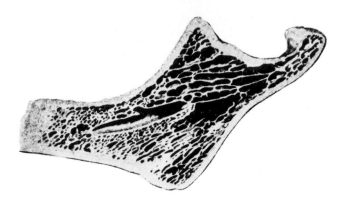

Figure 3–6 Section through the right mandibular ramus to show the trabecular alignment. (From Sicher, H., and Tandler, J.: Anatomie für Zahnärtze. J. Springer, 1928.)

Thus, it is easy to see that while bone may be hard, while it appears to be unyielding, while it remains long after the rest of the body disappears, it most decidedly is not a "dead" tissue. Its basic structure is designed to meet the demands of a lifetime of varied functional activity. Millions of years of evolution, with favorable and unfavorable genetic and epigenetic mutations, have developed an osseous skeleton that is extremely well qualified to meet the manifold demands of life. Although the functional matrix hypothesis of van der Klaauw, Moss and others has been discussed in the previous chapter under *Growth,* it is quite obvious that it applies equally in any discussion of the dynamics of bone.[11, 12] The growth of the oral viscera—the mere presence or absence of soft tissue structures as shown in macroglossia or congenital aglossia (see Chap. 6)—produces a profound response in the bone and affects its ultimate morphology. The student is advised to read the Guided Reading List at the end of the text. The neurotrophic influence on growth, the functional and capsular matrices, the growing spaces which maintain patency of the airway and provide for "air-conditioning"—here lie the exciting frontiers of our present day knowledge of craniofacial form and function.

One of the strongest forces absorbed by the cranial and facial superstructures is the force of mastication. Since the strength and direction of functional forces may be reflected in changes in the internal architecture and external form of the bones receiving the stresses, it is obvious that what the dentist does or does not do to establish and perpetuate a normal occlusion for the patient can affect areas rather far removed from the oral cavity.[13]

MYOLOGY

To propel his skeleton, man has 639 muscles, composed of 6 billion muscle fibers. Each fiber has 1000 fibrils, which means that there are 6000 billion fibrils at work at one time or another (Fig. 3–7).

Certain basic laws govern muscle activity. Muscle has two physical properties that are important in its kinetic activity. These are (1) elasticity and (2) contractility.

ELASTICITY

Normally, the inert elasticity of a body is related to its length, to the cross section, to the force being exerted and to a certain constant coefficient, which is

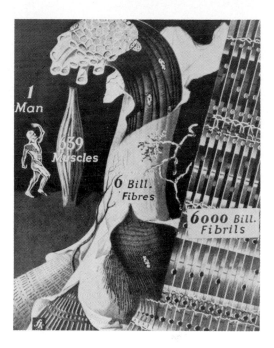

Figure 3–7 The power units of man. (From Kahn, F.: Man in Structure and Function. Alfred A. Knopf, 1943.)

determined by the nature of the body. For the simplest uni-axial case, the ratio is

$$\frac{F}{\Delta} = \frac{AE}{L}$$

where F is force, Δ is deformation, A is cross-sectional area, L is length and E is the modulus of elasticity.

The linear elastic range or extent of elasticity as expressed in Hook's law is dependent upon the nature of the material involved. With muscle, however, Hook's law is valid and linear only at the very beginning of increase in length or load. Normal relaxed muscle withstands only a certain amount of elongation (about six tenths of its natural length) before rupturing. This is only an approximation and, of course, is dependent on the muscle involved, the type of stress, the individual resistance, age and possible pathologic conditions which have produced fibrotic changes that would markedly limit extensibility of the muscle.[14] Extensibility within certain limits is quite easily accomplished by an external force, but the muscle returns to its exact original shape after being stretched, illustrating the quality of elasticity.

CONTRACTILITY

Another important quality of muscle, preventing it from following an arithmetical proportion (as expressed by Hook's law for inert objects), is inherent contractile force.

Contractility is the ability of a muscle to shorten its length under innervational impulse. Although the elasticity of the muscle influences contractility, this phenomenon is quite different.[15] The complex biochemical changes that induce muscle contraction are not completely known. A simplified version of current evidence indicates that a muscle is first stimulated by an electric action potential, causing a contraction. Energy for the muscle is provided, for the most part, by breakdown of the high energy bonds in adenosine-triphosphate (ATP). Fatigue in a muscle is produced when lactic acid, an energy breakdown by-product, collects in the tissues, lowering the pH to a level at which the muscle can no longer function efficiently.[16]

In any definition of contractility it is important to differentiate between the muscle as a whole and the reaction of individual muscle fibers. Sherrington has pointed out that individual fibers have no variable contraction status, but are either relaxed or going into maximum contraction by virtue of adequate stimulus (his "all or none law").[17] The strength of the contraction of a particular muscle depends on the number of fibers engaged in this activity at a particular time. Even during rest a certain number of peripheral fibers are being called on by the nerve system for maintenance of posture. Maximum contractility of a muscle brings into action all available muscle fibers. Each fiber that is active contracts with the same amount of force each time, as long as the action potential is adequate to start the contraction cycle. A good analogy here would be pulling the trigger of a pistol. Up to a certain point the pressure applied by the trigger finger brings no response. At the critical moment when the spring resistance of the trigger is exceeded, the hammer springs forward with maximum force to explode the charge. It does not matter how much force is used beyond this critical point; the reaction of the trigger spring is the same.

How much muscle will shorten during contraction again depends on a number of factors (striated or smooth muscle, number of fibers, cross section, frequency of discharge, muscle fiber length, etc.). Some muscles may contract as much as 50 to 75 per cent of their natural length. The temporalis muscle, because of its relatively longer fibers, has a greater contraction length than the masseter muscle. While it is relatively easy to measure the work load of a muscle that is doing work directly, such as lifting a heavy weight or swinging a bat, another function — stabilizing — is less obvious and less measurable but, nonetheless, deeply important. Indeed, muscles are used most of the time in stablizing or counter-balancing action rather than in carrying out a visible motion.

As we analyze contractility it is essential to distinguish between isometric and isotonic contraction. Isometric contraction occurs when a muscle is simply resisting an external force without any actual shortening. In an isotonic contraction, such as flexing the biceps, there is an actual shortening.

The dentist must know that the greatest strength of contraction is elicited when the muscle approximates its resting length (Fig. 3–8). The strength diminishes as muscles shorten or lengthen beyond their optimal or resting length. For example, as the mandible closes from physiologic or postural position to occlusion, there is reduction in the strength of the contraction from the resting position to the occlusal position. If mandibular closure continues on beyond what would normally be an occlusal level, there is a rapid diminution of contractile power. However, in a recent study in which a gnathodynamometer was used on open and closed bite cases, just the opposite results were observed.[18] Open bite cases averaged 97 lbs. of force, while closed bite cases averaged 118 lbs. (females only 96 to 104 lbs.). This is attributed to the fact that the mouth is propped open 2½ to 3 centimeters anteriorly by the gnathodynamometer, preventing overclosure of closed bite cases, and opening the open bite cases to a greater distance from postural resting maximum contractile-power position. When overclosure is permitted, to full but deficient occlusal position, opposite tendencies are observed. (See Chap. 6, Cleft lip and palate.)

A muscle develops its maximum force when all of its fibers are repeatedly stimulated to "fire." This summation of contractions of the muscle fibers produces muscle tetany and develops four times that of the normal "single contraction" strength in the muscle. A muscle's strength is proportional to its cross-sectional area, i.e., from 3 to 10 kg. per square centimeter of cross-section.[16]

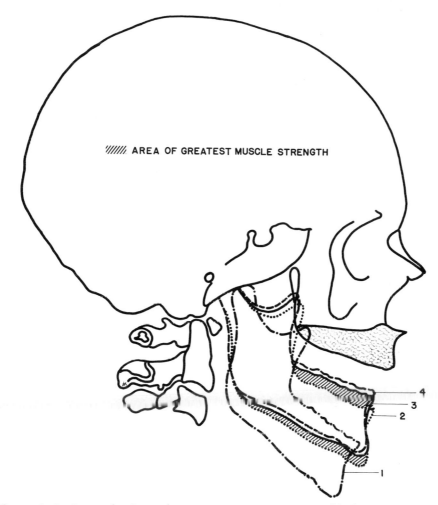

Figure 3–8   Strength of muscle contraction in various mandibular positions. 1, Open mouth. 2, Postural resting position. 3, Occlusal position. 4, Overclosure. Shaded area is region of greatest strength. Strength falls off more rapidly between 3 and 4 than between 2 and 1.

PRINCIPLES OF MUSCLE PHYSIOLOGY

In addition to an understanding of elasticity and contractility, the dentist must appreciate the importance of other concepts of muscle physiology. These may be formulated as guiding principles or "laws."

The best way to visualize the innervation of a muscle is by the use of an electromyogram. Einthoven discovered in 1918 that a muscle in contraction gives off an idiomuscular current. This is referred to as an action current. Apparently, only the contraction of the muscle produces this electrical phenomenon. The current generated is so small that it must be amplified many thousands of times to be recorded. By means of the electromyogram one can get a relatively accurate picture of muscular activity under diverse functional conditions (Fig. 3–9). For example, it can be determined whether motion is free or directed, whether it is fast or slow, or strong or weak.

ALL OR NONE LAW.   (See discussion under Contractility.) The intensity of the contraction of any fiber is independent of the strength of the exciting

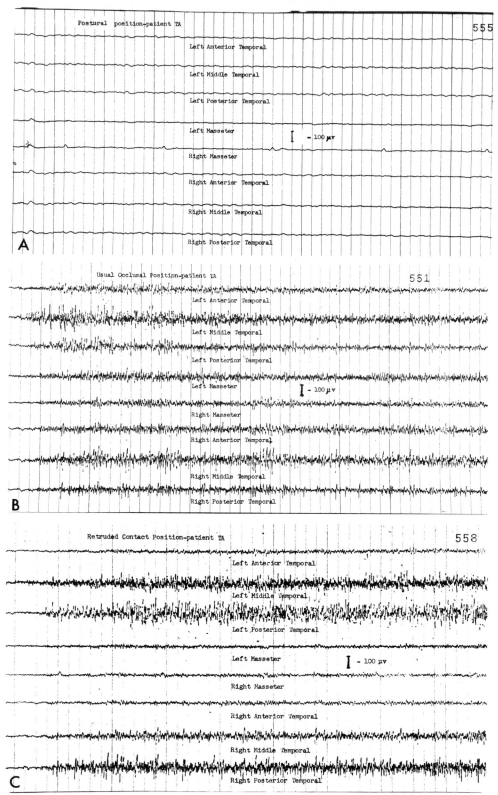

Figure 3–9 A, Electromyograph of left and right anterior, middle and posterior temporalis muscles, in postural resting position. B, Usual occlusal (habitual) position with synchronous but increased activity noted. C, Retruded contact position. Both temporalis and masseter recordings have been made. Note dominance of middle and posterior fibers. This is similar to the pattern in a functional retrusion, deep overbite case. (From Moyers, R. E.: Postnatal development of orofacial musculature. ASHA Reports, No. 6, 38–47, 1971.)

stimulus, provided that the stimulus is adequate. Stimuli below threshold strength elicit no response; if they are over threshold strength a contraction of maximal intensity is made by the muscle fiber. The strength of a muscle contraction depends on two major factors: (1) the frequency of the stimuli—and (2) the number of fibers involved. The force of the contraction automatically adjusts to the load. The tension varies directly with the load, within normal limits.

It should be stressed, however, that the all or none law applies only when muscle is in a physiologic reacting state. When muscles are fatigued, Merton notes that the activity action potentials no longer trigger classic all or none contractions from the muscles.[19] In some temporomandibular joint disturbances this probably has significant clinical application, judging from the aberrant electrical activity elicited.

MUSCLE TONUS.   Muscle tonus is a state of slight constant tension which is characteristic of all healthy muscle and which serves to obviate the muscle taking up slack when it enters upon contraction. In addition to this, tonus is the basis of reflex posture. It is purposive and coordinated in the maintenance of various positions. The constant minimal contraction of antigravity muscles to maintain a standing position is a good example.

RESTING LENGTH.   The resting length of a muscle is a rather constant and predeterminable relationship, permitting the maintenance of postural relations and dynamic equilibrium by contraction of the minimal number of fibers, consistent with the demands of the particular moment (muscle tonus).

STRETCH, OR MYOTATIC, REFLEXES.   The reflex contraction of a healthy muscle which results from a pull on its tendon is called the stretch, or myotatic, reflex (Achilles tendon reflex for example).

RECIPROCAL INNERVATION AND INHIBITION.   The inhibition of the tonus or contractility of the muscle may be brought about by the excitation of its antagonist. Without reciprocal innervation and inhibition, the myotatic or stretch reflexes would make flexion and extension simultaneously antagonistic. Action current that is measured can be discerned not only in a muscle which is in action but in the antagonist as well. It is through antagonistic action that the motion of the primary mover is controlled. This law of reciprocal innervation like the "all or none law," is attributed to Sherrington.[17]

THE BUCCINATOR MECHANISM

The first section of this chapter indicates that there is strong interdependence of bone and muscle. Although bone is the hardest tissue in the body, it is one of the most responsive to change when there is an alteration in the environmental balance. The major factor in this environmental balance is the musculature. Muscles are a potent force, whether they are in active function or at rest. As we have seen from a study of the laws of muscle action, a resting muscle still is performing a function—that of maintaining posture and a relationship of contiguous parts.[20, 21]

The teeth and supporting structures are constantly under the influence of the contiguous musculature. The integrity of the dental arches and the relations of the teeth to each other within each arch and with opposing members are the result of the morphogenetic pattern, as modified by the stabilizing and active functional forces of the muscles. Environmental factors are the contact relationship and resistance afforded by the buttressing effect of contiguous teeth, occlusal interdigitation and the bone building-resorption balance maintained in the periodontal membrane. The actual shape and size of the roots of the teeth and the total amount of periodontal fibers may be contributory. Stability is thus dependent on the sum total of *all* elements—genetic, epigenetic, environmental, morphologic and physiologic. Winders[23] has shown that during mastication and deglutition, the tongue may exert two to three times as much force on the dentition as the lips and cheeks at any one time (Fig. 3–10); but the net effect is one of balance as tonal contraction, peripheral fiber recruitment of the buccal and labial muscles and atmospheric pressure team up to offset the momentarily greater functional force of the tongue (Figs. 3–11, 3–12). Lear and Moorrees substantiate the imbalance of buccolingual forces, but point out that limitations, such as measuring equipment, hydraulic nature of response, size of sample and even geometry of the dental arch do "not permit definitive form-function conclusions to be reached at the moment. . . . The enigma between dental form and muscle function remains. Its solution will not come from the continuous

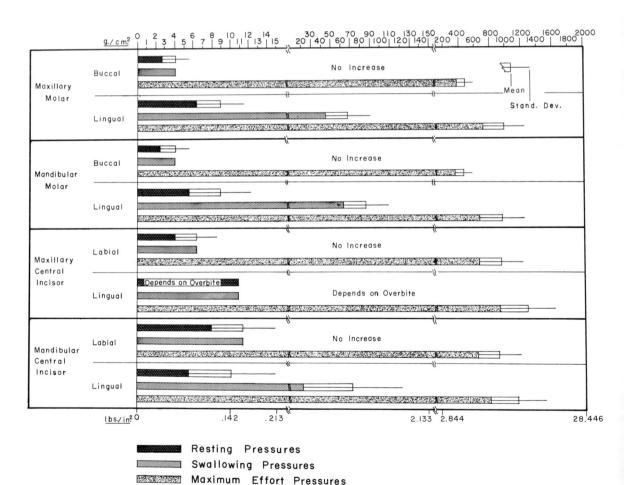

Figure 3–10 Magnitude of lip, cheek and tongue pressures in molar and incisor areas, as measured by Winders with strain gauges and transducers. Pressures were obtained on subjects with excellent dentition. Resting, swallowing and maximal-effort pressures are graphed for buccal, labial and lingual components. Lingual pressures are significantly greater during postural rest and deglutition but little more during maximal effort. Resting pressure appears greater only on the labial aspect of the mandibular incisors. (Adapted from Winders, R. V.: Recent findings in myometric research. Angle Orthodont., 32:38–43, 1962.)

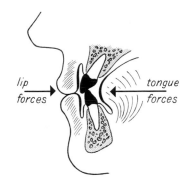

Figure 3–11 Lip, tongue and cheek balancing forces on the teeth and supporting bony structures.

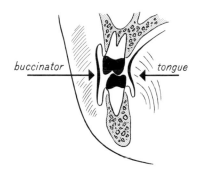

lepeuuon of sweeping generalizations, even though they are philosophically attractive and clinically comforting."[9]

Proffit, a primary researcher in this field notes, "Labial pressures are easier to measure than lingual pressures because the problem of the subject's consciously or unconsciously avoiding the pressure transducer is less likely. Under the best of circumstances, data for lingual pressure must be regarded with some suspicion because of the possibility of such 'physiologic reactance' (Fry, 1960),"[30] The fact that we do not know all the answers does not prevent us from recognizing the obvious role of muscle and its influence on the tooth and bone systems (see Chap. 2, functional matrix theory). Aberrations of muscle function can and do produce marked malocclusions (see Chap. 6). The restrictive, guiding role of the buccinator mechanism (Fig. 3–13) must be recognized and emphasized.[24]

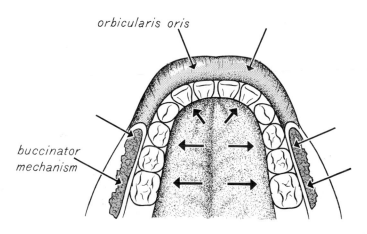

Figure 3–12 The molding pressures on the dental arch, exerted by the contiguous musculature.

THE BUCCINATOR MECHANISM

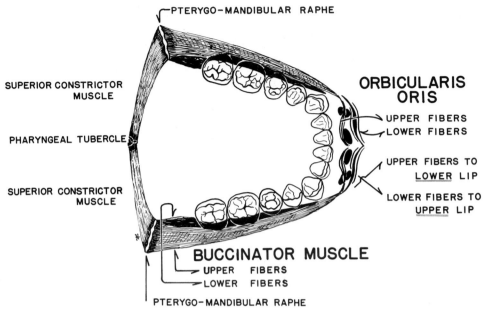

Figure 3–13   The buccinator mechanism. Note continuous muscle band that encircles the dentition and is anchored at the pharyngeal tubercle. (Modified from J. Jarabak.)

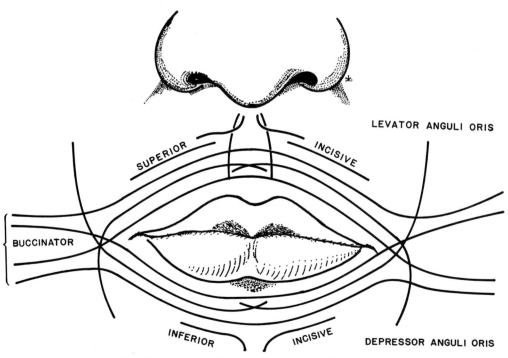

Figure 3–14   The decussating fibers of the orbicularis oris muscle, the anterior component of the buccinator mechanism. Note the sphincter-like or "purse-string" functional possibilities.

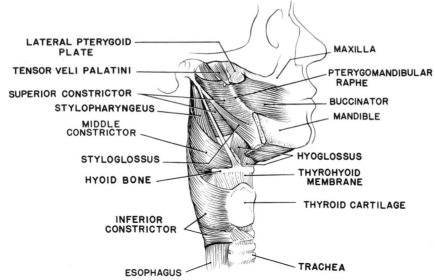

Figure 3–15 Muscles of the face and neck, functioning in maintaining posture, in speech, mastication, deglutition and respiration. (Redrawn after Spalteholtz.)

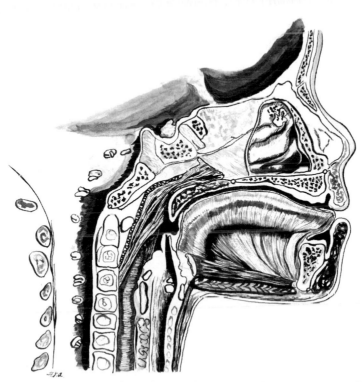

Figure 3–16 Drawing to show habitual posture of tongue in newborn and in infant, with tip occupying the space between the gum pads both during postural resting position and during function. (After Bosma, J. F.: Comparative physiology of the pharynx, *in* Pruzansky, S. [ed.]: Congenital Anomalies of the Face and Associated Structures. Springfield, Ill., Charles C Thomas, 1961.)

Starting with the decussating fibers of the orbicularis oris muscle, joining right and left fibers in the lips (Fig. 3–14), the buccinator mechanism runs laterally and posteriorly around the corner of the mouth, joining other fibers of the buccinator muscle which insert into the pterygomandibular raphe just behind the dentition. At this point it intermingles with fibers of the superior constrictor muscle and continues posteriorly and medially to anchor at the origin of the superior constrictor muscles, the pharyngeal tubercle of the occipital bone. There are 13 muscle attachments to the mandible alone, with elasticity, contractility and tonus making the analogy of the rubber bands acting on the bone system not too far-fetched.

Opposing the buccinator mechanism is a very powerful muscle—the tongue. The tongue begins its manifold activities even before birth, when it functions in the swallowing of amniotic fluid. It is relatively one of the best developed structures in the human body at birth. Not only is the tongue advanced in function because of its important role in nursing, but it is also relatively larger than contiguous structures and thus assumes a posture interposed between the gum pads, rather than completely contained within them, as might be expected[28-30] (Fig. 3–16).

THE TONGUE

The prenatal development of the tongue has already been outlined in Chapter 2. Actual study of postnatal growth and development of the human tongue, and even the muscles of mastication, is most inadequate. But an analysis of its physiology is important, if we are to talk about swallowing patterns, tongue thrust, open bite, and so forth.

In infancy, the extrinsic, suspensory muscles attach the tongue to various osseous structures and are largely responsible for the gross movements, mostly in the horizontal plane (suckle-swallow, etc.) The hyoglossus attaches to the hyoid bone, the styloglossus to the styloid process, the genioglossus to the mandible, and the palatoglossus to the palative aponeurosis. Kawamura attributes protraction, retraction and lateral deviation to these muscles, with the genioglossus probably most involved in the plunger-like suckle-swallow.[27] There are four intrinsic muscles, named because of their direction of fibers in superior longitudinal, inferior longitudinal, vertical and transverse. All but the palatoglossus are innervated by the twelfth cranial nerve. With fine, detailed movements attributed to intrinsic muscles, the presence or absence of proprioceptive nerve endings is important. Until recently, researchers were not able to locate such nerve endings. Muscle spindles have been found, but they are probably sparse in distribution and limited more to extrinsic muscles. Yet, because of the highly skilled activity, proprioceptive information is transmitted directly to the hypoglossal nucleus in the brain stem.[24] (See Functions of the stomatognathic system, later in this chapter.)

The tongue has amazingly versatile functional possibilities by virtue of the fact that it is anchored at only one end. This very freedom permits the tongue to deform the dental arches when function is abnormal. Whether the abnormal tongue activity is the result of a compensatory response to an abnormal morphogenetic pattern or is retained from the infantile "visceral swallow," the balance between outside and inside forces may be disturbed, accentuating maxillary incisor protrusion, creating an open bite tendency and fostering a narrowing of the maxillary arch. Compensatory mentalis muscle activity may exacerbate this process and exert a strong retracting force on the mandibular incisors. This will be discussed in greater detail in Chapter 6, Etiology of Malocclusion. Even with a malocclusion and perverted and compenstory perioral muscle function, a state of balance of all factors, muscular and others, is reached. It is important for the student to realize that a malocclusion represents nature's attempt to establish a balance between all morphogenetic, functional and environmental components. A *malocclusion is in dynamic balance at that particular time.*

It is relatively easy to assign certain functions and to measure the forces involved in muscle activity in the extremities. Muscle units are clearly defined and the origins and insertions quite evident. This is not true in the craniofacial complex. In addition to the basic balancing or postural duties of the musculature (Fig. 3–9) are the manifold activities associated with mastication, deglutition, respiration and speech. And, to make the picture even more complicated, there are the activities of the muscles of facial expression. It is difficult to analyze the function of one muscle, without including the associated or reciprocal activities of another. Most functions are a net result of the activity of two or more muscles. Sometimes the intimate intermingling of fibers and the decussating of these fibers around the mouth and orbital cavities conceal the particular activity that should be attributed to a specific muscle. Yet the laws of muscle physiology are inviolate. If we dig deeply enough and analyze carefully enough, it becomes abundantly clear that all these muscles follow the same basic laws that the skeletal muscles obey, despite their complex, subtle and sophisticated activity.[31-35]

FUNCTIONAL MOVEMENTS

At first glance an analysis of muscle physiology in the head and neck does not seem too difficult. The mandible is the only movable bone in the head and face, and it can only be moved in certain directions because of the limitations of morphology and of the structure of the temporomandibular articulation. An analysis of the precarious balance that the head maintains on the vertebral column illustrates the constant demand for activity in holding the head erect (Figs. 3–17 to 3–20). The postural function must be effective enough to permit

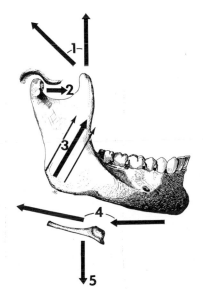

Figure 3–17 Muscles primarily responsible for mandibular functional movements. 1, Anterior and posterior fibers of temporalis; 2, lateral pterygoid; 3, anterior, middle and posterior components of masseter; 4, suprahyoid; 5, infrahyoid. Medial pterygoid not shown. In forced retrusion, electromyographic records show a dominance of posterior temporalis, posterior masseter and posterior suprahyoid muscles. Resistance to posterior condylar displacement by the lateral pterygoid muscles (2) is apparently insufficient, since primary function is that of opening, not closing, and secondary stabilizing assignment on closure can result in excessive forward movement of the articular disk on maximum contraction. (After Posselt, U.: The Physiology of Occlusion and Rehabilitation. F. A. Davis Co., 1968.)

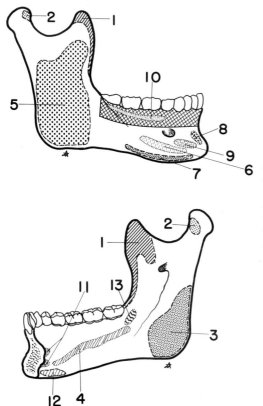

Figure 3–18 The functional matrix for this movable element of the craniofacial complex has 13 attachments. These controlling muscles provide stability of PRP (postural resting position). Thus, the dentist must harmonize the abnormal OVD (occlusal vertical dimension) with the normal PVD (postural vertical dimension) if he is to achieve success in any orthodontic or rehabilitative therapy.

the muscle activity associated specifically with mastication, deglutition, respiration and speech. At times it must augment the specific activity; at other times the postural function may be directly antagonistic. Thus, a number of functions are superimposed on the primary and postural function. We can understand these functions better if we start with an analysis of the various movements of the mandible.

The mandible responds to a number of muscular stimuli. Starting with the teeth in occlusion, the mandible is opened by the condyle being brought downward and forward as the chin point drops downward and backward (Figs. 3–21, to 3–22). Gravity and also the primary contraction of the lateral pterygoid muscles are largely responsible for the opening movement. Stabilizing and adjusting activity is seen in the suprahyoid and infrahyoid groups, in the geniohyoid, mylohyoid and digastric muscles. The stylohyoid muscle changes in length. The hyoid bone itself moves downward and backward with the opening movement of the mandible. The temporal, masseter and medial pterygoid muscles show a controlled relaxation as the mandible opens. This controlled relaxation serves to make the opening movement smooth. It has been shown that paralysis of one or more of these basic mandibular closers may make the opening movement jerky and uncontrolled. During the opening movement of the mandible, the articular disk is brought forward by the lateral pterygoid muscle and intimately related capsular ligaments as the condyle rotates against the inferior surface of the disk and as the disk itself glides forward on the articular eminence.[36, 37]

The closing movement of the mandible is also a closely coordinated activity of the closing and opening muscles. Considerably more power is elicited on mandibular closure due to the bilateral activity of the masseter and temporalis muscles, assisted by the smaller medial pterygoid muscles. The hyoid bone moves upward and forward during mandibular closure. The lateral pterygoid muscles, through their controlled relaxation, help effect a smooth and uninterrupted activity. If resistance is met during the closure, greater activity is generated in the lateral pterygoid, suprahyoid and infrahyoid muscles.[38] This may extend to the postvertebral and prevertebral postural muscles and to the facial musculature, if the functional demands are great enough.

To protrude the mandible, the lateral and medial pterygoid muscles contract in unison, in conjunction with controlled stabilizing relaxation of the opening muscles.

The retruding action of the mandible is less definite and less efficient. Retrusion is accomplished largely by the contraction of the posterior fibers of

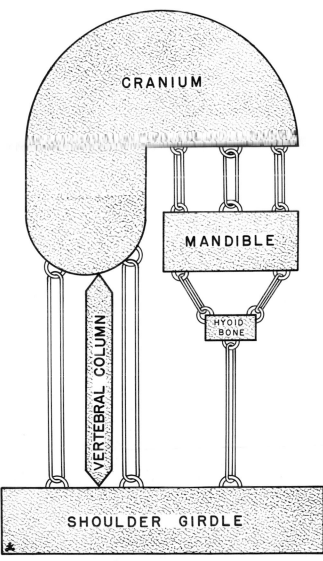

Figure 3-19 Diagrammatic representation to show muscle groups concerned with maintaining the balance of the head on the vertebral column.

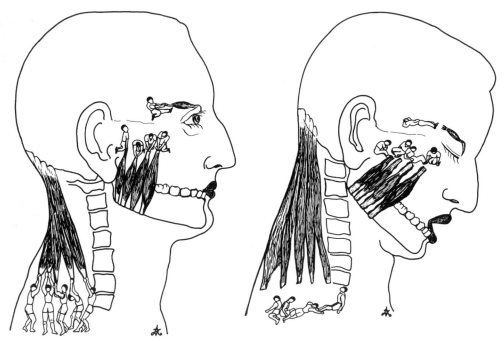

Figure 3–20   The head is balanced, eyes open and mandible suspended in postural rest during the waking hours. Sleep or lack of consciousness reduces muscle activity to a minimum, allowing the head, mandible and eyelids to drop. (Redrawn from Kahn, F.: Man in Structure and Function. Alfred A. Knopf, 1943.)

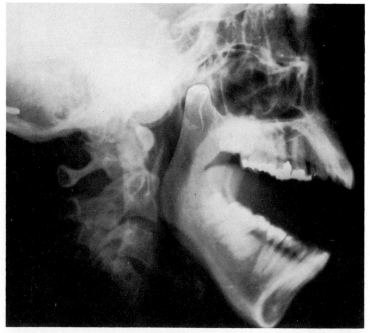

Figure 3–21   Lateral cephalometric roentgenogram showing the open mouth position with the condyle forward on the articular eminence.

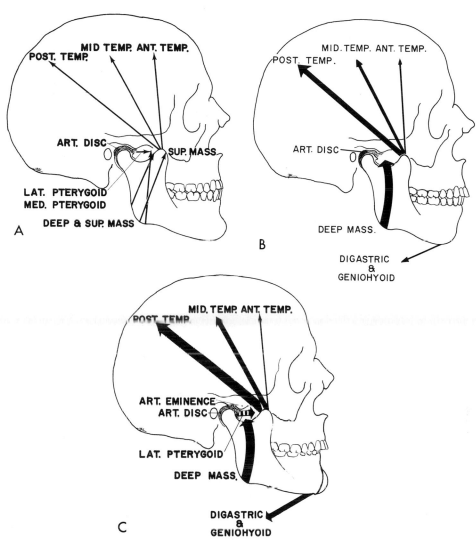

Figure 3–22 A, Drawing to show normal muscle activity associated with normal jaw relationship and normal occlusion. Electromyographic recordings would show even distribution of anterior, middle and posterior temporalis and deep and superficial fiber activity (see Fig. 3–9). B, Where there is a Class II malocclusion, mandibular retrusion and excessive apical base difference, middle and posterior temporalis and deep masseter fibers show greater magnitude of contraction. This adapts to and enhances the mandibular retrusion. C, With Class II malocclusion and deep overbite, the functional retrusion tendency is increased. In addition to dominance and posterior and deep masseter activity, stretch reflex may be elicited for the lateral pterygoid fibers which insert into the articular disk. This serves to pull the disk forward as the condyle is functionally retruded (see arrow). Condyle may then impinge on retrodiskal pad.

the temporalis muscles, with some assistance from the geniohyoid, digastric and mylohyoid muscles. The hyoid bone also moves posteriorly, indicating some action of the infrahyoid muscle group. Electromyographic research indicates that the deep fibers of the masseter muscle assist in retrusion of the mandible.[39-43] It should be remembered that the ligaments that make up the stabilizing elements of the temporomandibular joint tend to restrict any retruding action.

To establish a "working" bite, the mandible must be moved to the right or left. This lateral movement is initiated by the combined activity of the lateral pterygoid muscle on one side with controlled relaxation on the other side and by the contraction of the temporalis muscle on one side and controlled relaxation on the opposite side. In other words, if the mandible is being moved to the left to masticate a bolus of food, there is a contraction of the right lateral pterygoid muscle and a controlled relaxation of the right temporalis muscle. On the left side there is a definite contraction of the left temporalis muscle and a controlled relaxation of the lateral pterygoid muscle on that side. As the teeth are brought closer to an end-to-end relationship, the masseter contracts on the left side, assisting in the ipsilateral activity. As the teeth are brought closer together, strong activity is elicited in both the masseter and temporalis muscles on both sides. The magnitude of contraction is greater on the working side than on the balancing side, however.

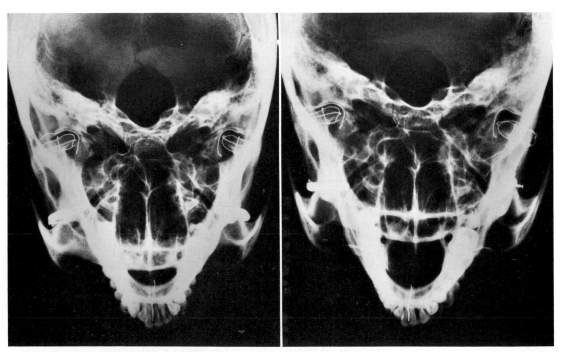

Figure 3–23   (Left) Oriented roentgenogram of skull, taken from above. Wire markings show the outline of the condyles and their relation to the glenoid fossa in centric occlusion. Postcondylar space would permit retrusion. Note that the long axes of the condyles meet in the foramen magnum, and perpendiculars to the long axes at the center of the condyle roughly parallel the buccal surfaces. (Right) Oriented roentgenogram of skull with mandible related in right lateral working bite. There is an increase in postcondylar space on the opposing side, a slight reduction in postcondylar space on the working side, and a slight shift to the working side. (From Posselt and Graber.)

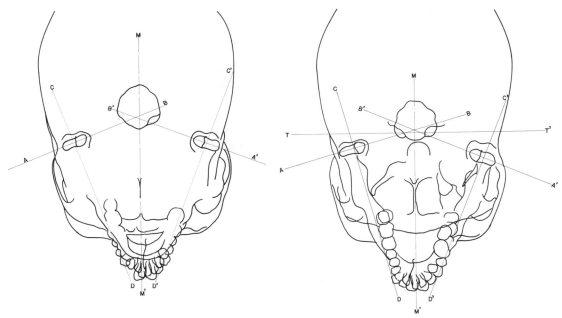

Figure 3–24 (Left) Cephalometric tracing of Figure 3–23 (left), showing angular relationships of condylar axes AB and A′B′ with midsagittal plane MM′. Note that the perpendiculars CD and C′D′, established at the midcondylar point, are roughly parallel with the maxillary buccal segments. Also, the long axes intersect in the foramen magnum almost in the midsagittal plane. (Right) Cephalometric tracing of Figure 3–23 (right), demonstrating changes effected by moving the mandible into a right lateral working bite. The right condyle moves a bit farther into the postglenoid fossa as the left condyle glides downward and forward on the articular eminence. Coupled with these movements is a slight lateral shift of both condyles to the right (Bennett movement). (From Posselt and Graber.)

An interesting observation may be made concerning the intersection of the long axes of the mandibular condyles (Fig. 3–24). From an engineering point of view, this arrangement of the long axes would seem ideal, inasmuch as the head is balanced on the vertebral column at this point. The long axes usually intersect at or near the midline—a favorable mechanical advantage for synchronous bilateral activity.

In the lateral shift of the mandible the articular disk moves toward the side of the working bite. This is known as "Bennett movement."[44] The condyle moves slightly laterally and rotates on the working side. On the balancing side, the condyle and disk move downward and forward on the articular eminence. (Figs. 3–23, 3–24). Muscle activity on the balancing side consists largely of primary lateral pterygoid contraction and controlled relaxation of the masseter, temporalis and suprahyoid group during the lateral excursive movement. On the working side, there is primary contraction in the middle and posterior fibers of the temporalis muscle and in the posterior fibers of the masseter, and some evidence of the increased activity in the hyoid group. Stabilizing relaxation also seems to occur in the anterior fibers of the temporalis and masseter muscles and, at one stage, in the suprahyoid and infrahyoid muscles. Despite the complexity of these interrelated primary moving and secondary balancing activities, the function is smooth and uninterrupted. The activity on the working side depends on the size and nature of the bolus of food and on the position of this bolus anteroposteriorly in the working buccal segment. Interesting myographic studies have been done showing the marked change in magnitude and frequency of muscle fiber activity as a result of a change in the type of food being masticated.

COMPENSATORY MUSCLE FUNCTIONS

While mastication may call for the most potent effort from the associated muscles, the most frequent demands are made by deglutition, respiration, speech and posture. At times two or more of these functions are carried on simultaneously. Such complex activity naturally brings into function associated muscle elements, and this makes an analysis of the role of any individual muscle quite difficult. A good motto for the cranial, facial, masticatory, suprahyoid and infrahyoid muscles plus the prevertebral and postvertebral muscles is "team work." This team work means that adjusting or compensatory muscle activity is available as the functional demands vary. This also means that where there is a malocclusion or abnormal morphologic relationship, *certain compensatory or adaptive muscle functions may arise, either to restrain the dental malocclusion or to actually increase the discrepancy.* This will be discussed in greater detail in the balance of this chapter and in Chapters 6 and 7.

POSITIONS OF MANDIBLE

To better understand variations from the normal, let us first outline the basic sagittal plane positions of the mandible with respect to the maxilla and cranium. These basic positions are:

1. Postural resting position (physiologic rest)
2. Centric relation
3. Initial contact
4. Centric occlusion
5. Most retruded position (terminal hinge position)
6. Most protruded position
7. Habitual resting position
8. Habitual occlusal position.

This arbitrary listing is based on the work done by many men since the first comprehensive study of Bennett in 1908.[44] Posselt has recorded graphically the various positions and movement area in the sagittal plane, as shown in Figure 3–25.

Because of the manifold demands on the muscles associated with mandibular movements, coordination is essential in both synergistic and antagonistic groups.

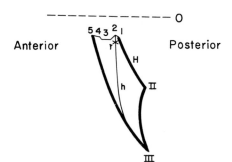

Figure 3–25 Average movement area in median plane (left profile). Approximately natural size. H, The terminal hinge movement; 1, the retruded contact position; 2, the intercuspal position; 3, the edge-to-edge occlusion; 4, anterior biting to a reversed vertical overlap; 5, the protruded contact position; h, the habitual (automatic) closing movement; II, transition from terminal hinge to further posterior opening, III, the maximal opening; O, line parallel with the occlusal plane. (Redrawn after Posselt, U.: The Physiology of Occlusion and Rehabilitation. Philadelphia, 2nd ed. F. A. Davis Co., 1968.)

POSTURAL RESTING POSITION (PVD).   In the infant, those muscles associated with suckling or the intake of food are relatively well developed from the
start. But when a child is not engaged in taking food, the mandible assumes a
position of rest, whether teeth are present or not (Fig. 3–26). The smooth function of the perioral musculature and the return to a rather constant resting
position is in marked contrast with the akimbo and jerky movements of the
extremities of the infant. Thus, the mandibular resting position is one of the
earliest postural positions to be developed.[42] The mandible is literally suspended from the cranial base by the cradling musculature (Fig. 3–19). The
jaws are not clamped together, but they are separated by a rather constant
distance, even before there are any teeth in the mouth (Fig. 3–26). Electromyographic and cephalometric studies have demonstrated the relative constancy of
this postural resting position from infancy to senility.[45] Even though the muscles
are not in active function, a limited number of fibers are apparently still contracting to maintain the relaxed position of the mandible and posture of the
head (Fig. 3–27). It should be stressed, however, that postural resting position,
like all physiologic phenomena, is subject to variability. As Posselt[46] observes,
"The postural position can be altered by conditions in the masticatory system
as well as by systemic factors. Factors influencing the postural position are the
following: (1) body and head posture, (2) sleep, (3) psychic factors influencing
muscle tonus, (4) age, (5) proprioception from the dentition and muscles,
(6) occlusal changes, such as attrition, (7) pain, (8) muscle disease and muscle
spasm, and (9) temporomandibular joint disease."

CENTRIC RELATION.   The term "centric relation" has been widely used by
the prosthodontist for some time. It has many shadings and variations of definition. Generally speaking, centric relation refers to the position of the mandibular
condyle in the articular fossa. (This is discussed at some length at the end of
Chap. 4.) As far as muscle physiology is concerned, however, centric relation
may be defined as the unstrained, neutral position of the mandible in which
the anterosuperior surfaces of the mandibular condyles are in contact with the

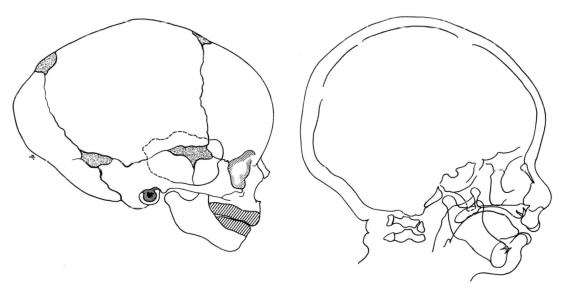

Figure 3–26   (Left) Concept of relation of jaws at birth, as portrayed in some anatomy texts.
(Right) Relation of structures as revealed by oriented lateral cephalograms, with the jaws apart.
Note the tongue interposed between the dental arches. (After Brodie and Thompson.)

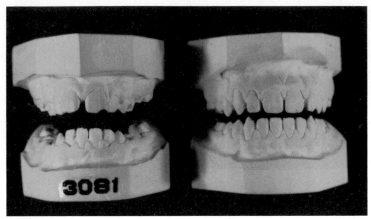

Figure 3–27   Severe Class II, Division 1 malocclusion, before and after orthodontic treatment. Casts on left are related in postural position, showing the original 11 mm. interocclusal clearance in this deep overbite case. Casts on right show 4 mm. interocclusal clearance after therapy, harmonizing OVD (occlusal vertical dimension) with PVD (postural vertical dimension).

concavities of the articular disks as they approximate the posteroinferior third of their respective articular eminentia. This means that the mandible is deviating neither to the right nor to the left and is neither protruded nor retruded. Such a relation can be the same as the postural resting position, the point of initial occlusal contact and centric occlusion. As has been shown, condyle and disk movement is negligible as the mandible closes the 3 to 4 mm. interincisal clearance from postural rest position to centric occlusion. But centric occlusion requires the contact of the teeth, in addition to an unstrained position of the condyles in their articular fossae, while centric relation does not require occlusal contact. The term is obviously more generic. Any complete definition of centric relation should convey the impression of normality, balanced relations, bilateral symmetrical activity and the state of being "unstrained."

INITIAL CONTACT.   As the mandible moves from physiologic rest, or the postural resting position, toward occlusion of the teeth, if all is normal, it maintains a centric relation position as far as the articular fossae are concerned. The movement that occurs in the temporomandibular joint is almost completely the rotation of the condyle in the lower joint cavity. If there is a normal occlusion, the point of initial contact produces no change in the function of the temporomandibular joint, and all inclined planes are brought together simultaneously in the maxillary and mandibular teeth. Initial contact in the ideal individual is usually synonymous with centric occlusion. The same connotations of balanced, unrestrained, normal and bilaterally symmetrical relationships apply here. If, however, there is a malocclusion or a premature contact of one or more teeth in each jaw, initial contact is no longer the same as centric occlusion. Premature contacts are, unfortunately, quite frequent. They can and do initiate deflections in the mandibular path of closure. (See Chaps. 9 and 14.) They cause traumatic forces to be exerted on the teeth and environmental tissues and, in extreme cases, can produce severe temporomandibular joint symptoms of crepitus, asymmetrical activity and pain. It is the duty of the dentist to reduce these premature contacts. He must restore normal function to the temporomandibular joint and eliminate any pathologic lateral, anterior or posterior displacement of the condyles in the articular fossae, in the movement from postural resting position to full occlusion. This will be discussed in greater detail in Chapters 14 and 16.

CENTRIC OCCLUSION (OVD).   As just pointed out in the previous discussion, the definition of centric occlusion in orthodontics also implies a state of balance. With maximal contact of the inclined planes of the opposing teeth, there must be bilaterally symmetrical activity, a balanced and unstrained relationship of temporomandibular structures, etc.[45-49] Centric occlusion is a static position and can be easily reproduced by having the patient bring the teeth together, if there is no malocclusion or malfunction present. This may seem confusing to the student who has been taught elsewhere that centric occlusion is maximum contact of opposing teeth. But to the orthodontist, this is habitual occlusion, and not necessarily centric. Centric occlusion must be harmonious with centric relation. Habitual occlusion need not be, and often is not. As a dentist knows, there are few patients who can show a centric occlusion. Premature contacts, loss of teeth, overeruption of teeth, overextension of artificial restorations, malpositions of individual teeth—all these mitigate against the establishment of a centric occlusion. The dentist must maintain a constant vigil to prevent any of these factors from operating and jeopardizing the integrity of this optimal occlusal position.

MOST RETRUDED POSITION (TERMINAL HINGE POSITION).   Since we are discussing demonstrable sagittal mandibular positions, we must include the reproducible "retruded" position of the mandible with the teeth in occlusion. To many prosthodontists this "terminal hinge axis position" is essential to establish the mandibular and maxillary casts in their proper positions on the

C.R. position = Terminal hinge axis.

POSTERIOR   SUPERIOR   DISPLACEMENT

Figure 3–28 Tracing of lateral cephalometric headplate showing: 1, open mouth position; 2, postural resting position; 3, premature initial contact; 4, retruded occlusal position. Tooth guidance from point of premature initial contact has changed the path of closure from upward and forward to upward and backward.

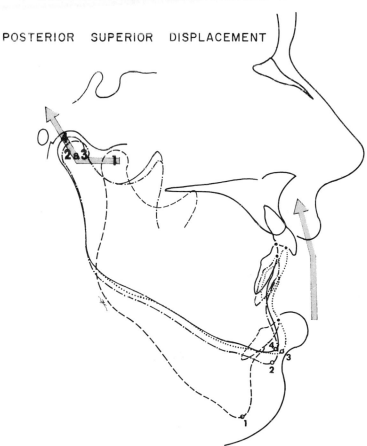

articulator. The controversy that exists here is discussed in Chapter 4 and is common knowledge to most dentists. Much of the problem is due to semantic limitations. Since it is possible to reproduce this most retruded position fairly easily and to train the patient to assume this position with regularity, it has become a common starting point in occlusal analysis and rehabilitation. Because premature contacts frequently disturb the occlusal relationship of upper and lower teeth, many dentists believe that by forcing the mandible into its most posterior position it is easier to eliminate occlusal prematurities that exist. For the physiologist, however, some of these mechanical interpretations and machinations are not in accord with basic physiologic concepts. There is a range of movement in any joint in the body. The multitude of functional demands on the temporomandibular joint makes it obvious that a closely machined ball and socket fit is impossible. Thus, it is possible for any person to move the mandible a millimeter or more posteriorly from a position of centric relation and centric occlusion. Such movement frequently elicits a stretch of myotatic reflex, clearly evident in electromyographic records. This can hardly be called "normal." As with any physiologic phenomenon, there is considerable range among individuals. There are individuals who cannot retrude at all from habitual occlusion, while others can move 1 to 2 mm. To the gnathologists this may sound like sacrilege, but to the orthopedic surgeon, who deals with a great number of joints in the body, this is just plain human variation.

In attempting to establish the proper relationship of the jaws, the dentist is desirous of obtaining the most retruded unstrained position of the mandible—the normal position of the condyles in the articular fossae. The natural tendency for the patient, however, is to protrude the mandible as the dentist attempts to record the "retruded position." The dentist, in "guiding" the patient's bite, must avoid forcing the mandible past the "unstrained" point that he is seeking. It is often too easy to force retrusion of the condyle to the point at which it can no longer compress the postarticular tissues any further. To record the jaw position at this point would certainly not be in accord with the definition of terminal hinge axis, i.e., the habitual, normal, bilaterally symmetrical and *unstrained* position of the condyles in the articular fossae. At the very least it would be unbiologic. Fortunately, as Ramfjord and Hiniker have shown, both anterior and posterior displacement of the mandible is temporary, despite erroneous prosthetic manipulation. Functional matrix domination through the 13 muscle attachments on the mandible is clearly evident (Fig. 3–18).[50]

MOST PROTRUDED POSITION.   The most protruded position in the mandible is more variable from individual to individual than the retruded position. Within the same individual, however, it is reproducible. It has not been used clinically to orient the prosthodontist or the dentist attempting a full month rehabilitation as much as the retruded position. Any functional analysis, however, must take into consideration the range of movements of the mandible. The inclination of the condylar path is considered more important than the actual terminal protrusive position.

Where there is an inherent flaccidity to the capsular structures, some patients can dislocate their mandibles in the extreme protrusive position. The condyle is drawn anterior to the lowest point of the articular eminence. No longer is there harmony in the combined action of the articular disk and mandibular condyle. In some cases the condyle rides over the anterior margin of the disk in dislocation. In others the disk is drawn too far anteriorly and the condyle rides over the posterior periphery of the articular disk, even though it is in a most protrusive position. When the condyles are "locked" anterior to the articular eminence, the stretch reflexes of the associated musculature are elicited. These muscles go into partial tetanic contraction and a fatigue syndrome is set up. The posterior surface of the mandibular condyle is drawn strongly against the anterior convexity of the articular eminence by the contracting musculature. In attempting to reduce a mandibular dislocation, the dentist must be very careful to pad his thumbs before placing them on the occlusal surfaces of the mandibular molars. As the mandible is moved forcibly downward and backward, there is a sudden and convulsive retraction as the condyle rides over the articular eminence. The molar teeth are brought into occlusion with a good deal of force.

HABITUAL RESTING POSITION.   No listing of the basic positions of the mandible can be complete without recognizing that the habitual resting position may not be the same as the true physiologic postural position. For example, there are certain types of malocclusions that prevent the patient from achieving a physiologic resting position. In a severe Class II, Division 2 malocclusion with the maxillary incisors markedly inclined to the lingual, there is a tendency to force the condyles posteriorly and superiorly in the articular fossae (Fig. 3–22).

Electromyographic studies seem to show greater activity in the muscles associated with mandibular posture than would be normal for an unstrained position at rest (Fig. 3–9). In many cases the removal of the abnormal guiding force of the lingually inclined maxillary incisors allows the mandible to come forward, and a demonstrable reduction in electrical activity at this new resting position can be seen. Certain other pathologic conditions can interfere with

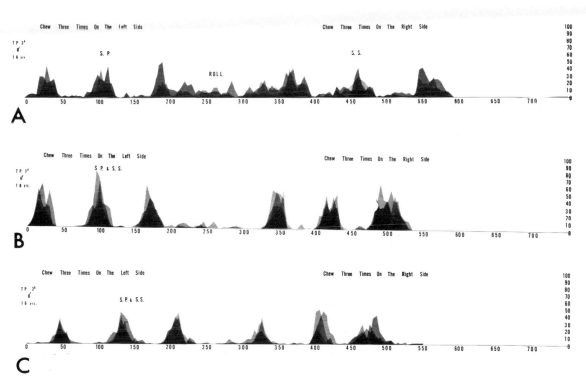

Figure 3–29   Converted electromyographic tracings of severe Class II, Division 1 malocclusion (A) before orthodontic treatment, (B) after treatment and (C) after equilibration (see Fig. 3–30). Note the progressive synchrony of muscle activity after orthodontics and occlusal adjustment. In each sequence, the patient is chewing a homogenous bolus of food, three times each on left and right sides. Electrodes were placed on right and left masseter and temporalis muscles. (Courtesy H. T. Perry, Jr.)[39]

the establishment of a normal postural position of the mandible. Abnormal atmospheric pressure in the oral cavity, selective paralysis induced by poliomyelitis, markedly enlarged adenoids, pain, temporomandibular joint pathology, certain systemic diseases, psychic trauma and confirmed mouth breathing are possible conditioning factors. (See Chap. 6.) Acute mental disturbances and even day-to-day occurrences and fatigue may set up certain circumstances that modify the physiologic resting position, or postural position. It should be emphasized that none of these variations endanger the patency of the airway, which remains relatively inviolate except to sudden accidental assaults. It is the duty of the dentist, of course, to eliminate all conditions that might prevent the establishment of a normal postural position if the habitual resting position is not one and the same.

HABITUAL OCCLUSAL RELATION (OVD).   In a normal occlusion the centric occlusion and habitual occlusion should be the same. But the occlusal relationship is much more susceptible to environmental assaults, to functional aberrations, to changes induced by improper restoration of carious teeth, to tooth loss, and so forth. The habitual occlusal position, or intercuspal position, can be, and often is, an abnormal one. Malposition of individual teeth and tooth guidance due to premature contacts produce traumatic disturbances that are injurious to the teeth and investing tissues. *It is vitally important that the dentist make sure that the habitual occlusal position and the centric occlusal position are*

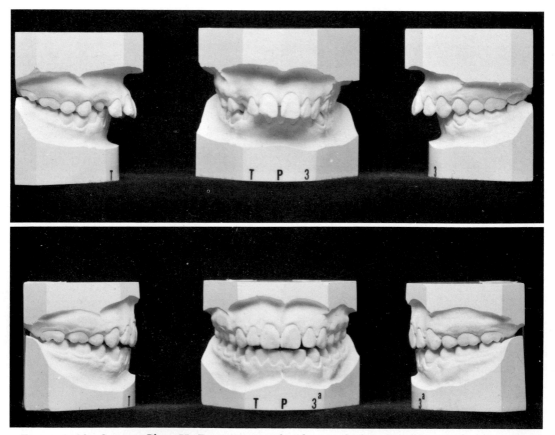

Figure 3–30   Severe Class II, Division 1 malocclusion, before treatment and one year out of retention. Converted electromyographs demonstrate establishment of synchronous muscle activity as a result of correction of malocclusion. (Courtesy H. T. Perry, Jr.)[39]

the same and that they are in harmony with centric relation and the postural resting position of the mandible.[51] In malocclusion, there is asynchronous activity of the closing muscles in habitual and working bite occlusions. Perry demonstrates the change that can be effected by orthodontic correction of the malocclusion, in addition to occlusal equilibration (Figs. 3–29, 3–30).

THE TEMPOROMANDIBULAR JOINT

Since we are dealing with a dynamic system and since the functions of mastication, deglutition, speech, respiration and postural maintenance depend in a large measure on the movement of the mandible and its relationship to the stable cranial and facial base, a knowledge of the workings of the temporomandibular joint is important. This articulation between the condyle of the mandible and the inferior surface of the squamous portion of the temporal bone, or glenoid fossa, is classified as a compound movable articulation. A sagittal section through the temporomandibular joint would show the anterosuperior portion of the condyle approximating the inferior third of the convex articular eminence (Figs. 3–31 to 3–35). Interposed between the head of the condyle and the articular eminence is the articular disk. The glenoid fossa, articular disk and mandibular condyle are enclosed in the articular capsule. This is often referred to as a capsular ligament, since it is thickened on its lateral aspect by the temporomandibular ligament. The capsular ligament has a synovial membrane lining; synovial fluid is present. The head of the condyle is tubular or ellipsoidal. This cannot be seen in sagittal section, but a superior view shows the contours (Figs. 3–23, 3–24).

A rather unique feature of the temporomandibular articulation is that it is really two joints (Figs. 3–31, 3–36). The attachment is made in such a way that the articular disk between the condyle and articular eminence serves to separate the structures into two separate joint cavities. An injection of radiopaque-disclosing solution into either cavity remains confined and will not spread into

Figure 3–31 Sagittal section drawing of temporomandibular joint. Note that there are two distinct joint cavities. Lateral pterygoid fibers extend into the retrodiskal pad in embryonal development, but cannot be found there after birth. They insert into the leading edge of the disk (and capsule) and neck of the condyle. In older persons, the presence of islands of cartilage may be seen in the meniscus. Hence, the designation as fibrocartilage in some texts. Retrodiskal tissue is loose and compressible, in contrast with the noncompressible meniscus. Cartilage in condylar head is covered by a dense layer of fibrous connective tissue, unlike any other joint in the body. Recent research indicates that the two heads of the lateral pterygoid muscle may have different contraction patterns. This might account for some of the condyle-disk-eminence disharmonies seen in TMJ (temporomandibular joint) problems (clicking, crepitus, etc.).

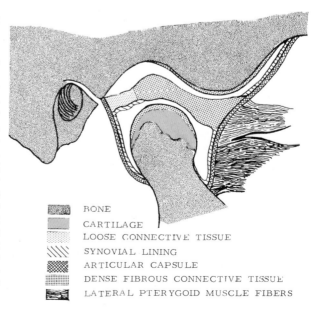

BONE
CARTILAGE
LOOSE CONNECTIVE TISSUE
SYNOVIAL LINING
ARTICULAR CAPSULE
DENSE FIBROUS CONNECTIVE TISSUE
LATERAL PTERYGOID MUSCLE FIBERS

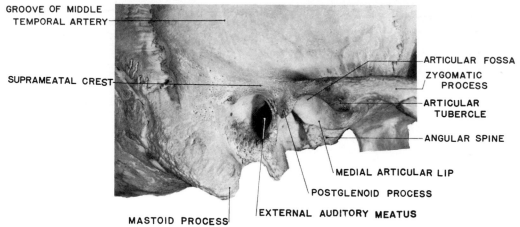

GROOVE OF MIDDLE
TEMPORAL ARTERY

SUPRAMEATAL CREST

ARTICULAR FOSSA
ZYGOMATIC
PROCESS
ARTICULAR
TUBERCLE
ANGULAR SPINE

MEDIAL ARTICULAR LIP
POSTGLENOID PROCESS
EXTERNAL AUDITORY MEATUS
MASTOID PROCESS

Figure 3–32 Lateral view of glenoid fossa. Note the well-developed postglenoid process. (Courtesy H. Sicher.)

the remaining cavity unless there is a performation of the disk. The great importance of this dual joint cavity system lies in the dual functional duties.

In the inferior joint between the head of the mandibular condyle and the articular disk, the movement is almost totally of a rotary or hinge type. This rotary movement occurs by itself when opening from occlusion to physiologic resting position. It continues in conjunction with the translatory movement of the upper joint as the mandible opens beyond physiologic rest and goes into functional excursions. In the superior joint between the temporal bone and the articular disk, movement is gliding or translatory.

When the mandible is opened beyond the physiologic resting position,

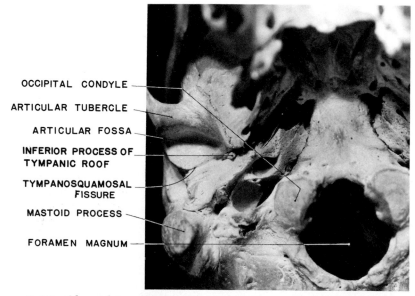

OCCIPITAL CONDYLE

ARTICULAR TUBERCLE

ARTICULAR FOSSA

INFERIOR PROCESS OF
TYMPANIC ROOF

TYMPANOSQUAMOSAL
FISSURE

MASTOID PROCESS

FORAMEN MAGNUM

Figure 3–33 Glenoid fossa from below. There is a well-developed inferior process of the tympanic roof. In front of it, the petrosquamosal fissure; behind it, the petrotympanic fissure. (Courtesy H. Sicher.)

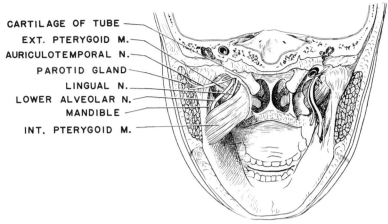

CARTILAGE OF TUBE
EXT. PTERYGOID M.
AURICULOTEMPORAL N.
PAROTID GLAND
LINGUAL N.
LOWER ALVEOLAR N.
MANDIBLE
INT. PTERYGOID M.

Figure 3–34   Drawing of temporomandibular articulation from behind. (Courtesy H. Sicher.)

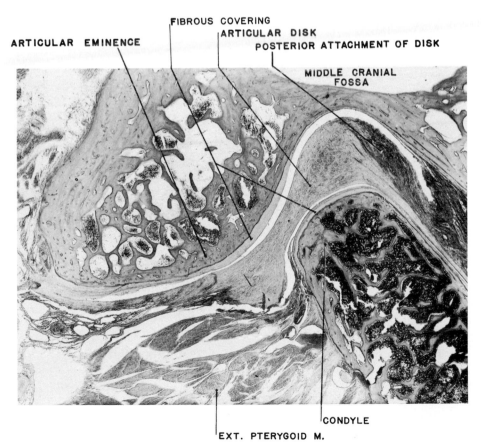

ARTICULAR EMINENCE

FIBROUS COVERING
ARTICULAR DISK
POSTERIOR ATTACHMENT OF DISK

MIDDLE CRANIAL FOSSA

CONDYLE

EXT. PTERYGOID M.

Figure 3–35   Sagittal section through temporomandibular articulation of 28-year-old man. (Courtesy Chase, Orban and Sicher.)

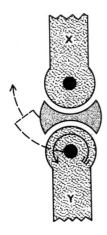
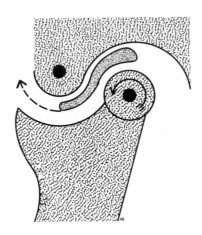

Figure 3–36 Left, Diagram of a grinding joint into which a disk has been inserted. Right, Lateral view of same. (After C. H. Hjortsjo.)

the articular disk (bound rather closely to the condyle, but loosely to the temporal bone) glides downward and forward on the articular eminence of the temporal bone, while the condyle rotates against the inferior portion of the articular disk in the lower joint cavity. The lateral pterygoid muscle helps move the disk anteriorly by virtue of fibers which arise from infratemporal surface of the greater ring of the sphenoid, medial to the infratemporal crest. Other fibers arise from the lateral surface of the lateral pterygoid plate and insert into the anterior margin of the condylar neck and the articular capsule. These fibers (sphenomeniscal) serve to stabilize the disk during mastication and deglutition. Pterygoid fibers have actually been seen extending into the retrodiskal structures, through the retrodiskal zone and attaching as a ligament to the malleus in fetuses. Fibers also attach to the walls of the tympanic fissure.[38]

In so-called Bennett movement, the condyle rotates and moves slightly laterally on the working side. According to Posselt, this rotation is usually not more than 1.5 or 2 mm. and never more than 3 mm. in magnitude. He has been able to distinguish Bennett movement during both habitual lateral motion and border movements. The border type of Bennett movement is more posterior than the habitual Bennett movement.[46] All persons have a Bennett shift in at least one condyle, but that considerable variability exists. At least three factors contribute to the variability. These are lack of harmony in condylar size and fossa, little consistency of the form of the articulating bodies and variation in condylar position.

While the lateral pterygoid muscle serves as the protractor for the disk, moving it forward by virtue of insertion of fibers into the capsule and disk, only the retrodiskal tissue and capsule, and integrity of the ligaments serve to retract the disk. There is no articular disk retracting muscle. In other words, the lateral pterygoid has no opposing stabilizing and antagonistic muscle force, as far as the disk is concerned.

A small change in any of the variables affecting the temporomandibular joint (TMJ) may cause pathology. For example, when there is lack of harmony of postural vertical dimension (PVD) and occlusal vertical dimension (OVD), with mandibular overclosure, electromyography shows a change in muscle habit patterns during the closing cycle. Normally, the anterior, middle and posterior fibers of the temporalis muscle and the superficial and deep elements of the masseter muscle exhibit relatively equal magnitude of contraction in the closing maneuver from PVD to OVD (Fig. 3–22). Excessive interocclusal space and overclosure, or "deep bite," may change this harmonious, stabilizing, balancing and smooth action. With overclosure comes a retrusive activity of the dominant posterior temporalis fibers, often joined by deep masseter fibers, exerting a posterior thrust on the mandibular condyle (and disk). The lateral pterygoid muscle is placed under tension causing a repeated stretch reflex and subsequent muscle contractions or spasms.[52] This holds the disk in a forward position, while the condyle is being forced upward and backward by posterior temporalis muscle action. The condyle, riding over the posterior periphery of the disk, produces a discernible click, and then impinges on the postarticular connective tissue. The postarticular tissue is supplied by nerve fibers from the auriculotemporal nerve and is less adapted to stresses of mandibular function. Joint structures may adapt to deviate activity for a time, but with constant stimulation of stretch reflex, forward pull of the disk, impingement on postarticular connective tissue, muscle spasm and overclosure, these structures may not continue to adapt indefinitely. Proprioception cannot handle the aberrant feedback signals issued by the neural system. Irritation and lack of harmony of the structures is clinically observed in the form of clicking and crepitus. This condition can be mistaken for arthritic changes and treated improperly with meniscectomies and injections.[53]

Shore feels that the clicking or "popping" in the temporomandibular joint is due to the jumping forward of the condyle a fraction of a second ahead of the disk.[54] Yet, muscle physiology seems to substantiate the analysis by the present author that repeated stretch reflex of the lateral pterygoid muscle, causing muscle spasm, literally pulls the rug (disk) out from under the retruded condyle as the posterior temporalis fibers either move or hold the condyle in a retrusive position. Pain can be caused either by impingement on retrodiskal tissues, or by pterygoid spasm (MPD).[55] Whatever the sequence of events, there is broad agreement on the lack of harmony of condyle, disk and eminence during the opening and closing movements.

While abnormal translatory condylar movement may be seen with overclosure (Figs. 3–37, 3–38), this is only part of the story. An important part of the temporomandibular joint malfunction syndrome (called myofascial-pain-dysfunction, or MPD by Laskin and co-workers) is the neurogenic or psychogenic background. The mouth serves as an erotogenic zone, an area of emotional expression for the infant. It also serves to gratify tensional stresses in the adult. The widespread phenomena of bruxism and clenching show positive correlation with the increasing levels of nervous excitability. There is a psychogenic superstructure imposed on the functional and morphologic abnormalities. Temporomandibular joint disturbances are very real and are encountered frequently. Vertical dimension problems, occlusal interferences, functional abnormalities, muscle spasm and psychogenic elaboration on the organic complaint are variable in degrees but usually present in every patient. Chapter 16 discusses correction and control of these problems.

The therapeutic challenge to the dentist as a result of temporomandibular joint malfunction is obvious. The potential preventive and interceptive service that he can render is significant indeed! The elimination of traumatic occlusion and abnormal tooth guidance, and restoration of a normal path of closure and a normal occlusal vertical dimension, will often halt the objective symptoms. As Laskin points out, the muscles that control the action of the temporomandibular joint have a high innervation ratio, with a high degree of sensitivity.[55] Alterations of one millimeter or less can lead to clinical problems — and their solution. In some cases the relief occurs very dramatically. In others, where there has

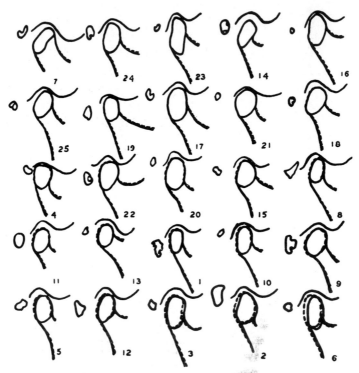

Figure 3–37 Superimposed tracings of 25 patients with normal occlusion, demonstrating the primarily rotary movement of the condyle from postural resting position to full occlusion. (Courtesy V. Boman and D. Blume.)

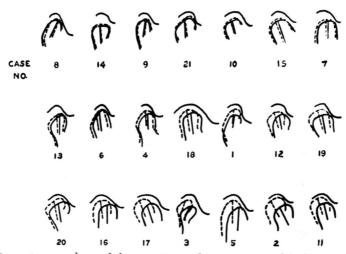

Figure 3–38 Superimposed condylar tracings of temporomandibular joint roentgenograms of 21 patients with Class II, Division 1 malocclusions. There is considerably more translatory movement in evidence in the range from postural rest to habitual occlusion. (Courtesy V. Boman and D. Blume.)

been damage to the tissues (sometimes compounded by injection of sclerosing solution, cortisone or Novocaine), recovery may be much slower and only partial.[37, 56-59]

The dentist must be fully aware that there is no other joint in the body that is used more than the temporomandibular joint. It is beautifully engineered and usually serves a lifetime without any trouble. But, because of the manifold functional demands made on it and because of the magnitude of force exerted, abnormal function and malocclusion of the teeth can elicit marked repercussions in the temporomandibular joint. It is vital that the dentist have a thorough appreciation of the dynamics of the stomatognathic system.[60-62]

FUNCTIONS OF THE STOMATOGNATHIC SYSTEM

It has already been pointed out that any study of physiology of the stomatognathic system would be quite incomplete if it discussed only the phenomenon of mastication. Equally important are the functions of swallowing, respiration and speech. Although each will be discussed separately, it must be emphasized that these functions are intimately related and occur simultaneously.

The orofacial musculature is relatively the most sophisticated in the newborn, so that the patency of the airway breathing and nutritional demands may be met.[15, 29, 30, 63-65] Already present as unconditioned reflexes—for there is no time to learn these life-saving activities—are oropharyngeal reflexes for mandibular posture, respiration, tongue position, deglutition, suckling, gagging, coughing, sneezing and vomiting.

Tactile sensation is extremely well-developed for the newborn, as Hooker and Humphrey have shown. By 11 weeks in utero, stimulation of lips causes the tongue to move; stimulation of upper lip may cause mouth closure and even deglutition. Gag reflex starts at about 18½ weeks; respiration at 25 weeks is possible, and the suckle can be elicited at 29 weeks, with both suckling and swallowing by 32 weeks.[29, 66-68] At birth, the mouth is almost the sole avenue of communication with the outside world, and the tactile acuity of this area continues as the child brings all objects to the mouth first. Sensory guidance for all activities, including jaw movements, covers a large area and includes multiple contacts for sensory input (tongue, lips, soft palate, posterior pharyngeal wall and the temporomandibular joint).

MASTICATION

In the infant, food is taken in first by suckling. This is an unlearned or automatic reflex in *Homo sapiens*. It would seem from an analysis of the suckling phenomenon that at no time of life are more muscles involved in the intake of food than in the newborn. An infant suckles as if his whole life depended on what he does at that moment. There is a rhythmic "caving in" of the cheeks, bobbing of the hyoid bone, snake-like movement of the tongue, anterior mandibular thrust, sphincter-like activity of the lips and an actual nodding movement of the entire head.

The classic suckle-swallow position in the newborn, as outlined by Bosma, shows the head extended, tongue elongated and low in the floor of the mouth, jaws apart and lips pursed around the nipple. The mandible is somewhat protruded (no articular eminence has as yet developed). During function, i.e., deglutition, the rhythmic contraction of the tongue and facial muscles aids in the stabilization of the mandible.[15]

As the infant learns to take solid food, the intensity of the act of satisfying hunger is reduced, but most of the muscles of the cheeks, tongue and floor of the mouth are involved. There is less activity of the lips and less mandibular thrust. The infant quickly learns to use his lips primarily to keep the food from being forced out of the mouth during the peristaltic-like action of the tongue and cheeks as the bolus of food is forced back toward the pharynx. The ingested food is mixed with the saliva by active tongue function. In the infant, as the bolus takes up the saliva it is forced between the gum pads or the occlusal surfaces of the erupting teeth. At the same time the rhythmic action of the muscles of the cheek serves to force the food back toward the tongue, which mashes the bolus of food against the hard palate. To permit the bolus of food to interpose between the gum pads or teeth, the mandible is depressed by gravity and the hyoid and lateral pterygoid muscles, with a simultaneous deflection toward the working side. The lateral shift of the mandible is more apparent in hard-to-chew foods. After a portion of the bolus of food is accommodated between the occlusal surfaces, the mandible is forcibly closed, primarily by temporal and masseter muscle activity.

Fletcher summarizes recent work on the masticatory stroke in the adult, using the six phases outlined by Murphy.

1. The preparatory phase, in which food is ingested and positioned by the tongue within the oral cavity, and the mandible is moved toward the chewing side. Murphy observed a slight, constant deviation to the non-food side an instant before the masticatory stroke began and used this point to identify the "precise beginning" of the preparatory phase.

2. Food contact, characterized by a momentary hesitation in movement. This he interpreted to be a pause triggered by sensory receptors concerning the apparent viscosity of the food and probable transarticular pressures incident to chewing.

3. The crushing phase, which starts with high velocity then slows as the food is crushed and "packed." Gibbs (1969) observed that when the central incisor is approximately 0.24 in. from closure, the jaw motion is stabilized at the condyle on the working side and the final closing stroke thereafter is guided by this "braced condyle." Ahlgren (1961) reported that the first three or four strokes in mastication typically emphasize the crushing phase and that they usually display equal and synchronous activity on both sides.

4. Tooth contact, accompanied by a slight change in direction but no delay. According to Murphy all reflex adjustments of the musculature for tooth contact are completed in the crushing phase before actual contact is made. This observation is supported by Møller (1966), who demonstrated decreases in electromyographically recorded activity of the mandibular elevator muscles before molar contact. Conversely, Beaudreau, Daugherty, and Marland (1969) reported a "distinct and discrete motor pause" consistently elicited in the temporalis and masseter following tooth contact.

5. The grinding phase, which coincides with transgression of the mandibular molars across their maxillary counterparts and is therefore highly constant from cycle to cycle. Messerman (1963) termed this phase the *terminal functional orbit*. Ahlgren (1961) noted that during this phase the bilateral muscular discharge becomes unequal and asynchronous, indicating that the person is chewing unilaterally.

6. Centric occlusion, when movement of the teeth comes to a definite and distinct stop at a single terminal point, from which the preparatory phase of the next stroke begins. Gibbs (1969) found that the jaw of subjects with normal occlusion remained in this position for "a considerable time" whereas the pause was rather brief for those with malocclusion.[34]

Masticatory frequency is variable, but appears to be one to two strokes per second with a normal bolus of food.[14] The number of masticatory strokes before swallowing seems to be characteristic of the individual and is relatively constant.

DEGLUTITION

Moyers lists the characteristic of the infantile swallow as follows:

(1) The jaws are apart, with the tongue between the gum pads.

(2) The mandible is stabilized primarily by contraction of the muscles of the VIIth cranial nerve and the interposed tongue.

(3) The swallow is guided, and to a great extent controlled by sensory interchange between the lips and the tongue (see Fig. 3–39).[29]

As stated above, the gum pads are not usually in contact during the act of swallowing. With liquid foods particularly, a "clucking" is frequently heard. The instinctive and rhythmic peristaltic-like muscle activity steers the liquid or bolus of food back into the pharynx after it leaves the oral cavity. The food is then propelled through the pharynx by the superior, middle and inferior pharyngeal constrictors past the epiglottis into the esophagus. The epiglottis closes off the pharynx as its posterior peripheral portions are forced backward against the superior constricting ring.[70]

With the change to semisolid and solid food and the eruption of teeth there is also a modification of the swallowing act. The tongue no longer is forced into the space between the gum pads or incisal surfaces of the teeth, which actually

INFANTILE (VISCERAL) SWALLOW

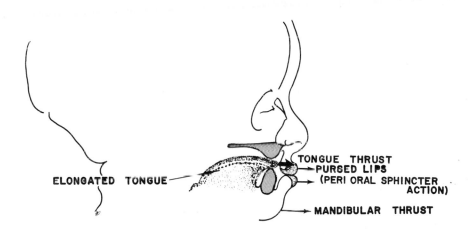

ELONGATED TONGUE

TONGUE THRUST
PURSED LIPS
(PERI ORAL SPHINCTER ACTION)

MANDIBULAR THRUST

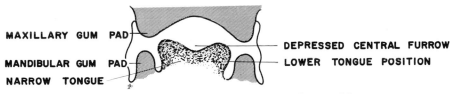

MAXILLARY GUM PAD

MANDIBULAR GUM PAD

NARROW TONGUE

DEPRESSED CENTRAL FURROW

LOWER TONGUE POSITION

Figure 3–39 Infantile swallowing mechanism. Plunger-like action is associated with nursing. Cheek pads flow between posterior gum pads during nursing, unopposed by peripheral portions of tongue. Associated with the tongue thrust is the anterior positioning of the mandible. The condyle may be felt gliding rhythmically forward and backward in the nursing act. Note concave midline contour of dorsum of tongue.

contact momentarily during the swallowing act. Mandibular thrust diminishes during a transitional period of 6 to 12 months. The mandibular closing muscles take over more of the role of stabilizing the mandible as the cheek and lip muscles reduce the strength of their contraction. The spatula-like portion of the tongue collects the food and forces it posteriorly. The tip of the tongue is no longer moving in and out between the anterior gum pads but assumes a position near the incisive foramen at the moment of deglutition. This "somatic swallow" contrasts with the relatively immature "visceral swallow" of the newborn (Fig. 3–40).

As Fletcher points out, the infantile swallow is attributable to a significant difference in oral cavity morphology and to large tongue size, orientation and suspensory system. Whereas general bodily dimensions change in the neonate on a ratio of five to one, the infant tongue only doubles in size. The expansion of peripheral attachments continues well into the postnatal period. The change

MATURE (SOMATIC) SWALLOW

HUMPED UP TONGUE

PERISTALTIC TONGUE PALATE APPROXIMATION

REDUCED PERI-ORAL SPHINCTER

MOMENTARY INCISOR CONTACT

NO MANDIBULAR THRUST

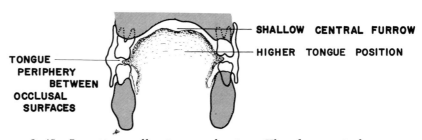

SHALLOW CENTRAL FURROW

HIGHER TONGUE POSITION

TONGUE PERIPHERY BETWEEN OCCLUSAL SURFACES

Figure 3–40 Somatic swallowing mechanism. The dorsum is less concave and approximates the palate during deglutition. The tip of the tongue is contained behind the incisors; peripheral portions flow between opposing posterior segments. Anterior mandibular thrust has disappeared.

to the adult swallow pattern occurs gradually in what has been called the transitional period.[34] Neuromuscular maturation, change in head posture, gravitational effect on mandible are conditioning factors. Usually, by 18 months of age, the mature swallow characteristics listed by Moyers are readily observable.

(1) The teeth are together.

(2) The mandible is stabilized by contractions of the mandibular elevators, which are primarily Vth cranial nerve muscles.

(3) The tongue tip is held against the palate, above and behind the incisors.

(4) There are minimal contractions of the lips during the mature swallow.[29]

Fletcher divides the deglutitional cycle into four phases, highly integrated and synergistically coordinated.[34] These are the preparatory swallow, the oral phase of swallowing, the pharyngeal phase of swallowing and the esophageal phase of swallowing. The preparatory phase starts as soon as liquids are taken in, or after the bolus has been masticated. The liquid or bolus is then in a swallow-preparatory position on the dorsum of the tongue (in the infant, bolus accumulation may be seen also between the base of the tongue and the epiglottis). The oral cavity is sealed by lip and tongue.

During the oral phase the soft palate moves upward and the tongue drops downward and backward. At the same time the larynx and the hyoid bone move upward. These combined movements create a smooth path for the bolus as it is pushed from the oral cavity by the wave-like rippling of the tongue. While solid food is "pushed" by the tongue, liquid food flows ahead of the lingual constrictions. The oral cavity, stabilized by the muscles of mastication, maintains an anterior and lateral seal during this phase (Fig. 3–41).

The pharyngeal phase of swallowing begins as the bolus passes through the fauces. The pharyngeal tube is raised upward *en masse*, and the nasopharynx is sealed off by closure of the soft palate against the posterior pharyngeal wall (i.e., Passavant's ridge). The hyoid bone and the base of the tongue move forward as both the pharynx and the tongue continue their peristaltic-like movement of the bolus of food.

The esophageal phase of swallowing commences as food passes the cricopharyngeal sphincter. While peristaltic movement carries the food through the esophagus, the hyoid bone, palate and tongue return to their original positions. Thus, as Figure 3–44 shows, the four phases smoothly flow from one into the next, making it difficult to determine the actual phase change.

The average individual swallows about once a minute between meals and as frequently as 9 times a minute during eating. Even during sleep the swallowing act is performed at infrequent intervals (Fig. 3–41). There are various estimates of the frequency of deglutition, which range as high as 2400 somatic and visceral swallows per 24-hour period.[14, 71, 72] Lear, Flanagan and Moorrees, using a combined pneumatic and electronic recording harness, tested 20 young adults and checked results by means of visual observation and an acoustic apparatus.[73] An overall mean of 7.5 swallows per hour was found, but the range was wide—2.8 to 15.6 per hour. During eating the mean swallowing rate rose to 296 per hour, ranging from 202 to 376. During supine and sitting positions mean values per hour were 31.4 and 36.5, respectively. Among 20 subjects who were tested over a 24-hour period, total number of swallows per day ranged from 233 to 1008. The mean value was 585—considerably less than previously indicated by other investigators. It should be remembered, however, that the group tested was a sample of young adults. Since there is evidence that children show a

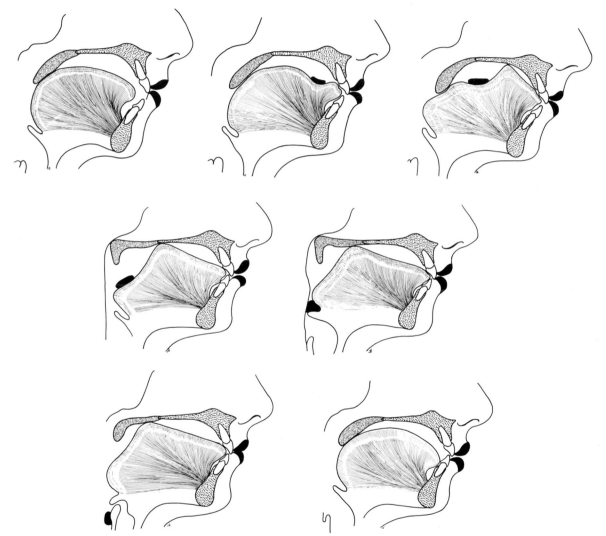

Figure 3–41   Drawings to show representative stages of tongue position during normal degluti-tion. Note the peristaltic-like activity. (After Björk and Lundström.)

more frequent swallowing pattern, it would be expected that a group whose range was 800 to 1200 swallows per 24-hour period might include the largest number of children between 5 and 12 years of age.

Some observers feel that patients with certain types of malocclusion (i.e., Class II, Division 1 and open bite problems) swallow more frequently. The level of nervous irritability and the use of the swallowing cycle as a tensional release mechanism may also enhance deglutitional frequency.

TONGUE THRUST. It is obvious that the act of swallowing, repeated so frequently, may have a profound effect on the maxilla or mandible, particularly if there is an abnormal swallowing pattern (Fig. 3–42). Moyers thinks that the prolonged retention of the infantile swallowing mechanism can be a matter of some concern and may well contribute to the creation of a malocclusion.[29] Some clinicians have observed malocclusion in over 80 per cent of persons with abnormal swallowing habits. To the orthodontist, who has learned how a powerful tongue and improperly functioning perioral muscles can deform a delicately responsive dentition, such high percentages are possible.[74, 75] The physiologist is less certain. Clinical implications will be discussed in Chapter 6.

The tongue thrust pattern of oral activity has been given many titles, some of which are the following: perverted or deviate swallow, reverse swallow, retained infantile swallow, tooth apart swallow, and so forth. Yet, because no single characteristic of tongue thrust activity is constant, all such terms become too restrictive. Even the use of "normal" versus "abnormal" swallow has been criticized. There is no "norm" for the pattern of tongue thrust.[76] Malocclusion may or may not be present. Teeth may or may not be brought together. Labial pressures may or may not be "normal." Speech defects may or may not be observed. Even arch form may or may not be affected, in spite of all evidence that tongue force is greater than opposing lip and cheek pressures. D'Arcy Thompson explained that many biologic structures follow engineering principles.[77] The Brader hypothesis pictures the dental arch as an ellipsoidal curve with three centers of rotation, governed in form by the engineering principles of an elastic membrane, i.e., that there is an inverse relationship between force and curvature of the arch. That would mean that where pressure is greatest the curve is

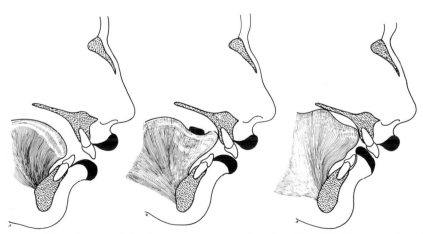

Figure 3–42 Abnormal deglutition associated with a Class II, Division 1 malocclusion. Note the thrusting forward of the tip of the tongue and sucking in of the lower lip. (After Björk and Lundström.)

tightest.[78] This introduces suspension geometry and volume as further arch form conditioning factors. Proffit and Norton feel that at our present level of knowledge, they can draw two conclusions (Fig. 3–43):

1. Influences on horizontal dimensions, exemplified by dental arch form, and vertical dimensions, by swallowing, speaking, breathing, etc., have not been proven. Rest relationships may provide the key to form-function relationships at this level.

2. Influences on vertical tooth and jaw relationships, as in open bite malocclusions, have not been considered carefully enough as yet. Relationships between tongue and lip activity probably do exist but are poorly defined. Studies must be designed to test the pertinent variables.[30]

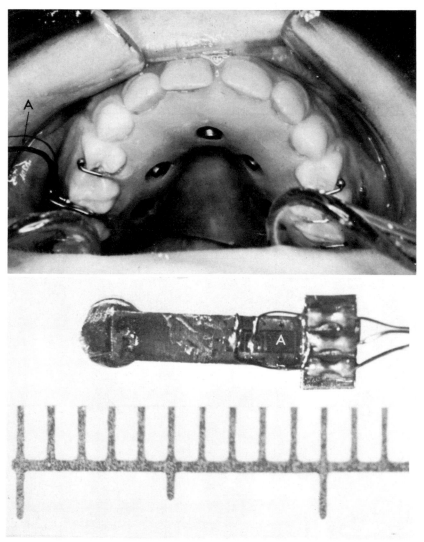

Figure 3–43   Lingual pressure transducers used by Proffit and co-workers to measure tongue pressures during function. Transducers are mounted in palate covering device, allowing simultaneous pressure recording at five locations. A-wire leads from transducers, passes behind the last molar and emerges via the vestibule. Lower photograph is an enlarged pressure transducer. Scale markings are 1 mm. A is the strain gauge. Transducer designed and built at the University of Kentucky. (From Proffit, W. R., and Norton, L. A.: The tongue and oral morphology: influences on tongue activity during speech and swallowing. ASHA Reports, No. 5, 106–115, 1970.)

RESPIRATION

The phenomena of mastication and deglutition seem complex and demanding enough for the postural and masticatory muscles and the unattached muscles of facial expression. But we must superimpose on these the function of respiration. The physiology of the stomatognathic system is truly remarkable when we realize that all three phenomena are frequently occurring simultaneously. Respiration, like mastication and swallowing, is an inherent reflex activity. The demands on the musculature are subtle and more difficult to observe. A wonder to behold is the fantastically efficient split-second opening and closing of the epiglottis, keeping out the food but permitting the entry of life-giving air.

Bosma and his co-workers have analyzed respiration in the infant and found that quiet respiration is typically carried out through the nose, with the tongue in proximity to the palate, obturating the oral passageway.[31, 32, 70] Both the pharynx and the larynx are active during respiration and it is in this area that the infant differentiates between respiration and associated activities, such as the grunt, cough, cry or sneeze.[63] Posture also has a significant effect on respiration.[79]

Initial responses to environmental stimuli are seen in the respiratory function, with emphasis on exhalation. Respiration maintains the patency of the pharyngeal area, since there is a collapse of the pharynx in the tracheotomized infant. Development of respiratory spaces and maintenance of the airway are significant factors in orofacial growth (see Chap. 2, functional matrix theory). The mechanism of crying is intimately tied up with respiration, and the laryngeal and pharyngeal coordination of muscles is seen quite early. Only after this coordination develops may he embark on the more mature and discriminate neuromuscular demands of articulate speech.

SPEECH

Speech, like breathing, also makes no gross demands on the perioral muscles. Although all mammals apparently masticate, swallow and breathe, speech is limited to the human being. Unlike mastication, deglutition and respiration, which are reflexive in nature, speech is largely a learned activity dependent on the maturation of the organism. Speech is to be distinguished from the reflexive sounds that are associated with physiologic states. Coming late in the evolutionary development of man, speech makes use of muscles which have many other functions. West lists the "other than speech functions" as follows: (a) those that are *innate,* automatic, vegetative reactions, such as swallowing, gagging, breathing, vomiting and suckling; (b) those that are *learned,* automatic, vegetative reactions, such as biting, chewing and sucking; (c) those that are *learned,* automatic, *emotional* reactions, such as grimaces, mannerisms and tics; (d) those that are *innate,* automatic, *emotional* reactions such as laughing, sobbing and smiling; (e) those that are learned, *nonautomatic, discriminatory* and specially *voluntary* reactions, such as exploratory movements of the tongue, spreading of the lips, kissing and blowing; (f) those that are learned, automatic *practical* reactions, such as whistling, playing a wind instrument and humming a tune.[80]

It is easy to see why a large number of muscles are involved. The muscles of the walls of the torso, the respiratory tract, the pharynx, the soft palate, the tongue, the lips and face, and the nasal passageways are all concerned in the production of speech sounds. Simultaneous breathing to provide a column of air is essential to produce vibrations necessary for sound. The lips and tongue and velopharyngeal structures modify the outgoing breath stream to produce variations in the sound. Assuming the presence of normal structures, speech production is dependent on the coordinated action and precise activity of muscles that may be performing other functions at the same time. If the structures are not normal, as with cleft palate, normal speech sounds may not be possible, despite the compensatory muscle activity (Fig. 3–44). (See Chap. 6.)

Current research links the parameters of volume of air flow, oral and nasal breath pressure and the neuromuscular physiology seen in the orofacial complex.[81] Even though the mechanisms for producing sounds involve at least parts of the same systems used for mastication, respiration and speech, actions used in producing language differ considerably. The speech mechanism. acts on the breath stream in a number of ways, controlling the air mechanism, air direction, air flow, air release, air pressure, general air path and lingual air path. These actions involve muscle groups and call for compensatory interaction if abnormality exists in one area. In cleft palate, with palatal insufficiency, the inability to control the air path direction may elicit adaptive reaction elsewhere, e.g., greater postpharyngeal wall (Passavant's pad) activity, enlargement of turbinates, mandibular postural position change, contraction of the nares, enlargement of tonsils and adenoids, and so forth.[64]

With respect to the tongue, which fills the oral cavity at birth, only the extrinsic muscles which largely control horizontal movement needed for the suckle-swallow are well-developed. Those intrinsic muscles needed for speech are poorly developed. The transition from gross movements of the tongue to precise and finely controlled ones extends over the first several years of life, through the infantile and transitional swallowing periods, into the mature deglutitional pattern era. The speech therapist is concerned with residual infantile tongue posture and function, since lisp, open bite, anterior air escape and substitute speech sounds are possible sequelae of residual infantile swallowing habits.[82]

The lips, as well as the tongue, undergo maturational changes preparatory to speech. In infants, suckling and rooting reflexes are dominant. The first sounds actually make no demands on the lips, e.g., "aa." The degree of lip protrusion is considered significant in varying the length of the vocal tract. With reduction of purse-string suckle-swallow activity, more delicate peripheral lip movements are seen, coinciding with tongue maturation.[82–85]

Of particular importance to the dentist is the velopharyngeal valve. In children with cleft palate, inadequate valving seems to be the rule, not the exception, even in rehabilitated cleft cases. Upward and backward movement of the soft palate in such problems does not emulate the normal pattern, as shown in Figures 3–45 and 3–46. Normally, the third quadrant of the soft palate contacts the postpharyngeal wall with sounds like "P," "B," "F" and "W."[83]

Jensen studied the anterior teeth relationship and speech in normal and Class II, Division 1 malocclusions.[88] The evidence is quite substantial that there is compensatory tongue and lip activity, adapting to the abnormal overjet and dental arch morphology. How much of this is cause and how much is effect cannot be determined. But it is not unreasonable to assume, in this era of working hypotheses, that compensatory muscle activity can at least maintain existing dento-alveolar relationships, even if it does not accentuate the deformity. As an associated factor in potential arch deformation, speech assumes some importance. References 80–88, at the end of this chapter, will help the reader to understand more about the physiology of speech. A full discussion of the effects of abnormal muscle function is given in Chapter 6.

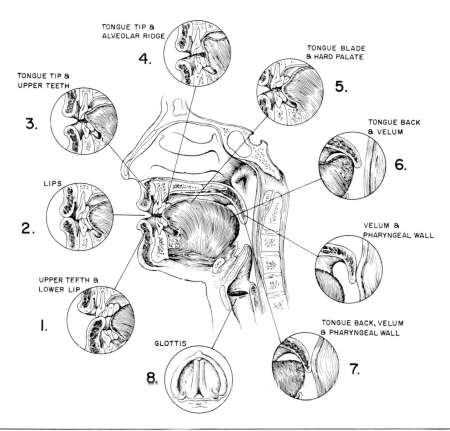

STRUCTURAL COMPONENTS OF THE ARTICULATORY VALVE	CLOSED VALVE		CONSTRICTED VALVE		VOICED NASALS
	VOICELESS	VOICED	VOICELESS	VOICED	
1. Labio–dental (upper teeth & lower lip)			"f" [f]	"v" [v]	
2. Bi–labial (lips)	"p" [p]	"b" [b]		"w" [w]	"m" [m]
3. Linguo–dental (tongue tip & upper teeth)			"th" [θ]	"th" [ð]	
4. Linguo–alveolar (tongue tip & alveolar ridge)	"t" [t]	"d" [d]	"s" [s]	"z" [z] "l" [l]	"n" [n]
5. Linguo–palatal (tongue blade & hard palate)	"ch" [tʃ]	"j" [dʒ]	"sh"[ʃ]	"zh" [ʒ] "r"[r] "y"[j]	
6. Linguo–velor (tongue back & velum)					"ng" [ŋ]
7. Linguo–velor–pharyngeal (tongue back, velum & pharyngeal wall)	"k" [k]	"g" [g]			
8. Glottal (glottis)			"h" [h]		

Figure 3–44   Chart shows kinesiologic positions for the oral and pharyngeal mus-culature during articulation of consonantal sounds. Note particularly that sections 6 and 7 of chart show the tongue in an incorrect position in order to emphasize that the entire medial dorsal aspect of the tongue is normally found in contact with the soft palate during the production of sounds "ng," "k," and "g." (From Sloan, R. F., Brummett, S. W., Westover, J. L., Ricketts, R. M., and Ashley, F. L.: Recent cinefluorographic advances in palatopharyngeal roentgenography. Am. J. Roentgenol., 42:977–985, 1964.)

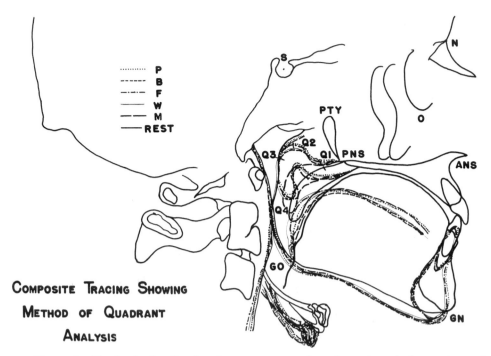

Figure 3–45 Analysis of soft palate movement from lateral cephalometric tracings to show elevation and pharyngeal wall contact. Soft palate is ordinarily divided into four quadrants (Q1, Q2, Q3, Q4) for study. Normally, there is little posterior pharyngeal wall movement. Observe the hyoid bone positional change from postural rest to speaking function in this tracing. (From Graber, T. M., Bzoch, K. R., and Aoba, J. T.: A functional study of the palatal and pharyngeal structures. Angle Orthodont., 29:30–40, 1959.)

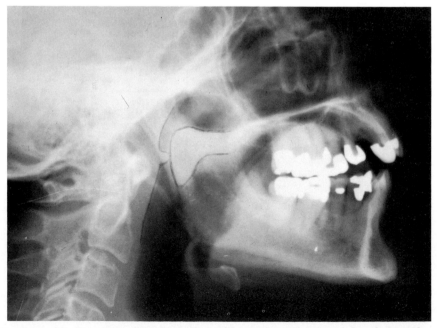

Figure 3–46 Dramatic "Passavant's pad" activity; white female adult with normal speech. This unusual anterior bulging of the postpharyngeal wall is seen more commonly as a compensatory mechanism in cleft palate speech.

REFERENCES

1. Meyer, H. V.: Die Architekturen der Spongiosen. Arch. Anat. Physiol. Wissensch. Med., 1867.
2. Wolff., J.: Ueber die innere Architekturen des Knochens. Virchow Arch. Path. Anat., 50:389–453, 1870.
3. Roux, W.: Beiträge zur Morphologie der functionellen Anpassung. Arch. Physiol. Anat., 9:120–158, 1885.
4. Weinmann, J. P., and Sicher, H.: Bone and Bones. 2nd ed. St. Louis, C. V. Mosby Co., 1955.
5. Epker, B. N., and Frost, H. M.: Biomechanical control of bone growth and development. J. Dent. Res., 45:364–371, 1966.
6. McElhaney, J. H.: Load and electrical charge relationships for cortical bone. In Moyers, R. E., Krogman, W. M.: Craniofacial growth in man. Oxford, Pergamon Press, 1971.
7. Frost, H. M.: Tetracycline bone labeling in anatomy. Am. J. Phys. Anthrop., 29:183–195, 1968.
8. Graber, T. M., Chung, D. D. B., and Aoba, J. T.: Dentofacial orthopedics versus orthodontics. J.A.D.A., 75:1145–1164, 1967.
9. Lear, C. S. C., and Moorrees, C. F. A.: Buccolingual muscle force and dental arch form. Am. J. Orthodont., 56:379–393, 1969.
10. Benninghoff, A.: Form und Bau der Gelenkknorpel in ihren Beziehungen zur Funktion. Z. Zellforsch., 2:783–862, 1925.
11. Klaauw, C. J., van der: Cerebral skull and facial skull. A contribution to the knowledge of skull structure. Arch. Neerl. Zool., 9:16–36, 1946.
12. Moss, M. L.: Functional cranial analysis and the functional matrix. ASHA Reports, no. 6, 5–18, 1971.
13. Enlow, D. H.: Wolff's law and the factor of architectonic circumstance. Am. J. Orthodont., 54:803–822, 1968.
14. Kawamura, Y.: Dental significance of four oral physiological mechanisms. J. Canad. Dent. Ass., 34:582–590, 1968.
15. Bosma, J. F.: Symposium on Oral Sensation and Perception. Springfield, Ill., Charles C Thomas, 1967.
16. Ganong, W. F.: Review of Medical Physiology. Los Altos, Lange Medical Publishers, 1971.
17. Sherrington, C. S.: The Integrative Action of the Nervous System. New Haven, Yale University Press, 1947.
18. Yildirim, F., and DeVincenzo, J. P.: Maximum opening and closing forces exerted by diverse skeletal types. Angle Orthodont., 41:230–235, 1971.
19. Merton, P. A.: Problems of muscle fatigue. Brit. Med. Bull., 12:219–221, 1956.
20. Jacobs, R. M.: Muscle equilibrium, fact or fancy. Angle Orthodont., 39:11–21, 1969.
21. Jacobs, R. M.: Treatment objectives and case retention: cybernetic and myometric considerations. Am. J. Orthodont., 58:552–564, 1970.
22. Winders, R. V.: Recent findings in myometric research. Angle Orthodont., 32:38–43, 1962.
23. Winders, R. V.: Forces exerted on the dentition by the perioral and lingual musculature during swallowing. Angle Orthodont., 28:226–235, 1958.
24. Cox, R. L.: Muscular development and maturation of the dentofacial complex: Normal and abnormal. ASHA Reports, no. 5, 20–32, 1970.
25. Werner, H.: Measuring of lip pressure. Acta Odont. Scand., (Suppl. 40) 22:40–49, 1964.
26. Weinstein, S., Haack, D. C., Morris, L. Y., Snyder, B. B., and Attaway, H. E.: On an equilibrium theory of tooth position. Angle Orthodont., 33:1–26, 1963.
27. Kawamura, Y.: Neuromuscular mechanisms of jaw and tongue movement. J.A.D.A., 62:545–551, 1961.
28. Cleall, J, F.: Deglutition: a study of form and function. Am. J. Orthodont., 51:560–594, 1965.
29. Moyers, R. E.: Postnatal development of orofacial musculature. ASHA Reports, no. 6, 38–47, 1971.
30. Proffit, W. R., and Norton, L. A.: The tongue and oral morphology: influences of tongue activity during speech and swallowing. ASHA Reports, no 5, 106–115, 1970.
31. Bosma, J. F.: Evaluation of oral function of the orthodontic patient. Am. J. Orthodont., 55:578–584, 1969.
32. Bosma, J. F., and Brodie, D. R.: Cineradiographic demonstration of pharyngeal area myotonia in myotonic dystrophy patients. Radiology, 92:104–109, 1969.
33. Milne, I. M., and Cleall, J. F.: Cinefluorographic study of functional adaptation of the oropharyngeal structures. Angle Orthodont., 40:267–283, 1970.
34. Fletcher, S. G.: Processes and maturation of mastication and deglutition. ASHA Reports, no. 5, 92–105, 1970.
35. Weinberg, B.: Deglutition: a review of selected topics. ASHA Reports, no. 5, 116–131, 1970.
36. Perry, H. T., Jr.: Relation of occlusion to temporomandibular joint dysfunction: the orthodontic viewpoint. J.A.D.A., 79:137–141, 1969.
37. Coleman, R. D.: Temporomandibular joint: relation of the retrodiskal zone to Meckel's cartilage and lateral pterygoid muscle. J. Dent. Res., 49:626–630, 1970.
38. Griffin, C. J., and Munro, R. R.: Electromyography of the jaw-closing muscles in the open-close-clench cycle in man. Arch. Oral Biol., 14:141–149, 1969.

39. Perry, H. T., Jr.: Kinesiology of the temporal and masseter muscles in chewing a homogeneous bolus. Northwestern University, Doctoral thesis, 1961.
40. Perry, H. T., Jr.: Functional electromyography of the temporal and masseter muscles in Class II, Division 1 malocclusion and excellent occlusion. Angle Orthodont., 25:49–58, 1955.
41. Perry, H. T., Jr.: The physiology of mandibular displacement. Angle Orthodont., 30:51–69, 1960.
42. Perry, H. T., Jr., and Harris, S. C.: Role of neuromuscular system in functional activity of the mandible. J.A.D.A., 48:665–673, 1954.
43. Brill, N., Lammie, G. A., Osborne, J., and Perry, H. T., Jr.: Mandibular positions and mandibular movements: a review. Brit. Dent. J., 106:391–400, 1959.
44. Bennett, N. G.: A contribution to the study of movements of the mandible. Proc. Roy. Soc. Med., 1:79–95, 1908.
45. Perry, H. T., Jr.: Static and dynamic orthodontics. Am. J. Orthodont., 48:900–910, 1962.
46. Posselt, U.: The physiology of Occlusion and Rehabilitation. 2nd ed., Philadelphia, F. A. Davis Co., 1968.
47. Perry, H. T., Jr.: Principles of occlusion applied to modern orthodontics. D. Clin. North America, 13:581–590, 1969.
48. Glickman, I., Pameijer, J. H. N., Roeber, F. W., and Brion, M. A. M.: Functional occlusion as revealed by miniaturized radio transmitters. D. Clin. North America, 13:667–679, 1969.
49. Pameijer, J. H. N., Glickman, I., and Roeber, F. W.: Intraoral occlusal telemetry. III. Tooth contacts in chewing, swallowing and bruxism. J. Periodont., 40:253–258, 1969.
50. Ramfjord, S. P., and Hiniker, J. J.: Distal displacement of the mandible. J. Prosth. Dent., 16:491–502, 503–512, 1966.
51. Perry, H. T., Jr., Lammie, G. A., Main, J., and Teuscher, G. W.: Occlusion in a stress situation. J.A.D.A., 60:626–633, 1960.
52. Graber, T. M.: Overbite, the dentist's challenge. J.A.D.A., 79:1135–1145, 1969.
53. Kelikian, H.: A method of mobilizing the temporomandibular joint. J. Bone Joint Surg., 32:113–131, 1950.
54. Shore, N. A.: Educational program for patients with temporomandibular joint dysfunction (ligaments). J. Prosth. Dent., 20:77–82, 1970.
55. Laskin, D. M.: Etiology of the pain-dysfunction syndrome. J.A.D.A., 79:147–153, 1969.
56. Burton, R. C.: The problem of facial pain. J.A.D.A., 79:93–101, 1969.
57. Sarnat, B. G.: Developmental facial abnormalities and the temporomandibular joint. J.A.D.A., 79:108–117, 1969.
58. Bell, W. E.: Clinical diagnosis of the pain-dysfunction syndrome. J.A.D.A., 79:154–160, 1969.
59. Blackwood, H. J. J.: Pathology of the temporomandibular joint. J.A.D.A., 79:118–124, 1969.
60. Perry, H. T., Jr.: The symptomology of temporomandibular joint disturbance. J. Prosth. Dent., 19:288–298, 1968.
61. Sarnat, B. G.: The Temporomandibular Joint. 2nd ed., Springfield, Charles C Thomas, 1964.
62. Swenson, H. M.: ABC's of periodontics—"T" is for the temporomandibular joint, J. Indiana Dent. Ass., 49:144–146, 1970.
63. Lind, John (ed.): Newborn infant cry. Acta Paediat. Scand. (Suppl. 163), 1965.
64. Graber, T. M.: Oral and nasal structures in cleft palate speech. J.A.D.A., 53:693–706, 1956.
65. Graber, T. M.: The three "M's": muscles, malformation and malocclusion. Am. J. Orthodont., 49:418–450, 1963.
66. Hooker, D.: The Prenatal Origin of Behavior. New York, Lawrence Kansas & Hafner, Inc., 1969.
67. Humphrey, T.: Reflex activity in the oral and facial area of human fetuses in Bosma, J. F.: Second Symposium on Oral Sensation and Perception. Springfield, Ill., Charles C Thomas, 1969.
68. Humphrey, T.: Human prenatal activity sequences in the facial region and their relationship to postnatal development. ASHA Reports, no. 6, 19–37, 1971.
69. Ahlgren, J.: Mechanism of mastication: a quantitative cinematographic study of masticatory movements. Acta Odont. Scand. (Suppl. 44), 24, 1966.
70. Bosma, J. F.: Maturation of function of the oral and pharyngeal region. Am. J. Orthodont., 49:94–104, 1963.
71. Straub, W. J.: Malfunction of the tongue. Am. J. Orthodont., 46:404–424, 1960.
72. Hanson, M. L., Logan, W. B., and Case, J. L.: Tongue thrust in pre-school children. Am. J. Orthodont., 57:15–22, 1970.
73. Lear, C. S. C., Flanagan, J. B., and Moorrees, C. F. A.: The frequency of deglutition in man. Arch. Oral Biol., 10:83–99, 1965.
74. Bell, W. A.: Muscle pattern of late fetal tongue tip. Angle Orthodont., 40:262–265, 1970.
75. Hopkins, G. B.: Neonatal and adult tongue dimensions. Angle Orthodont., 37:132–133, 1967.
76. Fishman, L. S.: Postural and dimensional changes in the tongue from rest position to occlusion. Angle Orthodont., 39:109–113, 1969.
77. Thompson, D.: On Growth and Form. London, Cambridge Press. 1942.
78. Brader, A.: Dental arch form in relation to intra-oral forces. Essay. Edward Angle Society, Denver, 1969.
79. Rasmus, R. L., and Jacobs, R. M.: Mouth-breathing and malocclusion: quantitative technique for measurement of oral and nasal air-flow velocities. Angle Orthodont., 39:296–302, 1969.

80. West, R. *in* Travis, L. E. (ed.): Handbook of Speech Pathology. New York, Appleton-Century-Crofts, Inc., 1971.
81. Lubker, J. F.: Aerodynamic and ultrasonic assessment techniques in speech-dentofacial research. ASHA Reports, no. 5, 207–223, 1970.
82. Subtelny, J. D.: Malocclusions, orthodontic corrections and orofacial muscle adaptation. Angle Orthodont., 40:170–201, 1970.
83. Graber, T. M., Bzoch, K. R., and Aoba, J. T.: A functional study of the palatal and pharyngeal structures. Angle Orthodont., 29:30–40, 1959.
84. Bzoch, K. R.: Assessment: radiographic techniques. ASHA Reports, no. 5, pp. 248–270, 1970.
85. Cole, R. M.: Speech. ASHA Reports, no. 6, 79–95, 1971.
86. Björk, L.: Velopharyngeal function in connected speech. Acta Radiol., (Suppl. 202), 1–94, 1961.
87. Nylen, B. O.: Cleft palate and speech. Acta Radiol. (Suppl. 203), 1–124, 1961.
88. Jensen, R. Anterior teeth relationship and speech. Acta Radiol. (Suppl. 276), 1968.
89. Nagy, L., and Denes, J.: Electromyographic analysis of the temporal and masseter muscles activity in persons with normal occlusion and deep bite. Fogorv Szemle, 61:235–238, 1968.
90. Møller, E.: The chewing apparatus. An electromyographic study of the action of the muscles of mastication and its correlation to facial morphology. Acta Physiol. Scand. (Suppl. 280), 69, 1966.
91. Perry, H. T., Jr.: Muscle Contraction patterns in swallowing. Angle Orthodont., 42:66–80, 1972.

chapter 4

NORMAL OCCLUSION

The positions of the teeth within the jaws and the mode of occlusion are determined by developmental processes that interact on the teeth and their associated structures during the periods of formation, growth and postnatal modification. Dental occlusion varies among individuals according to tooth size and shape, tooth position, timing and sequence of eruption, dental arch size and shape and patterns of craniofacial growth.

The study of occlusion is concerned with more than morphologic description; it delves into the nature of variations in components of the masticatory system and considers the effects of age changes, functional modifications and pathology. Variability in the dentition results from the interplay of genetic and environmental factors which affect both prenatal development and postnatal modification.[1]

If we define normal as "the usual," then a beautifully straight alignment of 16 teeth in each jaw does not qualify (Fig. 4–1). There are few such alignments except in prostheses. Even when the teeth are perfectly aligned in each jaw, this is no guarantee that the occlusion is normal. Perfect interdigitation is the ideal and is routinely possible only in the artistic, full-denture creations of the prosthodontist. For the orthodontist, ideal occlusion is an admirable goal but is usually a therapeutic impossibility.

A cardinal axiom to begin with is that *the normal in physiology is always a range, never a point*. Twenty-eight teeth in proper arrangement and in balance with all environmental and functional forces may conceivably be normal. A balanced, stable, healthy and esthetically attractive occlusion is also conceivably normal, even if minor rotations are present. It may be equally normal for one child to have a marked overbite and overjet and procumbent incisors and for another to have little or no overbite and overjet, coupled with upright incisors. The curve of Spee, compensating curve, cusp height and facial relation of each tooth to its antagonist, and other characteristics of occlusion may all vary within a broad range and still be normal. And yet, what may be abnormal for one age may be normal for another. Good examples of the time-linked nature of normalcy are such transient malocclusions, as crowding during eruption of incisors, the "ugly duckling" flaring of the maxillary lateral incisors, the Class II first molar relationship tendencies before the loss of the deciduous second molars and the lingual inclination of erupting mandibular second molars before the tongue has had a chance to influence the erupting teeth (see Chap. 2). *It is vitally important that the dentist recognize these transient conditions for what they are,*

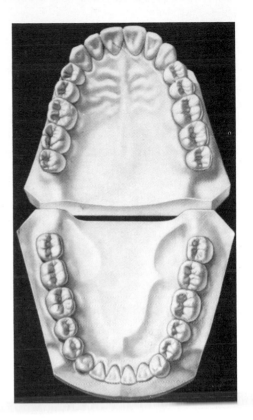

Figure 4–1   An ideal arrangement of 32 teeth seldom duplicated in the natural dentition. (Courtesy Columbia Dentoform Corp.)

and not interfere with nature's attempt to achieve what will later be a normal pattern and a normal arrangement of teeth. This is stressed because orthodontists as well as dentists in general practice have been guilty of utilizing orthodontic appliances at the wrong time, interfering with what often is a normal developmental pattern. Too often the net result has been minimal or actually damaging to the teeth and investing tissues. An iatrogenic malocclusion results.

Any definition of normal occlusion should no longer be static and descriptive merely of tooth relationships. A dynamic definition is essential. Not only the teeth themselves, but the investing tissues, the contiguous and motivating masticatory musculature, the curve of Spee, the interocclusal clearance, and the temporomandibular joint morphology and action are essential considerations in the modern concept of occlusion. The recognition of these fundamentals of occlusion did not come overnight, however.

Although this chapter is allocated arbitrarily to the development of the total concept of occlusion, there is no intention of placing any less emphasis on the important growth and developmental details and physiologic background found in Chapters 2 and 3, which are so very essential for the establishment and preservation of that occlusion. In the truest sense, there can be no compartmentalizing of knowledge into chapters; this is done only for the sake of organization of reading material and for convenience.

THE DEVELOPMENT OF THE CONCEPT OF OCCLUSION

Historically, much of the early development of dentistry was inductive, reasoning from the particular to the general. The development of the idea of occlusion can be traced through fiction and hypothesis to fact. The fictional approach, in a philosophical sense, was a convenient arrangement of a series of observations and thoughts more or less logically arranged. All too often these observations were sporadic, interrelated only by chance, bound together by a single tenuous thread.

The hypothetical attack on the problem of occlusion was based on a provional acceptance of certain logical entities. These were to fill in the gaps in empirical knowledge and thus tentatively complete the picture. There was a distinct understanding, however, that other discoveries and future experiences must verify them. As Simon said, a hypothesis can be finally maintained only if it does not contradict the facts of experience.[2] This is just the opposite of fiction. Another difference between the hypothetical and fictional approaches is that the building of a hypothesis is predicated on plausibility; the selection of an inductive or fictional explanation is based on the usefulness of the concept.

Fact is reality, what has really happened. Fact is a truth known by actual experience or observation. Both the fictional and hypothetical approaches are necessary preludes to the establishment of fact but must give way wherever contradiction arises. The development of the concept of occlusion thus can be divided into three periods: the fictional period, prior to 1900; the hypothetical period, from 1900 to 1930; the factual period, from 1930 to the present. Obviously, this is a division of convenience. The impression is given that there is a distinct cleavage into three entities, whereas the transition was gradual, with considerable overlapping. But the trend is undeniable. Fictions and hypotheses still form convenient "crutches" where our knowledge on certain aspects of stomatognathic function is still sketchy. There is less and less need for them, however, as definitive research and advances in biometric analysis provide an ever-expanding compendium of factual information.

There is another trend in the development of the concept of occlusion—the trend from the static to the dynamic. Original concepts of occlusion were those of a completed act—literally an anatomic approach, a description of how the teeth meet when the jaws are closed. "Clusion" means "closing," the prefix "oc" means "up"—thus, a "closing up." This static approach lasted well into the hypothetical period. With more emphasis on physiology, and recognition of functional disorders, a much broader interpretation of occlusion has developed.

FICTIONAL PERIOD

The first of the three periods in the development of a concept of occlusion—the fictional period—like Topsy, "just growed." Pioneers like Fuller, Clark and Imrie talked of "antagonism," "meeting" or "gliding" of teeth.[3-5] Others relied on anatomic descriptions of the morphology of the teeth as individual units. The creation of a normal standard, a typical relationship, a basis on which to compare departures from the normal, was lacking. Definitions that seemed most useful for the particular problem at hand were formulated. In discussing the "norm," Kingsley[6] wrote in 1880:

> Peculiarities of the permanent teeth are recognized by everyone of extended observation . . . because they are a greater or less departure from a normal standard. . . . Such a standard cannot . . . be one shape to which all must conform. . . . The standard of normality of the dental arch is a curved line expanding as it approaches the ends, and all teeth standing on that line.

While much of what Kingsley said was later to serve as a working hypothesis, or subsequently became established fact after definitive research, there were contributors to this fictional period of orthodontic development whose flights of fancy quietly passed away with the beginning of the 20th century. Eugene Talbot's text, *Irregularities of the Teeth and Their Treatment,* went through five editions, the last in 1903, before succumbing to progress. The book makes fascinating reading, as the author attributes facial deformities to maternal impressions, and delineates in great detail the adolescent neuroses of nasal and facial bones, developmental neuroses of the eye, the maxillary bones, the palate, tooth position, and so forth. The chapter on "the degenerate teeth," depicting the deteriorating, degenerating status of mankind in general and the dentition in particular, is frightening.[7] The Talbot concept of normal occlusion was that it was a historical event, long since passed in the decline of the species, and possible only with an atavism or "throwback" to our primitive ancestors. This hardly served as an inspiration for those to follow who were hopeful of preventing, intercepting and treating developing malocclusions.

HYPOTHETICAL PERIOD

EDWARD H. ANGLE

Undoubtedly it was Edward Hartley Angle, in 1899, who crystallized the orthodontic thinking on occlusion and brought the concept out of the realm of fiction" (see Chap. 1, Angle vignette). He did much to organize the existing concepts and formulate definite principles of diagnosis and treatment. In 1907, summarizing his views to that date, he wrote:[9]

Occlusion is the basis of the science of orthodontia. The shapes of the cusps, crowns and roots, and even the very structural material of the teeth and attachments are all designed for the purpose of making occlusion the one grand object. . . . We shall define occlusion as being the normal relations of the occlusal inclined planes of the teeth when the jaws are closed.

He describes the illustration, "Old Glory" (Fig. 4–2):

. . . in (Old Glory) which represents all the teeth in normal occlusion, it will be seen that each dental arch describes a graceful curve, and that all the teeth in these arches are so arranged as to be in harmony with their fellows in the same arch, as well as those in the opposite arch. . . . Each tooth . . . helps to maintain every other tooth in these harmonious relations for the cusps interlock and each inclined plane serves to prevent each tooth from sliding out of position.

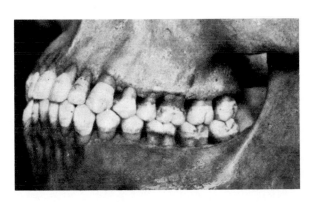

Figure 4–2 "Old Glory," which Angle used to exemplify normal occlusion (prognathic).

After discussing in detail the anatomic relations of the teeth, Angle furnished us with one of the best examples of a hypothesis—his "key to occlusion." He noted that:

... all teeth are essential, yet in function and influence some are of greater importance than others, the most important of all being the first permanent molars. ... They are by far the most constant in taking their normal positions . . . especially the upper first molars . . . which we call the keys to occlusion. We believe that nature so rarely errs in the location of the upper first molars—the very cornerstones, as it were, in the foundation of the structure of an organ so essential to the whole physical economy as the dental apparatus—as to make it a matter of little or no concern to us except, possibly, in research work.

This hypothesis was the basis of Angle's classification of malocclusion, and it was immediately branded as dogma by contemporary adversaries. Yet, perhaps more than any of Angle's contributions, this has withstood the test of time. The universality of his categorizing of malocclusion is complete, over 70 years after its introduction. Modifications and interpretations have been made, but the anteroposterior basis for classifying occlusion remains. Occlusion of teeth as the sole criterion of normality is now joined by anteroposterior relationship of the jaws, with the teeth reflecting this relationship—or malrelationship. Again, Angle noted:

Writers on orthodontia have long been in the habit of making use of an imaginary line, known as the "teeth in alignment" and the "line of the arch," from which to note regular and irregular alignment of the crowns of the teeth. Two lines are inferred, one for each arch. In the sixth edition the author (Angle) referred to the line of occlusion as "the line of greatest normal occlusal contact." He would now define it as being the line with which, in form and position according to type, the teeth must be in harmony, if in normal occlusion. The line of occlusion is more than the tangible and material. It may be regarded as the basic ideal of the dental apparatus, the comprehension and appreciation of which will grow in proportion as our knowledge of the science of occlusion unfolds.

This definition created the impression of a static relationship. Terminology had been greatly strengthened and was more precise, but ambiguity, especially in the concept of "normal," was still present. From the hypothesis of the constancy of the first molar and the line of occlusion, Angle developed the philosophy that it was essential to have all the teeth present in the arches if normal occlusion was the goal, and that normal facial features were possible only then. Under the influence of Wuerpel, the artist, he developed an affinity for the artistic approach. Facial beauty demanded all the teeth in normal occlusion. Orthodontics either created or destroyed facial contour. To Angle, the orthodontist molding the facial form through occlusion was an artist, even a sculptor.

MATTHEW CRYER AND CALVIN CASE

Cryer and Case, Angle's two most formidable contemporary adversaries, were quick to leap to the attack.[10, 11] Cryer had pointed out that Angle showed the straight profile of Apollo Belvedere (Fig. 4–3) as his ideal, and that the "Old Glory" skull which he chose to exemplify ideal occlusion was taken from Broomell and was the skull of a Negro male (Fig. 4–2). How could one mix a prognathic denture with an orthognathic profile? The norm concept of occlusion, then, would have to take into consideration individual variation. Case, in 1905, also took Angle to task for considering bimaxillary protrusions as normal

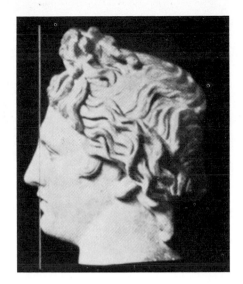

Figure 4–3 Apollo Belvedere. The ideal profile: the straight face. (Angle)

and for not recognizing individual variation (see Chap. 1, Case vignette). That Cryer and Case were correct is seen when the Broomell skull is compared with the illustration of normal occlusion used by Turner (Fig. 4–4). Wheeler shows this quite well with prognathic and retrognathic skulls, both normal (Figs. 4–5 to 4–7). But, like Angle, Case's concept of occlusion was static.[43] He wrote:

> Occlusion refers to the closure of the teeth, one upon the other; and normal dental relations, normal occlusion, and typical occlusion refer to the standard anatomical occlusion; the word normal means "according to the rule" or "that which is in conformity with the natural law."

Case accepted Angle's hypothesis of the constancy of the first molar as strongly as he rejected the fiction that "normal occlusion and normal facial lines are inseparable." He was aware of dentofacial relations, or the relations which the teeth in occlusion bear to the physiognomy. Case introduced the use of plaster casts of the face to illustrate the different kinds of facial features that go with each type of malocclusion, and particularly the profile differences that can be seen. Also, his concept of apical base was an early one, as he divided

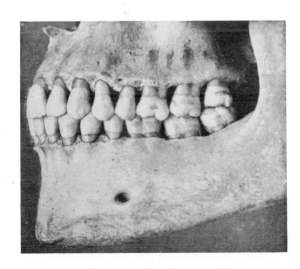

Figure 4–4 Normal occlusion (retrognathic). Such an occlusion would suit the straight face of Apollo better than Figure 4–2, the "Old Glory" of Angle. (From Anthony, L. P.: American Textbook of Prosthetic Dentistry. 7th ed. Lea & Febiger, 1942.)

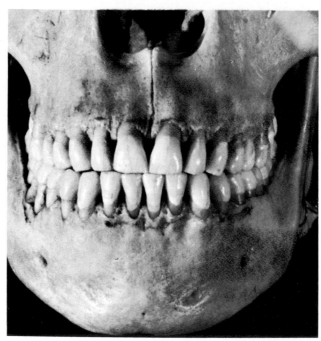

Figure 4-5 Frontal view of adult skull with normal occlusion. Considerable occlusal wear has resulted in optimal occlusal contact and a minimum of overbite. Note midline deviation and cross-bite tendency on right of skull. There is apparently more mandibular alveolar bone loss on the same side. (From Wheeler, R. C.: Textbook of Dental Anatomy and Physiology. 4th ed. W. B. Saunders Co., 1965.)

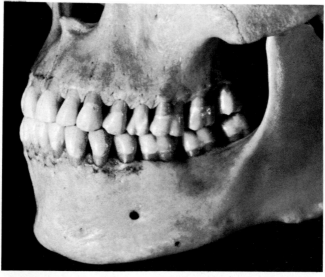

Figure 4-6 Lateral view of Figure 4-5. Overjet is practically nonexistent, a characteristic of the paleolithic dentition. Both this and the previous figure of a paleolithic dentition are considered "normal" and a treatment goal for modern man by disciples of the Begg technique. (From Wheeler, R. C.: Textbook of Dental Anatomy and Physiology. 4th ed. W. B. Saunders Co., 1965.)

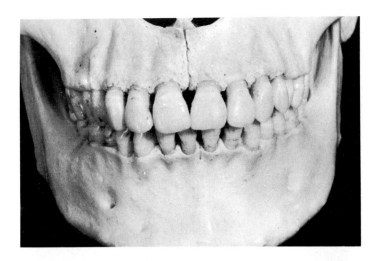

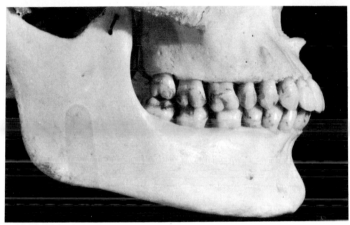

Figure 4-7   Frontal and lateral views of an adult normal occlusion. In contrast with the skull in Figure 4-6, where the teeth are quite upright, the long axes of the central incisors meet in a more acute angle. Overbite and overjet are greater here. The question to be asked here is, "Which is more normal—this skull with overjet and overbite or that of the previous illustration with neither?" Both skulls are from approximately the same time period. (From Wheeler, R. C.: Textbook of Dental Anatomy and Physiology. 4th ed. W. B. Saunders Co., 1965.)

the dentofacial area into four segments or zones of movement (Fig. 4-8). He was well aware of the role of the nose and the chin button and called attention to these features and their influence on the profile. Case advised that the terms "protrude" and "retrude" when used in reference to the relative position of the teeth should always refer to the relation they bear to the normal dentofacial position, not to the normal occlusal position. In 1908 Case again emphasized the static empiric nature of the concept of occlusion.[12] He commented:

There has been a recent effort among a certain class of orthodontists to make the word occlusion stand for a far wider scope of meaning than any of the lexicographers would think of claiming for the word. The claim is: that when the jaws are in masticating closure, it is improper to say that the teeth are in occlusion unless they close in absolute normal occlusion. And further: it is improper to say that the teeth are in normal occlusion unless the facial outline, supported by the teeth and alveolar arches, are in absolute dentofacial harmony. . . . Normal is a useful word because slight variations from the

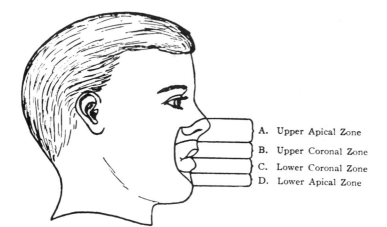

A. Upper Apical Zone

B. Upper Coronal Zone

C. Lower Coronal Zone

D. Lower Apical Zone

Figure 4–8   Zones of permanent dentition in relation to the face. Current emphasis on lip line and lip contour by Holdaway, Burstone and others, in analyzing treatment objectives, shows the importance of harmonizing tooth, bone and neuromuscular systems. (Case, C. S.: A Practical Treatise on the Technics and Principles of Dental Orthopedia. Reprinted Leo Bruder. New York, 1963.)

typical anatomical are "the rule" rather than the exception, as is well known by the difficulty which some authors find in an endeavor to find a perfect illustrative specimen of what they are pleased to term "normal occlusion" but which, per se, is an ideal anatomical occlusion.

This differentiation between normal and ideal has cropped up repeatedly since Case first mentioned it, and the question is far from being resolved today. It makes an important point. Normal is always a range in physiology and anatomy, while the ideal is a rigidly circumscribed entity that finds few examples in nature.[13, 14]

Van Loon, the Dutch physician who studied in Chicago, served as the bridge between Calvin Case and Paul Simon.[15] Van Loon used the plaster casts of the face and teeth in an anthropologic manner which Simon developed further.

Some of our greatest leaders in orthodontics at present were trained in the Angle school. But some of his categorical observations, bordering on dogma, failed the test of a good hypothesis—verification by subsequent experience and discoveries. Notable among these observations was the concept that all the teeth must be present to obtain normal facial contour.

The first suggestion of a functional analysis or a dynamic approach to occlusion came with some experiments by Bennett in 1908.[16] Bennett wrote, "Now the normal position of rest of the mandible is with the teeth slightly separated, but with the lips easily closed." He noted that the condylar movement was primarily rotatory on opening from occlusion to rest position, "and (that) it is after passing this point that the movement of the condyle seems to become rather suddenly considerable" (in other words, translatory). In 1913 Turner, writing from the standpoint of a prosthodontist, again mentioned the concept of physiologic rest.[17]

B. E. LISCHER AND PAUL SIMON

After the stimulus supplied by Case and Bennett,[9, 11] Lischer[18] and Simon tried hard to broaden the concept of occlusion by relating the teeth to the rest of the face and cranium. While Lischer's definition of occlusion was less precise than Angle's, Lischer did introduce the act of mastication as a requisite part of the definition. This was definitely a more functional approach. Simon and Lischer also related the teeth in occlusal contact to cranial and facial planes outside the denture proper. The concept of the orbital plane as a basis for

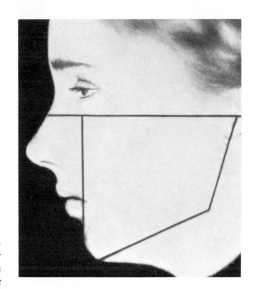

Figure 4–9 Photographs of models and facial profile, gnathostatically oriented to Frankfort horizontal plane and to Simon's orbital plane. (From Simon, P.: Fundamental Principles of a Systematic Diagnosis of Dental Anomalies. Stratford Co., 1926.)

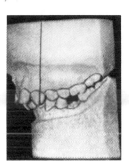

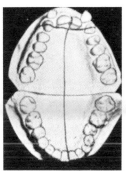

determining anteroposterior position of the denture in the face did not stand up. Stanton wrote, "The orbital law of the canine has no foundation in fact." Hellman wrote much the same thing.[19] It was not so important whether the perpendicular to the Frankfort plane at orbitale really passed through the distal third of the maxillary canine in normal occlusion. But the use of a plane outside the teeth, oriented to the anthropologic plane of Frankfort horizontal, illustrated the facial ramifications of malocclusion, outside the dental area (Figs. 4–9, 4–10). Recognition of the interdependence of teeth and occlusion, jaw relationships, craniofacial morphology and their effect on the ultimate concepts of occlusion formed the basis of the science of gnathostatics. Simon made strong representations against the acceptance of an arbitary norm standard in occlusion.[2]

Figure 4–10 Bilateral and midsagittal palatal contour of Figure 4–9 as compared with dotted outline representing predetermined "norm." (Simon)

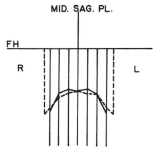

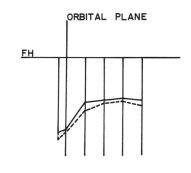

A widely prevalent attitude regards the normal as something real, or natural, something provided for us by the outer world of things. (Angle and his followers.) This is a naïve attitude, the product of a primitive mode of thought. It is also dogmatic; conclusions are reached and accepted without hesitation or verification. Another view is that of the skeptic, who also recognizes the need and justice of a norm concept. Anomalies are found everywhere . . . hence there must also be a normal. . . . But this, alas, is a delusion—all we ever find are variations; an exact, ideal normal does not exist, cannot exist. And this is our enigma; in theory we will never find the normal, in practice we forever feel its need and apply it constantly. . . . After we fully understand the constitutional and environmental influences that form the individual denture; which of these are helpful and which are injurious; which of these may be altered and which are unchangeable—then the fiction of the conception of a normal will of itself become historically useless.

Even as Bennett and Turner had been a step ahead of current dental thought, so Simon, in 1922, was to find that, while his recommended mechanical diagnostic procedures were accepted in many circles, his philosophical considerations were passed over altogether, to be resurrected 25 years later. It is well to reread his prophetic words, written over fifty years ago.

A wide experience has taught us that orthodontics does not occupy itself to any great extent with function but only with the form of dentures. . . . The part which function plays is somewhat platonic. Function is always regarded as dependent on structure, and orthodontists generally consider it as secondary. An orthodontist may urge his patients to use their dentures, especially after the corrective treatment, but he does not subject them to a functional test. He never speaks of articulation, but always of occlusion—his subject is a denture at rest, not one in action. . . . It appears as if our norm concept were undergoing a transformation—a change for the better. Heretofore we have regarded it as a fiction. But the functional norm, as the physiologist would consider it, is empirically demonstrable; it approaches reality. Here is the stepping stone to a concept of dynamic occlusion.

Simon saw an approach to a norm concept of occlusion only through biometry, or biologic statistics of variability. He outlined the anthropometric approach which makes use of biometrics. "We must grasp and employ anthropologic methods," wrote Simon. "Orthodontic methods of investigation must then approach those of craniometry and cephalometry."[2]

MILO HELLMAN

Hellman[19] saw in anthropology the same promise for method and interpretation of fact as did Simon (see Chap. 1, Hellman vignette). He drew on a wealth of material to study growth and development (Figs. 4–11, 4–12). He showed the racial variations in so-called normal occlusions. Hellman and others studied the prognathism of the human denture in relation to a cranial base. The study of selected skulls, however, despite its recognition of interdependence of the denture and the supporting craniofacial superstructure, was still primarily a static approach as far as occlusion was concerned. The anatomic description of matter-of-fact relationships and involved tables of craniometric measurements on dried skulls exploited none of the functional implications of Bennett, Turner and Simon.

Friel, at the first International Orthodontic Congress in 1926 again called attention to function. Speaking of the objectives of orthodontic treatment, he observed, "I would like for you to distinctly understand that the real objective is function, whatever that function may be, and that each orthodontist, as far

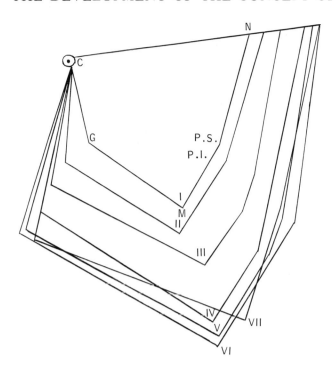

C-Condyle. G-Gonion. M-Mentum. N-Nasion. P.I.-Prosthion inferior.
P.S. - Prosthion superior

Figure 4–11 Diagrammatic representation of profile changes as the face emerges from beneath the cranium. (Hellman)

as I can determine, must decide this for himself."[20] Quite obviously, even as normal occlusion was primarily an articulator-oriented, prosthetic concept, so function was similarly conditioned in the minds of most orthodontists, with cuspal contact, interdigitation and balancing contact the most important ingredients of both. Although much lip service was being paid to facial balance and harmony, or lack of the same, it was assumed that establishment of a normal occlusion would automatically bring about proper facial contour.

FACTUAL PERIOD

There are good reasons for picking 1930 as the dividing line between the hypothetical and factual periods, between static and dynamic concepts, between ambiguous and more precise terminology. The death of Angle in this year removed a powerful sustaining influence for a concept open to some question from factual and functional points of view. In addition, B. Holly Broadbent and Hans Planer emerged in 1930, bringing a new tool of research and a broader, more physiologic approach. Broadbent introduced an accurate technique of roentgenographic cephalometry (Fig. 4–13), which eliminated most of the disadvantages of anthropologic cephalometry.[21] For the first time investigators were

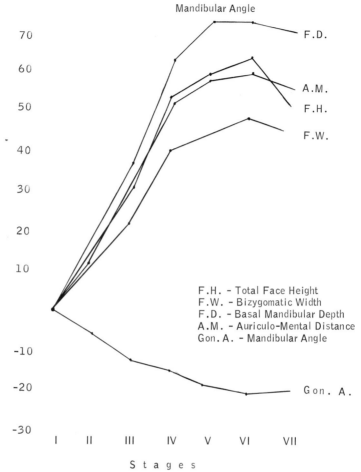

Percentage Addition and Reduction of Composite Maxima

in Height, Width, Depth, Position of Face and

Mandibular Angle

F.H. - Total Face Height
F.W. - Bizygomatic Width
F.D. - Basal Mandibular Depth
A.M. - Auriculo-Mental Distance
Gon. A. - Mandibular Angle

Stages

Figure 4–12   Dimensional changes in the face on the same time scale. Facial depth increases most, height less rapidly, and width the least. Note time-linked basis of change with concentration on Stages V and VI for greatest activity. (Hellman)

able to follow longitudinally the orofacial developmental pattern and the intricacies of tooth formation, eruption and adjustment. No longer did they have to depend on dried skulls of unknown history and of dubious ethnic origin, age and health backgrounds.

Together with the introduction of this improved method of study came a rebirth of those half-buried, prophetic words of Bennett, Turner and Simon. The factual period was to become the functional period. Planer of Vienna pointed out in 1930 that mere occlusal contact of teeth was not enough.[22] The efficiency of the masticating mechanism and its health depended on certain other fundamental considerations.

First of all, the concepts of physiologic rest position (or occlusal position) must be understood. Physiologic rest position means the resting position which is determined by muscle tone. It is constant throughout life. On the other hand, the physical or

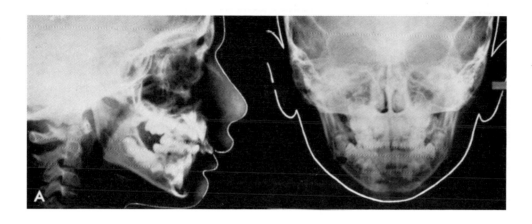

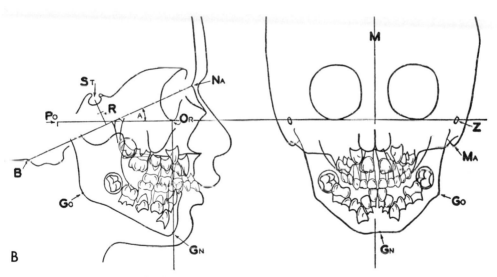

Figure 4–13   A, Standardized lateral and frontal orthodiagraphic roentgenograms oriented for tracing and measuring dentofacial structures. B, Tracings of salient structures and some of the more important landmarks. B, Bolton point; GN, Gnathion; GO, Gonion; M, Median plane; NA, Nasion; OR, Orbitale; PO, Porion; R, Registration point; ST, Sella turcica; Z, Zygomatic arch. (Courtesy B. H. Broadbent.)

occlusal position (vertical dimension) is variable and may become smaller. If all opposing teeth are lost it may disappear entirely. When the occlusal position is still normal and the bite height is therefore normal, one finds that during physiologic rest position the teeth, which otherwise meet, are slightly out of occlusion. In a normal bite the difference between the height of the bite of the two positions is slight. The amount of difference is of great diagnostic importance. When physical (or occlusal) bite height has been reduced . . . patients often complain about tiredness in chewing muscles, etc. . . . . This happens because the points of insertion of the masticating muscles are closer together. These patients often complain, too, about breakage of prosthesis (usually at the same joint), breakage of facets, and clicking of the joint.

Planer then told when bites should be opened and when they should not, depending on the amount of space between two positions. Occlusion now meant the interdigitation of teeth plus the status of the controlling musculature and functional factors. The factual period is replete with research in depth on tooth and jaw development, exemplified by the work of Moorrees, Garn, Meredith, Massler, Sicher, Dahlberg, and others.[23] A whole generation of orthodontists has been weaned on roentgenographic cephalometry, after Broadbent's 1931 report. Longitudinal assessment by objective criteria is now the theme. Chapters 2 and 3 provide fitting progress reports in this factual period. Chapter 8 describes some of the current research tools for dental arch and cephalometric studies. Electromyography, since its pioneer dental application by Moyers, brings a host of names like Carlsöö, Ahlgren, Møller, Bosma, Perry, Jarabak and others. The space-age electronic contributions of micro-miniature telemetry have stimulated literally dozens of projects by researchers like Glickman, Pameijer, Ramfjord, Cleall, Lear, Kawamura, Winders, Weinstein and others. More sophisticated radiographic techniques such as laminagraphy, with new grids, screens and films, now help break down the working hypotheses into fact or fiction. We have not reduced the unknown, but we have increased what we know, which is a healthy state of affairs for a dynamic dental profession.

The Guided Reading List, which follows Chapter 18, provides subject-headed groups of writings by those cited above, and by others. This gives the serious student an opportunity to extend his horizons of knowledge. The factual period, indeed, like a good meal, almost speaks for itself.

In the past 40 years, or since 1930, a third element of occlusion has received more attention—*the temporomandibular joint.* Through the efforts of many investigators the importance of the role of the temporomandibular articulation in relation to occlusion has been established (see Chap. 3). There is an intimate relationship between the interdigitation of the teeth, the status of the controlling musculature and the integrity of the temporomandibular joint. This relationship makes it impossible to exclude any component in the development of the present total concept of occlusion. Considerable controversy exists over the relationship of the condyle to the articular eminence and the influence on occlusion. But wide agreement exists on the concept of occlusion as a dynamic process—one which requires the aforementioned triumvirate of factors in proper relationship to each other.[41, 42]

Panoramic radiographic techniques now available should help to resolve some of the conflict by virtue of their greater ability to portray condyle-articular eminence-fossa relations more accurately than the previously nonstandardized, distorted views made with nonprofile roentgenographic techniques. These have been doomed to limited diagnostic value because of their inability to screen out superimposing and intervening structures and still show accurate anatomic relationships.[24] (Fig. 4–14).

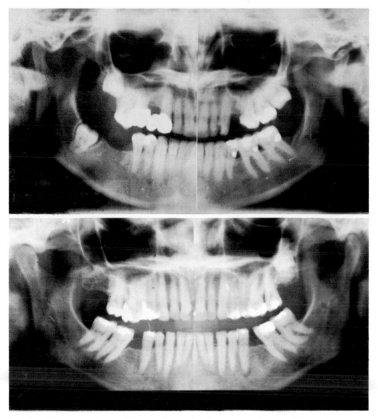

Figure 4–14 Panoramic radiographs which present excellent images of temporomandibular joints, as well as the dentition and bony support. Intervening superimpositions are eliminated by the laminagraphic process.

DYNAMIC OCCLUSION

Because of the rapid development of a broader concept of occlusion in the last 40 years, the original trends have been somewhat accentuated. Factual knowledge has largely replaced the fictional or hypothetical approach. Recognition of the roles played by muscle physiology and the temporomandibular joint has firmly entrenched the dynamic, functional concept. Controversy over a so-called "normal condylar position" is largely resolved despite the strong emphasis on gnathology and some attempts to reproduce the human jaw kinetics on the articulator. There are die-hards, of course, who neither read the current lieature nor understand muscle physiology and telemetry and who still adhere to the outdated "force it back, shove it back, drive it back" concepts. For them, the "most retruded position" in the fossa for the condyle is "normal." But Glickman, Ramfjord and co-workers, Posselt, Perry and a host of other researchers have shown conclusively that the 13 muscle attachments to the mandible provide a high degree of stability of position that occlusal equilibration and full mouth reconstruction can't change permanently, in most cases.[25-33] We have only to turn back to Chapter 3 and refresh our thought on bone and muscle conflict in the growing, living patient to know that the most likely stable position in the fossa for the condyle is that determined by those same 13 attachments, in addition to the articular capsule and tendons, the morphogenetic pattern and vertical dimension considerations. In this complex framework, overly simplified, tooth-oriented working hypotheses (working on the articulator, at least) simply do not belong in this factual age. Normality again implies a range, recognizes individual differences morphologically and functionally and is subject to modification, compensation, homeostasis and adaptation in its time-linked and developmentally linked history (see Chap. 3).

This does not mean that the accommodation is always in teeth and bone, never in muscle. Tooth contacts can cause lateral shifts and abnormal *occlusal* relationships. Tooth malpositions in addition to vertical dimension problems can cause functional protrusions or retrusions, when the teeth are brought together in habitual occlusal contact.[32] But, as Glickman's telemetry shows, since the teeth are in contact only 2 to 6 per cent of the time in 24 hours, this is a transient abnormality that often demonstrates functional compensation for a considerable period of time.[26] Centric relation, determined by the muscles, must be the dominant consideration. The challenge for the dentist is to make sure that habitual occlusion is truly centric occlusion, still in balance with the motivating musculature in three planes of space. Articulators, even the most complex ones, can provide only part of the answer. Hinge axis is a convenient starting point and a reproducible maneuver. But the applied biologist considers this only a starting point.

It has become increasingly difficult to maintain an isolated orthodontist's, periodontist's or prosthodontist's point of view. The factual knowledge of occlusion has developed so far, especially in the last decade, as to make the mechanistic concept of occlusion untenable without contributions from each field.

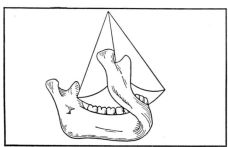

Compensating curvatures of the dental arches (curved occlusal planes).

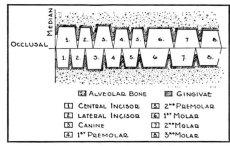

Facial relations of each tooth in one arch to its antagonist or antagonists in the opposing arch in centric occlusion.

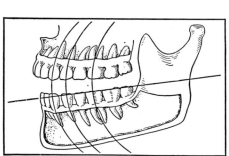

Compensating curvatures of the individual teeth (curved axes).

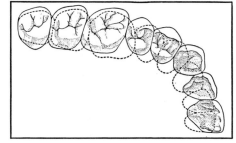

Occlusal contact and intercusp relations of all the teeth of one arch with those in the opposing arch in centric occlusion.

Figure 4–15   (From Wheeler, R. C.: Textbook of Dental Anatomy and Physiology. 4th ed. W. B. Saunders Co., 1965.)

Returning to Glickman and co-workers, the concept of centric occlusion itself has been overemphasized.[26] In their study, involving patients with and without centric pathway prematurities, telemetric monitoring showed infrequent use of centric occlusion most retruded position. Even when prematurities were eliminated, there was no increase in centric contact, either during mastication or during swallowing. Thus, the traditional concept of habitual occlusion as a detour position due to occlusal prematurities is not validated. "More of the tooth contacts during chewing were single thrusts, not glides. Side-to-side contacts along the buccal and lingual cusps and central fossa of the maxillary teeth were not regular features of chewing, but occurred consistently in bruxism." Contrary to expectations, tooth contacts were of longer duration during swallowing than chewing. However, Graf has shown that parafunctional occlusal stress (bruxism, clenching) is of even greater duration. From this type of analysis then, prematurities are of more importance in parafunctional than normal functional activities.[33]

Dempster, Adams and Duddles have made a detailed study of the arrangement of the roots of the teeth in the jaws.[34] Figures 4–16 through 4–19 show the diversity of axes of single and multirooted teeth. So called "ideal" dental arches simply do not exist. Gnathologists who glibly talk of "normal" curves of Spee, curves of Monson or the Bonwill patterns, whether it is a plane or spherical surface, should restudy their concepts in the light of this qualitative and quantitative analysis of the "hidden" parts of the dentition by Dempster and his co-workers. Like the concept of the "hinge axis," empiric and mechanistic concepts are most fallible in anatomy and physiology—though this is too often not apparent on the articulator. The variable axial inclinations should be recognized with respect to tooth migration and positional change subsequent to contiguous tooth loss. As explained in Chapter 15, the degree of autonomous adjustment in guided extraction cases is dependent in part on apical position and axial inclination. With minimum apical movement, ultimate positional changes can be predicted with reasonable accuracy, using this series of drawings.

As we seek to develop criteria for "normal" occlusion, many ingredients must be weighed. Size, shape and number of teeth, spacing, crowding, axial inclination, overbite and overjet all offer possible avenues of departure, and yet have a range, permitting compensation, if one or more factors, by themselves, are out of harmony with the overall pattern. Nature's attempt to adapt, or adjust, is dramatically evident in different facial types.

In convex profiles with prominent midface and relatively retruded upper and lower face, there is a greater anteroposterior jaw discrepancy. This is normal for this type of face and so is the labial inclination of upper and lower incisors normal, as they meet in a more acute angle. In the concave facial profile, the limits of normality are no less broad, but they encompass a range of anteroposterior jaw relationship with the maxilla seldom ahead of the mandible, and often actually behind. Axial inclinations of incisors in this type of face are more vertical, with mandibular incisors often showing lingual, axial inclination tendencies. For the concave facial type, this is "normal." Which "normal" is more "normal?" It may be that our society prefers the flat Hollywood face to the convex profile. But this is a social, not a natural standard. Equally, dental arch shape varies, even as does tooth inclination. Brachycephalic faces with broad arches are often characteristic of middle European stock. Is this more normal than the dolichocephalic facial type, the long, lean drink of water,

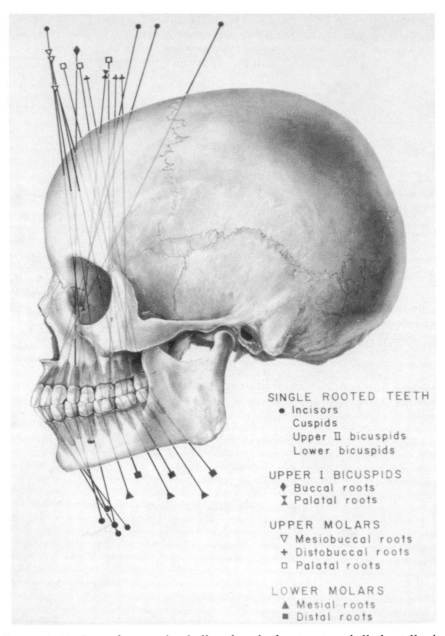

SINGLE ROOTED TEETH
- Incisors
  Cuspids
  Upper Ⅱ bicuspids
  Lower bicuspids

UPPER I BICUSPIDS
- ◆ Buccal roots
- Ⅰ Palatal roots

UPPER MOLARS
- ▽ Mesiobuccal roots
- + Distobuccal roots
- ▫ Palatal roots

LOWER MOLARS
- ▲ Mesial roots
- ▪ Distal roots

Figure 4–16   Lateral view of a skull with orthodontic wires drilled axially through the roots of the teeth and on through to the exterior, showing the variable orientation of the different axes. The code for the wires refers to the different roots. (From Dempster, W. T., Adams, W. J., and Duddles, R. A.: Arrangement in the jaws of the roots of the teeth. J.A.D.A., 67:779–797, 1963.)

epitomized by the Englishman, with long, narrow arches? As Altemus has shown (see Chap. 5) racial and ethnic variations are profound.[35] The normal occlusions of a young Black and a young Oriental differ greatly according to position in the face, shape, size and position of the jaws, draping of the musculature, size and function of the tongue, size, shape, position of the teeth and so forth.

If we introduce age and sex variables, this is still another assault on our attempt to set up arbitrary standards of normality. Deciduous teeth are more upright and have more anterior overbite. Early mixed dentition shows more labial inclination and more overbite in many cases. By 12 years of age, most girls have achieved a relatively stable occlusion, not likely to be affected materially by significant increments of lower face growth. This is not true for boys, who

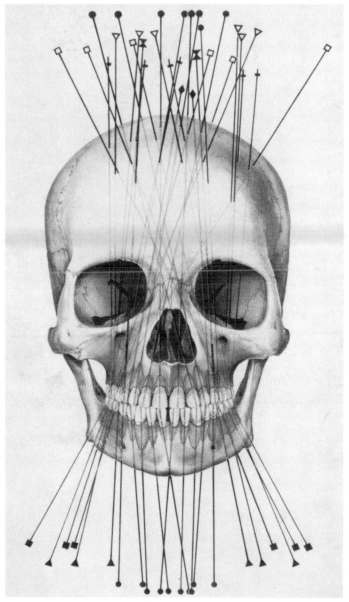

Figure 4–17   The relative orientation of the long axes of the roots of the teeth as seen in an anterior view of the same skull as shown in Figure 4–16. Coding for roots is same as previous illustration. (From Dempster, W. T., Adams, W. J., and Duddles, R. A.: Arrangement in the jaws of the roots of the teeth. J.A.D.A., 67:779–797, 1963.)

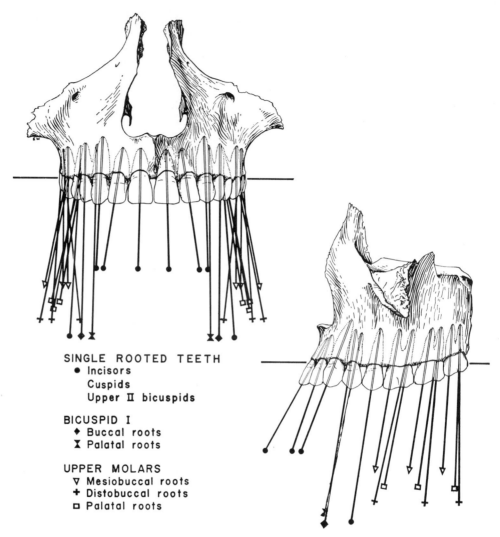

Figure 4-18 Composite illustration of the maxilla and the upper teeth as seen from the anterior and lateral aspects, showing the average arrangement of teeth. As with the mandible, the axial inclinations are of average values, derived from the means of right and left sides of 11 jaws. The long axes of the roots of the teeth have been extended beyond the crowns and are shown in orthographic projection. Same code for roots as in Figure 4-17. (From Dempster, W. T., Adams, W. J., and Duddles, R. A.: Arrangement in the jaws of the roots of the teeth. J.A.D.A., 67:779–797, 1963.)

still have major horizontal growth potential for the mandible, with further reduction of overbite and likelihood of mandibular incisor retropositioning and crowding (see Chap. 2). The mesial change in molar occlusion is twice that of girls.[44]

Since the habitual occlusal relationship is so variable, despite the historically evident attempts to use it solely to establish stomatognathic normality, it is obvious that the remaining components of orofacial integrity should be analyzed. The teeth are in occlusal contact only 2 to 6 per cent of the time (and even then, not in centric occlusion). Therefore, 94 per cent of the time, at least, they are apart. The largest segment of time is in postural rest position, determined by the musculature. This relationship is relatively less variable and less likely to reflect the vagaries of environmental assault (see Chap. 3). Postural rest position is a good place to start in an assessment of the *vertical* status and harmony of orofacial features.[36] The three dimensionality of normality is apparent. Plaster casts, clasped together in habitual occlusion, allow only sagittal and transverse study, and are incomplete.[44]

If a central occlusal position is so variable and if vertical maxillomandibular relationship is as important as anteroposterior relationship, what further role does the musculature play? Teeth may appear to meet properly, but if there is hypermobility, if the periodontal membrane is thickened, if the labial and

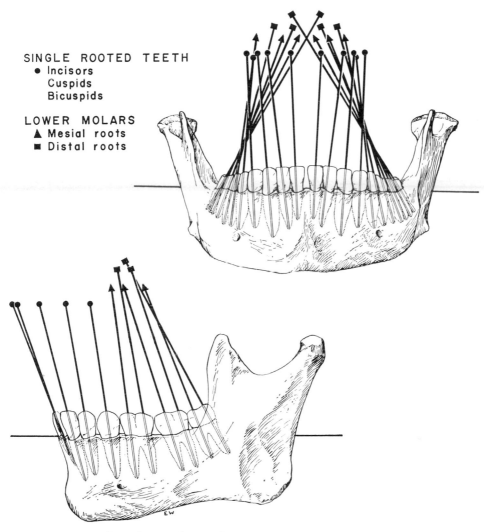

SINGLE ROOTED TEETH
● Incisors
  Cuspids
  Bicuspids

LOWER MOLARS
▲ Mesial roots
■ Distal roots

Figure 4–19 Complete orthographic projection of the mandibular teeth as seen has been averaged. The root axes have been extended beyond the crowns to emphasize the alveolar bone. The angulation of the roots of the left and right sides of 11 jaws have been averaged. The root axes have been extended beyond the crowns to emphasize the angular pattern. (From Dempster, W. T. Adams, W. J., and Duddles, R. A.: Arrangement in the jaws of the roots of the teeth. J.A.D.A., 67:779–797, 1963.)

lingual muscle forces are jiggling the teeth and if there are parafunctional stresses like bruxism, this is not a normal occlusion. A thorough muscle or functional analysis is essential. It may be difficult if not impossible to distinguish between normal and abnormal because of the ability of nature to adapt, compensate and adjust.

Completion of the functional analysis requires a status check of the temporomandibular joint. This subject is covered in more detail in Chapter 3, and temporomandibular joint disturbances are outlined and discussed from a therapeutic standpoint in Chapter 16. It would be a serious omission to leave out an examination of the temporomandibular joint from a functional point of view, if we wish to include most important contributing elements of normal occlusion. Clicking, crepitus, limited opening, muscle spasm, compensatory muscle activity, asymmetrical opening and closing maneuvers and pain are all possible, singly or in combination and affect the occlusion.[38] In this "factual era" of development of the concepts of occlusion, in which we use sophisticated armamentaria and make a functional analysis, it is important to see that there is no temporomandibular joint pathology.

As with so many things, progress has taken us farther from the answer than we seemed to be 70 years ago, How easy it was to look at "Old Glory" and say, "Ah, this is normal!" Now we arbitrarily set up at least three components of occlusion and know that there are at least twice that in modifying factors.

1. The occlusal position, or tooth contact position. Centric occlusion is not seen in nature as often as on the articulator or in the mounting of the orthodontists pretty white plaster models on the shelf. Masticatory habit patterns, tooth inclinations and malpositions, size and shape of teeth, functional premature contacts, faulty restorations, tooth loss, basal bone dysplasias, and the inherent stability or instability of the periodontal structures all affect the occlusal position.

2. The postural resting position. The status of the controlling musculature is important in all three dimensions and a significant factor in occlusal dynamics a major part of the time.

3. The temporomandibular joint. It is a part of the functional complex, with long-range as well as immediate effects on the integrity of the stomatognathic system.

The designation of normal depends on assessment of each of the three elements, singly and in combination. The "clincher" is the health of each element. Teeth that are healthy, even if malaligned, with healthy investing tissues, normally functioning musculature and no temporomandibular joint pathology go a long way toward being normal.[14, 37] Anything less than this is hard to defend.

REFERENCES

1. Brown, T.: Developmental aspects of occlusion. Ann. Aust. Coll. Dent. Surg., 2:61–67, 1969.
2. Simon, P.: Fundamental Principles of a Systematic Diagnosis of Dental Anomalies. Translated by B. E. Lischer. Boston, Stratford Co. 1926.
3. Fuller, J.: Popular Essay on the Structure, Formation and Management of the Teeth. London, Sherwood, Neeley & Jones, 1810.
4. Clark, J. P.: A Practical and Familiar Treatise on Teeth and Dentism. London, A. W. Webster, 1836.
5. Imrie, W.: The Parents' Dental Guide: Being a Succinct Treatise on the Diseases of the Teeth and Gums. London, Churchill, 1841.
6. Kingsley, N.: A Treatise on Oral Deformities, with Appropriate Preventive and Remedial Treatment. New York, D. Appleton & Co., 1880.
7. Talbot, E. S.: Irregularities of the Teeth and Their Treatment. Philadelphia, S. S. White Manufacturing Co., 1903.
8. Angle, E. H.: Classification of malocclusion. D. Cosmos, 41:248, 1899.

9. Angle, E. H.: Treatment of Malocclusion of the Teeth. 7th ed. Philadelphia, S. S. White Manufacuring Co., 1907.

10. Cryer, M.: Typical and atypical occlusion of teeth. D. Cosmos, 46:713, 1904.

11. Case, C.: Principles of occlusion and dentofacial relations. D. Items Int., 27:489, 1905.

12. Case, C.: A Practical Treatise on the Technics and Principles of Dental Orthopedia. Chicago, C. S. Case & Co., 1908.

13. Poulton, D. R.: An orthodontic view of normal occlusion. J. Calif. Dent. Ass., (Spring Scientific Issue) 27:2–10, 1969.

14. Hopkins, J. B., and Murphy, J.: Variations in good occlusions. Angle Orthodont., 41:44–65, 1971.

15. Van Loon, C.: Neue Method zur Festellung normaler Bezeihungen der Zähne zu den Gesichtslinien. Z. Zahnheilk. 18:18–39, 1916.

16. Bennett, N. G.: A contribution to the study of movements of the mandible. Proc. Roy. Soc. Med., 1:79, 1908.

17. Turner, C. R.: American Textbook of Prosthetic Dentistry. Philadelphia, Lea & Febiger, 1913.

18. Lischer, B. E.: Principles and Methods of Orthodontics. Philadelphia, Lea & Febiger, 1912.

19. Hellman, M.: The face and teeth of man. J. Dent. Res., 9:179, 1929.

20. Friel, S.: Occlusion. Observations on its development from infancy to old age. Int. J. Orthodont., 13:322–334, 1927.

21. Broadbent, B. H.: A new x-ray technique and its application to orthodontics. Angle Orthodont., 1:45, 1931.

22. Planer, H.: Die Bisshöhe. Z. Stomatol., 28:284, 1930.

23. Moorrees, C. F. A., Burstone, C. J., Christiansen, R. L., Hixon, E. H., and Weinstein, S.: Research related to malocclusion. Am. J. Orthodont., 59:1–18, 1971.

24. Graber, T. M.: Diagnosis and panoramic radiography. Am. J. Orthodont., 53:799–821, 1967.

25. Glickman, I., Pameijer, J. H. N., Roeber, F., and Brion, M. A. M.: Functional occlusion as revealed by miniaturized radio transmitters. D. Clin. North America, 13:667–679, 1969.

26. Glickman, I., Pameijer, J. H. N., and Roeber, F.: Intraoral occlusal telemetry. II. Registration of tooth contacts in chewing and swallowing by intraoral electric telemetry. J. Prosth. Dent., 19:151, 1968.

27. Scharer, P., Stallard, R. E., and Zander, H. A.: Occlusal interferences and mastication: an electromyographic study. J. Prosth. Dent., 17:438, 1967.

28. Scott, I., and Ash, M. M.: A six-channel intraoral transmitter for measuring occlusal forces. J. Prosth. Dent., 16:56, 1966.

29. Ramfjord, S. P., and Hiniker, J. J.: Distal displacement of the mandible. J. Prosth. Dent., 16: 491–502, 503–512, 1966.

30. Posselt, U.: The Physiology of Occlusion and Rehabilitation. 2nd ed. Philadelphia, F. A. Davis Co., 1968.

31. Perry, H. T. Jr.: Principles of occlusion applied to modern orthodontics. D. Clin. North America, 13:581–590, 1969.

32. Beyron, H.: Optimal occlusion. D. Clin. North America, 13:537–554, 1969.

33. Graf, H.: Bruxism. D. Clin. North America, 13:659–666, 1969.

34. Dempster, W. T., Adams, W. J., and Duddles, R. A.: Arrangement in the jaws of the roots of the teeth. J.A.D.A., 67:779–797, 1963.

35. Altemus, L. A.: A comparison of cephalofacial relationships. Angle Orthodont., 30:123–140, 1960.

36. Garnick, J. J., and Ramfjord, S. P.: Rest position. An electromyographic and clinical investigation. J. Prosth. Dent., 12:895–911, 1962.

37. Fastlicht, J.: Crowding of mandibular incisors. Am. J. Orthodont., 58:156–163, 1970.

38. Crum, R. J., and Loiselle, R. J.: Temporomandibular joint symptoms and ankylosing spondylitis. J.A.D.A., 83:630–638, 1971.

39. Leighton, B. C.: Cases illustrating spontaneous changes in the dental arches during the first nine years of life. Dent. Pract., 14:86, 1963.

40. Leighton, B. C.: The value of prophecy in orthodontics. Dent. Pract., 21:359–372, 1971.

41. Corbett, N. E., DeVincenzo, J. P., Huffer, R. A., and Shryock, E. F.: The relation of the condylar path to the articular eminence in mandibular protrusion. Angle Orthodont., 41:286–292, 1971.

42. Droel, R., and Isaacson, R. J.: Some relationships between the glenoid fossa position and various skeletal discrepancies. Am. J. Orthodont., 61:64–78, 1972.

43. Jacobsen, A.: Attrition of teeth in the South African Bantu. Am. J. Orthodont. (in press).

44. Paulsen, H. U.: Changes in sagittal molar occlusion during growth. Tandlaegebladet, 75:1258–67, 1971.

45. Sanin, C., and Savara, B. S.: The development of an excellent occlusion. Am. J. Orthodont., 61:345–352, 1972.

46. Andrews, L. F.: The six keys to normal occlusion. Am. J. Orthodont., 62:296–309, 1972.

47. Storey, E.: Growth and remodelling of bone and bones. Am. J. Orthodont., 62:142–165, 1972.

chapter 5

INCIDENCE AND RECOGNITION OF MALOCCLUSION

While dental caries has been regarded as the major dental disease throughout the world, malocclusion is a close runner-up. With fluoridation, there is a good chance for significant reduction or even elimination of caries as a problem. The morphogenetic nature of most malocclusions assures us that this dentofacial problem will continue to demand the best that dentistry can offer for a long time, indeed.

Various studies have been done in an attempt to make an epidemiologic registration of malocclusion.[1-5, 9, 10, 44] Myllärniemi has compiled the reported prevalences in mixed or permanent dentitions in Table 5–1, the Angle classification distribution in mixed and permanent dentitions in Table 5–2 and the prevalence of malocclusion in deciduous dentitions in Table 5–3.[6] The diversity of figures is obvious. The criteria for normal occlusion are highly variable. Angle's classification, which is described in detail later on in this chapter, seems to be the only common denominator, and it is admittedly circumscribed and perhaps too idealistically oriented for a broad population study. It is interesting to note, however, that in 1609 children studied, 20 per cent of the deciduous dentitions had malocclusion, 39 per cent of the mixed dentitions were in the malocclusion category, and 58 per cent of the sample in the permanent dentition had malocclusion. No difference was noted according to sex. The most prevalent type of malocclusion in the deciduous dentitions was anterior open bite, tied in with tongue thrust and finger habits, and Class II, Division 1 (mandibular retrusion) was next. In the mixed dentitions, crowding was most common, with mandibular retrusion second. In the permanent dentitions, Class II, Division 1 and crowding were equally distributed.

Björk and Helm found that about half of over 5000 Danish school children needed treatment, with the incidence of malocclusion greater, or about 75 per cent. In a related study, they compiled seven young adult male ethnic groups—Danish, Chinese, Bantu, Australian aborigine, Quechua, Japanese and Navajo.[4, 7–9] The frequencies of specific malocclusion characteristics are summarized in Table 5–4. The significant differences in various malocclusion traits

TABLE 5–1 REPORTED PREVALENCES OF MALOCCLUSION IN MIXED DENTITION OR IN PERMANENT DENTITION

AUTHOR(s)		SAMPLE			MAL-OCCLUSION PREVALENCE (per cent)
		Nationality	*Size*	*Age*	
Hellman	1921	American Long Beach	546	10–15	69.6
Korkhaus	1928	German Bonn	1000	14	55.4
Taylor	1935	Australian	129	12–15	66.6
Massler and Frankel	1951	American Cicero, Ill.	2758	14–18	78.8
Newman	1956	American Newark, N.J.	3355	6–13	51.9
Mills	1966	American Suitland, Md.	1455	13–14	82.5
Popovich and Grainger	1959	Canadian Burlington	300	12	88.0
Goose et al.	1957	English, urban and rural children	1588	7–15	urban 49.8 rural 37.9
Miller and Hobson	1961	English Manchester	199	14	38.5
Biljstra	1958	Dutch Groeningen	940	school children	66.5
Andrik	1954	Slovakia Bratislava	2509	10–15	49.0
Gergely	1958	Hungarian 3 towns	3087	15–20	48.0
Telle	1951	Norwegian Hedmark	2349	7–8	58.7
Helm	1968	Danish North Zealand	1700	9–18	boys 79.1 girls 77.9
Tewari	1966	Indian Chandigarh	2124	6–12	38.0

TABLE 5–2 REPORTED PREVALENCES OF ANGLE'S THREE MALOCCLUSION CLASSES IN MIXED AND IN PERMANENT DENTITIONS

AUTHOR(s)		CLASS I	CLASS II	CLASS II$_1$	CLASS II$_2$	CLASS III
		Prevalences (per cent)				
Korkhaus	1928	26.8	25.8	—	—	1.0
Anti-Wuorinen	1932	66	13.5	—	—	3.5
Taylor	1935	48	—	10.1	5	2.9
Brandhorst	1946	46.9	31	—	—	3.1
Seipel	1946	—	10	—	—	4
Björk	1947	—	—	14.6	4.5	2.8
Telle	1951	30.1	21.3	—	—	7.3
Massler and Frankel	1951	51.2	—	16.7	2.7	9.4
Andrik	1954	34.0	14.4	8.4	2.3	1.2
Haralabakis	1957	36.3	23	—	—	2.5
Gergely	1958	35.9	—	6	7	1.1
Popovich and Grainger	1959	56.2	29	—	—	1.8
Tewari	1966	14	15	—	—	9
Helm	1968	58	24	—	—	4.2

—indicates no figure reported.

TABLE 5–3 REPORTED PREVALENCES OF MALOCCLUSION IN THE DECIDUOUS DENTITION

AUTHOR(S)		SAMPLE			MALOCCLUSION PREVALENCE (per cent)
		Nationality	*Size*	*Age*	
Chiavaro	1915	Italian	1000	3–6	28.9
Ainsworth and Young	1925	English	2170	2–6	32.5–19.4
Plaetschke	1938	German	1000	2–6	50.2
Pedersen	1944	Danish	720	2–5	14.6–21.0
Cohen and Green	1954	American	443	4–5	34.5
Popovich and Grainger	1959	Canadian	300	3	66.1
Miller and Hobson	1961	English	291	4–5	20.0–18.5
Moller	1963	Icelandic	486	2–5	17.2–20.0–17.4

(Tables 5–1, 5–2, 5–3 from Myllärniemi, S.: Malocclusion in Finnish rural children. An epidemiological study of different stages of dental development. Doctoral thesis, Center for Study of Child Growth and Development, University of Helsinki, 1970.)

TABLE 5–4 REPORTED PREVALENCES OF MALOCCLUSION IN DIFFERENT ETHNIC GROUPS AND PEOPLES LIVING UNDER PRIMITIVE CONDITIONS

AUTHOR(S)		SAMPLE			MALOC-CLUSION	CLASS I	CLASS II	CLASS III
		Nationality	*Size*	*Age*	*Prevalences (per cent)*			
Newman	1952	Greenland Eskimos	55	adults	41.8	36.4	0	5.4
			40	6–17	56.4	53.8	0	2.6
Thomsen	1955	Tristan da Cunha	117	adults	15	—	9	6
Moorrees	1957	Aleuts	107	adults	—	—	0	13.2
Sweeney and Guzman	1966	Guatemala Highland Indians	442	6–14	37	—	—	—
Grewe et al.	1968	Red Lake Reservation Indians, Minn., USA	651	6–18	66.4	54	9.5	2.9
Mehta	1969	Shell mound Indian skulls Al., USA	25	adults	some crowding, no occlusal anomalies			
Coulin	1956	New Guinea Papua Negrids	1085	3–50	62	—	5.5	—
Davies	1956	Puka-Puka Polynesians	472	3–70	35.6	19.7	3.8	12.1
Monzon et al.	1965	Filipinos males	522	adults	8	—	—	—
Houpt et al.	1967	Ghana Negroes	271	4–18	38.6	—	1.2	1.3
Begg	1965	≫Stone Age Man≫ skulls Australian aborigines	800	adults	70	54	13	2.3
Jacobson	1967	South African Bantu skulls	460	adults	—	—	2.7	0.7

—indicates no figure reported.

emphasizes the broad diversity of categories of malocclusion. The Danes, for example, showed the deepest overbite, the most frequent Class II pattern and the greatest occlusal anomalies in the incisor region. The Japanese, however, were not far behind, actually showing more maxillary incisor protrusion. Generally, the primitive groups showed the least malocclusion characteristics.[43] Very little Class III tendencies were seen, and then only in the Chinese and Danes. Crowding afflicted Navajo and Japanese most, but the Danes showed the highest incidence of the dentitional type of malocclusion, as well as basal malocclusion groups. From the various epidemiologic studies, it seems valid to conclude that the Caucasian segment of the population in the United States would show approximately the same percentages as those of the Danes. In the United States a greater incidence of mandibular retrusion is seen, and there are fewer cases of mandibular prognathism. It has been estimated by orthodontists in this country that approximately two thirds of the patients that undergo treatment have mandibular retrusion characteristics. Only 2 to 3 per cent exhibit mandibular protrusion. However, it should be emphasized that this dominance of mandibular retrusions in orthodontic practices does not reflect the total population ratio of malocclusion types. From all indications, the majority of malocclusions seem to be Class I, with crowding as the major malocclusion characteristic.[10] Problems of crowding or spacing of teeth, however, occur in patients with normal jaw relationship as well as those with retruding or protruding mandibular relationships. One of the biggest problems in making a precise estimate of the percentage of malocclusion in our population is the fact that no definitive criteria have been established for normal occlusion, as opposed to ideal occlusion. If by normal we mean "the usual," then there are many characteristics that create a malocclusion by combination with other characteristics, or as only a matter of degree. (Overjet, overbite, basal relationship, crowding, cross-bite, functional prematurities, etc., are discussed in more detail in Chap. 4.) The complexities of hereditary transmission of the characteristics of malocclusion and the exact results of racial admixtures are fertile fields

Figure 5–1 Proportionality of the average Caucasian face expressing the harmony of parts. (After A. M. Schwarz.)

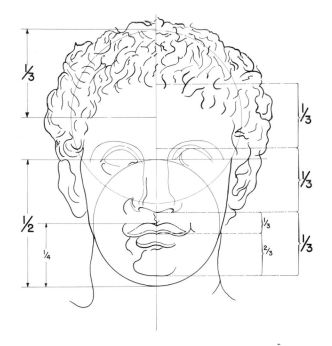

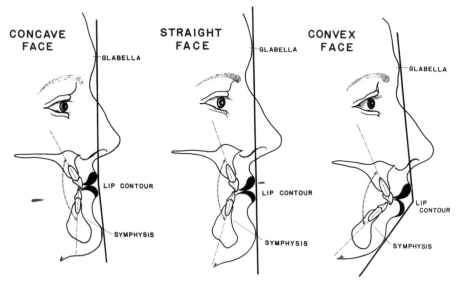

Figure 5–2 Concave, straight and convex profiles. The anterior limits of maxilla and mandible form a straight line that parallels the forehead-lip-chin profile line in the straight face in the center. In the convex face on the right, the maxilla is protruded and mandible retruded in their relationships. The incisor axial inclinations reflect this basal relationship change and are more procumbent.

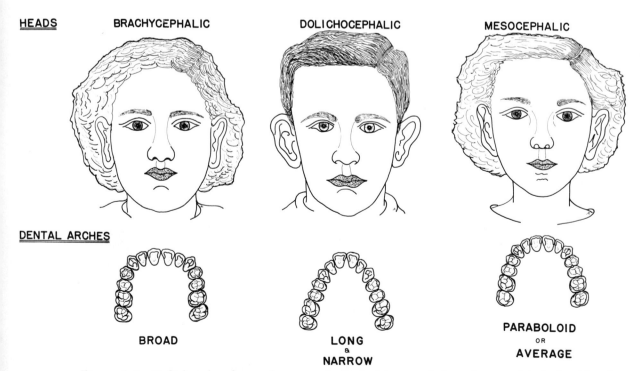

Figure 5–3 Dolicho-, brachy- and mesocephalic facial types; below, the most likely dental arch form that goes with each facial type.

for further study before any exact information can be given. The role of heredity will be discussed in greater detail in Chapter 6, Etiology of Malocclusion.

Facial type as well as racial type must be considered. To the artist, the average Caucasian face has a definite proportionality (Fig. 5–1). In the concave or straight face, arch or jaw relationship is less frequently of concern than problems of arch length deficiency (Fig. 5–2). When there is a maxillomandibular malrelationship in the straight face, it is more frequently mandibular prognathism. In the convex or forward divergent face, an anteroposterior basal discrepancy is more frequently present, and there is a higher incidence of mandibular retrusion. Dolichocephalic individuals have long narrow faces and relatively narrow dental arches (Fig. 5–3). Brachycephalic individuals have very broad and relatively short faces and broad, round dental arches. Meso-

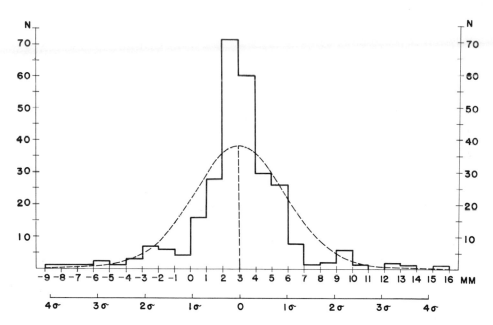

Figure 5–4 Distribution of overjet in a young male population sample compared with the normal probability curve. (From Bjork, A.: The Face in Profile. Svensk. Tandlak, T., Suppl. 40, 1947.)

cephalic individuals fit somewhere in between these two. Malocclusions may vary with the facial type. However, it must not be assumed that narrow arches inevitably go with narrow faces and broad arches with broad faces. Despite the general trend in this direction, clinical examination frequently will reveal exceptions and gradations in the degree of narrowness or broadness of dental arches, as correlated with facial type. Some anthropologists would claim that there are so many exceptions to this trend that the observation has only limited value.

It can be assumed, however, that, in a large population sample, a specific characteristic of occlusion, such as overbite, will show a normal statistical distribution. The greatest percentage of individuals will be clustered around the mean. A graphic illustration is that of Björk, showing the amount of overjet in 281 Swedish conscripts, as compared with the normal probability curve.[11] Obviously, by far the greatest number is clustered around the mean (Fig. 5–4). Statistically, it is rather easy to predict where a person will most likely fit with respect to the rest of the population. For instance, the width of the maxillary central incisors varies from 6.5 to 10.5 mm. in a large group. If the population distribution is normal, most individuals will cluster around the mean of 8.5 mm. If the sample is analyzed statistically and a standard deviation is worked out for the group, two thirds of the entire sample will fall within a range of one standard deviation on either side of the mean. In this particular instance, then, two thirds of the people would have central incisors measuring from 8 to 9 mm. And even though the range may be from 6.5 to 10.5 mm., 95.5 per cent of all the people will have central incisors measuring from 7.5 to 9.5 mm. in width.

ARCH FORM

As has been indicated, there is apparently some relationship between facial type and dental arch form. But what is "normal" for a particular individual? This question has interested dentists since 1885 when Bonwill attempted to establish certain postulates for constructing artificial dentures. He noted that the tripod shape of the mandible formed an equilateral triangle, with the base between the condyles and the apex between the central incisors. The average length of the sides was 4 inches, with a variation of never more than ¼ inch. Bonwill emphasized the principle that human anatomy is in "perfect consonance with geometry, physics and mechanics . . . . If nature is given a fair chance to right herself, she will return to the normal standard of mathematical and mechanical precision; to do otherwise would annihilate creation."[12] Hawley, in 1904, modified the Bonwill approach, and recommended that the combined widths of the six anterior teeth serve as the radius of a circle, and the teeth be placed on that circle. From this circle, he constructed an equilateral triangle, with the base representing the intercondylar width.[13] This construction was to serve as a guide for establishing arch form, though not an absolute orthodontic treatment objective. Angle recognized the parabolic curve of the arch, but considered the Hawley arch predetermination only an approximation. "The best the orthodontist can do is to secure normal relations of the teeth and correct general form of the arch, leaving the finer adjustment to individual typal form to be worked out by Nature through her forces which must, in any event, finally triumph."[14]

Other attempts have been made since then to establish methods of arch predetermination by Williams, Stanton and Gilpatric.[15-17] Stanton concluded, after years of investigation that he could define normal occlusion as follows:

1. Outer cusps and incisal edges lie on a smooth curve.
2. Arch forms are open and closed curves, that is, ellipse, parabola, cubic parabola, "horseshoe" and parallel sides.
3. Most human arches vary within 5 mm. in width (one side from midpalatal suture).
4. Most human arches vary within 13 mm. in length (from buccal groove to upper incisal edge).[16]

Izard felt that existing arch predetermination methods did not take into account the natural variability of the arch and that occlusion does not govern arch form.[18] He advocated use of facial dimensions, setting up a constant ratio of arch width and facial depth. Seventy-five per cent of arches could be described by an ellipse, 20 per cent by a parabola, and only 5 per cent by a "U" or square shape. Izard used bizygomatic width and auriculo-incisal distance to establish ellipses for arch form. Meredith and Higley, however, could not confirm this facial width and arch form conclusion.[19] Descriptions of arch form have been validated by subsequent research of MacConnaill and Scher, Wheeler, Sved, Scott, Burdi and Lillie, and others[20-24] The catenary chain or curve seems to express the basic form of the human arch.

Currier using radiographs of plaster casts, delineated the dental arch morphology with the aid of a computer.[25] His analysis showed that the ellipse provided a better fit (smaller variance) for the maxillary arch and mandibular circumferences than a parabola. The parabola served better for the maxillary and mandibular middle curve than an ellipse. Since the outer (facial) or circumference of buccal and labial surfaces is of greater concern to orthodontists, the ellipse was considered a better guide for arch form than the parabola. Neither parabola nor ellipse exhibited a significant fit to the inner or lingual curve of upper and lower dental arches.

It would appear from mathematical interpretation that the dental arch is amenable to computerized analysis. This, together with the development of computerized cephalometrics, promises increased accuracy and objectivity in diagnosis and greater likelihood of attaining the greatest potential of orthodontic therapy.

VARIATIONS IN SIZE, FORM, NUMBER AND POSITION OF TEETH

Unfortunately, the classic illustrations of a skull with perfect occlusion or an artificial plastic reproduction of teeth set in perfect alignment are only infrequently duplicated in nature. If we accept as one definition of "normal" the implication of predominance, we might justifiably say that malocclusion is normal. Certainly, minor irregularities (such as rotated teeth, excessive overbite or overjet) exist in most individuals. Why is this so? There are a number of possibilities. These will be discussed in greater detail in Chapters 6 and 7.

SIZE OF TEETH

The most common and most obvious possibilities are variations in the size and shape of the teeth themselves. Teeth, like individuals, vary in size. A large

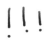

person will usually have large hands, large feet and a large head, but the same correlation does not necessarily follow as far as the teeth are concerned. Tooth size does not seem to be tied to stature. It is sex-linked, however, with males having larger teeth than females.

The orthodontist is often impressed by the fact that a young and rather smallish patient may come in with maxillary central incisors that are obviously much too large for the face. In most instances, if the incisors are large the rest of the teeth are likely to be larger than normal, but this does not always follow. There are many patients who have large central incisors and small and even peg-shaped maxillary lateral incisors, and who may or may not have large premolar teeth. Even as there is no marked correlation between the size of the teeth and the size of the individual, there often seems to be no correlation between the size of the teeth and the size of the jaws. The incisor teeth usually appear to be too great for the face. However, it should be noted that although the teeth do not change in size after they have erupted, a child of 8 years still has ahead of him considerable facial growth, particularly growth in facial height.

Racial variations in tooth size do exist, as Altemus has shown.[26] Eighty Negro children, 40 boys and 40 girls, were analyzed with regard to maxillary and mandibular tooth size, amount of tooth material, premolar coronal and basal arch width, and arch length. As the table below shows, the amount of tooth material is greater, the first premolar basal and coronal arch width is greater, and the basal arch length longer for the Negro children when compared with Caucasian children of the same age.[27] The analysis and mean measurements, developed by Ashley Howes, serve as the basis for comparison.[28]

Many an orthodontist will tell his patient, "you have large teeth and small jaws." Or, "you have a five room house on a four room foundation." Undoubtedly, complex hereditary factors are involved here and it is not possible to ascertain all the reasons for these discrepancies at present. Quite probably it is possible to inherit tooth size from one parent and jaw size from another. Certainly it is possible to inherit facial characteristics, and it would seem that dental morphology relationships are often associated. Large teeth and small jaws or small teeth and large jaws can create malocclusions.

Through the years orthodontists and now, more and more dentists in general practice uninformed in basic growth and developmental principles have learned by bitter experience that it is not possible to expand the dental arches and "straighten" the teeth, disregarding the amount of bone supporting the

TABLE 5–5.   RACIAL VARIATION IN TOOTH SIZE*

	TOOTH MATERIAL (TM)	1st BICUSPID CORONAL ARCH WIDTH (BCAW)	BCAW TM	1st BICUSPID BASAL ARCH WIDTH (BBAW)	BBAW TM	BASAL ARCH LENGTH (BAL)	BAL TM
Maxillary Arch							
Howes	91.7	41.6	45.5	43.8	47.7	32.4	35.4
Altemus	106.1	44.1	41.6	46.8	44.2	40.0	37.9
Mandibular Arch							
Howes	84.1	33.9	40.5	39.9	47.1	31.4	37.1
Altemus	97.6	36.2	37.1	40.5	41.5	38.3	39.2

*Howes' data is for Caucasian children; Altemus' data is for Negro children.

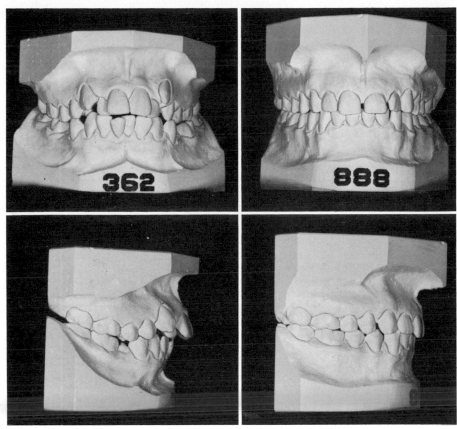

Figure 5–5   Plaster casts of two 12-year-old girls with the same size teeth. The two girls are approximately the same size, weight and build. Both are of Scandinavian ancestry. The occlusion of both parents is within normal limits; although, in the cast on the right, the mother of the girl has small dental arches and smaller teeth.

teeth. Inevitably, muscular and functional forces start to work immediately and re-establish tooth positions that are in harmony with available space in the jaw and with function. A good illustration of the importance of size is seen in Figure 5–5 where two individuals of the same age and with the same size teeth show a marked difference in the position of the teeth. In the cast on the left, there is not enough supporting bone to accommodate the teeth in their normal position. In most instances it is futile to expect growth and development to change this situation significantly. Changes in muscle function, where there has been abnormal lip and tongue activity associated with mastication and deglutition, may permit certain changes. But if muscle function is already normal, any therapeutic change in arch form or arch size after 12 years of age should be looked upon with trepidation.

FORM OF TEETH

Intimately related to the size of the teeth is their shape. As we know, incisors, like shoes, come in all shapes and sizes. The role of heredity is again important. The shape of things to come is determined at the moment of conception. Difference in race may mean differences in tooth shape. For the child of Japanese parents it is likely that the upper centrals will be strongly concave on the lingual side, with marked marginal ridges and an accentuated cingulum. For the youngsters born of native parents in central Africa it is likely that the central incisors will be broad and flat with a smooth lingual surface. Because of the heterogeneity of our American population many possibilities in tooth shape exist. The central incisors may be flat or partly curved, with the labial surface ridged or smooth, have marked mamelons (incisal notching), etc. The incisors may be widest at the incisal margin or they may be widest at the middle third, tapering down toward the incisal. Sometimes the incisors contact at the gingival margin and taper toward the incisal (Fig. 5–6).

Maxillary lateral incisors are notoriously variable. They may be thin and flat, with or without pronounced cingulum, or they may be blunt and short or actually conical. Frequently the left and right lateral incisors vary in size and shape. Bilateral symmetry in tooth shape and size is not to be assumed, as many orthodontists know from their ineffectual struggle to establish proper interdigitation, maxillary and mandibular midline harmony and, in particular, correct canine position. There is more harmony in canine size within the same individual, but canines vary greatly from person to person. Particularly, there is a difference in the amount of labial convexity and the length and inclination of the cuspal inclined planes. Root lengths of the cuspids show equally great variations. The shape of the premolar teeth is not only variable from individual to individual but within the same person. Mandibular second premolars are particularly prone to variability in shape. With some, the lingual cusp is practically nonexistent and the tooth diminutive. In others, the mesiodistal dimension is elongated, with the lingual cusp high, and the tooth simulates a deciduous molar. Still other mandibular second premolars may be very wide buccolingually. They may or may not interdigitate properly with the opposing premolar teeth.

Garn, Lewis and Kerewsky have noted that the more distal a tooth in each morphologic class is, the more likely it is to be subject to greater numerical variation than the tooth nearer the midline.[29] Thus, the lateral incisor is more

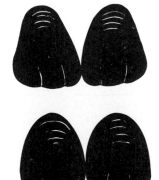

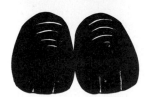

Figure 5–6 Varying shapes and contact relationships of maxillary central incisor teeth.

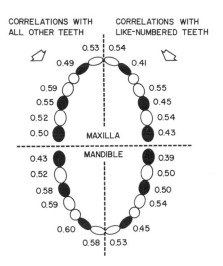

Figure 5–7 Size intercorrelations of the more mesial teeth (white) and the more distal teeth (black) in each morphological class. Whether the mean values of *r* pertain to all correlations involving the teeth in question (left) or correlations involving like-numbered teeth alone (right), it is clear that the most distal tooth in each class is generally characterized by lower size interrelationships, with the possible exception of I_2. (From Garn, S. M., Lewis, A. B., and Kerewsky, R. S.: Size interrelationships of the mesial and distal teeth. J. Dent. Res., 44:350–354, 1965.)

frequently missing than the central incisor, and the second premolar is more frequently missing than the first premolar. There is also more variability in size (Fig. 5–7). The more distal teeth tend to exhibit fewer size interrelationships (or communalities) than the more mesial teeth of the same morphologic class. A comparison of size variance is shown in Table 5–6.

This study confirms the observations of Lundström who noted the greater variability of lateral incisors and second premolars.[30] Moorrees and Reed[31] write, "Considerable discordance can occur in the relations of mesiodistal crown diameters among permanent or deciduous, successional, as well as maxillary and mandibular teeth and tooth groups. These findings serve to explain favorable and unfavorable factors influencing the alignment and occlusion of the permanent teeth. The lack of perfect correlation between maxillary and mandibular teeth warrants considerable attention in clinical diagnosis."

One word of caution: remember that the permanent teeth as they erupt are not going to change in size. Frequently the erupting maxillary central incisors seem enormous to a concerned parent. He does not realize that the face will "grow up" to these teeth as the child himself grows and matures. In our modern society it is often difficult to determine the original size of premolar and molar teeth of the average 16-year-old. Dental caries has necessitated the placing of artificial restorations. These often do not establish the original shapes, contours and dimensions of the tooth. Thus, the dentist introduces another variable in size and shape that is bound to have its effect on the ultimate occlusion of the teeth. The importance of restoration of normal contour and dimensions of all carious teeth is emphasized in Chapter 13.

Another consideration of importance is the comparison of the size and shape of deciduous teeth and their permanent successors. Frequently the mother will say to the orthodontist, "His baby teeth were so beautiful and so straight. Look at him now with all those crooked teeth and no room for others that have not even come in yet." Clinical examination all too frequently bears out this lay observation. The deciduous teeth may be harmonious in size and shape and very evenly placed in the maxilla and mandible (Fig. 5–8); but if there are no spaces between them by the time they are ready to be lost, look out! The dentist can do just that by making a radiographic examination and determining the size of the permanent teeth. It is possible for him to predict from dental radiographs

TABLE 5–6   COMPARATIVE TOOTH SIZE VARIANCE OF MESIAL AND DISTAL TEETH

TOOTH	VARIANCE (σ^2)	F-RATIO σ_1^2/σ_2^2	SIGNIFICANCE
	MAXILLARY		
I^1	0.3588 ⎱		
I^2	.4134 ⎰	1.152	NS
P^1	.2052 ⎱		
P^2	.1971 ⎰	1.041	NS
M^1	.3271 ⎱		
M^2	0.3893 ⎰	1.190	NS
	MANDIBULAR		
I_1	0.1568 ⎱		
I_2	.1806 ⎰	1.152	NS
P_1	.2079 ⎱		
P_2	.1874 ⎰	1.109	NS
M_1	.4369 ⎱		
M_2	0.4462 ⎰	1.021	NS

(From Garn, S. M., Lewis, A. B., and Kerewsky, R. S.: Size interrelationships of the mesial and distal teeth. J. Dent. Res., *44*:350–354, 1965.)

and a mixed dentition analysis the approximate size and shape of the permanent successors. The discrepancy in tooth size between deciduous and permanent incisors is called *incisor liability*. This, together with the amount of interdental spacing, intercanine arch length increase and slight arch length increase by more anterior eruption of permanent incisors, allows the clinician to predict whether or not there will be enough room. With his knowledge of growth and development and an appreciation of the available space, he may be able to tell the parent just what to expect. This is discussed in detail in Chapters 8, 13, and 15.

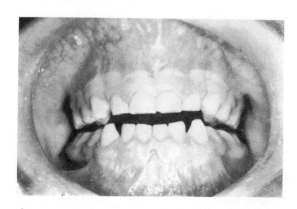

Figure 5–8 Apparently harmonious occlusion in the deciduous dentition. Actually, the lack of spacing between the teeth makes this mouth a potential orthodontic problem, with tooth sacrifice a distinct possibility.

NUMBER OF TEETH

It hardly seems necessary to state that if the proper number of teeth are not present in the maxilla and mandible a malocclusion is the likely result. Yet teeth are frequently missing, either congenitally or because they have been removed as the result of caries. Teeth most likely to be missing are the third molars, the maxillary lateral incisors (Fig. 5–9), the maxillary or mandibular second premolars, the mandibular central incisors and the maxillary first premolars, in that order of frequency. As mentioned previously, the more distal tooth of each morphologic class is more likely to be missing. But any tooth, including the first and second molars and canines, may be absent. Estimates by various investigators indicate that one person in four is likely to have a third molar that is missing or abnormally shaped. Three people out of every 100 will have one or two maxillary lateral incisors malformed or congenitally absent. (See illustrations in Chapter 7.) Muller *et al.* studied 14,940 children, 11 to 15 years of age, finding 521 with missing permanent teeth, excluding third molars. Girls showed a higher incidence of missing teeth than boys did. Negro girls showed less congenital absence, however. More permanent teeth were missing in the maxillary arch, but no differences were noted on the right and left sides.[33] Here again, the dentist by periodic radiographic examination can and must determine the status of the developing occlusion (Fig. 5–10). The presence, size, shape and position of the developing permanent teeth cannot be determined by a dentist with merely a good pair of eyes, a sharp explorer and mouth mirror. Routine radiographic examinations are essential to guide the child patient through the critical formative years.

TOOTH POSITION

A description of the position of teeth, or teeth and jaws, requires a frame of reference—a so-called norm. "Normal occlusion" too often means one thing to the prosthodontist, another thing to the periodontist and something else to the orthodontist. As has been pointed out in Chapter 4, the historical development of our concepts of occlusion has led us from a narrow mechanical appreciation of surface and plane contacts to the present knowledge that there are a number of other equally important factors, such as axial inclination, depth of cusps, root-crown ratio, arch form, temporomandibular joint activity, perioral muscle function, basal jaw relationship, etc. Experience has shown us that what may be a normal occlusion for one man may be abnormal for another. Recog-

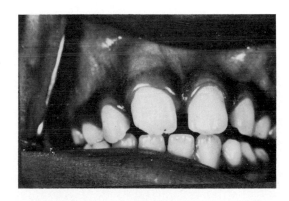

Figure 5–9 Congenital absence of maxillary lateral incisors.

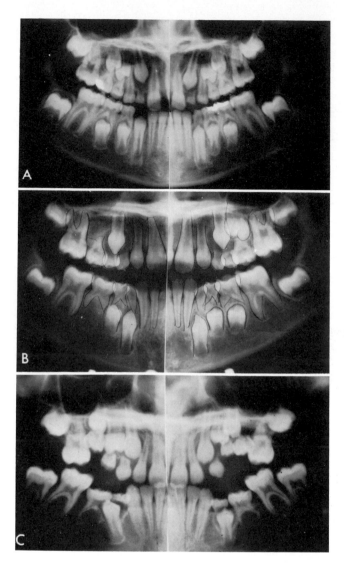

Figure 5–10 Effect of congenital absence on contiguous teeth. A, Congenital absence of maxillary lateral incisors, with canines erupting mesially into lateral position. B, Maxillary first premolars missing, with canines erupting distally into premolar space. C, Ankylosis of second deciduous molars and congenital absence combined. Both direction and amount of eruptions are affected.

nizing the broad base and functional implications, one must develop a reasonably firm concept of where the teeth should be for a particular individual with certain physical propensities. This is the *individualized norm.*

We must always be careful not to accept this norm as an absolute and arbitrary standard that can be used as a general goal for all othodontic problems. Norman Kingsley[34] admonished us against this easy fallacy in 1880 when he wrote, "Symmetry and harmony do not imply uniformity and the dental arch may be developed up to the highest type of perfection, and yet there exists as great a variety of form as there would be in the faces of the aggregated beauties of the world: races, nations and families are thus represented without deformity." And as Simon[35] has said, "All we ever find are variations, endless variations; an exact, ideal norm does not exist, cannot exist. And this is our enigma; in theory we will never find the normal, in practice we forever feel its need and apply it constantly." Thus, the concept of a "conditioned norm" has been developed, to serve us until that time when our knowledge of constitutional and environmental factors is so profound that we no longer need a standard. We have not yet developed our understanding to the point where we can discard this crutch.

MALOCCLUSION GROUPS

Malocclusions may involve four tissue systems: teeth, bones, muscles and nerves. In some cases only the teeth are irregular; jaw relationship may be good and muscle and nerve function normal. In other cases teeth may be regular in their alignment, but an abnormal jaw relationship may exist, so that the teeth do not meet properly during function. Or again, the malocclusion may involve all four systems, with individual tooth malpositions, abnormal jaw (or bone) relationship and abnormal nerve and muscle function. Because of the intimate interplay between nerve and muscle, i.e., nerves actually "wire" the muscles, some biologists combine these two systems into one "neuromuscular" system. Another way to categorize malocclusions is to divide them into three groups: (1) dental dysplasias, (2) skeletodental dysplasias and (3) skeletal dysplasias. Prior to a discussion of these groups, however, it is necessary to define some terms about which there has often been considerable confusion and mis-understanding.

GLOSSARY OF TERMS CONCERNING MALPOSITION

In the history of orthodontics, many terms have been used to describe the malposition of the individual teeth. Some of these terms are ambiguous and etymologically incorrect. The word "occlusion" in medicine means a blocking or closing up. The etymology is *ob* and *claudere*, which literally means "to close up." "Malocclusion" would then mean abnormal closing up and would not be completely appropriate when employed as a term descriptive of indi-vidual tooth positions per se. Carabelli probably is one of the first to systemat-ically analyze occlusion, around the middle of the 19th century. Terms like *overbite* and *edge-to-edge* bite are attributed to his classification.[36] The follow-ing terms are approved by the American Association of Orthodontists as accepta-ble and recommended, but not mandatory.

Orthodontics—a noun indicating the science which has for its object the prevention and correction of dental and oral anomalies.

Orthodontic—adjective describing or referring to orthodontics.

Orthodontically—adverb, implying manner or action.

Anomalies, or Abnormalities—those fundamental aberrations of growth and function which the orthodontist strives to establish in normal and anatomical balance.

Dental Anomalies, or Dental Abnormalities—those aberrations in which the teeth have deviated from the normal in form, position and relationship.

Oral Anomalies, or Oral Abnormalities—those aberrations which include other structures in addition to the teeth.

Eugnathic Anomalies, or Eugnathic Dental Abnormalities—those aberrations which are limited to the teeth and their immediate alveolar supports.

Dysgnathic Anomalies, or Dysgnathic Abnormalities—those aberrations which extend beyond the teeth and include the maxilla, the mandible or both.

Dentofacial Anomalies, or Dentofacial Abnormalities—terms which indicate a dysgnathic anomaly.

Macrognathia—a term indicating a definite overgrowth of the jaw or jaws.

Micrognathia—a term indicating marked undergrowth of the jaw or jaws.

Macroglossia—a term indicating definite overgrowth of the tongue.

Microglossia—a term indicating abnormally small tongue.

Myofunction and Myodysfunction—terms which refer to the normal function or malfunction of the muscles.

Normal Relationships and Malrelationships—terms which apply to the conjoining structures as they should be or to their relationship when disturbed or disrupted.

Normal Dental Function and Dental Malfunction—terms which indicate the correct or incorrect action of opposing teeth in the process of mastication, often incorrectly referred to as a "normal occlusion."

Normal Occlusion of the Teeth, and Malocclusion of the Teeth—terms which indicate the relations of the opposing dentures when brought into habitual opposition.

Anterior, Posterior—terms which describe the relative positions in a forward or backward direction.

Unilateral, Bilateral, Maxillary, Bimaxillary and Mandibular—terms which indicate the part or extent of the jaws affected.

Symmetrical, Asymmetrical—terms which indicate the manner of their involvement (teeth and jaws).

Contraction and Distraction—terms which indicate teeth or other maxillary structures too near the median plane, or too far in an outward direction from it.

Protraction and Retraction—terms which indicate teeth or other maxillary structures too far forward or too far backward.

Attraction and Abstraction—terms which indicate teeth or other maxillary structures too high up or too low down in the face.

Intraversion and Extraversion—terms which indicate teeth or other maxillary structures which are too near or too far from the median plane.

Anteversion, Retroversion—terms which indicate teeth or other maxillary structures too far forward or too far backward.

Supraversion, Infraversion—terms which indicate teeth or other maxillary structures above or below their normal vertical relationships.

If a choice is to be made between the "traction" and "version" endings, the "version" ending is preferred.

In actual usage, certain of these terms have found relatively limited application. For example, the terms "eugnathic" and "dysgnathic," while etymologically correct, are seldom encountered in the literature. The series of terms introduced by Simon, "contraction" and "distraction," "protraction" and "retraction," "attraction" and "abstraction," "intraversion" and "extraversion," and "anteversion" and "retroversion," are seen infrequently and need not be learned. "Supraversion" and "infraversion" are in common use for teeth that have either overerupted or have not erupted sufficiently. Individual teeth malpositions are described as seen in the accompanying illustrations (Figs. 5–11, 5–12). Anterior teeth may be in labioversion or linguoversion or torsiversion. The molars, premolars and canines may be in torsiversion, mesioversion or distoversion. The molars and premolars may be in linguoversion or buccoversion. The canines may be in mesioversion and labioversion. Of course, it is possible for a molar or premolar to be in more than one position. For example, a first premolar may be in mesiobuccoversion and in torsiversion.

In the literature, the reader will often encounter the prefix "labial," "lingual," "mesial," "distal" and "buccal" instead of the "labio-," "linguo-," "mesio-," "disto-," and "bucco-" used in the diagram. The British Society for the Study of Orthodontics prefers the use of the term "medial" to "mesial." If a tooth is tipped or tilted, it is said to be medially, distally, labially, lingually or buccally inclined. If a tooth is bodily malposed, then it is referred to as "displaced" instead of "inclined."

Describing the position or malposition of individual teeth, there are other terms with which students should be familiar (Fig. 5–13). The term "overbite" applies to the distance which the maxillary incisal margin closes vertically past the mandibular incisal margin, when the teeth are brought into habitual or centric occlusion. "Overjet" is a horizontal measurement referring to the distance between the lingual aspect of the maxillary incisors and the labial

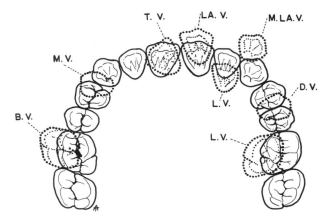

Figure 5–11 Malpositions of individual teeth. (Adapted from Anderson, G. M.: Practical Orthodontics. 9th ed. C. V. Mosby Co., 1960.)

LA. V. = LABIOVERSION
L. V. = LINGUOVERSION
T. V. = TORSIVERSION
D. V. = DISTOVERSION
M. V. = MESIOVERSION
B. V. = BUCCOVERSION
M. LA. V. = MESIOLABIOVERSION

surface of the mandibular incisors when the teeth are in habitual or centric occlusion. "Open bite" is descriptive of a condition where a space exists between the occlusal or incisal surfaces of maxillary and mandibular teeth in the buccal or anterior segments, when the mandible is brought into habitual or centric occlusion (Fig. 5–14). The term "closed bite" or "deep bite" describes a condition of excessive overbite, where the vertical measurement between the maxillary and mandibular incisal margins is excessive when the mandible is brought into habitual or centric occlusion. "Cross-bite" refers to a condition where one or more teeth may be abnormally malposed buccally or lingually or labially with reference to the opposing tooth or teeth (Fig. 5–14). "Scissors bite" applies to total maxillary buccal (or mandibular lingual) cross-bite, with the mandibular dentition completely contained within the maxillary dentition in habitual occlusion.[45]

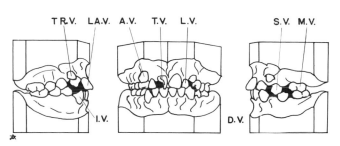

Figure 5–12 Side and front drawings of plaster casts of a dental malocclusion illustrating the possible individual tooth malpositions. (After Salzmann, J. A.: Practice of Orthodontics. J. B. Lippincott Co., 1966.)

TR. V. = TRANSVERSION   T. V. = TORSIVERSION
LA. V. = LABIOVERSION   L. V. = LINGUOVERSION
A. V. = AXIVERSION   S. V. = SUPRAVERSION
M. V. = MESIOVERSION   I. V. = INFRAVERSION
D. V. = DISTOVERSION

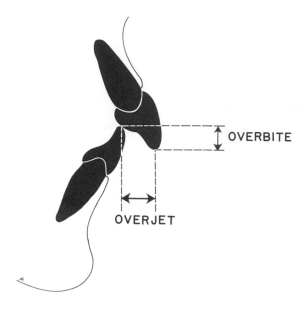

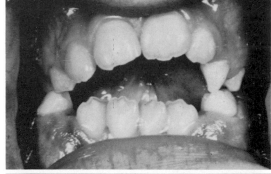

Figure 5–13   Overbite and overjet.

Figure 5–14 Problems of anterior open bite, with concomitant narrowing of maxillary arch and cross-bite. Adaptive and deforming musculature tends to perpetuate the malocclusion.

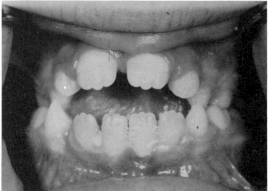

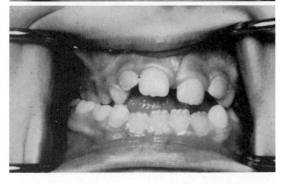

DENTAL DYSPLASIAS

A dental malocclusion exists when the individual teeth within one or both jaws are abnormally related to each other. Only the tooth system is involved. This condition may be limited to a couple of teeth or it may involve the majority of teeth present (Fig. 5–15). The relationship of the upper and lower jaws is considered normal, facial balance is almost always good, and muscular function is also considered normal. In dental or dento-alveolar dysplasias there is usually lack of space to accommodate all the teeth. This may be due to certain local factors such as premature loss of deciduous teeth, prolonged retention of deciduous teeth or improper restorations, but it is more likely to be due to a basic hereditary pattern, perhaps a tooth size discrepancy, that may or may not have been modified by environmental factors. In dental or dento-alveolar dysplasias the inclined plane relationship and conformation of the teeth to the arch form dictated by the configuration of upper and lower jaws is imperfect. Incisors may be rotated, canines may have insufficient room to erupt into their normal place in the dental arch, premolars may be partially impacted or may be erupting buccally or lingually to the normal positions in the dental arches. Molar segments may have drifted mesially, forcing teeth anterior to them into positions of malocclusion. The concept that the student must have is that facial development and skeletal pattern and muscle development and function may be good although there is a disharmonious relationship between the teeth and their immediate supporting bone, resulting in individual tooth irregularities.

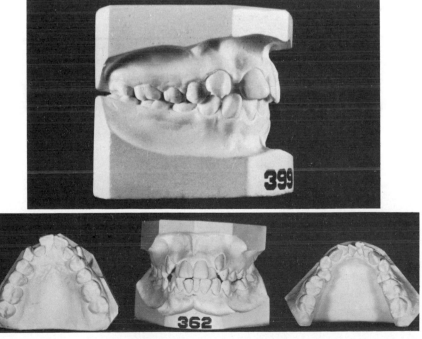

Figure 5–15 Examples of dental dysplasias: (upper) involving only one tooth primarily; (lower) involving a number of teeth. Jaw relationship is normal.

The time is long past when the dentist thought of orthodontic problems as involving only the teeth. It is now recognized that the anteroposterior relationship of the maxilla and mandible to each other and to the cranial base is of vital concern. Individual tooth irregularities may or may not be present in this particular category but the relationship of the maxilla to the mandible and of both the maxilla and the mandible to the cranium have a profound influence on the orthodontic objectives and ultimate therapeutic achievements (Fig. 5–16). Frequently, the bone system, neuromuscular system and tooth systems are involved, with adaptive or compensatory muscle activity to fit the skeletal dysplasia. Relatively few malocclusions are skeletal involvements exclusively.

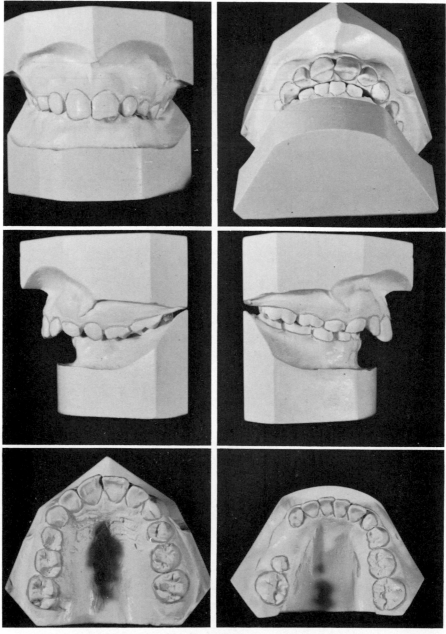

Figure 5–16 Skeletal dysplasia. Teeth are regular in each arch, but upper and lower dental arches are improperly related to each other or to the cranial base.

SKELETODENTAL DYSPLASIAS

This category describes those malocclusions where not only are the teeth, singly or in groups, in malposition, but where there is an abnormal relationship of the maxilla and the mandible to each other or to the cranial base (Fig. 5–17). In addition to irregularly positioned teeth, the mandible may be too far forward or backward with respect to the maxilla or cranial base, or the maxillary denture itself may be too far forward or backward with respect to either or both the cranial base and mandible. As might be expected, skeletodental dysplasias are more involved and require a different therapeutic approach than dental dysplasias. Muscle function usually is not normal in this group. All four tissue systems are involved. Much depends on the type and degree of skeletal malrelationship. In an orthodontic practice this group makes up the largest percentage of patients.

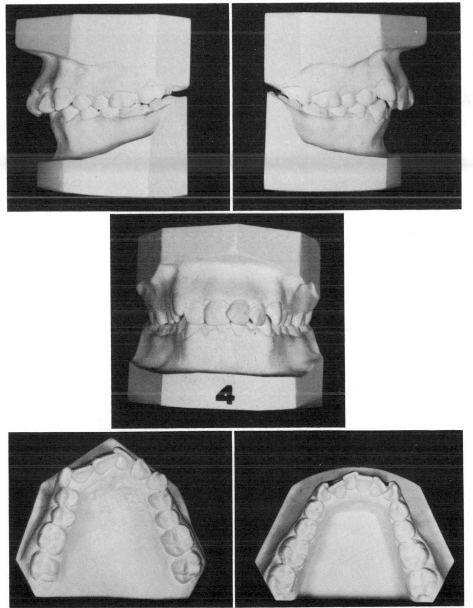

Figure 5–17 A skeletodental dysplasia. Both jaw relationship and tooth positions are abnormal.

CLASSIFICATION OF MALOCCLUSION

The classification of these skeletal or jaw and face relationships is not new and has been attempted frequently. One of the best classification efforts has been made by Simon, using the gnathostatic approach and orienting the dentition to anthropometric landmarks in an attempt to better show the actual relationship of the dentition in the face (Fig. 5–18). Simon took the suggestion made by Bennett in 1912 that malocclusions be categorized in three planes of

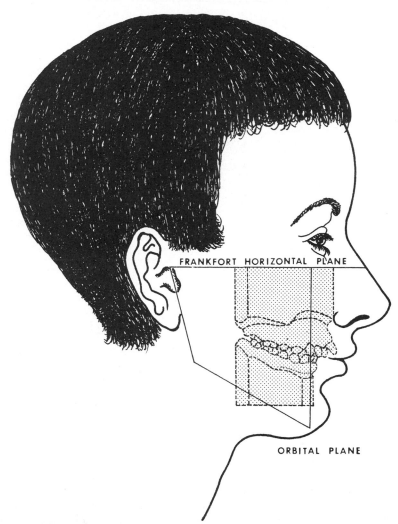

Figure 5–18 Gnathostatic approach used by Simon to orient plaster models in each patient's face. The top of the maxillary study model was made parallel with the eye-ear plane (Frankfort horizontal). The occlusal plane on the plaster models established the same angle to the maxillary cast base as the natural occlusal plane established with the eye-ear plane in the patient proper. This cast orientation permitted a more precise appraisal of jaw relationship. Simon's claim (now generally discredited) was that the perpendicular to the Frankfort horizontal plane at orbitale, creating his orbital plane, passed through the distal third of the maxillary canine in normal occlusion. Malocclusions with anteroposterior discrepancies were categorized by their relationship with the orbital plane.

space—horizontal, vertical and transverse. The gnathostatic diagnostic approach is described and illustrated in more detail in Chapter 4.[35] Other classification systems have been suggested but have found only limited application because the infinite variations of oral and occlusal anomalies make such a description difficult, complex and unwieldy. Perhaps the most universally used classification was introduced by Edward H. Angle in 1899. As noted in Chapter 4, the basis of Angle's[14] classifications was his hypothesis that the first molar is the "key to occlusion." (See p. 184.)

It is now apparent to most orthodontists that the maxillary first permanent molar relationship is not quite as inviolate as Angle thought. Cephalometric studies have shown considerable variation in the relationship of all structures.

Moorrees and Grøn[37] write:

> In orthodontics, a great many classifications have been proposed, but in spite of their merits, none has replaced the Angle system. This method has already received universal acceptance primarily because its characterization of malocclusion in terms of the sagittal plane established a clear-cut descriptive symbolization of occlusal anomalies and facial disharmony. Yet Angle's classification with connotations as to crowding, overbite, etc., can never be more than a labeling and overgeneralization of the malocclusion owing to the great variability of the clinical manifestation from patient to patient within each of the three classes of Angle's system.

Angle's classification still serves a very useful purpose in describing the anteroposterior relationships of the maxillary and mandibular dental arches which usually reflect the jaw relationship. Modified by our broader knowledge of growth and development and the role played by function, the Angle classification is an important tool of diagnosis for the dentist. Together with the terms on the previous pages describing individual tooth positions, it is possible to scientifically categorize malocclusions and communicate this information accurately to others.

Angle[37] divided malocclusions into three broad classes (Fig. 5–19): Class I (neutroclusion), Class II (distoclusion), and Class III (mesioclusion). What Angle actually did was to categorize malocclusion syndromes, creating a mental picture of groupings of certain malocclusion characteristics in each class. That there is an overlapping of these characteristics is obvious; yet the same lack of homogencity exists for so-called normal. Thus, malocclusion as well as normal occlusion is a range, not a fixed point.

CLASS I

The most important consideration here is that the anteroposterior relationship of the maxillary and mandibular molars is correct, with the mesiobuccal cusp of the maxillary first molar occluding in the mesiobuccal groove of the mandibular first molar. Since Angle assumed that the maxillary first molar was essentially normal in its position, this would mean that the lower dental arch, as represented by the mandibular first molar, is in normal anteroposterior relationship with the maxillary dental arch. By inference, the supporting maxillary and mandibular bony bases are in normal relationship (Figs. 5–23, 5–24). The malocclusion is essentially a dental dysplasia. (See first part of this chapter.) Rotations, individual tooth malpositions, missing teeth and tooth size discrepancies fall under this classification (Fig. 5–25). There is usually normal muscle function associated with this type of problem. A large sampling of our population would show that a majority of the malocclusions are Class I

(Text continued on page 232)

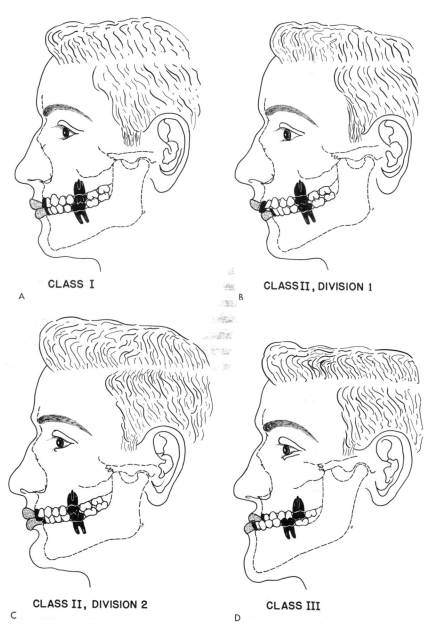

Figure 5–19 Angle's Classification of Malocclusion. A, Class I: mesiodistal first molar relationship normal; tooth irregularities elsewhere. B, Class II, Division 1: lower first molar distal to upper first molar. Mandibular retrusion usually reflected in patient profile. C, Class II, Division 2: lower first molar distal to upper first molar. Deep overbite often reflected in patient profile. D, Class III malocclusion: lower first molar mesial to upper first molar. Mandibular prognathism usually reflected in patient profile.

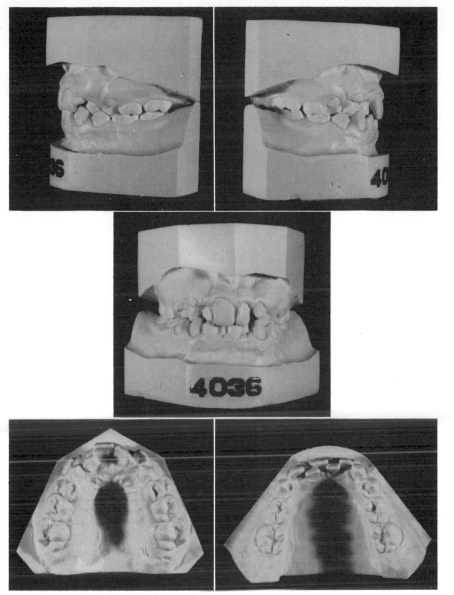

Figure 5–20 Class I malocclusion. Mesiodistal relationship of upper and lower first molars to each other is correct. Individual tooth irregularities and arch length problems exist elsewhere.

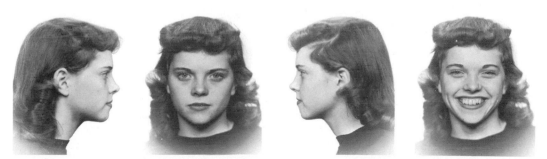

Figure 5–21 Class I malocclusion (Fig. 5–20). Facial profile within normal limits.

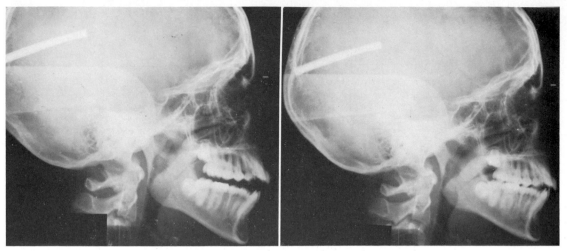

Figure 5–22   Class I malocclusion (Figs. 5–20, 5–21). Cephalogram shows normal maxillomandibular relationship.

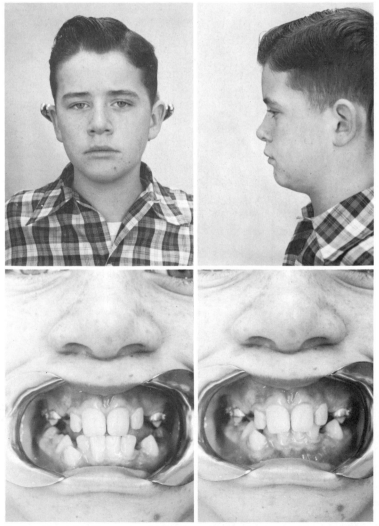

Figure 5–23   Facial balance is good, jaw relationship normal, as is to be expected in most Class I malocclusions.

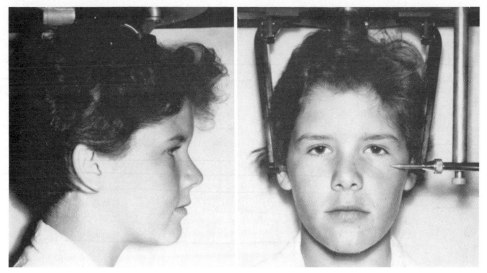

Figure 5–24   Profile and frontal photographs show beautiful facial balance, yet there is a Class I malocclusion present. (Courtesy W. R. Mayne.)

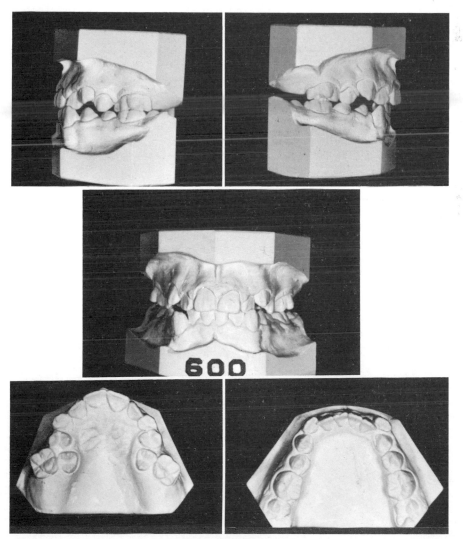

Figure 5–25   Class I malocclusion, but facial balance is normal (Fig. 5–24).

231

(Angle).[10] Occasionally, the mesiodistal relationship of the upper and lower first molars may be normal, the interdigitation of the buccal segments correct, with no overt tooth malpositions; but the entire dentition is forward with respect to the facial profile. The orthodontist calls this a bimaxillary protrusion (Figs. 5–26 to 5–28). With normal anteroposterior jaw relationship, the teeth are forward on their respective bases. Bimaxillary protrusions usually fall in the Class I category (Fig. 5–28).

A malocclusion may exist in the presence of abnormal perioral muscle function, with a normal mesiodistal first molar relationship, but with the teeth anterior to the first molars completely out of contact even during full habitual occlusion. This is called an "open bite" (Figs. 5–14, 5–29). Open bite conditions usually are seen in the anterior part of the mouth, but may occur in the posterior segments. Frequently the first molar relationship is Class II or Class III (Angle).

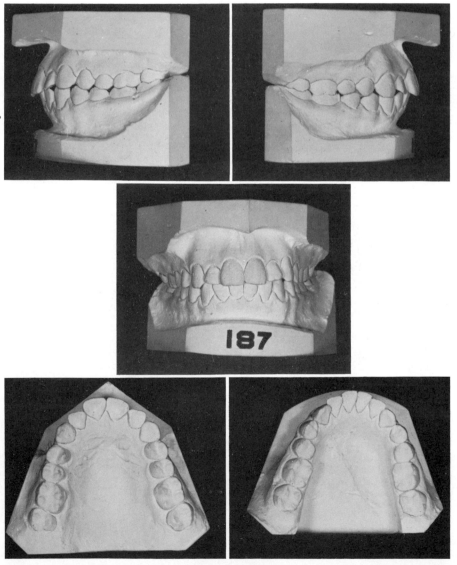

Figure 5–26 Class I malocclusion, bimaxillary protrusion, Caucasian female. Mesiodistal first molar relationship is normal, but entire dentition appears to be too far forward in the face as in Figure 5–28.

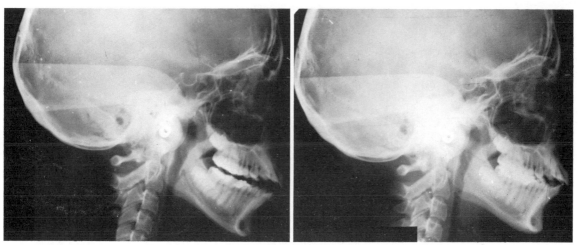

Figure 5–27 Lateral postural rest and occlusion cephalograms illustrating the maxillary and mandibular incisor procumbency seen in Figures 5–26 and 5–28.

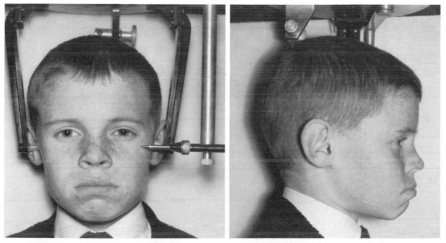

Figure 5–28 Lateral and frontal photographs of a patient with a Class I bimaxillary protrusion. Hyperactive mentalis muscle activity exists when the lips are brought into contact. (Courtesy W. R. Mayne.)

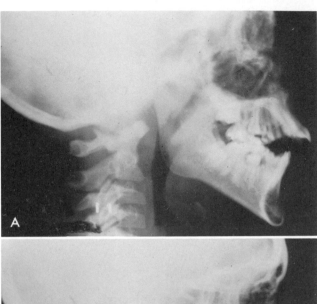

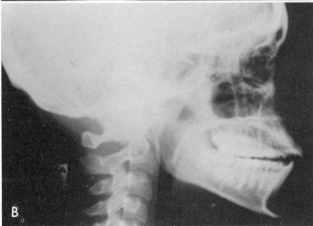

Figure 5–29   Open bite malocclusions that are still Class I (Angle), despite excessive overjet in A and bimaxillary protrusion in B. Deforming musculature exacerbates the open bite relationship. Muscle control appliances plus orthopedic force in a vertical vector are often necessary to eliminate the tooth-muscle-bone involvement. Decisions for tooth sacrifice must be arrived at carefully because of role of tongue.

CLASS II

In this group the lower dental arch is in a distal or posterior relation to the upper dental arch, as reflected by the first permanent molar relationship. The mesiobuccal groove of the mandibular first molar no longer receives the mesiobuccal cusp of the maxillary first molar but usually contacts the distobuccal cusp of the maxillary first molar, or it may be even farther posterior. The interdigitation of the remaining teeth reflects this posterior relationship so that it is proper to say that the mandibular denture is "distal" to the maxillary denture. There are two divisions to Class II malocclusion.

DIVISION 1 (FIGS. 5–30 TO 5–32).   In Class II, Division 1 malocclusions, the molar relationship is as just described above (distoclusion) and there are certain other associated characteristics. The mandibular denture may or may not be normal with respect to individual tooth position and arch form. Frequently the lower anterior segment shows supraversion or overeruption of the incisor teeth, a tendency toward "flattening" and some irregularities. The arch form of the maxillary denture is seldom normal. Instead of the usual rounded "U" shape, it assumes a morphology approaching that of a "V." A demonstrable narrowing in the premolar and canine regions is responsible for this, together with a protrusion or labioversion of the maxillary incisors. A significant difference here, comparing Class II, Division 1 malocclusions with

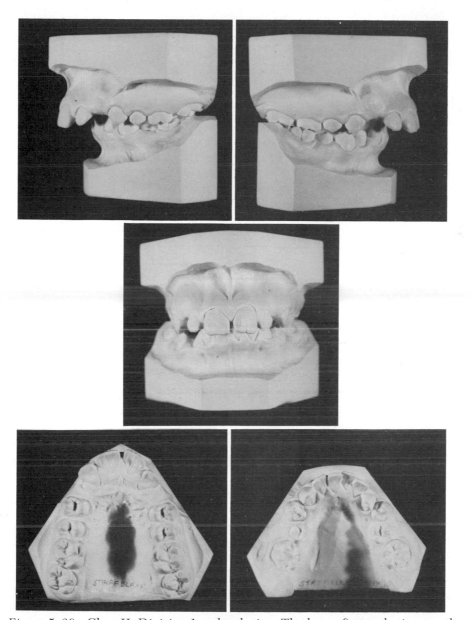

Figure 5–30 Class II, Division 1 malocclusion. The lower first molar is more than a half cusp distal in its relationship to the upper first molar. Overbite and overjet are excessive.

LABBOVERZUSA - ANTEUERZUSA

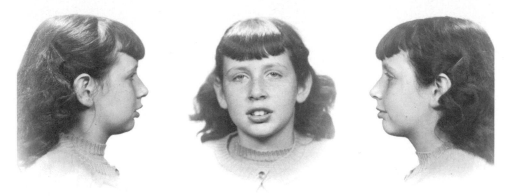

Figure 5–31   Class II, Division 1 malocclusion. The facial profile reflects the abnormally distal lower dentition relationship. Abnormal lip posture is associated with this type malocclusion.

those of Class I (neutroclusion), is the associated abnormal muscle function. Instead of the musculature serving as a balancing and stabilizing "splint," it can become a deforming force.[39] With the increase in overjet (horizontal protrusion of the maxillary incisor segment) the lower lip cushions to the lingual aspect of these teeth (Figs. 5–33 to 5–35). The habitual posture in the more severe cases is with the maxillary incisors resting on the lower lip. The tongue no longer approximates the palate at rest. During swallowing, abnormal mentalis muscle activity and aberrant buccinator activity, together with compensatory tongue function and changed tongue position, tend to accentuate the narrowing of the maxillary arch, the protrusion, labial inclination and spacing of the maxillary incisors, the curve of Spee and the flattening of the mandibular anterior segment (Fig. 5–36). Depending on the tongue position and tongue function, the mandibular incisors may or may not overerupt. They often do. The distal relationship of the mandibular molar and mandibular arch may be

(Text continued on page 240)

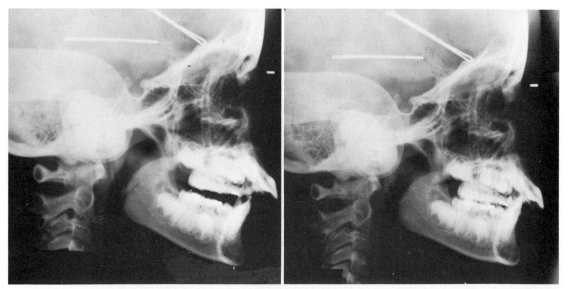

Figure 5–32   Lateral cephalograms in postural rest and occlusion to show excessive interocclusal clearance, excessive overbite and overjet in a Class II, Division 1 malocclusion.

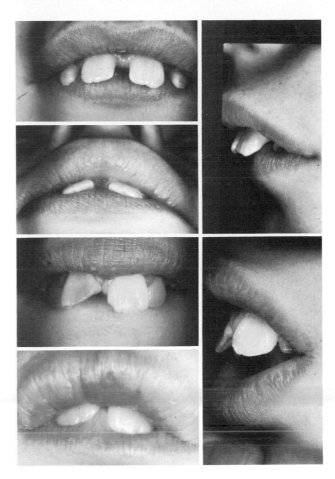

Figure 5-33 Typical lip postures associated with severe Class II, Division 1 malocclusion.

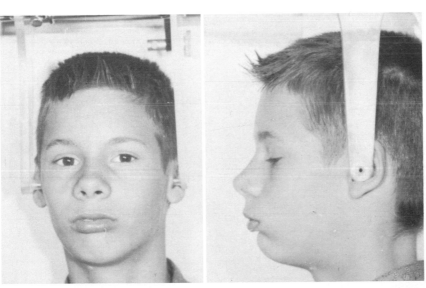

Figure 5-34 Facial photographs reflect skeletodental malocclusion. Note deficient lower face height and marked mentolabial sulcus. (Courtesy Department of Orthodontics, St. Louis University.)

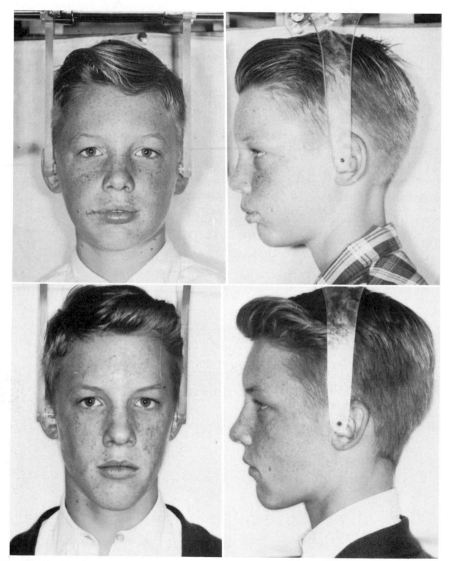

Figure 5–35   (Top) Abnormal perioral muscle function frequently accompanies Class II, Division 1 malocclusions of this type. (Bottom) Excellent correction of severe malocclusion eliminated basal dysplasia and abnormal functional pattern. (Courtesy Department of Orthodontics, St. Louis University.)

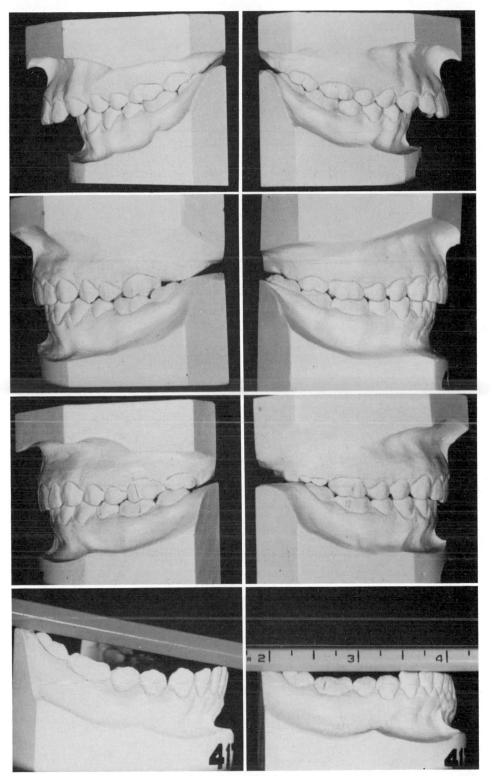

Figure 5–36   Severe Class II, Division 1 malocclusion, with deep overbite, marked overjet. Lower lip cushions to lingual side of maxillary incisors, perpetuating the discrepancy. Maxillary second molars were removed and the maxillary arch moved distally and held with orthopedic force. Note reduction in deep bite and reduction of Curve of Spee, despite fact that no mandibular appliances were used.

either unilateral or bilateral. Research on growth and development and numerous cephalometric studies point to the strong influence of hereditary pattern, as modified by compensatory functional factors as a basis for most Class II, Division 1 malocclusions.[40]

The careful diagnostician, however, does not stop with an appraisal of excessive overbite and overjet, with accompanying compensatory muscle activity, and then assume he is dealing with a Class II, Division 1 malocclusion. In some cases it is possible for the interocclusal clearance and overbite and overjet to be greater in a Class I than in a mild Class II malocclusion. A check of mesiodistal first molar relationship, and of anteroposterior maxillomandibular basal relations and interrelations of all four tissue systems is essential before arriving at a classification based on first impressions (Figs. 5–37, 5–38).

DIVISION 2 (FIGS. 5–39 TO 5–41). Even as the morphology of Class II, Division 1 creates a mental picture of the dental and facial relationships, so does Class II, Division 2. As with Division 1, the mandibular molars and the mandibular arch assume a posterior position with respect to the maxillary first permanent molar and maxillary arch. But here the image changes. The mandibular arch itself may or may not show any individual irregularities, but usually has an exaggerated curve of Spee, and the lower anterior segment

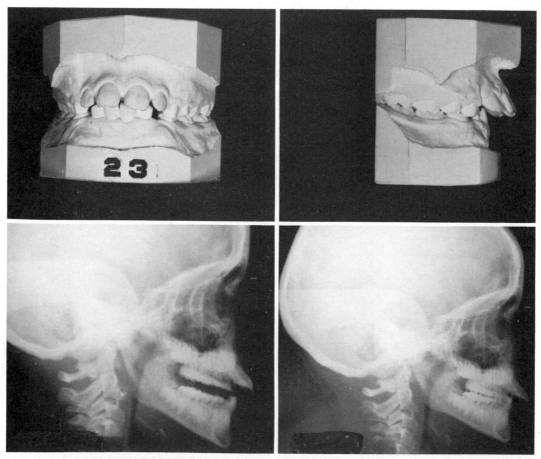

Figure 5–37   Class I malocclusion with excessive overbite, overjet and perverted perioral muscle activity. Interocclusal clearance is excessive (lower left). Mandible is not retruded in relation to maxilla.

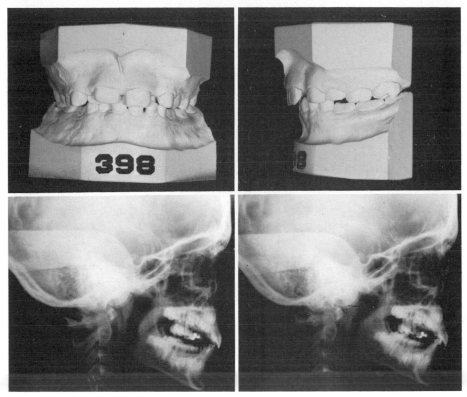

Figure 5–38   Class II, Division 1 malocclusion. Overbite and overjet excessive, but not to degree of case in Figure 5–37. Interocclusal clearance smaller than previous figure. Mandible is retruded in relation to maxilla.

is more frequently irregular, with supraversion of the mandibular incisors. The mandibular labial gingival tissue is often traumatized. The maxillary arch is seldom narrow, often wider than normal in the intercanine area, and a remarkably constant distinguishing feature is the excessive *lingual* inclination of the maxillary central incisors with excessive *labial* inclination of the maxillary lateral incisors. Overbite is quite excessive (closed bite). In some cases variations occur in the maxillary incisor positions. Both central and lateral incisors may be lingually inclined and the canines labially inclined. Such an occlusion is traumatic and may be quite damaging to the mandibular incisor segment supporting structure (Fig. 5–42). Cephalometric studies show that the apices of the maxillary central incisors are usually labially malposed. In contrast with Class II, Division 1, perioral muscle function is usually within normal limits as in Class I malocclusions. Because of the "closed bite" and the excessive interocclusal clearance, however, certain functional problems involving temporalis, masseter and lateral pterygoid muscle activity are common. As the mandible is brought from postural resting position to habitual occlusion, the combination of lingually inclined maxillary incisors and infraocclusion of the posterior teeth often results in the creation of an abnormal path of closure (Fig. 5–43). The mandible can be forced into a retruded position by tooth guidance[41] (Fig. 5–44). The condyle moves posteriorly and superiorly in the articular fossa creating a displacement. (See Chap. 9, Temporomandibular Joint Disorders for a fuller explanation of neuromuscular involvement.) This

(Text continued on page 246)

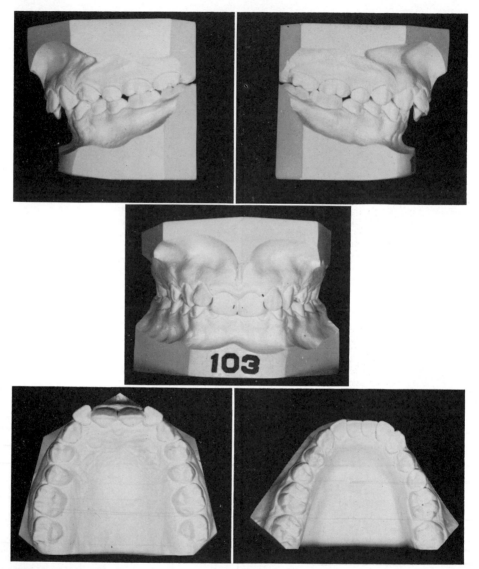

Figure 5–39 Class II, Division 2 malocclusion. This is the most characteristic form, with maxillary lateral incisors labially malposed, maxillary central incisors inclined excessively lingually, overbite very deep. Lower first permanent molar distal by more than half a cusp.

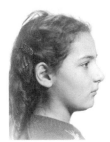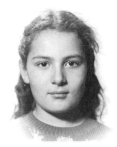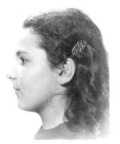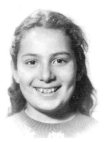

Figure 5–40   Facial photographs do not indicate a mandibular retrusion in this Class II, Division 2 malocclusion (Fig. 5–39).

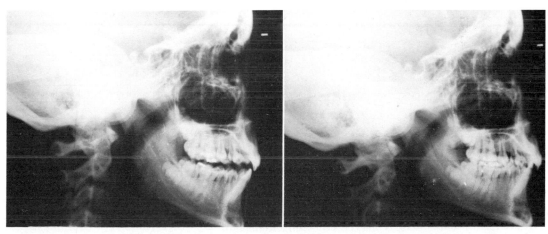

Figure 5–41   Lateral cephalograms show excessive interocclusal clearance, lingually inclined maxillary central incisors and excessive overbite.

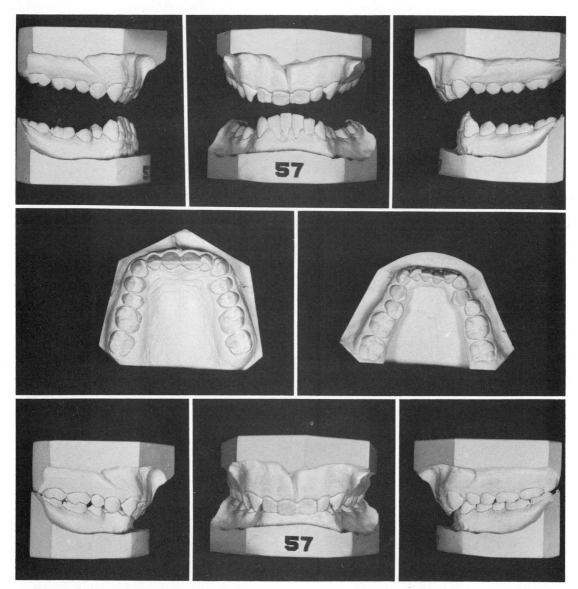

Figure 5–42   Severe Class II, Division 2 malocclusion with both maxillary central and lateral incisors lingually inclined and canines labially malposed. Note the stripping of the mandibular labial gingival tissue.

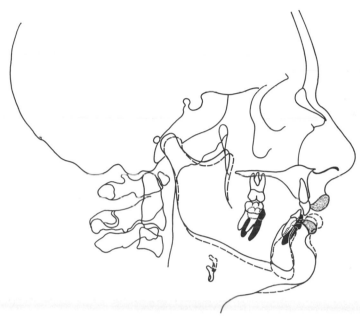

Figure 5–43   Cephalometric tracing of case illustrated in Figures 5–39 to 5–41 demonstrating posterior superior mandibular displacement as a result of incisal guidance combined with excessive overbite during closure from postural rest to occlusion.

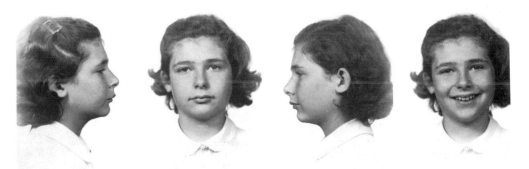

Figure 5–44   Class II, Division 2 malocclusion. Functional mandibular retrusion combined with mandibular overclosure increases the depth of the mentolabial sulcus and exaggerates the redundancy of the lower lip.

phenomenon emphasizes the interdependence of vertical and horizontal factors in the establishment of habitual occlusion and will be discussed in greater detail in Chapters 6 and 16. As with Division 1, the distal molar relationship of the mandibular arch may be bilateral or unilateral.

CLASS III

In this category the mandibular first permanent molar in habitual occlusion is mesial to normal in its relationship with the maxillary first molar. The interdigitation of the remaining teeth usually reflects this anteroposterior malrelationship. In contradistinction to Class II, Division 1, where the overjet is excessive, the mandibular incisors are frequently in total cross-bite, labial to

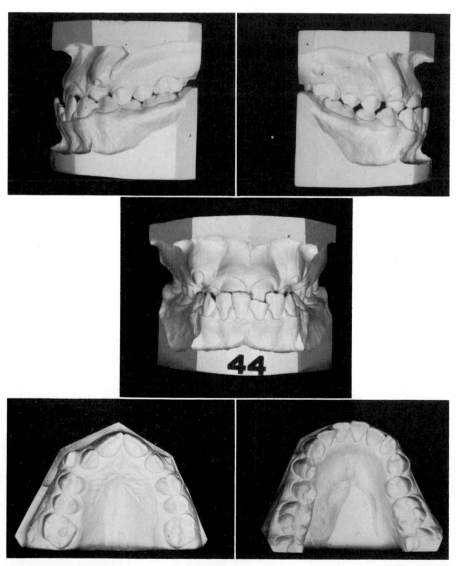

Figure 5–45   Class III malocclusion. The lower first molar is more than a half cusp mesial in its relationship to the upper first molar. The lower left central incisor has been fractured in an accident.

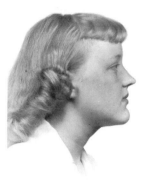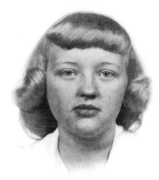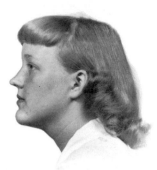

Figure 5–46 The facial profile reflects the abnormally mesial relationship of the mandibular denture seen in Figure 5–45.

the maxillary incisors (Fig. 5–48). In most Class III malocclusions, the lower incisors are inclined excessively to the lingual aspect, despite the cross-bite. Individual tooth irregularities are frequent. The space provided for the tongue appears to be greater and the tongue lies on the floor of the mouth most of the time. The maxillary arch is constricted, the tongue does not approximate the palate as it does normally, arch length is frequently deficient and individual tooth irregularities are common. As with Class II malocclusions the molar relationship may be unilateral or bilateral. Maxillary incisors are usually more lingually inclined than in Class I or Class II, Division 1 malocclusions, however (Fig. 5–49). In some instances this leads to a "pseudo Class III" malocclusion, with the lingually inclined maxillary incisors gliding down the lingual surfaces of the mandibular incisors on closure as the mandible is guided into an anterior displacement (Fig. 5–50). These problems respond dramatically to simple corrective orthodontic procedures and are not to be confused with true Class III malocclusions (Figs. 5–51, 5–52). Incidence of the pseudo Class III is low.

(Text continued on page 250)

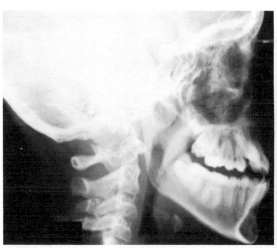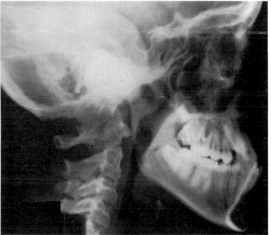

Figure 5–47 Lateral cephalograms of Class III malocclusion in postural rest and occlusion (Figs. 5–45, 5–46.)

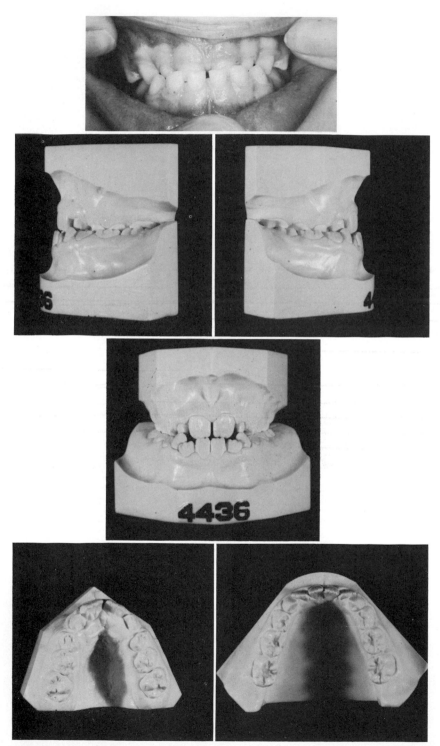

Figure 5–48   Class III malocclusion in deciduous dentition (3 years old) and 4 years later (7 years old). Early orthopedic guidance would have intercepted this perpetuating multi-system involvement (teeth, bone and muscle).

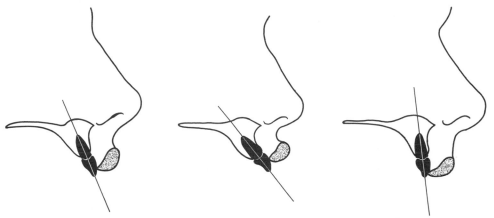

Figure 5–49 Typical maxillary incisor inclinations for Class I, Class II, Division 1 and Class III malocclusions.

Figure 5–50 Class III malocclusion as a result of maxillary incisor guidance. Mandible closes to point of initial contact (left) and is then guided into an anterior displacement as the posterior segments are brought into full occlusion (right). (A pseudo Class III malocclusion.)

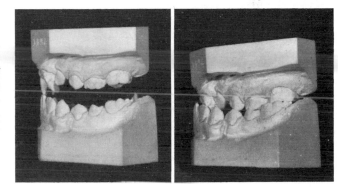

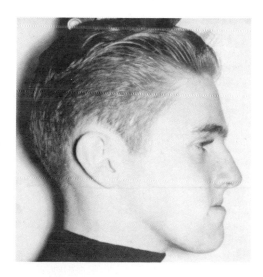

Figure 5–51 Basal Class III malocclusion. As with most Class III malocclusions, there is a steep mandibular plane. (Courtesy W. R. Mayne.)

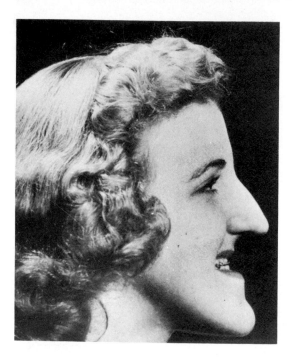

Figure 5–52   Severe Class III malocclusion.

ACKERMAN-PROFFIT CLASSIFICATION SYSTEM

Ackerman and Proffit, recognizing the primarily sagittal orientation, and the limitations of the Angle classification, have devised an all-inclusive method of diagramming and categorizing malocclusion. They point out that malocclusions having the same Angle classification may be only *analogous* malocclusions (having only the same occlusal relationships) and not necessarily *homologus* (having all characteristics in common).[36] Planning of diagnosis and treatment must depend on more than occlusal relationships. Any system that can group important variables is likely to provide better treatment guidance.

A classification system in which five characteristics and their interrelationships are assessed has been developed, using the Venn symbolic logic diagram as an organizing framework. It is known as the set theory. Venn proposed his diagram as a visual demonstration of interaction or overlap among parts of a complex structure. In other words, it deals with groups or collections of entities or characteristics (called sets). Figure 5–53 demonstrates how the set theory works, using two sets, or groups, with common properties. Using "x" and "y" as group designations, a graphic representation may be made. In A, the sets or groups have no overlapping qualities (like occlusion, facial type and tooth size in "x" set, versus blood chemistry, muscle fiber size, number of phalanges in "y" set). In B, the two groups share common qualities; in C, all y's have qualities of x, so that Y is called a sub-set. In D, it is shown that the elements of the universe are contained in sets X and Y, which in themselves have overlapping qualities in this instance. Ackerman and Proffit have represented malocclusions with a modified Venn diagram. In their scheme, a set is defined on the basis of morphologic deviations from the ideal (Fig. 5–53).

Since the degree of alignment and symmetry are common to all dentitions, this is represented as the outer envelope, or universe (Group 1). The profile is affected by many malocclusions, so it becomes a major set within the universe

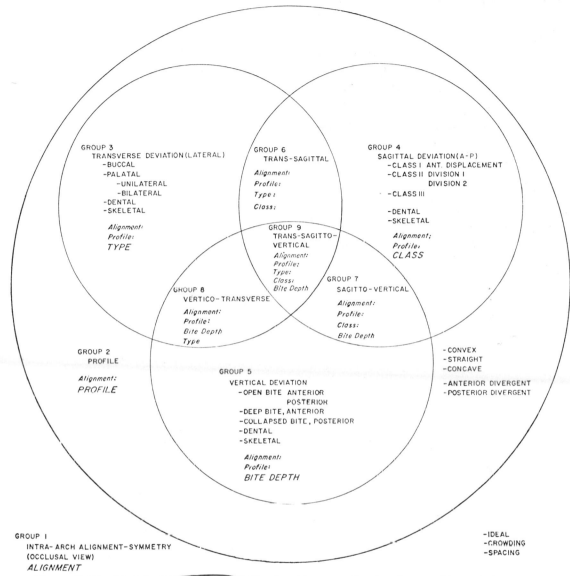

Figure 5–53 Modified Venn diagram for classification of malocclusion. (From Ackerman, J. L., and Proffit, W. R.: The characteristics of malocclusion: a modern approach to classification and diagnosis. Am. J. Orthodont., 56:443–454, 1969.)

(Group 2). Deviations in three planes of space, lateral (transverse), anteroposterior and vertical, are represented by Groups 3 to 9, which include the overlapping or interlocking sub-sets, all within the profile or Group 2 set.

Step 1, the first of five steps in the Ackerman-Proffit classification procedure, is an analysis of alignment and symmetry (Group 1). *Alignment* is the key word, and possibilities are ideal, crowded, spacing and mutilated. Individual tooth irregularities are described.

For Step 2, proceeding inward on the Venn diagram to Group 2, the *profile* is studied. As Figure 5–53 shows, this may be anteriorly or posteriorly divergent, with the lips being concave, straight or convex, with respect to the chin and nose.

Step 3 assesses lateral or *transverse* dental arch characteristics. The term *type* is used to describe various kinds of cross-bite. As the diagram indicates, an opinion regarding whether the problem is dento-alveolar or skeletal is recorded.

Step 4 requires an appraisal of *anteroposterior* sagittal relationships. The Angle classification is used, supplemented by the comment as to whether the malocclusion is dento-alveolar, skeletal or both.

In Step 5, the patient and dentition are viewed regarding the *vertical* dimension, with *bite depth* used as a descriptive term for vertical problems. Possibilities are anterior open bite, anterior deep bite, posterior open bite, posterior collapsed bite. Here, as in transverse and anteroposterior sets, the skeletal or dental nature of the problem is determined.

The overlapping of groups is seen in the center of the Venn diagram (Groups 6 to 9). These are the more severe problems, with characteristics from contiguous and enveloping groups. Group 9 would be the most severe, with involvement of criteria from all groups (Alignment, profile, transverse, anteroposterior and vertical problems). An example of this category is seen in Figure 5–53.

Group 9

Alignment	both arches crowded
Profile	posteriorly divergent, convex
Type	maxillary palatal cross-bite, bilateral, skeletal and dental
Class	Class I, excessive overjet, dental; Class II, skeletal
Bite depth	open bite, skeletal

This classification system is readily adaptable to computer processing and would require only a numerical scale in programming for automated data retrieval.

The limitations are recognized by the developers of the system. No account is taken of etiology, which is often vital treatment information. Since the analysis is essentially static, a functional analysis must still be made, as indicated in Chapters, 3, 4 and 8.

LIMITATIONS OF CLASSIFICATION SYSTEMS

There are a number of limitations to Angle's classification. The maxillary first permanent molar may vary in its position anteroposteriorly, as cephalometric studies have shown. In the mixed dentition, an end-to-end or flush terminal plane relationship of maxillary and mandibular permanent molars is considered normal and the occlusion often does not "settle in" until the exchange of the deciduous molars for the premolars. The Venn diagrammatic approach appears to aid in visualization of important facial implications which are often erroneously overlooked with the Angle classfication. Vertical and lateral dimensions and postural resting relationships must be understood to interpret any of the classification systems to greatest advantage. The dentist must be aware that the broad classes of malocclusion have etiologic, structural, functional and esthetic implications. Above all, function must always be considered, even though it is not "diagrammed." Form and function must mean more than semantic euphony or associated verbiage like "ham and eggs." Form and function are the very backbone of modern orthodontics.

REFERENCES

1. Chiavaro, A.: Malocclusions of the temporary teeth. Int. J. Orth., 1:171–189, 1915.
2. Hellman, M.: Variations in occlusion. D. Cosmos, 63:608–618, 1921.
3. Emrich, R. E., Brodie, A. G., and Blayney, J. R.: Prevalence of Class I, Class II and Class III (Angle) malocclusions in an urban population. An epidemiological study. J. Dent. Res., 44:947–953, 1965.
4. Helm, S.: Malocclusion in Danish children with adolescent dentition. An epidemiologic study. Am. J. Orthodont., 54:352–368, 1968.
5. Draker, H. L.: Handicapping labiolingual deviations. A proposed index for public health purpose. Am. J. Orthodont., 46:295–305, 1960.
6. Myllärniemi, S.: Malocclusion in Finnish rural children. An epidemiological study of different stages of dental development. Doctoral Thesis, Center for Study of Child Growth and Development, University of Helsinki, 1970.
7. Björk, A., and Helm, S.: Prediction of the age of maximum puberal growth in body height. Angle Orthodont., 37:134–143, 1967.
8. Björk, A., Krebs, A., and Solow, B.: A method for epidemiological registration of malocclusion. Acta Odont. Scand., 22:27–41, 1964.
9. Björk, A., and Helm, S.: Need for orthodontic treatment as reflected in the prevalence of malocclusion in various ethnic groups. Acta Socio-Med. Scand. (Suppl. 1), 1961. (Särtryck Ur).
10. Ast, D. B., Carlos, J. P., and Cons, N. C.: The prevalence and characteristics of malocclusion among senior high school students in upstate New York. Am. J. Orthodont., 51:437–445, 1965.
11. Björk, A., The face in profile. Svensk Tandlak. T. (Suppl. 40), 1947.
12. Bonwill, W. G. A.: Geometrical and mechanical laws of articulation. Trans. Odont. Soc. Penna., 119–133, 1885.
13. Hawley, C. A.: Determination of the normal arch and its application to orthodontia. D. Cosmos, 47:541–552, 1905.
14. Angle, E. H.: Treatment of Malocclusion of the Teeth. 7th ed., Philadelphia, S. S. White Manufacturing Co., 1907.
15. Williams, P. N.: Determining the shape of the normal arch. D. Cosmos, 59:695–708, 1917.
16. Stanton, F. L.: Arch predetermination and a method of relating the predetermined arch to the malocclusion to show the minimum tooth movement. Int. J. Orthodont., 8:757–778, 1922.
17. Gilpatric, W. H.: Arch predetermination—Is it practical? J.A.D.A., 10:553–573, 1923.
18. Izard, G.: New method for the determination of the normal arch by the function of the face. Int. J. Orthodont., 13:582–595, 1927.
19. Meredith, H. V., and Higley, L. B.: Relationships between dental arch widths and widths of the face and head. Am. J. Orthodont., 37:193–204, 1951.
20. MacConnaill, M. A., and Scher, E. A.: The ideal form of the human dental arcade, with some prosthetic application. Dent. Rec., 69:285–302, 1949.
21. Wheeler, R. C.: A Textbook of Dental Anatomy and Physiology, 4th ed., Philadelphia, W. B. Saunders Co., 1965.
22. Sved, A.: The application of engineering principles to orthodontics. Am. J. Orthodont., 38:399–421, 1952.
23. Scott, J. H.: The shape of dental arches. J. Dent. Res., 36:996–1003, 1957.
24. Burdi, A. R., and Lillie, J. H.: A catenary analysis of the maxillary dental arch during human embryogenesis. Anat. Rec., 154:13–20, 1966.
25. Currier, J. H.: A computerized geometric analysis of human dental arch form. Am. J. Orthodont., 56:164–179, 1969.
26. Altemus, L. A.: A comparison of cephalofacial relationships. Angle Orthodont., 30:223–240, 1960.
27. Altemus, L. A.: Comparative integumental relationships. Angle Orthodont., 33:217–221, 1963.
28. Howes, A. E.: Arch width in the premolar region—still the major problem in orthodontics. Am. J. Orthodont., 43:5–31, 1957.
29. Garn, S. M., Lewis, A. B., and Kerewsky, R. S.: Size interrelationships of the mesial and distal teeth. J. Dent. Res., 44:350–353, 1965.
30. Lundström, A.: Asymmetries in number and size of the teeth and their etiological significance. Trans. Europ. Soc. Orth., 1–19, 1960.
31. Moorrees, C. F. A., and Reed, R. B.: Correlations among crown diameters of human teeth. Arch. Oral Biol., 9:685–697, 1964.
32. Moorrees, C. F. A., and Chadha, J. M.: Crown diameters of corresponding tooth groups in the deciduous and permanent dentition. J. Dent. Res., 41:466–470, 1962.
33. Muller, T. P., Hill, I. N., Petersen, A. C., and Blayney, J. R.: A survey of congenitally missing permanent teeth. J.A.D.A., 81:101–107, 1970.
34. Kingsley, N. W.: Oral Deformities. New York, D. Appleton & Co., 1880.
35. Simon, P.: Fundamental Principles of a Systematic Diagnosis of Dental Anomalies (transl. B. E. Lischer). Boston, Stratford Co., 1926.
36. Ackerman, J. L., and Proffit, W. R.: The characteristics of malocclusion: a modern approach to classification and diagnosis. Am. J. Orthodont., 56:443–454, 1969.

37. Moorrees, C. F. A., and Grøn, A. M.: Principles of orthodontic diagnosis. Angle Orthodont., 36:258–262, 1966.
38. Angle, E. H.: Classification of malocclusion. D. Cosmos, 41:248–264, 350–357, 1899.
39. Graber, T. M.: The three "M's": muscles, malformation and malocclusion. Am. J. Orthodont., 49:418–450, 1963.
40. Proffit, W. R., and Norton, L. A.: Influences of tongue activity during speech and swallowing. ASHA Reports, no. 5, Washington, 106–115, 1970.
41. Graber, T. M.: Overbite—the dentist's challenge. J.A.D.A., 79:1135–1145, 1969.
42. Leighton, B. C.: The early signs of malocclusion. Trans. Eur. Soc. Orth., 1969.
43. Lavelle, C. L. B., Foster, T. D., and Flinn, R. M.: Dental arches in various ethnic groups. Angle Orthodont., 41:293–299, 1971.
44. Lindegard, B., Lindegard, L., Carlson, M., and Larsson, S.: Need and demand for orthodontic treatment. Tandlaegebladet, 75:1198–1210, 1971.
45. Grewe, J. M., and Hagan, D. V.: Malocclusion indices: A comparative evaluation. Am. J. Orthodont., 61:286–294, 1972.

chapter 6

ETIOLOGY OF MALOCCLUSION: GENERAL FACTORS

Of all the chapters in this book, this and Chapter 7 should be considered most provocative to the biologist or to anyone with a scientific bent. A pathologist has his job outlined for him as he implements Koch's postulates and sets out to find the causative factor for a specific abnormality, to isolate it, inject it and recover it. Following this lead, the orthodontist should pinpoint the most likely basis for a malocclusion, define it by stripping away associated or symbiotic conditions, study it carefully in broad population groups and then demonstrate its validity. Yet nothing of this sort has been done in orthodontics on an epidemiologic basis. The bulk of our knowledge is still based on retroactive reasoning. We are confronted with the clinical picture and by reasoning backward we attempt to establish the most likely causative agent. Retroactive reasoning may be a good didactic tool but it seldom serves as a basis for validating a scientific premise. Indeed, it is largely the manner in which we arrive at a hypothesis; the validation still remains to be done.

In the past, when a child had protruding upper front teeth and also breathed through his mouth, had enlarged tonsils and adenoids and a short, hypotonic, relatively functionless upper lip, any one of these factors might have been tabbed as the *causative* agent in the malocclusion. As we search the literature, it is not difficult to find many cases of protruding upper incisors attributed to mouth breathing alone, to enlarged tonsils, to abnormal swallowing habits alone, to a short upper lip, to finger sucking, etc. There is no question that all these characteristics may be *associated* with protruding upper front teeth. But the question of whether they are *causative* (primary) factors or merely related (symbiotic) factors that may also be attributed to an entirely different and unrecognized etiologic entity must be answered.

All too frequently, associated characteristics of malocclusion have been blamed for a specific condition when they belong on the "effect" end of the "cause and effect" relationship. In our search we are not unlike the man who starts a trip from one city to another. He comes to a fork in the road and must choose one road or the other. He makes his decision and proceeds, only to find after a short distance that he comes to another fork in the road; but this time there are five or six possible roads ahead. They may all seem identical at the beginning but we can be sure that all roads do not "lead to Rome"— or to the primary basis of the dentofacial deformity. The paucity of our present knowledge of etiology in orthodontics compels us to attack the cause and effect relationship from the wrong end—that of effect. By working backward we shall undoubtedly arrive at the beginning, someday. How nice it would be to approach it from the other end.

No longer can conscientious orthodontists look at a child's mouth, observe a space deficiency and then glibly attribute it to the premature loss of deciduous cuspids, deciduous first molars, or prolonged retention of deciduous incisors. Yet, in the past, local "causes" were stressed in the literature as the primary concern. Many of the answers in the future may come from scientists in other fields. Right now we recognize the transcending importance of the field of genetics. As more knowledge is accumulated in the complex behavior of genes, particularly those determining characteristics in our area of endeavor, we shall be better able to pinpoint the actual causes of dental malocclusion. Furthermore, we should not neglect a study of evolutionary changes in *Homo sapiens*, for anthropologists, by studying the changes that have occurred in the past millenniums, can project future changes with reasonable accuracy. This information will not come overnight and it would be most unwise to go overboard on any one likely "suspect."

As the philosopher Frederick Jensen[1] has said, "What we think we know today shatters the errors and blunders of yesterday and is tomorrow discarded as worthless. So we go from larger mistakes to smaller mistakes—so long as we do not lose courage. This is true of all therapy; no method is final."

SYSTEMS OF CLASSIFICATION OF ETIOLOGIC FACTORS

It must be recognized at the outset that any arbitrary division of causes is purely for the sake of analysis. It is fairly certain that the interdependence of form and function and the ability of the organism to make a homeostatic (adaptive) response to a given situation introduce a number of modifying factors that are responsible for the "status quo."

Heretofore, in an attempt to categorize the etiologic factors, several methods have been used. One classification refers to *inherited* and congenital causes as one group and lists such factors as characteristics inherited from the parents, problems of tooth number and size, congenital deformities, conditions affecting the mother during pregnancy, and fetal environment. The second group, *acquired* causes, includes such factors as premature loss and prolonged retention of deciduous teeth, habits, abnormal function, diet, trauma, metabolic and endocrine disturbances, etc.

Another approach is to divide the causative factors into *indirect* or *predisposing* causes and *direct* or *determining* causes.[2] Under such a classification, the predisposing causes would be heredity, congenital defects, prenatal abnormalities, acute or chronic infectious and deficiency diseases, metabolic disturbances, endocrine imbalance and unknown causes. McCoy lists the following as determining causes: missing teeth, supernumerary teeth, transposed teeth, malformed teeth, abnormal frenum labium, intrauterine pressure, sleeping habits, posture, pressure, abnormal muscular habits, malfunctioning muscles, premature shedding of deciduous teeth, tardy eruption of permanent teeth, prolonged retention of deciduous teeth, premature loss of deciduous teeth, loss of permanent teeth and improper dental restorations.

Moyers lists seven "causes and clinical entities."[3]

1. Heredity
   a. Neuromuscular system
   b. Bone
   c. Teeth
   d. Soft parts (other than nerve and muscle)
2. Developmental defects of unknown origin
3. Trauma
   a. Prenatal trauma and birth injuries
   b. Postnatal trauma
4. Physical agents
   a. Prenatal
   b. Postnatal
5. Habits (thumb and finger sucking, tongue sucking, lip biting, etc.)
6. Disease
   a. Systemic diseases
   b. Endocrine disorders
   c. Local diseases
7. Malnutrition

A modification of Salzmann's diagrammatic representation of the etiologic factors in malocclusion embodies prenatal and postnatal factors.[4] It shows well the genetic, differentiative and congenital factors that make up the prenatal elements of causation which can influence any one or all of the postnatal components—developmental, functional, environmental (Fig. 6-1).

Another method of classifying etiologic factors is to divide them into two groups, the *general* group—those factors that operate on the dentition from without, and the *local* group—those factors that are immediately associated with the dentition. Although there are drawbacks to this approach it is the easiest one to use. It works well if at all times the student remains aware of

PRE- AND POST- NATAL ETIOLOGIC FACTORS
OF MALOCCLUSION

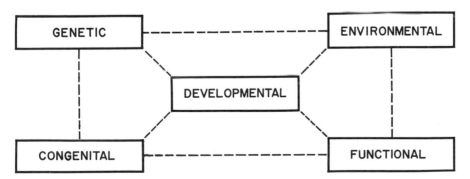

Figure 6-1   Diagrammatic representation of interdependence of etiologic factors in malocclusion. The interdependence of etiologic factors is obvious. The influence may be direct or reflect a homeostatic adjustment. (After Salzmann, J. A.: Practice of Orthodontics. J. B. Lippincott Co., 1966.)

the interdependence of general and local factors. Thus, there are few local factors that are not modified by one or more general influences. These correlations will be pointed out in the discussion of specific causes of malocclusion.

Classifications of Etiologic Factors

General Factors
1. Heredity (the inherited pattern)
2. Congenital defects (cleft palate, torticollis, cleidocranial dysostosis, cerebral palsy, syphilis, etc.)
3. Environment
   a. Prenatal (trauma, maternal diet, maternal metabolism, German measles, etc.)
   b. Postnatal (birth injury, cerebral palsy, TMJ injury, etc.)
4. Predisposing metabolic climate and disease
   a. Endocrine imbalance
   b. Metabolic disturbances
   c. Infectious diseases (poliomyelitis, etc.)
5. Dietary problems (nutritional deficiency)
6. Abnormal pressure habits and functional aberrations
   a. Abnormal suckling (forward mandibular posture, nonphysiologic nursing, excessive buccal pressures, etc.)
   b. Thumb and finger sucking
   c. Tongue thrust and tongue sucking
   d. Lip and nail biting
   e. Abnormal swallowing habits (improper deglutition)
   f. Speech defects
   g. Respiratory abnormalities (mouth breathing, etc.)
   h. Tonsils and adenoids (compensatory tongue position)
   i. Psychogenic tics and bruxism
7. Posture
8. Trauma and accidents

Local Factors
1. Anomalies of number
   a. Supernumerary teeth
   b. Missing teeth (congenital absence or loss due to accidents, caries, etc.)
2. Anomalies of tooth size
3. Anomalies of tooth shape
4. Abnormal labial frenum; mucosal barriers
5. Premature loss
6. Prolonged retention
7. Delayed eruption of permanent teeth
8. Abnormal eruptive path
9. Ankylosis
10. Dental caries
11. Improper dental restorations

GENERAL FACTORS

HEREDITY

Orthodontics, like behavioral psychology, has its "fashions." Certainly orthodontics has not escaped the ever-brewing controversy over the roles of heredity versus environment. Our early writers often stressed the predominant role of the inherited pattern, frequently with an air of helplessness about their inability to control this pattern. The pendulum swung strongly away from this approach on causation in the 1920's and 1930's, and the majority of writers attributed most dental malocclusions to local factors, paying only lip service to inheritance. In the last 20 years, because of a more concentrated and more scientific study of etiology of malocclusion from information that is a by-product of anthropologic and human genetic investigations, there has been a renaissance of the emphasis on hereditary pattern.

It is quite logical to start with heredity or the hereditary pattern in a discussion on etiology. After all, in the normal course of events it is not unreasonable to assume that the offspring inherits quite a few attributes from his parents. These factors, or these attributes, may be modified by prenatal and postnatal environment, by physical entities, by pressures, abnormal habits, nutritional disturbances and idiopathic phenomena. But the basic pattern is there, along with its tendency to go in a certain direction. We can say that there is a definite genetic determinant that influences the ultimate accomplishment of dentofacial morphology.[7,8] The pattern of accomplishment (growth and development) has a strong hereditary component.

There are certain racial and familial characteristics that tend to recur. Since the offspring is a product of parents of dissimilar heredity, cognizance must be taken of the inheritance from both sources. This means possibilities of a recapitulation of a hereditary trait from either parent or a combination of traits from both parents to produce a modified characteristic. The end product may be quite harmonious, or it may be disharmonious. A child may have facial features that markedly resemble those of his father or mother, or the net result may be a combination of features from each parent. He may inherit tooth size and shape, jaw size, shape and relationship, and similar muscle and soft tissue configuration from the father or the mother. But it is equally possible that he may inherit the tooth size and shape characteristics from one parent and the jaw size and shape from the other parent. The soft tissue draping may or may not approximate the maternal or paternal pattern. We just do not know enough about the complexities of combination and recombination of genes at the moment of conception to make an accurate prediction. But we do know what the ingredients are, even if we do not know the mixture ratios. It behooves us to study both parents carefully and to project the most likely pattern as a result of perpetuation of the dentofacial morphology of either the father or the mother, or the dentofacial morphology as a result of a combination of factors. Careful study of the parents will be most rewarding for the dentist interested in establishing a likely causative basis. Study of previous siblings is also rewarding because it often provides clues of hereditary tendencies, both normal and abnormal.

It must be understood that as we discuss the role which heredity plays in the etiology of any dental malocclusion we are dealing with probabilities. This is all we can do in genetics or physiology. We arrive at a clue, a hunch or a likely trend. Certain characteristics have greater hereditary likelihood, others less. We know from our study of the field of genetics that certain characteristics are dominant, others recessive. In the complex interplay of chromosomes and genes, two recessive factors may combine to become a dominant characteristic, or a dominant characteristic may be offset by a genetic potential from the other parent; and the characteristic may then disappear in the offspring. Certain genes seem to be more prone to recombination and mutation. Since most of our knowledge is deduced from extensive work done on the fruit fly (drosophila), which possesses only four sets of genes, the bulk of the answers awaits further definitive research. From what we know now, we may make certain broad observations concerning the role of heredity in the etiology of malocclusion.

HEREDITARY RACIAL INFLUENCE. Dental characteristics, like facial characteristics, show racial influence. In homogeneous racial groupings the incidence of malocclusion seems relatively low. In certain areas of the world—for example, some of the Philippine Islands—malocclusion is almost nonexistent. Population groups there are relatively pure genetically, and the occlusion of the natives "normal." Where there has been a mixture of racial strains the incidence of jaw size discrepancies and occlusal disharmonies is significantly greater. Stockard produced gross deformities with his crossbreeding of dogs.[5] Racial crossbreeding may emulate these experiments to a degree. Population studies regarding size seem to show that there may be a dominance of deficiency over excess as a result of these racial admixtures. For example, many more Class II malocclusions with mandibular underdevelopment are seen than Class III malocclusions where there may be excessive mandibular size. This observation must be conditioned by an overall purview of the evolution of man. Anthropologists show us that the jaws seem to be getting smaller, that there is a greater frequency of impaction of third molar teeth, a greater incidence of congenital absence of certain teeth and a retrognathic tendency in man as he ascends the evolutionary scale.

HEREDITARY FACIAL TYPE. The facial type, if not the individual characteristics, of the offspring probably is heavily influenced by heredity. Facial typing is three dimensional. Different ethnic groups and mixtures of ethnic groups have differently shaped heads. There are three general types; the brachycephalic, or broad round heads; the dolichocephalic, or long narrow heads; and the mesocephalic, a shape in between the brachycephalic and the dolichocephalic. (See Fig. 5–3.)

This is admittedly an arbitrary division and there are many gradations. With broad faces usually go broad cranial and facial bony building blocks and broad dental arches. With long narrow faces usually go harmonious bony structures that house narrow dental arches. Hasund and Sivertsen point out the sex-linked nature of facial width and dental arch shape. Females demonstrate a positive correlation—the wider the face, the wider the arch.[6] Unless we can change cranial and facial superstructures and reorient bony trabeculae, stress trajectories and supporting pillars and buttresses, along with their muscle attachments, we cannot significantly alter the hereditary pattern determinant that furnishes the blueprint for arch form, arch size, arch shape, etc. Specifically this means to the orthodontist that nature harmonizes the dental structures according to facial type. He cannot impose preconceived ideas of facial form and beauty on structures whose foundation is built for something else. Call it human engineering or whatever you wish, but this predominance of the morphogenetic pattern profoundly influences orthodontic objectives and therapeutic results. The question of facial type and its role in orthodontic diagnosis will be discussed in greater detail in Chapter 8.

HEREDITARY INFLUENCE ON THE GROWTH AND DEVELOPMENTAL PATTERN. Recognizing that the ultimate morphogenetic pattern has a strong hereditary component, it is reasonable to assume that the accomplishment of that pattern is also at least partially under the influence of heredity. For example, a child patient is very slow in losing his deciduous teeth and the eruption of permanent teeth is equally slow. The mother will say, "His brothers and sisters are also very slow, and so was I when I was his age." Obviously the environmental influences are important here, too, and they can and do modify the hereditarily determined pattern. Corollary to the individually transmitted facial growth pattern may be a more basic racial maturation gradient. The onset of puberty varies with the different races and with geographic distribution. Making the picture even more complex is the influence of sex. Maturation in the female is different from that in the male. Usually puberty, with its attendant growth and developmental processes, is confined to a narrower age range and begins earlier in girls than in boys. In girls, we see the major changes between 10½ and 13 years of age; in boys, anywhere between 12 and 18 years. Time of maturation is considerably more unpredictable in the male sex. So it seems that even the *accomplishment* of a particular pattern is subject to manifold influences. To single out one factor and assess its precise role is practically impossible.

HEREDITY AND SPECIFIC DENTOFACIAL MORPHOLOGIC CHARACTERISTICS. No less elusive is the role of heredity in the accomplishment of specific dentofacial attributes. Lundström made an intensive analysis of these characteristics in twins, and he concluded that heredity could be considered significant in determining the following characteristics:[7]

1. Tooth size
2. Width and length of the arch
3. Height of the palate
4. Crowding and spacing of teeth
5. Degree of sagittal overbite (overjet)

To the above list may be added probable hereditary influence on:

1. Position and conformation of perioral musculature to tongue size and shape
2. Soft tissue peculiarities (character and texture of mucosa, frenum size, shape and position, etc.)

If hereditary influence is present and can be demonstrated in the enumerated areas, it is logical to assume that heredity plays a part in the following conditions:

1. Congenital deformities
2. Facial asymmetries
3. Macrognathia and micrognathia
4. Macrodontia and microdontia
5. Oligodontia and anodontia
6. Tooth shape variations (peg-shaped lateral incisors, Carabelli's cusps, mamelons, etc.)
7. Cleft palate and harelip
8. Frenum diastemas
9. Deep overbite
10. Crowding and rotation of teeth
11. Mandibular retrusion
12. Mandibular prognathism

CONGENITAL DEFECTS

CLEFT LIP AND PALATE

Congenital or developmental defects are usually assumed to have a strong genetic relationship. This is more true of some conditions than of others. Various studies have shown that from one third to one half of all cleft palate children have a familial history of this deformity. Other congenital defects such as facial clefts seem to show less hereditary predetermination. Congenital defects like cleft lip and palate, separately or in combination, are among the most frequent congenital deformities in mankind (Fig. 6–2). One child in every 700 live births is afflicted. This amounts to 100,000 young people under 21 years of age or 5000 children each year (in the United States). The incidence of cleft lip and palate may be increasing.[8] Compared with the total number of births, the incidence of this deformity is low. But when it does occur, the parents of these unfortunate children search eagerly for some way to prevent the mental anguish, the misery and distortion of personality, the facial deformity, malocclusion and pathetic functional inadequacy that can be associated with cleft lip and palate. Figure 6–3A and B illustrates the Veau and current American Cleft Palate Association classifications of the deformity.

The teratologist says that from the pathologic we learn much about the normal. Cleft lip and palate provide nature's laboratory and an opportunity for us to observe aberrations in growth and development—inherent and environmentally induced.

Historically, as with all forms of surgery, maxillofacial techniques have undergone fads and fashions. Traumatic uranoplasty procedures closed clefts by molding the separated parts together. But what was a surgical success at two years of age, when judged by an esthetic and functional yardstick, became a complete failure by the time the patient was 20 years old, or even younger (Figs. 6–4, 6–5, 6–8 to 6–10). The restrictive, unyielding, scarifying lip operations in the early days demonstrated the dominance of muscle over bone and the potential of modified functional matrix control when environmental forces could be applied against the orofacial complex. A survey of cleft lip and palate surgery on a longitudinal basis has highlighted a number of questions that have important implications in a noncleft normal sample. From the point of view of surgical timing, why do results vary significantly, when the age of operation varies? Can cicatricial tissue retard maxillary growth, alveolar growth

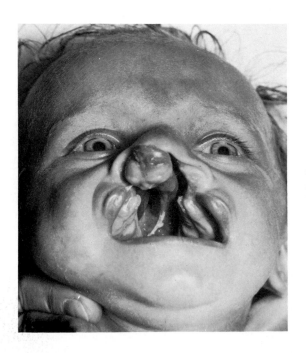

Figure 6–2 One child in every 700 has a cleft lip and/or palate. The entire premaxillary segment is fused to the nasal septum at the columella in the bilateral lip-jaw-palate cleft.

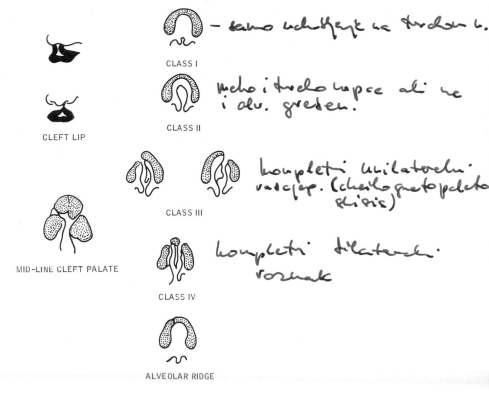

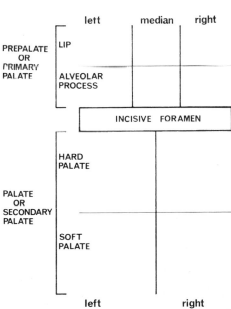

Figure 6–3 (Top) The most common cleft classification. Class I, soft palate with possible notching of hard palate. Class II, soft and hard palate, but no alveolar ridge. Class III, complete unilateral lip-jaw-palate cleft, right or left. Class IV, complete bilateral lip-jaw-palate cleft. Cases may also be categorized with alveolar ridge cleft only, lip cleft only and a true midline cleft. (From Graber, T. M.: A study of craniofacial growth and development in the cleft palate child from birth to six years of age *in* Hotz, R. (ed.): Early Treatment of Cleft Lip and Palate. Berne, Hans Huber, 1964.) (Bottom) Diagram of the basic cleft palate classification. (From Berlin, A. J.: Classification of cleft lip and palate, *in* Cleft Lip and Palate, Grabb, W. C., Rosenstein, S. R., Bzoch, K. R.: Little, Brown and Company, Boston, 1971.)

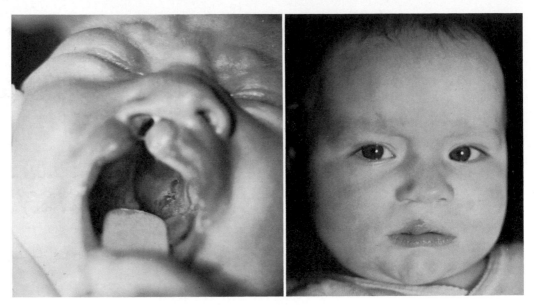

Figure 6–4   Right unilateral lip-jaw-palate cleft, complete; before and after lip surgery.

only, or can it merely deflect teeth from their normal eruptive path? What is the role of function? When and where does maxillary growth occur?

Studies by the author, and others have indicated that growth gradients are important, when planning surgical correction.[9–13] Too early surgical interference can, as shown in the illustrations already cited, produce bizarre deformities. But the type of original insult (partial cleft, complete unilateral, complete bilateral) influences the potential damage. As long as a bony bridge exists or is created early by bone graft, as illustrated by Monroe and Rosenstein, the chances for severe deformity are practically nil.[14] The type of surgery, the type of deformity and timing of intervention are equally critical. Nontraumatic procedures no longer duplicate the early uranoplasty results (Figs. 6–11 to 6–13).[79]

Cicatricial bands surely can restrict the horizontal maxillary anterior segment development. The present techniques specifically avoid constrictive pressures due to shortening of the buccinator mechanism. (See Chap. 3.) Collapse of buccal segments is reduced, particularly with a bony bridge present on one or both sides as a result of grafting procedures.

Restoration of normal function with proper lip closure produces dramatic molding effects on the premaxilla and is, again, applied physiology. The tightrope walked by the surgeon is to provide a functional matrix that restores normal soft tissue pressures and yet does not unduly restrict the contiguous tooth and bone parts. The lesson should not be lost for the functional orthopedic man, who might emulate the surgeon and create artificial functional matrix constricts. Apparently, this is the basis of the Fränkel philosophy and his use of functional correctors. (See Chap. 11.)

As our discussion of maxillary growth in Chapter 2 indicates, we have not yet resolved the question of pacemaker guidance, i.e., how much cranial base control, the exact role of the nasal septum, the possible contribution of fatty masses superiorly and posteriorly, the role of sutural growth, the contributions

(*Text continued on page 269*)

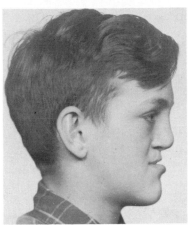

Figure 6–5 Growth restriction of middle face reflected in facial profile of a 13-year-old boy who has had 15 operations to close his lip and palate.

Case: M.S.

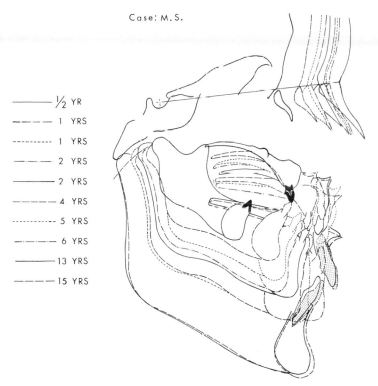

$\frac{1}{2}$ YR
1 YRS
1 YRS
2 YRS
2 YRS
4 YRS
5 YRS
6 YRS
13 YRS
15 YRS

Figure 6–6 Class IV cleft and Pierre Robin syndrome (see Fig. 6–7). Significant adjustive growth plus orthopedic guidance and surgery achieved the results shown over a 15-year period. A Kirschner wire between 4 and 6 years from vomer to premaxilla prevented horizontal maxillary growth, while the mandible continued to grow. Subsequent orthodontic therapy completed the correction. Note the changing directions of growth — horizontal, vertical, horizontal, and then vertical.

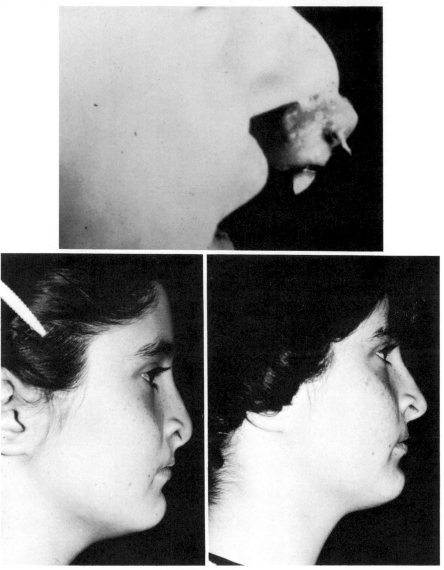

Figure 6–7 Patient in Figure 6–6, Pierre Robin syndrome, with bilateral cleft and premaxilla at tip of nose (top). Team effort of maxillofacial surgery and orthodontics, with orthopedic guidance to withhold premaxillary and maxillary growth, achieves profile improvement at 9 and 15 years (lower views). (Courtesy Rosenstein, S. W.: Pathological and congenital disturbances: the orthodontic viewpoint. J.A.D.A., 82:871–875, 1971.)

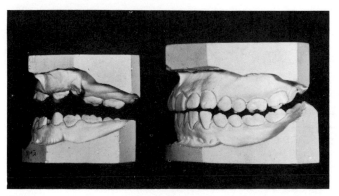

Figure 6–8 Casts of patient with repaired cleft lip and cleft palate related in postural resting position compared with a set of casts of a normal occlusion also related in postural resting position. The interocclusal clearance of the cleft patient is four times that of the normal subject.

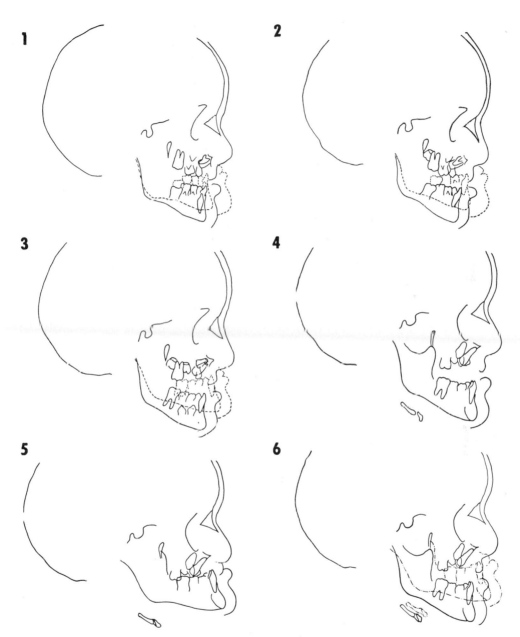

Figure 6–9   Cephalometric tracings in postural resting position and habitual occlusion of a victim of traumatic surgical closure of a complete lip-jaw-palate cleft. Note how the interocclusal clearance increases from 17 to 21 mm. over a four-year period. Downward and forward growth increments of the maxillary complex are negligible. 1, Six years of age, postural rest and occlusion tracings; interocclusal clearance 17 mm. 2, Seven years of age, postural rest and occlusion tracings; interocclusal clearance 18 mm. 3, Eight years of age, postural rest and occlusion; interocclusal clearance 20 mm. 4, Nine years of age, postural rest position; interocclusal clearance 21 mm. 5, Nine years of age, habitual occlusion. 6, Nine years of age, superimposed postural rest and occlusion tracings to show overclosure and mandibular prognathism on occlusion.

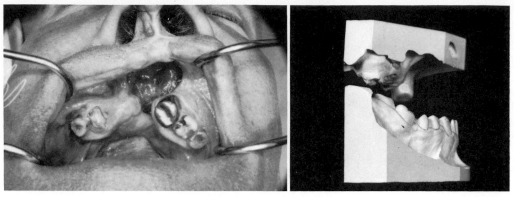

Figure 6–10 Early and traumatic surgical intervention in this complete lip-jaw-palate cleft resulted in the sloughing of the rudimentary premaxilla. Fibrous, unyielding scar tissue prevented normal expansion of the maxillary buccal segments.

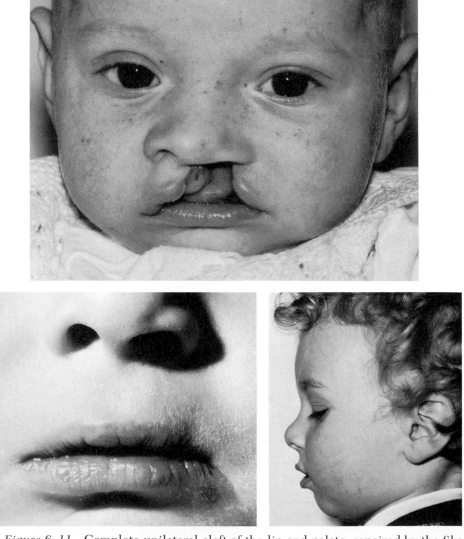

Figure 6–11 Complete unilateral cleft of the lip and palate, repaired by the Skoog technique at 3 months. (Top) Before operation, (bottom) one year after surgery. (From Skoog, Tord, *in* Grabb, W. C., et al. (eds.): Cleft Lip and Palate. Little, Brown, 1971.)

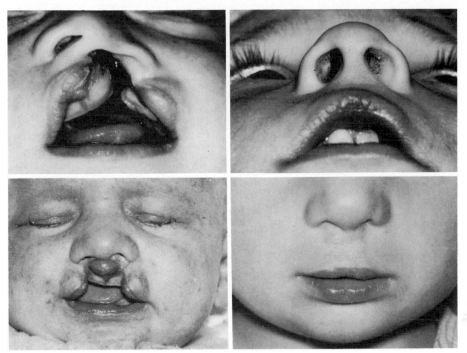

Figure 6–12 (Top, left) Unilateral complete cleft of the lip and palate in a three-month-old boy. Note the characteristic facial asymmetry due to underdevelopment of the maxillary segment on the cleft side. The top right picture was taken three years after repair, utilizing the technique for maxillary restoration by periosteal flaps. The bottom before and after pictures of a bilateral cleft show the small size of the prolabium at three months. Elongation of the columella by prolabial flaps and the Skoog technique provided ample height of the center of the lip and a most acceptable prolabium and free border of the lip. (From Skoog, Tord, *in* Grabb, W. C., et al. (eds.): Cleft Lip and Palate. Little, Brown, 1971.)

of the capsular and functional matrices, the actual growth of functioning spaces, the neurotrophic stimulus and nutritional influences, or even the intracellular DNA and RNA reactions in the total maxillary development. But we can study, as Enlow has done, when and where growth occurs.[13] With this knowledge, surgical procedures can be developed to coincide with the most favorable growth periods, just as orthodontic therapy can be properly timed. And techniques can be used which work with these growth processes, not against them. Even when a deformity has occurred, it is now possible to make a dramatic improvement eliminating morphogenetic and iatrogenic effects to a large degree.[76, 77]

To us as dentists, the malocclusion provides the greatest challenge. It is often not possible for the dentist to compensate for residual postsurgical abnormalities. In a unilateral cleft the teeth on the side of the cleft are usually in lingual cross-bite with the opposing lower teeth (Fig. 6–14). Many times the premaxilla is displaced anteriorly, or, because of a tightly repaired lip, the whole premaxillary structure is forced lingually. The maxillary incisors in this type of problem are frequently badly malposed with bizarre axial inclinations. In the area of the cleft, teeth are frequently jumbled (Fig. 6–15). The maxillary lateral incisor may be missing, atypical in shape or "twinned." To move the anterior teeth forward into correct overbite-overjet relationship (Fig. 6–17)

(Text continued on page 272)

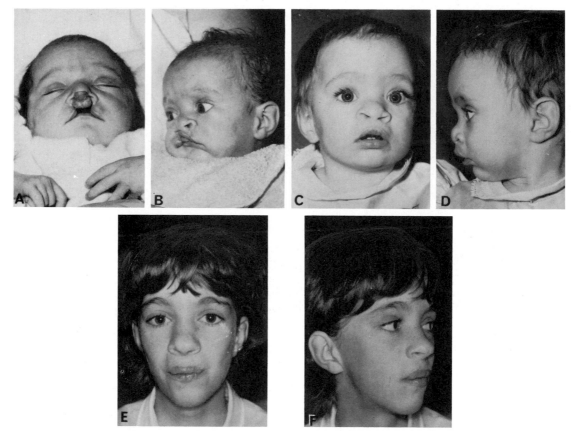

Figure 6–13   Bauer, Trusler and Tondra method of repair of bilateral cleft case with severely protruding premaxilla. (A & B) From two weeks of age, C & D, postoperative appearance. (E & F) At 13 years of age, elongation of columella has been done. (From Bauer, T. B., *in* Grabb, W. C., et al. (eds.): Cleft Lip and Palate. Little, Brown, 1971.)

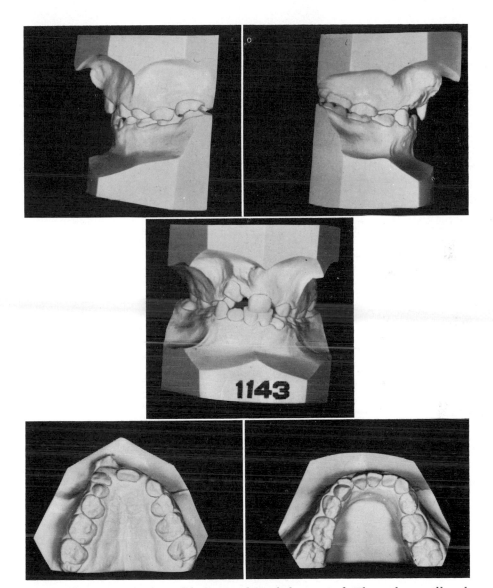

Figure 6–14 Complete unilateral lip-jaw-palate cleft repaired. The right maxillary buccal segment has collapsed toward the midline. Right maxillary lateral incisor is in line of cleft and very mobile.

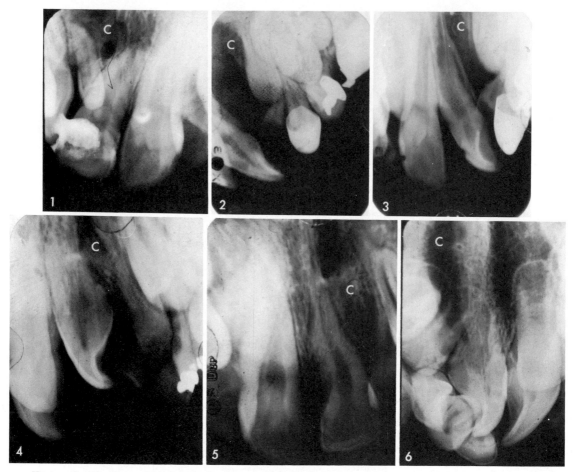

Figure 6–15 Dental radiographs of cleft areas of several patients show the effects of the cleft and cleft repair on contiguous teeth. The letter "C" marks each cleft area. 1, Note the peg-lateral and improperly formed upper right central incisor. 2, Lateral incisor is present on canine side of cleft. Usually it is in the premaxillary segment. 3, Central incisor badly rotated, lateral in cleft. 4, Cleft mesial to lateral incisor with deciduous lateral incisor in cleft. Left central incisor malposed and malformed. 5, Malformed central incisor. 6, Supernumerary tooth present.

often means forcing the teeth into a strongly resisting, repaired and partly scarred upper lip. Such procedures are unwise and can materially increase the likelihood of early loss of these teeth (Fig. 6–18). Whenever there is a struggle between muscle and bone, bone yields. The teeth and alveolar bone in this area are no exception. In an attempt to correct the lingual cross-bite (Fig. 6–19) frequently associated with repaired cleft palate, the problem is more than mere buccal movement of the maxillary teeth. Usually, the teeth are in relatively good relationship to their own basal bony support, but the entire palatal and alveolodental structure is displaced medially. Unless the orthodontist is prepared to move bony segments rather than just teeth, failure is likely (Fig. 6–20).

Treatment of the cleft palate individual is no longer left to any single specialist, whether he is a surgeon, pediatrician, prosthodontist, orthodontist or speech therapist. All coordinate their services to achieve the best overall result.

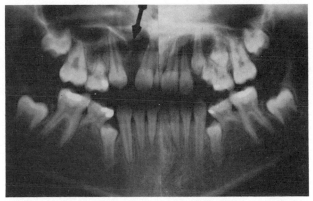

Figure 6–16 Cleft palate, combined with congenital absence of lateral incisor in cleft area and three missing second premolars. There is a much higher incidence of tooth abnormalities in patients with these problems.

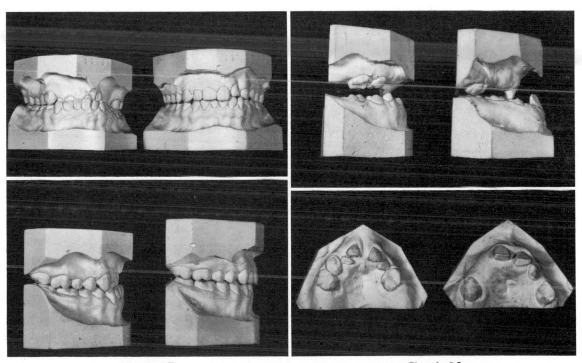

Fig. 6–17   **Fig. 6–18**

Figure 6–17 Anterior cross-bite corrected by orthodontic therapy. Since discrepancy was slight and mandibular protrusion due partly to tooth guidance, prognosis of correction is good.

Figure 6–18 Plaster casts of patient before orthodontic treatment (left) and after 3½ years' treatment (right). Anteroposterior discrepancy is greater despite therapy that has tipped maxillary incisors labially. This is due to mandibular growth increments unmatched by the maxilla. The problem is beyond orthodontic intervention.

Fig. 6–19

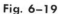

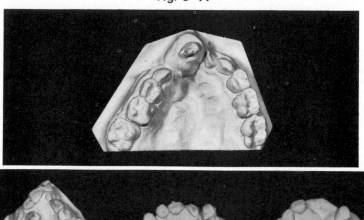

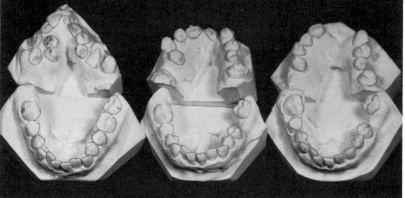

Fig. 6–20

Figure 6–19 Lip-jaw-palate cleft that has been repaired but with a mobile and diminutive premaxilla. Only one incisor will erupt into the mouth. Orthodontics is contraindicated.

Figure 6–20 Casts taken before, during and after orthodontic therapy which consisted of *en masse* movement of buccal segments with a split-palate removable appliance in conjunction with fixed orthodontic appliances. Maxillary anterior teeth had to be removed because of caries. Patient is now ready for a prosthesis.

OTHER CONGENITAL DEFECTS

Although cleft palate is the most common congenital defect to be of concern to the dentist as far as the creation of a malocclusion is concerned, such problems as tumors, cerebral palsy, torticollis, cleidocranial dysostosis, hemangiomas and congenital syphilis produce demonstrable abnormalities that require special dental guidance (Fig. 6–21).

CEREBRAL PALSY. Cerebral palsy is a paralysis or lack of muscular coordination attributed to an intracranial lesion. It is most commonly considered to be the result of a birth injury. The ramifications of this injury may be imperceptible or they may be extensive. As far as the dentist is concerned, effects of this neuromuscular disorder may be seen in the integrity of the occlusion (Fig. 6–22). Unlike cleft palate, where there are abnormal structures, the tissues are quite normal but the patient, because of his comparative lack of motor control, does not know how to use them properly. Varying degrees of abnormal muscular function may occur in mastication, deglutition, respiration and speech. The uncontrolled or aberrant activities upset the muscle balance that is necessary for the establishment and maintenance of a normal occlusion. (See Chap. 3.) Electromyographic studies on cerebral palsied children show a significant

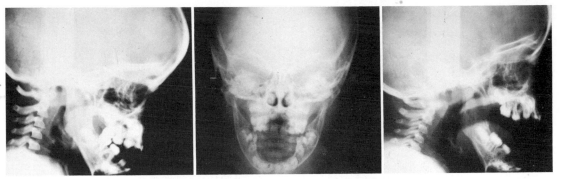

Figure 6–21   Hemangioma has literally "bent" the mandible, creating a severe open bite and basal deformation of the body of the mandible itself.

difference in the level of activity even when muscles are not in active function. It is obvious that abnormal pressure habits that result would create malocclusions. Severe deformities result when the muscles of the stomatognathic system are involved.[15] (See Abnormal Pressure Habits later in this chapter.)

TORTICOLLIS. The far-reaching effects of abnormal muscle forces are visible also in torticollis, or "wry neck." The foreshortening of the sternocleidomastoid muscle can cause profound changes in the bony morphology of the cranium and face, as studies have shown.[16] Torticollis provides an example of the thesis that in a struggle between muscle and bone, bone yields. Bizarre facial asymmetries with uncorrectable dental malocclusions may be created if this problem is not treated fairly early (Figs. 6–23, 6–24).

CLEIDOCRANIAL DYSOSTOSIS. Cleidocranial dysostosis is another congenital and frequently hereditary defect that may cause a dental malocclusion. There may be a unilateral or bilateral, partial or complete absence of the clavicle in conjunction with delayed cranial suture closure, maxillary retrusion and

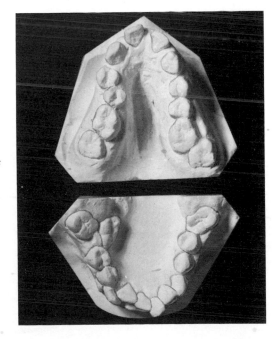

Figure 6–22   Malocclusion of hypertonic spastic girl 14 years of age. (Courtesy E. Trausch.)

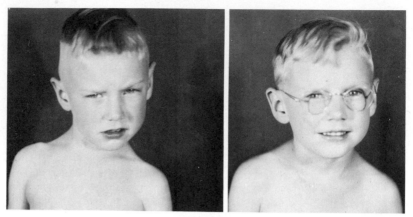

Figure 6–23 (Left) Preoperative torticollis, right side. Photograph shows marked facial asymmetry. (Right) Postoperative photograph. Mandibular posture has been improved, although the midline still deviates to the right. (Courtesy E. M. Sollar.)

possible mandibular protrusion. There is retarded eruption of the permanent teeth, and the deciduous teeth may be retained sometimes until middle age.[17] Roots of the permanent teeth are sometimes short and thin. Supernumerary teeth are common (Figs. 6–25 to 6–27).

CONGENITAL SYPHILIS. Although congenital syphilis has been greatly reduced in frequency, it still does occur. Abnormally shaped teeth and malposed teeth are considered characteristic disease phenomena.

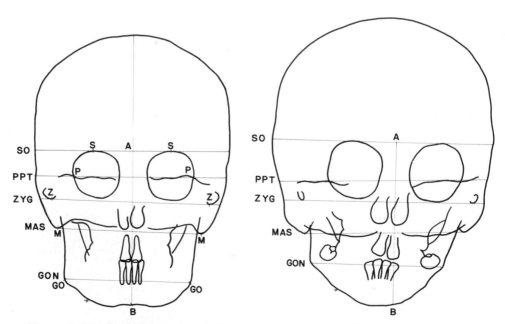

Figure 6–24 (Left) Frontal cephalometric tracing showing parallel and symmetrical relationship of paired structures in a normal individual. Transsectional planes are essentially parallel. (Right) Cephalometric tracing of patient in Figure 6–23. Mandibular outline is asymmetrical, gonial plane no longer parallel with facial and cranial planes. (After E. M. Sollar.)

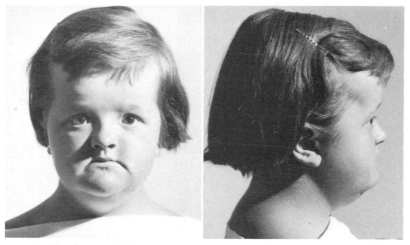

Figure 6–25   Cleidocranial dysostosis in a 12½ year old girl. (Courtesy J. Jensen.)

Figure 6–26 Lateral cephalometric headplate showing typical midface concavity, retention of deciduous teeth, noneruption of first permanent molars. (Courtesy J. Jensen.)

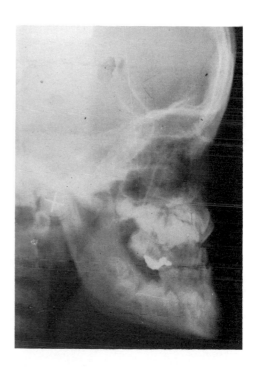

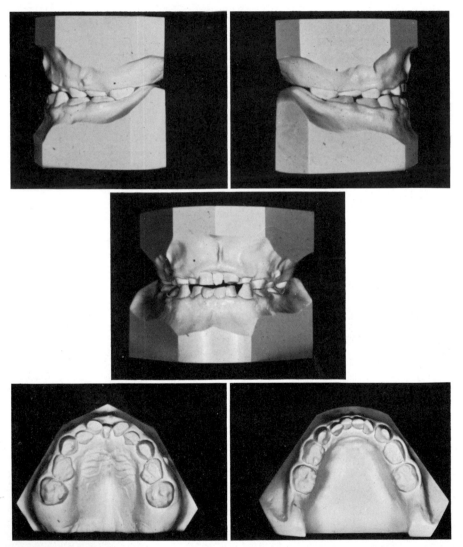

Figure 6–27   Plaster study models, Figures 6–25, 6–26. There is a Class III (Angle) tendency. Incisors show heavy abrasion. There is inadequate arch length to accommodate all the permanent teeth if they were to erupt. (Courtesy J. Jensen.)

ENVIRONMENT

It is relatively easy to discuss the role of heredity in the etiology of malocclusion and to see the effect of congenital defects on the integrity of the dental arches. It is far more difficult to categorize the remaining etiologic factors. For one thing, hovering over all specific disturbances is the guiding genetic determinant. Even in congenital defects like cleft palate, heredity plays a role in at least 35 per cent of the cases. It also has a significant place in problems of tooth number (supernumerary or missing teeth), actual accomplishment of pattern, tooth size and shape, arch form and so forth. We must always remember that where ontogeny recapitulates phylogeny and phenotypes are the product of genotypes, the ultimate product is a blend of the inheritance potential as it has been modified by a dynamic environment. T. Wingate Todd[18] has observed:

Faces differ, and most of us are content to assume that the differences are largely due to hereditary tendencies implicit in the genes. But as the face, like the rest of the body, is a plastic thing and since the adult contours are the end result of a growth pattern which in the course of its progress may be expedited, interrupted, retarded, warped, or inhibited by misadventures of health or by vagaries in the interplay of those organically organized influences by which the pattern is promoted, it is evident that environment, external and more particularly internal, must contribute in no small manner to the final result.

PRENATAL INFLUENCE.   The role of prenatal influences on malocclusion is probably very small. Uterine posture, fibroids of the mother, amniotic lesions, etc., have been blamed for malocclusions[19] (Fig. 6–28). Other possible causes

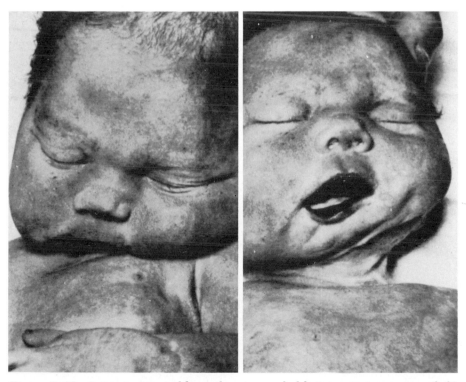

Figure 6–28   Intrauterine molding, showing probable intrauterine posture (left) and distortion and asymmetry in view on right. (By courtesy of Dr. Dermod MacCarthy. Walker, D. G.: Malformations of the Face. E. & S. Livingstone, 1961.)

of malocclusion are maternal diet and metabolism, drug-induced deformities, as with thalidomide, possible injury or trauma and German measles. Maternal nutritional and metabolic disturbances appear to be unlikely causes of developmental deformity.[20] Since the fetus is well cushioned by the amniotic fluid, minor injury to the mother is unlikely to affect the child. Abnormal fetal posture and maternal fibroids have caused marked cranial or facial asymmetries that are apparent at birth, but after the first year of life most of these have disappeared. Thus, the deformity is temporary. Even in cases of so-called micro-

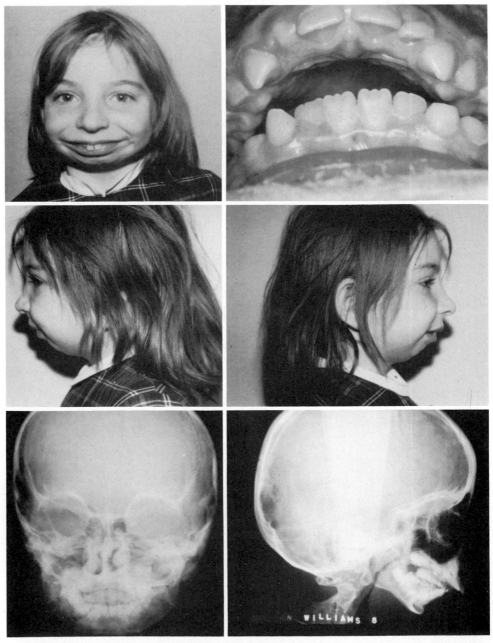

Figure 6–29 Eight-year-old twin, with birth injury and subsequent condylar ankylosis that allowed only 3 mm. opening (upper, right). Severe mandibular underdevelopment resulted.

mandible or Pierre Robin syndrome and Treacher-Collins syndrome[8] (mandibular dysostosis), there are tremendous increments of adjustive growth that largely eliminate the original malformation (Figs. 6–6, 6–7). German measles, as well as medications taken during pregnancy, causes gross congenital deformities including malocclusions.

POSTNATAL INFLUENCE.   To say that malocclusions are a result of birth injuries is to delve into retroactive reasoning in most cases. Birth is a tremendous shock to the newborn, but the cranial bones slide more and mold more than the facial and dental areas. The plasticity of the structures is such that any injury would be temporary except in rare instances. While it is certainly possible to injure the infant at birth with a high forceps delivery, this seldom occurs. A readier explanation is found usually by looking at the teeth and jaws of the parents—heredity. Authentic cases have been reported in the literature where the temporomandibular joint has been permanently damaged during birth (Figs. 6–29 to 6–33), but this is quite unusual. Malocclusions can be and frequently are associated with cerebral palsy (see Congenital Defects), which is usually attributable to birth injury. Depending on the damage, "spastics" may have bizarre, atypical dental malocclusions as the normal muscular balance is upset. Another possibility, though this is undocumented and again depends on retroactive reasoning, is the delivery-induced deformation of the upper jaw. Obstetricians frequently insert the forefinger and middle finger into the baby's mouth to ease passage through the birth canal. Because of the plasticity of the maxillary and premaxillary region, temporary deformation is quite likely and permanent damage may result.

Less frequent but more likely causes of malocclusion are disabling accidents that produce undue pressures on the developing dentition. Falls that produce condylar fractures may cause marked facial asymmetries (Fig. 6–34). Extensive scar tissue, for example, from a burn (Fig. 6–35), may also produce malocclusions. The delicate responsiveness of the dentition to environmental changes is shown in the case of a 13-year-old girl who has had to wear a plaster neck cast for four months as a result of a fractured cervical vertebra (Fig. 6–36). The strong elevating force on the mandible has forced the maxillary incisors

(Text continued on page 286)

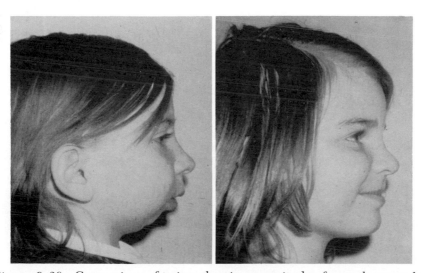

Figure 6–30   Comparison of twins, showing magnitude of growth arrest, left.

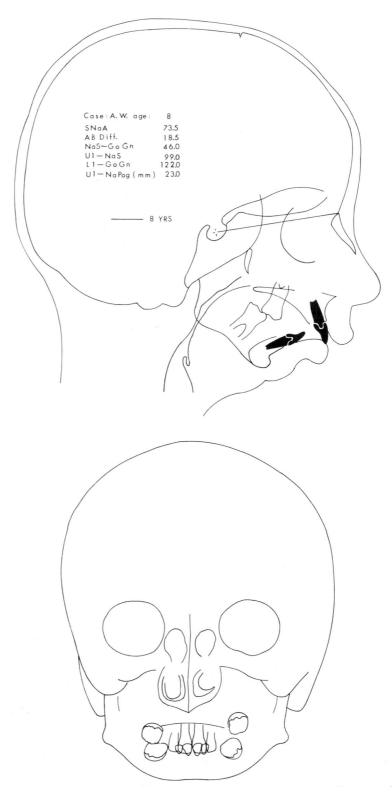

Case: A.W. age: 8
SNaA   73.5
AB Diff.   18.5
NaS—GoGn   46.0
U1—NaS   99.0
L1—GoGn   122.0
U1—NaPog (mm)   23.0

———— 8 YRS

Figure 6–31 Lateral and frontal cephalometric tracings that illustrate the severe anteroposterior and vertical mandibular deformity. A significant finding is that the bicondylar and bigonial width are within normal limits, despite the ankylosis. The implication is that ramus and condyle width growth are tied to cranial base growth, which is endochondral.

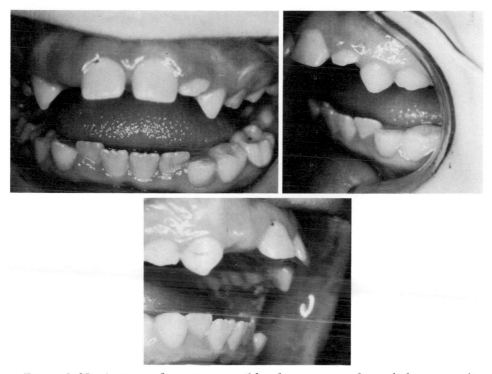

Figure 6–32 Amount of opening possible after surgery, after ankylosis was eliminated and a silastic wafer interposed between condyle and articular eminence.

Figure 6–33 Difficult breech delivery with fracture of mandibular condyle. Note facial asymmetry and deviation of midline to affected side.

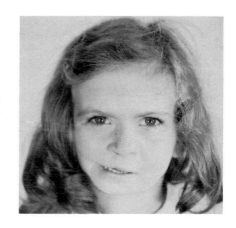

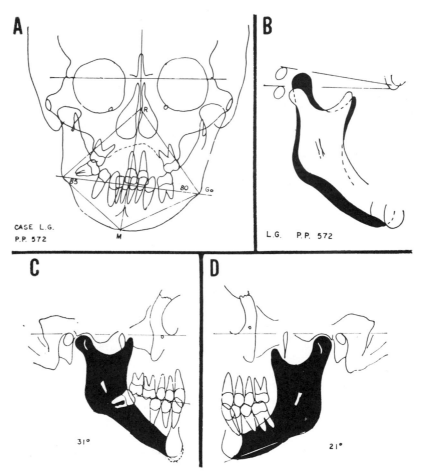

Figure 6–34   Patient with undergrowth of left mandibular condyle, causing facial asymmetry and deviation of chin to the same side. In frontal tracing (A), R-Go-M angle is 85° on the left and 80° on the right. (B), Superimposed outlines registered on mandibular canal show distal inclination of condyle and shorter neck and smaller ramus of left side, as compared with that of right side. (C), Tracing of left mandible, showing a mandibular plane angle of 31°. (D), Shows right mandible, with mandibular plane only 21°. (From Ricketts, R. A., *in* Sarnat, B. G. (ed.): The Temporomandibular Joint. Charles C Thomas, 1964.)

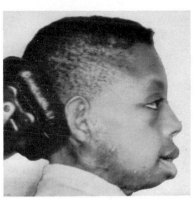

Figure 6–35   Extensive scarring of neck and lower face as a result of severe burns during infancy has restricted mandibular growth.

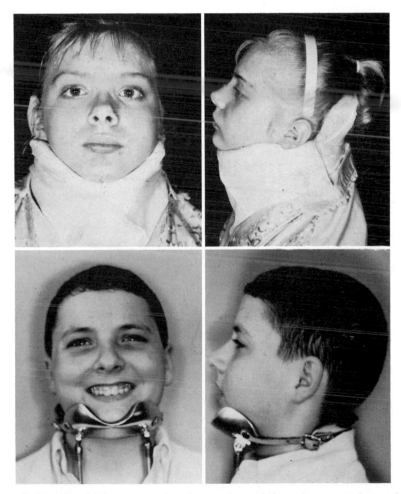

Figure 6–36   (Top) Plaster cast in place to immobilize the cervical vertebrae. The damage resulted from a "whip-lash" injury. The head is held in an extended position; there is constant pressure being maintained on the mandible. Similar deformation occurs with the Milwaukee brace or similar braces in the treatment of scoliosis (bottom). (See Fig. 2–84.)

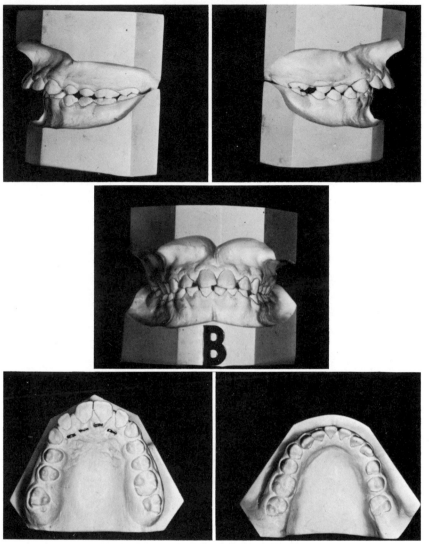

Figure 6–37   Plaster casts of patient in Figure 6–36 (top). Occlusion was normal before the accident. Constant upward pressure of the mandible and mandibular teeth has forced the maxillary incisors labially, and there are now deep depressions in the palatal tissue (lower left) to accommodate the mandibular incisal margins.

labially, and the mandibular incisors now fit into deep impressions in the palatal mucosa (Fig. 6–37). Prolonged Milwaukee brace wear produces similar deformity and malocclusion (Fig. 6–36).

PREDISPOSING METABOLIC CLIMATE AND DISEASE

A discussion of the effect of metabolic climate on malocclusion must deal primarily with diseases that affect that climate. Exanthematous fevers are known to upset the developmental timetable, and they often leave their permanent marks on the surface of the teeth. The exact effects of acute febrile disturbances on the development of occlusion, however, are not known. There is some recent evidence that acute febrile diseases may temporarily slow down the pace of growth and development. It is conceivable that a disturbance in the complex timetable of eruption, resorption, tooth loss, etc., might have permanent repercussions, but such concepts are based largely on retroactive reasoning. Some specific endocrinologic diseases may be potent makers of malocclusion. Diseases with a paralytic effect, such as poliomyelitis, are capable of producing bizarre malocclusions (Fig. 6–38). Diseases with muscle malfunction, such as muscular dystrophy and cerebral palsy, also have characteristic deforming effects on the dental arch (Fig. 6–23).[22] The effects of chronic diseases occasionally can be demonstrated, but here again exactitude is not the order of the day.

Endocrinopathies provide a more direct cause and effect basis. Frank pituitary and parathyroid disturbances are not common, but the effect on growth and development is striking when these disturbances occur[20] (Figs. 6–39 to 6–44). Less dramatic but more important to the orthodontist are thyroid problems which afflict an estimated 2 to 3 per cent of our population. Abnormal resorption patterns, delayed eruption patterns, and gingival disturbances go hand in hand with hypothyroidism. Retained deciduous teeth and individually malposed teeth that have been deflected from their normal eruptive path are frequent in these patients. Why is this so? We do not know as yet. The exact tie-in between reduced thyroid secretion, its effect on the other endocrine secretions, delayed endochondral bone formation, abnormal blood sedimentation and blood cholesterol, a low basal metabolic rate and dental abnormalities remains a good research project for the present, so that we may have the answer in the future.

The fact that we do not know the mechanism does not prevent us from recognizing and intercepting the effects. Many a subclinical case of hypothyroidism has been pointed out to an unknowing patient by an alert orthodontist looking at the patient's teeth and investing tissues, plaster casts, headplates and dental radiographs. Great benefit can come from early recognition of these prob-

(Text continued on page 292)

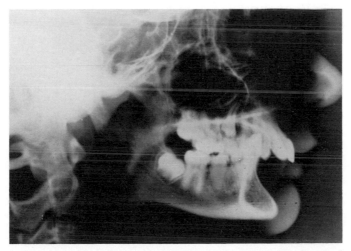

Figure 6–38   Lateral cephalometric headplate of patient who has had poliomyelitis. Anterior temporal muscle fibers, some facial muscles and suprahyoid muscles have been paralyzed, resulting in a strong retracting force on the mandible. In addition, the tongue is partly paralyzed and the soft palate completely inactive. Over a 2-year period since the onset of the disease, the anteroposterior discrepancy has increased despite orthodontic attempts at correction of the malocclusion.

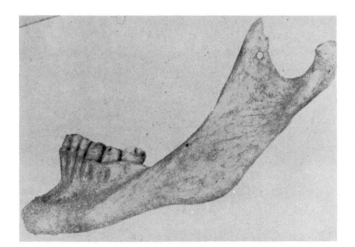

Figure 6–39 Acromegalic mandible showing tremendous post-developmental condylar growth, appositional growth at symphysis and modeling resorption at mandibular angle as a result of muscle forces. (From Weinmann, J. P., and Sicher, H.: Bone and Bones. 2nd ed. C. V. Mosby Co., 1955.)

Figure 6–40 Drawings of two 8-year-old dwarfs with marked endocrinopathies, as compared with a normal 2-year-old and a normal 8-year-old. The cretin or acutely hypothyroid dwarf has a thick neck, shorter extremities, large face and head, thick lips and large protruding tongue. The euthyroid or pituitary dwarf is harmoniously proportioned. In both instances the dentition is delayed, with all deciduous teeth still present. (Courtesy E. Grimm.)

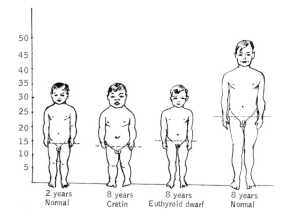

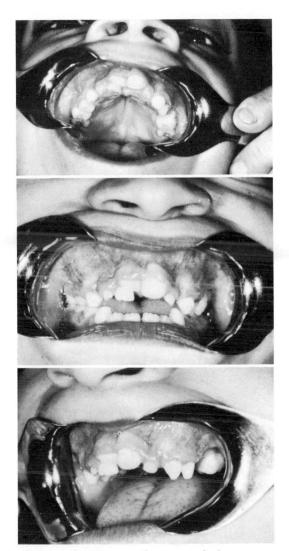

Figure 6–41   Occlusion of patient with cretinoid characteristics. Tongue is large; right maxillary deciduous central incisor is still retained despite eruption of permanent successor.

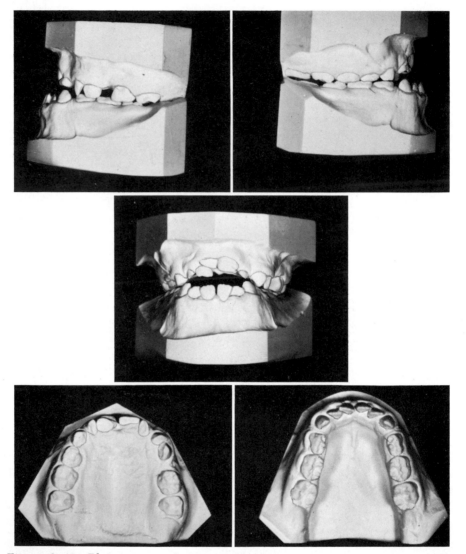

Figure 6–42   Plaster casts of 11-year-old patient in Figure 6–41. Upper left first deciduous molar has been lost due to caries. Anterior open bite and Class III relationship associated with cretinoid large tongue.

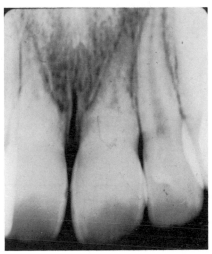

Figure 6–43 Spontaneous resorption of roots of maxillary central incisors. There is a history of a parathyroid tumor in this patient. (Courtesy J. Jarabak.)

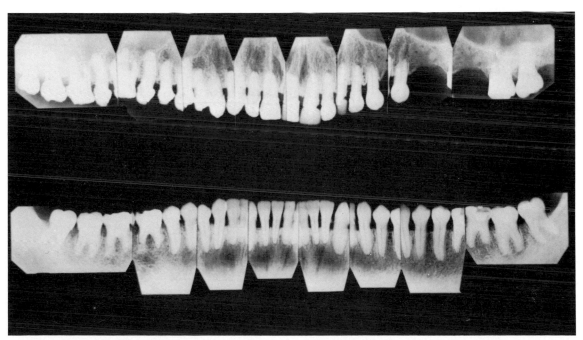

Figure 6–44 Multiple root resorptions in acromegaly (hyperpituitarism) in a 36-year-old adult. (Courtesy Herman Becks.)

lems and from therapy by a competent physician. Since the maintenance of a normal metabolic rate is essential for normal growth and development, everything possible should be done to eliminate the disease entity responsible for any upset in the timetable.

DIETARY PROBLEMS (NUTRITIONAL DEFICIENCY)

Nutritional deficiencies are relatively uncommon in the United States, but a visit to large areas of the world would show that as many as two billion people do not receive what we consider the essential elements of a minimum diet. Malnutrition in these areas of the world satisfies one definition of the word "normal," namely, "the usual." Disturbances such as rickets, scurvy and beriberi can produce severe malocclusions. So often the main problem is the upsetting of the dental developmental timetables. The resultant premature loss, prolonged retention, poor tissue health and abnormal eruptive paths mean malocclusion. Nutritional deficiencies that do occur in the United States and other countries with standards of living that make food readily procurable are usually due to faulty utilization of the ingested food, not insufficient intake. Hormonal or enzymatic imbalance may be such that the essential elements are excreted, to the detriment of the developing tissues.[22] Chronic alcoholism in the adult can produce a similar type of malnutrition. Patients suspected of having a metabolic disturbance that prevents utilization of ingested dietary essentials should be referred immediately to their physician. Damage can be irreparable.

ABNORMAL PRESSURE HABITS

Bone, as was discussed in Chapter 3, is a plastic tissue responsive to pressures that are continually acting on it. The dynamic role of the musculature is apparent. In the last few years the "plaster orthodontist" has been able to augment his artistic plaster facsimiles of the teeth and associated oral structures with cephalometric headplates. Information gained has been valuable. Some men have been so enthusiastic in the use of cephalometric x-ray pictures that they have been facetiously labeled "headplate orthodontists." Both plaster models and cephalometric headplates are static records, however—periodic records of initial morphology and subsequent changes in that morphology as influenced by the original hereditary pattern, metabolism, disease, growth and development, function and the dentist's efforts. Recent electromyographic research by Tulley, Lear, Gould and Picton, Doty, Bosma, Garrett, Powell and others, calls attention to the dynamic role of the musculature.[23-32] Electromyographic research by Moyers,[33] Perry,[34] Carlsöö[35] and Ahlgren[36] particularly, has infused new enthusiasm into orthodontic research on etiologic factors and the stability of post-treatment results. At the risk of being accused of adopting strong-arm tactics, I suggest that these men be called "muscle men," for their efforts may well bring into being a third type of orthodontist, the "myographic orthodontist." In a sense, the current interest in the effects of associated muscle action on the dentition is not new. Simon[37] wrote:

A wide experience has taught us that orthodontics does not occupy itself to any great extent with function, but only with the form of dentures. . . . The part which function plays is somewhat platonic. . . . Function is always regarded as dependent on structure, and the orthodontist generally considers it secondary. An orthodontist may urge his patient to use his dentures, especially after corrective treatment, but he does not subject them to a functional test. He never speaks of articulation, but always of occlusion — his subject is a denture at rest, not one in action.

Alfred Paul Rogers and his followers[38] also realized the importance of muscle function a long time ago, and they developed a series of exercises to assist in the elimination of muscle perversions associated with malocclusions. What electromyography does is to provide a more objective and definitive means of appraising muscle activity before, during and after orthodontic therapy. Our body of knowledge on etiology and post-treatment stability will be enlarged as present intensive research provides more information on muscle activity.

The electromyograph is an appraisal of the electrical activity of muscle. A minute amount of electric current is created with the contraction of muscles. Theoretically, we would like to measure this action potential, or action current, for one single motor unit. Actually, this is practically impossible, particularly with the use of surface electrodes. Since motor units do not act in harmony, greater work load means not only more frequent contraction but also more motor units acting in asynchrony to produce a smoother flowing muscle function. This masks the individual wave form, making recordings difficult to study at times. Nevertheless, the ability of modern electronic equipment to pick up, amplify and record electrical discharges from muscle activity with a minimum of distortion gives the physiologist a potent tool, if used carefully (Fig. 6–45). Current means of recording muscle activity are the crystographic ink writing recorder, the cathode-ray oscilloscope and the magnetic tape recorder. Surface, hook and needle type electrodes may be used in the area under study (Fig. 6–46). An interesting use made of the tape recorder has been its converting of the firing of muscle units into sound. It is thus possible to

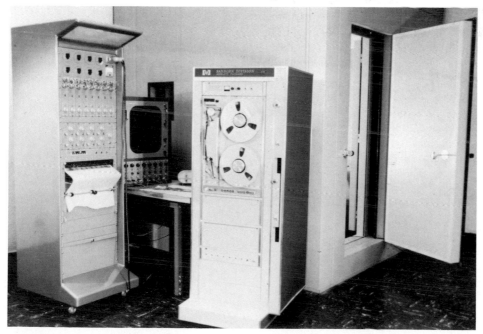

Figure 6–45   8 Channel Beckman EMG, with 8 channel oscilloscope and Sanborn tape recorder. Faraday Cage may be seen. (Courtesy Harold Perry, Northwestern University.)

ELECTRODE PLACEMENT

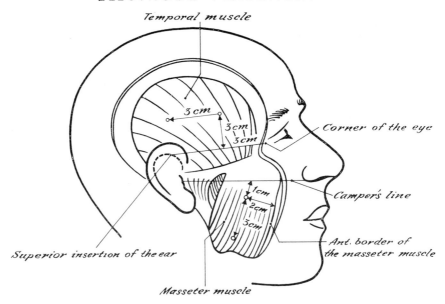

The HOOK ELECTRODE
Internal platina wire electrode (unipolar)
for masticatoy muscles

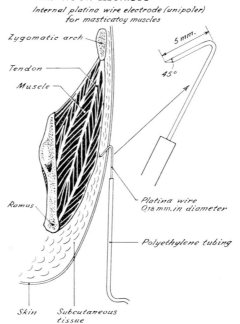

Figure 6–46   Electrodes. Electrodes should be relatively painless and lie as close as possible to the muscle being studied. Surface electrodes satisfied the first requirement but were inaccurate because they recorded from an ill-defined mass of tissue. Concentric needle electrodes lay within the muscle and recorded from a well-defined area. However, they were painful and might interfere with natural function. A thin, flexible wire placed under the skin close to the muscle made a good compromise to provide both an accurate and a painless recording of the muscle activity during mandibular movements. (Ahlgren, J.: Mechanism of mastication. Acta Odont. Scand. [Suppl. 44], 24:44–45, 1966.)

recognize the characteristic movements of muscle by the variations of the rumbling noise produced by the recorder.

Hotz, Tulley, Ballard, Subtelny, Bosma, Moorrees, Proffit, Winders, Cleall and many others have studied the role of musculature in malocclusion.[39-47] Their observations, in the light of objective myographic research, form the basis of our knowledge on this subject today. As dentists, we tend to think of certain of our muscles primarily as masticating elements. The dental student learns first that the masseter and temporal, external and internal pterygoid muscles are "muscles of mastication." This is only part of the picture. These muscles, as well as the other facial muscles with which they are intimately associated, have other functions that are equally important or more so, as is pointed out in Chapter 3. The average person eats three meals a day, but he swallows all day long, and he breathes constantly and talks a good part of that time. In addition to mastication, deglutition, respiration and speech, there is an even more important role of the musculature—that of posture. As electromyographic and cineradiographic studies have shown, even at postural resting position muscle is apparently in active function, maintaining a status quo of soft tissue and bony elements. The telltale modulated rumbling heard in a myographic tape recording of individuals with normal occlusion provides evidence of a certain level of constant activity even at postural rest. Tapes made on persons with malocclusion no longer record the even, synchronous recruitment of peripheral muscle fibers associated with normal occlusion. Often an erratic fibrillatory type of contraction is registered. Premature occlusal contacts and compensatory muscle activity during active function produce even greater departures from the normal. Such activity can change bony morphology, accentuating the malocclusion (Figs. 6-47, 6-48). How much of this is primary and how much secondary, adapting to the malocclusion, is difficult to determine.[43]

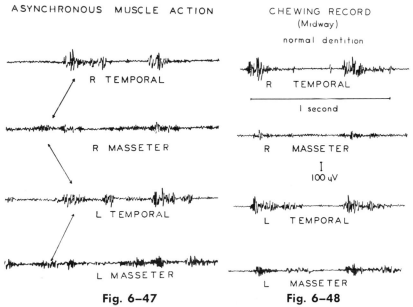

ASYNCHRONOUS   MUSCLE   ACTION

R TEMPORAL

R MASSETER

L TEMPORAL

L MASSETER

Fig. 6–47

CHEWING RECORD
(Midway)

normal dentition

R   TEMPORAL

I second

R   MASSETER

I
100 μV

L   TEMPORAL

L   MASSETER

Fig. 6–48

Figure 6–47   Asynchronous muscle action associated with a malocclusion. Contrast this with the even pattern of a normal occlusion (Fig. 6–48).

Figure 6–48   Normal electromyographic recordings of right and left temporal and masseter activity. (Figs. 6–47, 6–48 courtesy J. R. Jarabak.)

If there is a malrelationship between the maxilla and the mandible, making normal muscle function difficult, an adaptive activity of the muscles may occur. Nature usually tries to work best with what it has, so that a compensatory muscle functional activity is established to handle the demands of mastication, respiration, deglutition and speech. Good examples of this compensatory activity are seen in Class II and Class III malocclusions. Lischer's excellent drawings (Figs. 6–49 to 6–51) illustrate the point.[48] After orthodontic therapy, adaptation to the new morphologic relationship is clearly seen (Figs. 6–52 and 6–53).

Normally, at postural resting position there is a sort of balance of extraoral and intraoral muscle forces, with the buccal and perioral musculature passively restraining anterior displacement of the teeth. This can be illustrated by wrapping a piece of rubber dam over a skull or by drawing a diagram of the restraining muscle band (Fig. 6–54). This is admittedly oversimplified, for measurements show that force values alone do not balance. Lingual pressures are greater (Cleall and Winders). But hydraulic effect, tissue mass, cheek elastic index and morphogenetic pattern contribute to the total balance (Weinstein). (See Chap. 3.) The buccinator mechanism runs posteriorly to the pterygomandibular raphe, decussating with fibers of the superior constrictor muscle that carry on around

Fig. 6–49

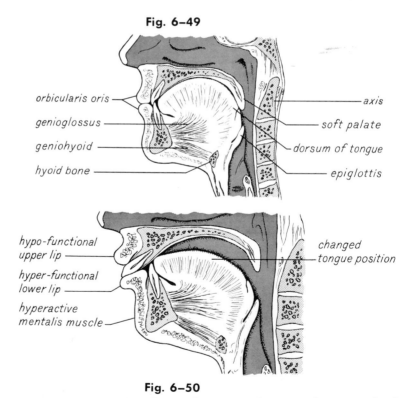

Fig. 6–50

Figure 6–49 Drawing of midsagittal section of a normal structural relationship. Note gentle, unstrained lip contact, balancing effect of external and internal muscle components and approximation of tongue and hard and soft palate.

Figure 6–50 Drawing of midsagittal section of an abnormal structural relationship such as associated with a Class II, Division 1 (Angle) malocclusion. Note lack of lip contact, cushioning of lower lip lingual to maxillary incisors, hyperactive mentalis muscle activity and changed tongue position—all contributing to an increase in the alveolodental dysplasia. (Figs. 6–49, 6–50 redrawn after B. E. Lischer.)

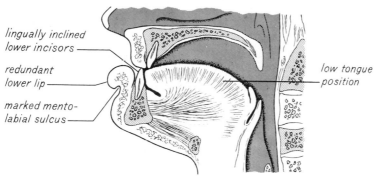

lingually inclined lower incisors

redundant lower lip

marked mento-labial sulcus

low tongue position

Figure 6–51 Drawing of midsagittal section of abnormal relationship associated with Class III (Angle) malocclusion. Observe redundant lower lip, deep mentolabial sulcus, lingually inclined mandibular incisors, tongue lower than normal with tip touching vermilion border of upper lip and maxillary incisor margin during deglutition. (Redrawn after B. E. Lischer.)

and anchor at the pharyngeal tubercle of the occipital bone. This bony attachment is not essential to maintain status quo, however, for all the facial muscles are intimately related to the postvertebral, prevertebral and cervical musculature, so that a change in one muscle would influence relationships with the other muscles (Figs. 3–17 to 3–20). In Class II, Division 1 malocclusions where there is excessive overjet, it is difficult to close the lips properly. No longer do the upper and lower lips contain the dentition. Rather, as part of the adaptive response, the lower lip cushions behind the maxillary incisors at rest and with every swallow (the frequency varies widely—according to Lear, Flanagan and Moorrees,[46] in their study of 20 normal adults—from 233 to 1008 swallows every 24 hours, with an average of 585); the abnormal contraction of the mentalis muscle and compensatory function of the other perioral muscles propel the maxillary incisors labially. The mandibular anterior segment is frequently flattened by

STAGE 1. INITIAL REST POSITION.
STAGE 2. TONGUE TIP ELEVATION.
STAGE 3. DORSUM MOVEMENT REACHING THE JUNCTION OF THE HARD AND SOFT PALATES.
STAGE 4. MAXIMUM SUPERIOR AND ANTERIOR HYOID POSITION.
STAGE 5. FINAL REST POSITION.

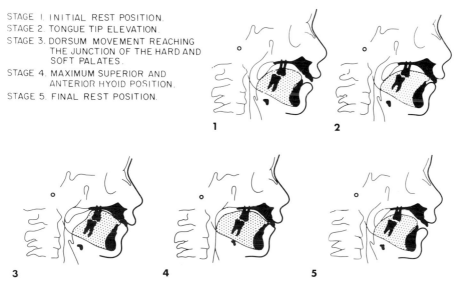

Figure 6–52 A series of tracings made from selected frames of a cinefluorographic sequence of swallowing of a patient with a Class II, Division 1 malocclusion. This recording was made prior to treatment and shows the movement of the tongue tip into the space between the upper and lower incisors. (Courtesy John Cleall.)

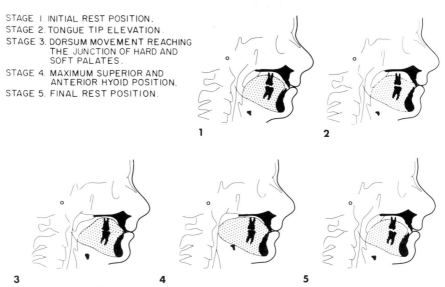

STAGE 1. INITIAL REST POSITION.
STAGE 2. TONGUE TIP ELEVATION.
STAGE 3. DORSUM MOVEMENT REACHING
         THE JUNCTION OF HARD AND
         SOFT PALATES.
STAGE 4. MAXIMUM SUPERIOR AND
         ANTERIOR HYOID POSITION.
STAGE 5. FINAL REST POSITION.

Figure 6–53 Following treatment, retention, and a post-retention period of two years, the same patient as shown in Figure 6–52 now demonstrates a lack of protrusive tongue activity. (Courtesy John Cleall.)

the postural and functional abnormality of the lower lip. Thus, the original malocclusion may have been the result of a hereditary pattern, but this has been made worse by the compensatory malposition and malfunction of the associated musculature. Unfortunately, this becomes a vicious circle. The greater the overjet, the more habitual the interposition of the lower lip nestled between the labial aspect of the mandibular incisors and the lingual aspect of the maxillary incisors. That these muscles function abnormally is clear, and electromyographic evidence only serves to record in black and white the departure from the normal (Fig. 6–55).

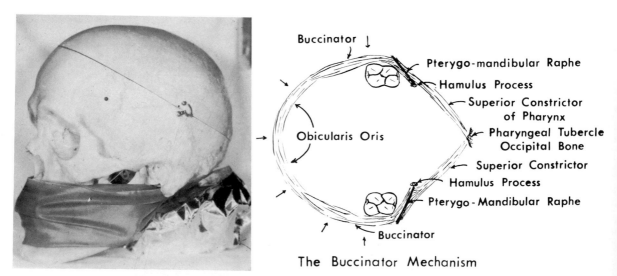

The Buccinator Mechanism

Figure 6–54 Buccinator, mechanism activity. Skull (left) has a band of rubber dam wrapped around dentition to illustrate restraining effect of contiguous musculature. In diagram (right), note the continuous band effect of the musculature anchored at the pharyngeal tubercle of the occipital bone. (Courtesy S. Weinstein.)

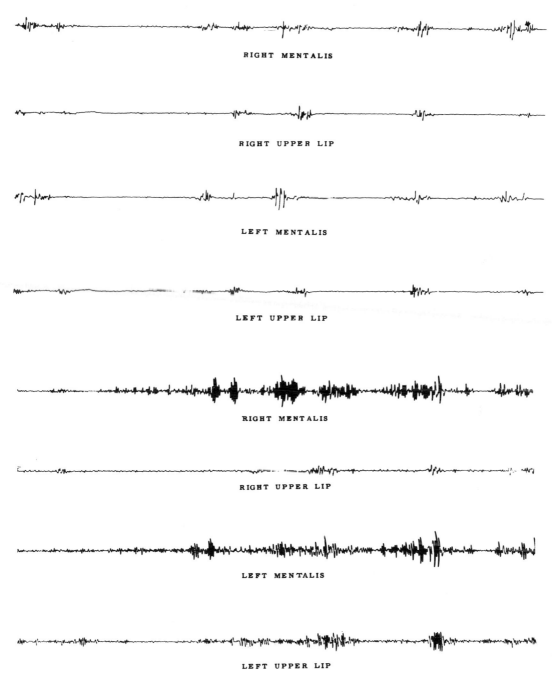

Figure 6–55   Normal lip and mentalis muscle activity in (A) contrasts with abnormal response in (B), as a result of compensatory, adaptive muscle activity associated with a Class II, Division 1 malocclusion. (Courtesy L. O. Schlossberg.)

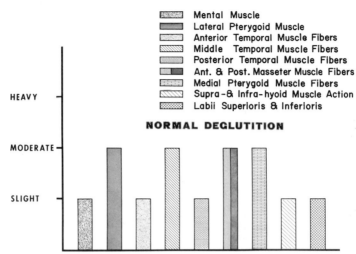

Figure 6–56 Bar graph illustrating comparative muscle pressures during the normal swallowing act. Only lateral and medial pterygoid, middle temporalis and anterior and posterior masseter fibers show moderate activity. The remainder demonstrate slight activity. (From Graber, T.: The "three M's": muscles, malformation, and malocclusion. Am. J. Orthodont., 49:418–450, 1963.)

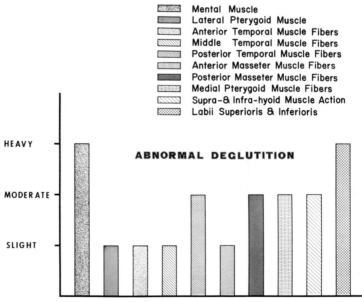

Figure 6–57 Bar graph illustrating comparative muscle pressures associated with abnormal swallowing. Note heavy mentalis and lip activity, dominance of posterior temporalis and masseter fibers, and increased hyoid muscle action. (See Fig. 6–56.) (From Graber, T.: The "three M's": muscles, malformation, and malocclusion. Am. J. Orthodont., 49:418–450, 1963.)

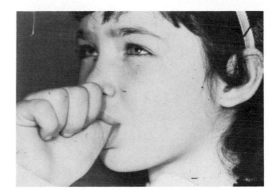

Figure 6–58 Thumb sucking—precursor to malocclusion.

In Class III malocclusions, by contrast, the lower lip is redundant and often hypofunctional (Fig. 6–51). With a severe mandibular protrusion or severe maxillary deficiency an interesting pattern of muscle activity may be observed during deglutition. The tongue lies lower in the mouth, but the tip reaches up and contacts the vermilion border of the upper lip as it drops partly behind the lower incisors. The oral seal is thus effected by tongue and upper lip. The lower lip may curl slightly on itself, with an increase in the depth of the mentolabial sulcus. Even in less severe maxillary deficiency cases or mandibular prognathism, the tongue posture is still low in the mouth. There is some tongue protrusion as the anterior portion curls back on itself to achieve a lingual dento-alveolar contact (Fig. 6–53). Sagittal sections of the maxilla in Class II and Class III malocclusions will show a marked difference in the anterior profile outline, largely attributable to the difference in muscle activity.

In the Class II, Division 1 malocclusion, the lower lip is constantly forcing the premaxillary segment upward and outward against a hypotonic, flaccid, relatively functionless upper lip. If there is a negative overbite (open bite), the tongue may actually assist in this deformation. In Class III malocclusions, the lower lip is impotent, while the upper lip is quite active as it lengthens and is drawn against the maxillary incisors and alveolar process by the contracting buccinator mechanism. This does not mean that the musculature has created the maxillary protrusion and mandibular retrusion in the Class II malocclusion, and the maxillary retrusion and mandibular protrusion in a Class III malocclusion. It may have accentuated the deformation by virtue of its adaptive functional activity.

This leads us directly into a discussion of habits as a causative element in malocclusion.

FINGER SUCKING HABIT

There are few phenomena confronting the dentist that are not open to controversy at one time or another. The delicate shading involved in a decision on just what is normal or abnormal and the dividing line between physiologic and pathologic are often established by the interaction of the training, clinical experience and philosophical bent of the dentist. "Within normal limits" is a broad canyon, not a narrow defile, and a dynamic, changing adaptive envelope of interacting components. If we agree with this observation, arbitrary opinions and pontifical writings should be suspect; yet in the literature there is no dearth of decidedly arbitrary and apparently definitive pronouncements on thumb sucking.

Newspapers are frequently fruitful sources of "the latest and best information." According to a popular poll, health and education are the two subjects impelling the greatest interest, with health first. Each newspaper has its column that discusses the assorted physical and mental problems of the reader. The by-lines under thumb sucking usually bear the names of physicians, pediatricians and psychiatrists, but only rarely dentists. Each "specialist" has his own pat package of facts, figures and recommendations, gleaned primarily from selected secondary sources. That the information given may conflict with equally authoritative columns that appear from time to time in the same paper, or other papers, often seems of no great concern to the press. The air of uncertainty of just what course to follow with respect to finger sucking pervades the pediatric literature, as the following paragraph shows:[50]

Thumb sucking and finger sucking are of importance because of the concern they cause in parents. The pediatrician to whom the alarmed parents come for advice is often as confused about the significance of the practice as are the parents themselves. He finds it difficult to help them or allay their fears. In order to do this successfully he is in need of a working knowledge of the significance of the habit at different age levels. He needs to know what harm, if any, may result; what factors lead to the development of the habit, and what measure should, or should not be taken to handle the situation adequately.[50]

William James,[51] the eminent psychologist, wrote:

An acquired habit, from a psychological point of view, is nothing but a new pathway of discharge formed in the brain, by which certain incoming currents ever after tend to escape. . . . Habits in relation to malocclusion perhaps should be classified as (1) useful, (2) harmful. Useful habits should include the habits of normal function, such as correct tongue position, proper respiration and deglutition and normal use of the lips in speaking. The harmful habits include all that exert perverted stresses against the teeth and dental arches as well as those habits such as open mouth habit, lip biting, lip sucking, thumb sucking. . . .

Haryett, Hansen, Davidson and Sandilands write:

Thumbsucking is a simple learned habit and contradicts the psychoanalytic theory which views the habit as a symptom of a deeper emotional disturbance.[52, 53]

The following quote is from a self-conscious Englishman, Dr. E. A. Barton[54] of London's University College Hospital.

Apart from the effect of constantly sucking the foul thumb, there is another side which demands consideration. The thumb is a hard body and, if frequently in the mouth, tends to pull forward the growing premaxilla together with their incisor teeth, so that the upper incisors project forward beyond the upper lip, giving the "dents des Anglais" appearance which the French so love to caricature. When the child has cut his second dentition, the dentist then reaps the harvest of extraction and plates with wired tensions to press into place the prominent incisors.

The dire predictions of Dr. Barton and many psychiatrists are not echoed in all quarters. It is obvious that everybody cannot be right, as a survey of over 800 articles written on the subject alone during the past 40 years will show.

Before we can attempt to analyze and understand the myriad opinions expressed, certain questions must be asked and answered as objectively as possible. (1) Are finger sucking habits with their associated muscular functional perversions damaging to the teeth and investing tissues or not? (2) If we grant that the creation of a dental deformity is possible, is the deformation of the developing teeth and jaws temporary or permanent? (3) Is thumb sucking an expression of infant sexuality, as it is called by Freud?[55] (4) Is inadequate or improper nursing a major factor? (5) Is the lack of love and affection the basis of the habit; do these children feel "rejected" by their parents and siblings and "lost" in our kaleidoscopic world? (6) Is thumb sucking evidence of a feeling of personal inadequacy, frustration, regression or insecurity; is it an attention-getting mechanism?[56-58] (7) Do attempts to intercept the habit create real psychic trauma and neuroses in later life? (8) Is the principle of learning theory applicable (i.e., is thumb sucking a simple learned habit, with no underlying neurosis)? The answers to all these questions will not be found in this or in any other discussion because much study remains before the veil of controversy can be lifted. But after spending more than 23 years gathering history and treatment data on more than 800 children, I believe I have found some of the answers. Other are partly uncovered, and some trends are emerging from clusters of factors as attempts have been made to analyze etiology, intensity, frequency, duration, chronology, mentality, associated abnormalities, sex, siblings, environment, response under stress, psychic superstructure, parental attitudes, previous habit breaking attempts, etc. It is likely that at least some of the views expressed herein will be at variance with opinions recorded elsewhere. Each "specialist," psychiatrist, pediatrician and dentist can find some support to substantiate his favorite thesis. But if objectivity is sought, certain contradictory and limiting factors should prove disconcerting to "all or none" philosophies nurtured by selected clinical material.

INCIDENCE AND DAMAGE.   Reports on the incidence of thumb sucking vary from 16 per cent to 45 per cent. Similarly, reports of malocclusion are variable, depending on the source, the original occlusion and the length of time the habit continued. Criteria are quite ill-defined and contrast from study to study. Kjellgren, in a study of 167 thumb suckers, found 87 per cent with a malocclusion; Popovitch, in the Burlington study, reported 52 per cent of the 689 children from 3 to 12 years of age with malocclusion that could be attributed to oral habits.[59, 60]

The question concerning whether the damage is temporary or permanent may be answered "yes" for both. Obviously, qualification is needed in many facets of the problem. Contributing to the problem are such entities as the original morphology, the suckle-swallow pattern, the maturational cycle of deglutition, the persistence, intensity and duration of the habit, the leverage produced by specific positions, and other factors. Since the tongue is such a potent deforming factor and since there is correlation between finger sucking and tongue thrusting, a differential diagnosis is essential to determine which is the primary factor. The diagnosis can be most difficult because of the intimate relation of form and function, and the adaptive activity of both. (See Chap. 3.) Perhaps it is best to analyze the finger sucking problem on a chronologic basis and bring in the various qualifying aspects as they occur.

FINGER SUCKING HABIT FROM BIRTH TO FOUR YEARS OF AGE

As is pointed out in Chapter 3, the newborn infant has a relatively well-developed mechanism for suckling, the means of his most important single exchange with the outside world. From it he receives not only his nutriment but his feelings of euphoria, or well-being, that is so essential in early life. A sense of security, a feeling of warmth of association and of being wanted, all these universally needed requirements are satisfied by the infant largely through suckling. Pediatricians and psychiatrists have recognized the importance of this channel of communication with the outside world. The lips of the infant are a sensory organ and the pathway to the brain is relatively well developed. Later on, as other synapses are developed and other pathways made available, the child does not need to rely so strongly on this avenue of communication.

While there are still a number of unanswered questions with respect to breast feeding versus bottle feeding, recent research shows that heretofore entirely too little attention has been paid to the sensory gratification associated with breast feeding. Infant sexuality and oral gratification are powerful kinesthetic, neuromuscular entities. Searching only for an efficient device for obtaining milk, nipple manufacturers have ignored the basic physiology of suckling. In breast feeding, the gum pads are apart, the tongue is brought forward in plunger-like fashion so that the tongue and lower lip are in constant contact, and the mandible moves up and down rhythmically and forward and backward by virtue of the flat condylar path as the buccinator mechanism alternately contracts and relaxes. The child feels the pleasant warmth of the breast not only in the tissues contacting the teat proper, but over an area extending well away from the mouth. The warmth and fondling of the mother's body undoubtedly enhance the feeling of euphoria. Man has yet to devise a substitute for love and affection and warmth of association. The conventional nipple contacts only the mucous membrane of the lips (the vermilion border) (Figs. 6–59, 6–60). The warmth of association conferred by the breast and the mother's body is largely lacking, and the physiology of suckling is not duplicated. Because of the poor design, the mouth is held open more widely and greater demand is made on the buccinator mechanism. The pumping action of the tongue, the raising and lowering and the rhythmic backward and forward movement of the mandible are reduced. Suckling becomes sucking; and frequently, with the enlarged hole at the end of the nipple, the child does not have to do much of this. To make the process of getting milk down the child's throat in the shortest possible time even more efficient, the use of a "squeeze bottle" of soft plastic permits the mother to accelerate the flow of fluid and further reduce the time needed for suckling.

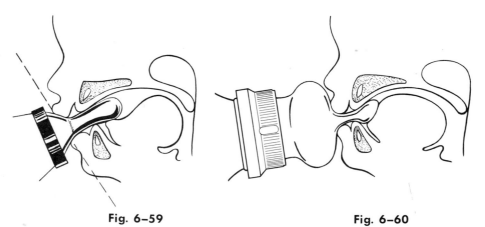

Fig. 6-59   **Fig. 6-60**

Figure 6–59   Nonphysiologic nursing with a conventional artificial rubber nipple. The mouth is propped open unduly and a lip seal difficult. Air intake with milk is likely. Abnormal muscle pressures are exerted as a compensatory response to the excessive opening movement required. (Courtesy Rocky Mountain Dental Products Co.)

Figure 6–60   Nursing action of Nuk Sauger nipple closely simulates natural activity. The entire perioral area is able to contact the warm nipple base which is flexible and adapts to the contours of the lips. (Courtesy Rocky Mountain Dental Products Co.)

A highly computerized and objective study of breast-fed, bottle-fed and mixed fed babies substantiated the observations of Anderson[70] that breast-fed babies are better adjusted and have less abnormal perioral muscle habits and less retained infantile mechanisms.[69] In a study comparing cup, bottle and breast feeding, a stronger sucking reflex was clearly evident in breast-fed babies.[61]

Balters and his associates in Germany concluded that although other factors were involved, improperly designed rubber nipples and harmful bottle nursing techniques caused many pediatric and orthodontic problems.[62] The conventional nursing nipple requires the child only to suck. He does not have to work and exercise the lower jaw as with suckling. With the conventional nipple the milk is more or less squirted into the throat, instead of being brought back by the peristaltic-like action of tongue and cheeks. Often the round nose nipple increases the amount of gulping of air; the infant must then be "burped" more frequently.

To provide as close a duplicate of the human breast as possible, a nipple was designed which incited the same functional activity as breast feeding (Figs. 6–60, 6–61). The functionally designed latex nipple largely eliminates the objectionable features of previous nonphysiologic counterparts. To satisfy the strong desire of the child to suckle and his dependence on this mechanism for euphoria, an "exerciser" or "pacifier" was developed (Fig. 6–62). It is hoped that the anatomic nipple together with the exerciser, if used properly, will greatly reduce the need and desire of the infant for supplemental sucking exercise—turning to the finger and thumb between meals and at bedtime. Most pediatricians feel the average mother does not spend enough time nursing her infant. A minimum of a half hour per nursing interval is recommended. Some children demand more attention and time, some less, depending on individual make-up and other avenues of sensory satisfaction. Thus, no hard and fast rule can be established. The mother must "feel her way" in this as in many relations with her offspring. But if she must err, let it not be on the side of inadequate attention and neglect of the minimal needs of nursing. The mouth is a major avenue of communication and a source of gratification. Weaning to the cup should be postponed until at least the first birthday. If nursing is done with the physiologically designed nipple in conjunction with fondling and maternal contact, there is reason to believe that the incidence of prolonged finger sucking habits will be significantly reduced. The development of abnormal tongue and lip habits that are the bane of every orthodontist's practice will be lessened considerably. It is quite possible that bruxism and clenching, so frequent in both children and adults, may also be reduced as gratification and sensory satisfaction are gained during the feeding act. Use of the physiologically designed pacifier is recommended for all children as they teethe and at other times as indicated to supplement the nursing exercise.

Gesell and Ilg of Yale's Child Development Laboratory contend that finger sucking is perfectly normal at one stage of a child's development.[63] I concur with this opinion and feel that most finger sucking and tongue sucking habits, which may be considered normal for the first year and a half of life, will disappear spontaneously by the end of the second year with proper attention to nursing. To advise a parent to break the child of the finger sucking habit during the time that it is normal to expect such action (the first year and one half of life) is to ignore the basic physiology of infancy. Since young children must continually adapt to their new environment, some infants will accept the restriction, sublimate their habit activities and turn to other environmental

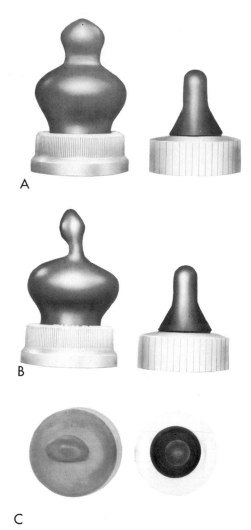

Figure 6–61   Comparison of conventional and Nuk Sauger nipples (A and B). Note longer shank on regular nipple and flat bakelite retaining cap as compared with shorter Nuk Sauger nipple shank and broad adaptive rubber base that can mold to lip contours. Side views of Nuk Sauger nipple and conventional nipple (C).

satisfactions or more mature forms of behavior. But many children will not, and the habit is made more pronounced so that it does not disappear autonomously as it would have if left alone. Failure of ill-advised or ill-devised attempts to break the habit, or constant badgering of the child by the parent to keep his finger out of his mouth, gives some children a potent weapon—an attention-getting mechanism. The child quickly learns how to attract the attention of his parents, and usually does. *No parent should call attention to the habit, regardless of the provocation.*[64] This observation holds true for children of all ages. In most persistent habit cases there is a clear history of early parental displays of displeasure and attempts to break the habit. This would seem to be one plausible explanation for the prolongation of the habit in many children beyond the time that it would normally be discarded along with other infantile mechanisms.

For the first three years of life, experience has shown that damage to the occlusion is confined largely to the anterior segment. This damage is usually temporary, *provided the child starts with a normal occlusion.* The original morphology is quite important because there is much controversy over the damage that may result from finger and thumb sucking habits. Because some of the damaging consequences of the habit are similar to the characteristics of a typical hereditary pattern type of Class II, Division 1 malocclusion, it is easy to assume that the retrognathic mandible, prognathic premaxillary segment, deep overbite, flaccid upper lip, high palatal vault and narrow dental arches are the result of finger sucking. Probably the morphology of the teeth and investing tissues varies relatively little in Class II, Division 1 malocclusion, whether or not there is a finger sucking habit. If the child has a normal occlusion and drops the habit by the end of the third year of life, seldom does he do more than reduce the overbite, increase the overjet and create incisor spacing in the maxillary arch. There may also be slight crowding or lingual malposition of the lower anterior teeth.

Theoretically, it is possible to draw a very neat sequence attributing a

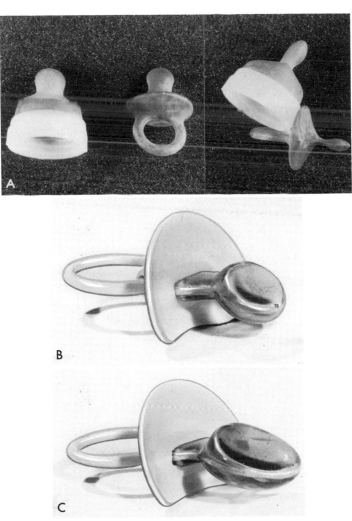

Figure 6–62 A, Edwall functional nursing nipple and physiologic pacifier. Note flat, thin contour. B, Primary exerciser (pacifier) designed to stimulate a normal nursing motion and a euphoric climate. C, secondary exerciser which is larger, for children after the first year of life. Palatal contact is such that it could stimulate all possible dental arch width growth. (B and C, Courtesy Rocky Mountain Dental Products Co.)

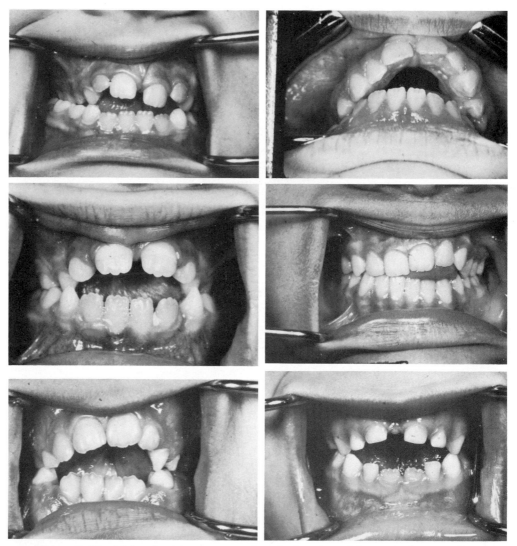

Figure 6–63   Malocclusions associated with thumb and finger sucking, and tongue thrust.

total maxillary protrusion to the sucking habit, with the increased pressure from the buccinator mechanism activating the pterygomandibular raphe just behind the dentition and forcing the maxillary teeth forward. In practice, while we see severe open bites, buccal cross-bites, protrusion of the maxillary anterior teeth and crowding of the mandibular incisors (Figs. 6–63, 6–64, 6–65), it is unlikely that the bilateral Class II buccal segment relationship can be attributed to the finger habit alone. More likely, compensatory tongue thrust, retained infantile suckle swallowing patterns and abnormal perioral muscle function are strong "assists," even in the unilateral Class II cases associated with thumb and finger sucking. Also, with a flush terminal plane that is normal in the deciduous dentition, along with a developmentally deeper-than-normal overbite, it takes less actual tooth movement to create a Class II molar relationship.[67]

These observations appear to be substantiated by the electromyographic research. Highly individualistic neuromuscular behavior prevents the assigning of a direct cause and effect relationship between muscle pattern and malocclusion. In one study, no biometric correlation between the visceral swallowing habit and the severity of the malocclusion was found; 10 out of 24 patients had retained visceral swallowing habits; 5 were in a transitional stage; and only 9 had reached the somatic swallowing state. However, 19 out of 24 demonstrated abnormal mentalis muscle activity.[49] Of the 13 open bite cases in the sample studied, 12 showed preponderant mentalis contraction, as illustrated by electromyograms taken by Baril and Moyers on the finger sucking group in postural position, and during swallowing, tapping, biting and sucking (Figs. 6–66 to 6–68). Mentalis muscle activity is discussed in detail later on in this chapter.

(Text continued on page 313)

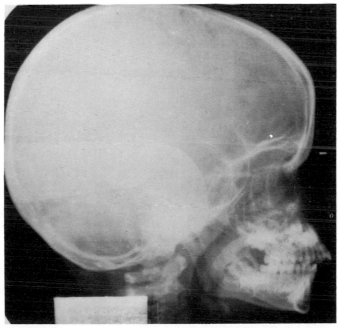

Figure 6–64   Lateral cephalogram of a 4-year-old girl with a confirmed thumb sucking habit. An anterior open bite and protrusion of the premaxillary segment have been created. This malocclusion is being made more severe now by adaptive but abnormal perioral muscle function.

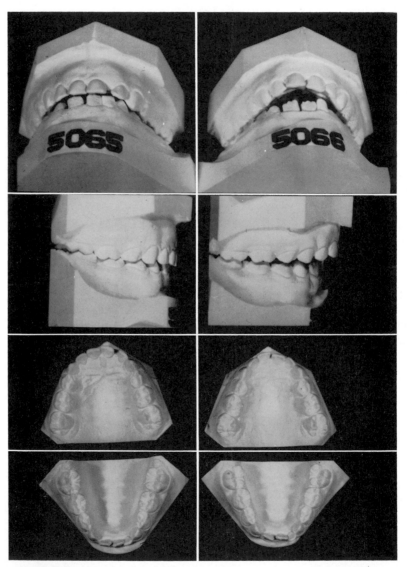

Figure 6–65   Identical twins, one with and one without a finger sucking habit. Notice overjet and buccal segment interdigitation differences.

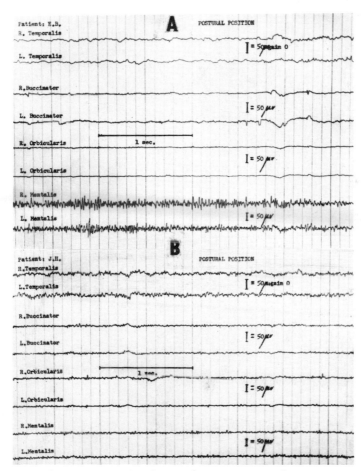

Figure 6–66   Electromyograms of two subjects in postural resting position. The gain is identical for the mentalis muscle in both A and B. (From Baril, C., and Moyers, R. E.: An electromyographic analysis of the temporalis muscles and certain facial muscles in thumb- and finger-sucking patients. J. Dent. Res., 39:536–553, 1960.)

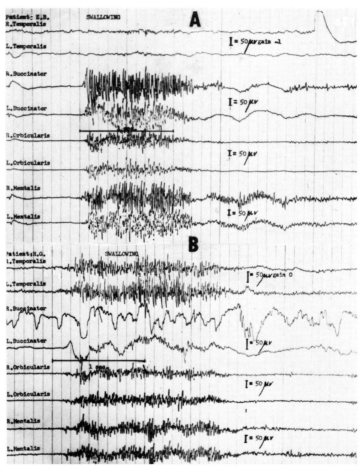

Figure 6–67 Electromyograms of two subjects during swallowing. A is a visceral swallower, and B is a somatic swallower. Note that the gain was decreased in A because of the great amplitude of contraction of the mentalis. The minimal contraction of the temporalis muscles in A is typical, and it is apparent that the seventh cranial nerve muscles are dominant during the act of swallowing. (From Baril, C., and Moyers, R. E.: An electromyographic analysis of the temporalis muscles and certain facial muscles in thumb- and finger-sucking patients. J. Dent. Res., 39:536–553, 1960.)

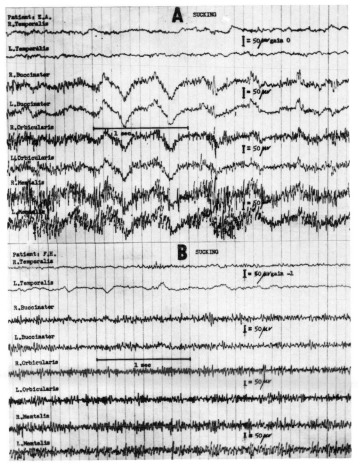

Figure 6–68   Electromyograms of two subjects during sucking. A shows a sucking pattern with preponderance of the mentalis muscles. B shows the dominance of the orbicularis oris muscles. Note also the minimal contraction of the temporalis muscles in both cases. (From Baril, C., and Moyers, R. E.: An electromyographic analysis of the temporalis muscles and certain facial muscles in thumb- and finger-sucking patients. J. Dent. Res., 39:536–553, 1960.)

ACTIVE FINGER SUCKING HABITS
AFTER AGE FOUR

As has already been indicated, most patients with a prolonged finger sucking habit come from homes in which ineffectual badgering attempts by the family to break the habit have ensured continuation beyond the time that it would have been dropped autonomously by the child. The prime offender is usually the father. He is most disturbed, least tolerant and most likely to try to break the habit by calling attention to it, showing obvious displeasure and resorting to admonition or actual punishment.

The permanence of the deformation of the occlusion can increase markedly in children continuing the habit beyond three and one half years of age (Fig. 6–69). As has been pointed out previously, this is not entirely due to the finger and thumb habit, but to an important assist from the associated perioral musculature. The increase in overjet that goes with so many finger habits makes normal swallowing procedures increasingly difficult. Instead of the lips containing the

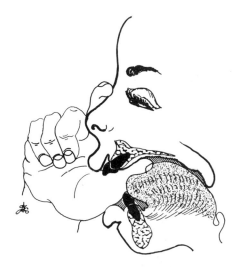

Figure 6–69   Finger habit opens mouth beyond postural resting position, exerting a labial and depressing vector on maxillary incisors and a lingual and depressing vector on the mandibular incisors. Observe that the tongue is also displaced by the habit. (After Moyers, R. E.: Handbook of Orthodontics. 3rd ed. Year Book Medical Publishers, 1972.)

dentition during deglutition, the lower lip cushions to the lingual of the maxillary incisors, forcing them farther forward (Fig. 6–70). Swallowing requires the creation of a "closing off"—a partial vacuum. Since we swallow at least once a minute all day long, lip muscle aberrations are often assisted by a compensatory tongue thrust during the swallowing act. There is good clinical evidence that deglutitional maturation is retarded in confirmed finger suckers. The infantile suckle-swallow, with its plunger-like function, continues, or the transitional period is greatly prolonged, with a mixture of infantile and mature swallowing cycles. This may be the most significant deforming mechanism. The finger habit in duration and intensity may be relatively innocuous (perhaps at bedtime only) but the tongue thrust continues to adapt to the morphology and the tongue does not drop back, hump up or spread out. The abnormal mentalis muscle function and lower lip activity serve to flatten the mandibular anterior segment. Of particular concern is the mentalis muscle, both at postural rest and during function (Fig. 6–71). Deformation thus proceeds in a more constant fashion than possible with the most confirmed digit habit. The real danger, then, is to change the occlusion sufficiently to allow the more potent deforming muscular forces to create full-fledged malocclusions. It is these perverted forces that create the unilateral and bilateral cross-bites so often associated with finger habits.[64–68]

Duration of the habit beyond early childhood is not the only determinant. Equally important are at least two other considerations. The *frequency* of the habit during the day and night affects the end-result. The child who sucks sporadically or just when going to sleep is much less likely to do any damage than one who constantly has his finger in his mouth. The *intensity* of the habit is important. In some children the sucking can be heard in the next room. The perioral muscle function and facial contortions are easily visible. In others the thumb habit is little more than a passive insertion of the finger in the mouth with no apparent buccinator activity. If the forefinger is a favorite digit, more damage may be expected with the dorsal surface of the finger resting fulcrum-like on the lower incisors than with the palmar surface hooked over the same teeth, with the tip of the finger innocuously placed in the floor of the mouth (Fig. 6–72). The finger itself may show the effects of the habit (Fig. 6–73).

This, then, is the trident of factors that must be recognized and evaluated

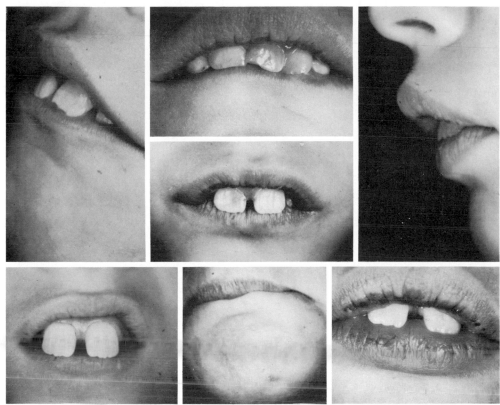

Figure 6–70 Protrusion of maxillary incisors coupled with open bite tendency in anterior segment results in short, hypotonic, functionless upper lip, with lower lip cushioning to lingual of maxillary incisors even at postural resting position (middle picture). On swallowing, the lip may be forced completely lingual to the maxillary incisors by strong mentalis muscle activity.

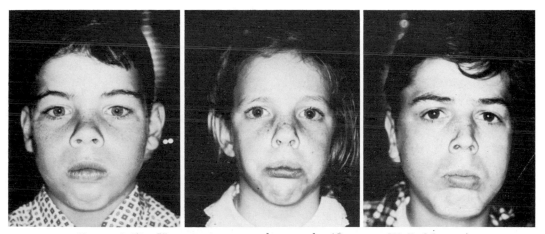

Figure 6–71 Hyperactive mentalis muscle. (Courtesy W. R. Mayne.)

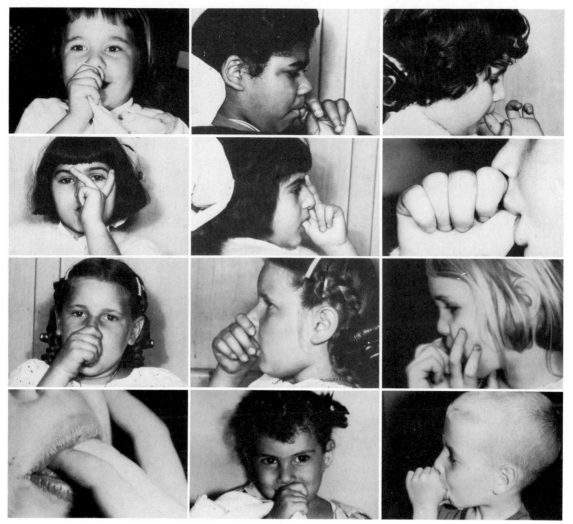

Figure 6–72   Various thumb and finger sucking positions. Note the leverage obtained by sucking the index and middle fingers when the palmar surfaces are facing upward.

before the question of degree of damage to the teeth and investing tissues can be properly answered. Duration, frequency and intensity—this trident of conditioning factors (Fig. 6–74)—must qualify conclusions of the psychiatrist, pediatrician and dentist.[68] The initial morphology and inherent dentofacial pattern further condition any predictions on the ultimate occlusion. If a child already has an inherent Class II, Division 1 malocclusion, damage from the finger habit and perioral muscle function may occur sooner and to a greater degree. We should remember that there is normally a flat terminal plane relationship of the first permanent molars, with the end-to-end cuspal relationship, until the loss of the deciduous molars and elimination of the leeway space. This is in reality a transitional Class II tendency. The chance always exists that confirmed finger habits, pulling forward on the maxillary denture, can provide just enough motivation for the creation of at least a unilateral Class II malocclusion in the permanent dentition. Prolonged finger, tongue and lip activity can only enhance this possibility.

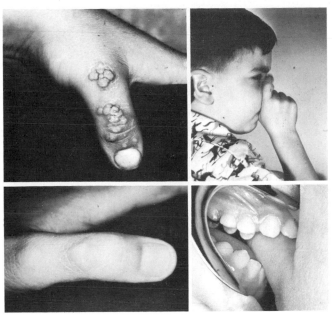

Figure 6–73 Low grade virus infection as a result of constant sucking and a damp environment (above); a callous formed (below) as a result of a thumb sucking habit.

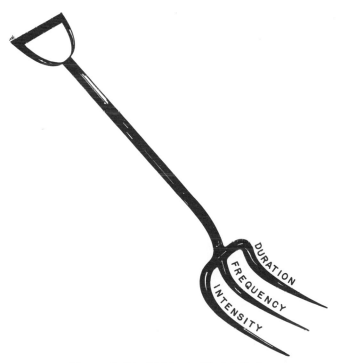

Figure 6–74 Trident of habit factors.

Physical damage is not the only consequence of persistent finger habits. In almost all these cases with the history of unsuccessful attempts to break the habit, the child is aware of the obvious displeasure of the parent or parents. Some children recognize finger sucking as an infantile mechanism and actually want to drop the habit. But, as with other habit patterns, they find that it is hard to do. Such a failure may put the child on the defensive and foster an attitude of defiance or frustration—hardly desirable mental hygiene. We need only examine our own failings in self-discipline and our reactions when "called on the carpet" to fully understand the child's attitude. With some children the retained infantile mechanism serves as an attention-getting weapon. This situation is not conducive to domestic equanimity, particularly when the parent is aware of the possibilities of permanent damage to the teeth and investing tissues. With still other children the finger habit may just be slow in disappearing. It is enjoyable; it is a habit ingrained by constant repetition, and the child has not transferred his pleasure-getting into the more mature, extrovertive activities expected of older children (Fig. 6–75).

Despite the concern by many Freudian-oriented psychologists and pediatricians that finger sucking is a symptom of a deeper neurosis and that breaking the habit will create adult problems, the clinical evidence of these well-worn claims just is not there. Perhaps here more than anywhere else has arm-chair psychology reveled in pseudoscientific interpretations and projections, unsubstantiated by objective research. Haryett, Hansen, Davidson and Sandilands have made an intensive multidisciplinary study of the problems and the dire warnings against the use of habit-breaking appliances, often based on case histories of two or three selected children.[52, 53] These authors find no evidence of the validity of the claims, substantiating my observations in over 800 cases, since 1947. Palermo suggests that thumb sucking rises out of a progressive stimulus-and-reward reaction and would spontaneously disappear unless it becomes an attention-getting mechanism.[74] Eysenck, in discussing learning theory and behavior therapy says categorically, "Learning theory . . . regards neurotic symptoms as simple learned habits; there is no neurosis underlying the symptom, but merely the symptom itself. *Get rid of the symptom and you have eliminated the neurosis.*"[71] In the Alberta study, 66 children were studied and divided into 6 groups of 11 subjects undergoing the following treatment: (1) control, (2) psychological treatment only, (3) palatal arch only, (4) palatal arch and psychological treatment, (5) palatal crib only, (6) palatal crib reinforced by psychological treatment. The arch followed the palatal contour. The crib is similar to that used by the author and described in Chapter 14. The palatal crib with spurs was found to be most effective; no habit transference such as masturbation (a frequent psychoanalytic claim) was observed. Associated habits like hair twisting, fondling, blanketing, etc., disappeared with the finger habit. The study supported the view of learning theorists—that thumb sucking is a simple learned habit and contradicts the psychoanalytic theory which considers thumb sucking as a symptom of a deeper emotional disturbance. Actual therapeutic measures are described in Chapter 14.

In any event, the dentist can render valuable assistance and improve mental hygiene for both the parents and the child. He can do this by guiding the patient past this roadblock along the road to maturity, by eliminating a source of conflict between the child and the parent and by preventing a permanent malocclusion with attendant unfavorable health and psychological implications.

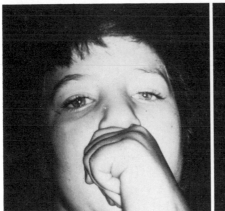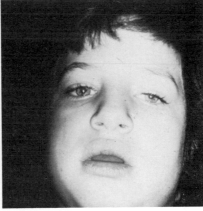

Figure 6–75   This patient has derived considerable pleasure in the past from the finger sucking habit. Confirmed habits are difficult to intercept, usually, but posing for this picture stopped the habit. (Courtesy P. E. Adams.)

OTHER PRESSURE HABITS (LIP AND TONGUE)

In the discussion of thumb and finger sucking, it was pointed out that abnormal lip and tongue activity frequently are associated with the finger habit. If the malocclusion is created by the initial assault on the integrity of the occlusion, i.e., finger sucking, compensatory muscle activity is developed which accentuates the deformity. With the increase in overjet it becomes increasingly difficult for the child to close his lips properly and create the negative pressure required for normal swallowing. The lower lip drops behind the maxillary incisors and is thrust against the lingual surfaces of the maxillary incisors by abnormal activity of the mentalis muscle to effect the closure (Fig. 6–76). The upper lip is no longer called upon to engage in sphincter-like activity in contact with the lower lip, as it must during normal swallowing; it remains hypotonic, functionless and appears retracted or short. This condition is referred to as incompetent resting lip posture in the literature. Because of the attempt to create an anterior lip seal, there is strong contraction of the orbicularis oris mentalis complex. Neurologically, there is undoubtedly a certain amount of feedback. Receptors (muscle spindles) have been demonstrated in the labial muscles. Tactile nerve endings in the lips receive general exteroceptive impulses, probably serving a proprioceptive and visceral function as well. The presence of proprioceptive fibers in the facial nerve has not been established. For exteroception, tactile impulses travel via the maxillary and mandibular branches of the trigeminal nerve. For enteroception, visceral impulses probably use the same pathway. With malocclusion and morphologic interference with normal lip activity, compensatory activity is probably initiated by sensory impulses, relayed to the motor cortex, which initiates volitional movement. Much of the activity is probably reflex-like, however, traveling from the sensory nucleus of the trigeminal nerve to the motor nucleus of the facial nerve in the pons.

The labial musculature is assisted by the tongue during deglutition, as described in Chapter 3.[72] Depending on the degree of deformation, the tongue thrusts forward to aid the lower lip in closing off during the swallowing act. Winders has demonstrated that tongue activity during normal swallowing is as much as four times as intense as the opposing force created by the lips in some

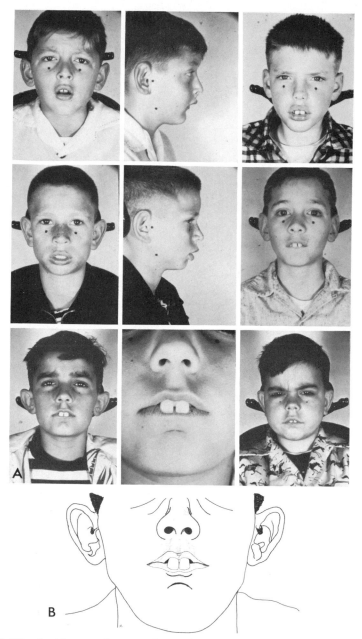

Figure 6–76   A, Abnormal perioral muscle function tending to accentuate the developing malocclusion. Such conditions must be eliminated during orthodontic therapy or the results will not be stable. (Courtesy E. H. Watkins.) B, Tooth movement by muscle force—in the wrong direction.

areas.[47] With the upper lip no longer serving as an effective restraining force and with the lower lip actually teaming up with the tongue to exert a powerful upward and forward vector of force against the premaxillary segment, the severity of the malocclusion is enhanced. With the increasing protrusion of the maxillary incisors and the creation of an anterior open bite, greater demands are made for compensatory muscle activity. The vicious circle repeats itself with each swallow. This means that a strong deforming force is being exerted against the dental arches as much as 1000 times a day. Finger sucking assumes a secondary role. Indeed, many children find that by sucking their lower lip or merely biting on it, they can achieve the same sensory satisfaction formerly obtained from the finger. They spontaneously drop the finger habit for the new, more convenient, but unfortunately more powerful lip habit (Fig. 6–77). Less frequently, they turn to tongue thrust and sucking for the pleasurable sensation. The plunger-like action is quite similar to the suckling act and is considered a reversion to, or a residual characteristic of, this infantile mechanism.

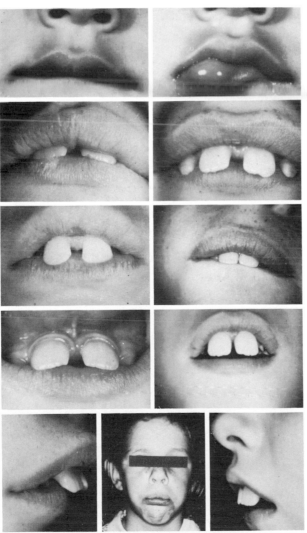

Figure 6–77   Abnormal lip habit that has replaced a confirmed finger sucking habit.

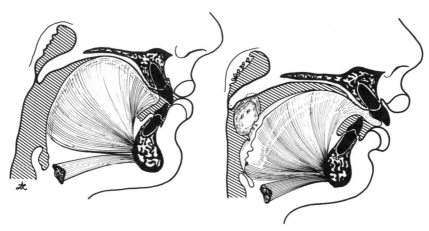

Figure 6–78   Normal and abnormal swallowing. In the normal section (A), incisors are momentarily in contact as the tip of the tongue touches the lingual interdental papillae of the maxillary arch. The dorsum of the tongue closely approximates the palate during the normal swallowing act; lips are tightly closed together. In the abnormal swallowing sequence (B), the teeth are often separated, the tongue thrusts forward into the excessive overjet, and the dorsum of the tongue drops away from the palatal vault. Enlarged tonsils may accentuate the tongue thrust habit. Instead of the lips creating a firm seal with each other, the upper lip remains relatively functionless while the mentalis muscles exert a strong forward and upward thrust of the lower lip against the lingual surfaces of the maxillary incisors. (After Moyers, R. E.: Handbook of Orthodontics. 3rd ed. Year Book Medical Publishers, 1972.)

There is a considerable amount of evidence that indicates that tongue thrust is merely a retention of the infantile suckling mechanism (Fig. 3–39). With the continuation of the finger habit as a "built-in" pacifier, the mature swallowing pattern does not develop on schedule. With the eruption of the incisors at five to six months of age, the tongue does not drop back as it should and it continues to thrust forward. Tongue posture during rest is also forward. Or, there is a prolonged transitional period, as shown by Baril and Moyers, with either the infantile or the mature swallowing pattern dominant at one time or the other.[65] The deforming force of the tongue as it thrusts continuously forward is obvious.

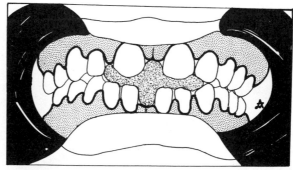

Figure 6–79   As the tongue thrusts forward between maxillary and mandibular teeth, the peripheral portions no longer lie between the occlusal surfaces of the buccal segment teeth. Overeruption of posterior teeth is thus possible, creating an open bite with identical occlusal and postural vertical dimensions.

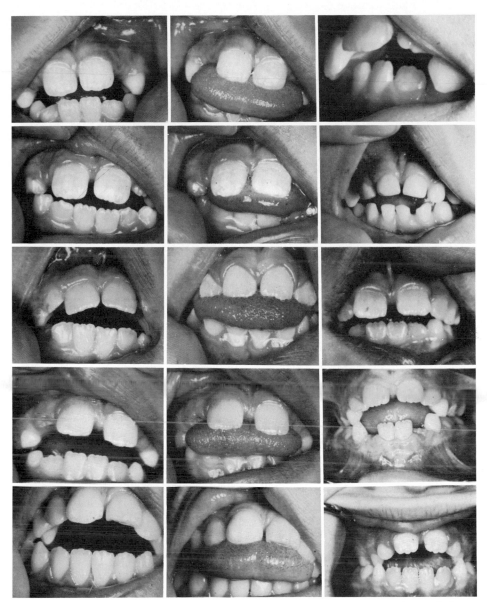

Figure 6–80 Anterior open bite, in conjunction with a tongue thrust habit and visceral swallowing pattern.

Anderson[70] corroborates the observations of the present author and of Moyers when he points out that tongue thrust is often a residuum of the finger sucking habit. In his study, 54.2 per cent of those with the habit of tongue thrust had a history of finger sucking. Among those without tongue thrust, only 25 per cent had prior thumb or finger sucking habits. On the question of breast feeding versus bottle feeding, the results again indicate a positive correlation with greater tongue thrust tendency in the bottle-fed group. In his sample, 83 per cent were bottle-fed and 17 per cent were breast-fed. In his tongue thrust positive sample, 91.7 per cent were bottle-fed, and only 8.3 per cent were breast-fed. In students without tongue thrust syndrome the findings were that 82.5 per cent were bottle-fed and 17.4 per cent were breast-fed. Obviously, this is not the only factor, but should be considered contributory.

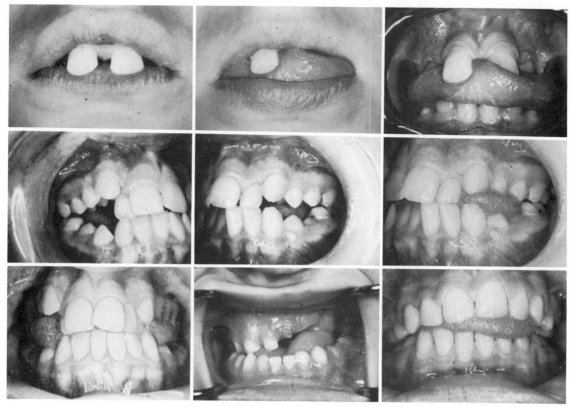

Figure 6–81   Atypical tongue habits. (Courtesy W. R. Mayne.)

Whatever the cause for the tongue habit may be (size, posture or function), it also serves as an effective cause of malocclusion. In some instances, as the tongue thrusts forward constantly, increasing the overjet and open bite, the peripheral portions no longer lie over the lingual cusps of the buccal segments (Figs. 6–78 to 6–85). Posterior teeth erupt and gradually eliminate the interocclusal clearance. The postural resting vertical dimension and occlusal vertical dimension become one and the same, with the posterior teeth in contact at all times. This is not a dentally healthy situation. One side-effect may be bruxism; another is the bilateral narrowing of the maxillary arch as the tongue drops

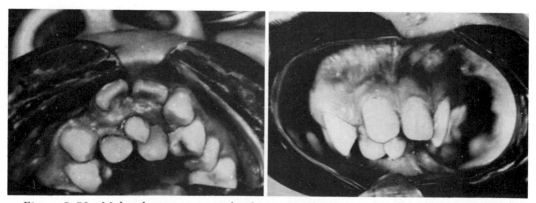

Figure 6–82   Malocclusion as a result of congenital aglossia. (Courtesy H. A. Eskew.)

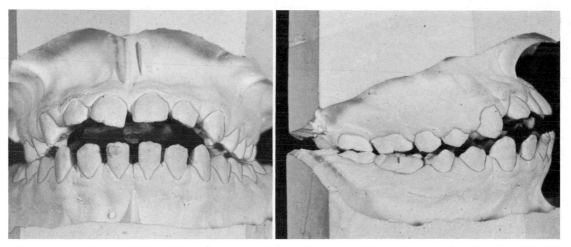

Figure 6–83   Malocclusion resulting from a condition of macroglossia.

lower in the mouth, providing less support for the maxillary arch. Clinically this may be observed as a unilateral cross-bite, with a convenience swing to one side or the other as the mandible is moved laterally under the influence of tooth guidance.

Tongue size as well as function is an important consideration. The effect of size on the dentition is shown dramatically in two cases—one patient with congenital aglossia, the other with macroglossia (Figs. 6–82, 6–83, 6–84).

Possibly contributing to the abnormal tongue position so often seen is the presence of enlarged tonsils and adenoids. As Moyers and Linder-Aronson show so well, tongue thrust may be a natural consequence of the forward displacement of the base of the tongue[72, 75] (Fig. 6–78).

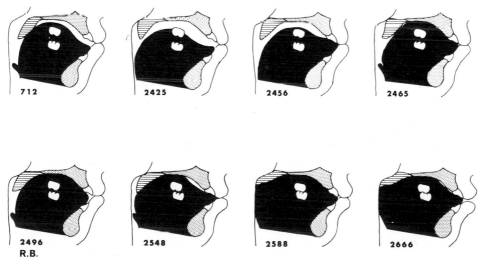

Figure 6–84   Tracings of the cineradiographic records obtained during swallowing in an individual with a disproportionately large tongue. Protrusive activity between the anterior teeth is clearly evident through most of the swallowing process, especially as the tongue begins to occupy the major area of the oral cavity. (Courtesy D. Subtelny.)

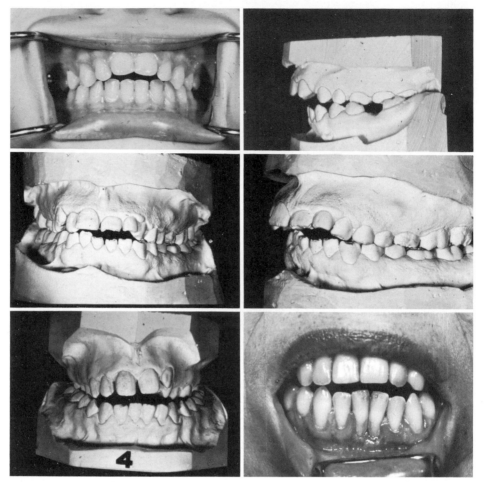

Figure 6–85   Adult open bite problems with history of finger sucking and tongue thrust habits. The prognosis of the health of the investing tissues in open bite cases is poor, as the picture in the lower right shows.

Whatever the cause, the end-result is often a permanent open bite malocclusion, with attendant supporting tissue pathology (Fig. 6–85).

The methods of coping with the tongue and lip habits are discussed in Chapters 13 and 14.

PSYCHOGENIC OR IDIOPATHIC FUNCTIONAL ABERRATIONS—CLENCHING AND BRUXISM

In any attempt to arbitrarily categorize a number of items there are always elements which could fit into more than one category and which overflow into other categories, or which somehow don't quite seem to fit into any category at all. In some instances, it is valid to ask the question, Which came first—the chicken or the egg? Specifically, do clenching and bruxism, the tetanic-like contraction of masticatory muscles and the rhythmic side-to-side grinding and gnashing of teeth during sleep, cause malocclusion or are they the results of a malocclusion? Very likely, cause and effect are not clear.[73] Unfavorable sequelae of a deep bite may be bruxism and clenching. But we also know that there is a psychogenic, kinesthetic and neuromuscular overlay or conditioning environment. Nervous tension finds a most gratifying release in clenching and bruxism. High-strung people are more prone to rend, grate, crack and wear down their teeth with a bruxing motion. Nocturnal bruxism cannot even be duplicated during the waking hours for most of them. The magnitude of the contraction is enormous and the deleterious effects on the occlusion are obvious (Fig. 6–86). A significant number of deciduous dentitions show the effects of bruxism. Clench-

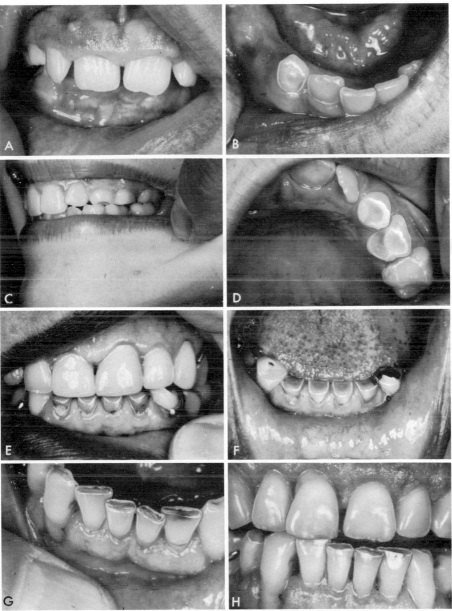

Figure 6–86 Bruxism, creating damage to occlusion, and enhancing the existing malocclusion. A and B, Deep overbite, usually associated with bruxing habit, with trigger area in lower right canine region. Entire labial surface has been ground away in this 10-year-old girl; C and D, Eleven-year-old girl, with lateral bruxing motion that produces excessive wear on upper left deciduous canine and first molar; E and F, Thirty-one-year-old woman with a protrusive bruxing motion and a high level of nervous irritability; G and H, Males in late 30's, with lateral and protrusive bruxing motions, causing excessive incisal wear and denudation of canine roots. (See Figure 9–5.)

ing cannot be checked clinically, but it is a likely concomitant activity. The correlation with erotogenic habits, if any, has not been established.

Probably there is a malocclusion or malfunction of occlusion in most cases as the "weak link" to be exploited by psychogenic demands. Usually it is a deeper than normal overbite, a "high" tooth or restoration, a malposed dental unit, etc. The process becomes a vicious circle as some of these malocclusion characteristics worsen under the traumatic onslaughts of bruxism and clenching. Much research remains to be done on the exact nature of the myositis-producing tooth-grinding phenomenon now seen so commonly in people of all ages in our complex, highly geared society.

POSTURE

From time to time, investigators purport to show that poor postural conditions can cause malocclusions. Many a stoop-shouldered child, with the head hung so that the chin rests on the chest, has been accused of creating his own mandibular retrusion. The majority of such accusations seem unfounded. Equally improbable is the creation of a full-fledged dental malocclusion by a child's resting his head on his hand for periods of time each day, or sleeping on his arm, fist or pillow each night. Poor posture and dental malocclusion may both be the result of a common cause. Poor posture may accentuate an existent malocclusion. But as the primary etiologic factor this remains to be proved or disproved conclusively. Until then, many orthodontists will see what they consider clinical substantiation of such factors.

ACCIDENTS OR TRAUMA

It is probable that accidents are a more significant factor in malocclusion than is frequently recognized. As a child learns to crawl and walk, the face and dental areas receive many blows that are not recorded in his history. Such undiscovered traumatic experiences may explain so-called idiopathic eruptive abnormalities (Figs. 7–31, 7–33). Nonvital deciduous teeth have abnormal resorption patterns, and as a result of an initial accident, they may deflect the permanent successors. These "dead" teeth should be examined radiographically at frequent intervals for comparative root resorption and possible apical infectious involvement. It is likely that a blow or traumatic experience is responsible for many of these cases.

REFERENCES

1. Jensen, F., as quoted in Graber, T. M.: The fundamentals of occlusion. J.A.D.A., 48:177–187, 1954.
2. McCoy, J. D., and Shepard, E. E.: Applied Orthodontics. 7th ed. Philadelphia, Lea & Febiger, 1956.
3. Moyers, R. E.: Handbook of Orthodontics. 3rd ed. Chicago, Year Book Medical Publishers, Inc., 1972.
4. Salzmann, J. A.: Practice of Orthodontics. Philadelphia, J. B. Lippincott Co., 1966.
5. Stockard, C. R.: The genetics of modified endocrine secretion and associated form pattern among dog breeds. Proc. Sixth Internat. Cong. Genetics, 1932.
6. Hasund, A., and Sivertsen, R.: Dental arch space and facial type. Angle Orthodont., 41:140–145, 1971.
7. Lundström, A.: Tooth Size and Occlusion in Twins. Stockholm. A. B. Fåhlcrantz Boktryckeri, 1948. (Abstr. in British D. J., 87:297, 1949.)
8. Pruzansky, S., and Aduss, H.: Prevalence of arch collapse and malocclusion in complete unilateral cleft lip and palate. Trans. Europ. Orth. Soc., 1–18, 1967.

9. Graber, T. M.: Cranio-facial morphology in cleft palate and cleft lip deformities. Surg. Gynec. Obstet., 88:359–369, 1949.

10. Pruzansky, S.: The growth of the pre-maxillary vomerine complex. Tandlaegebladet, 75:1157–1169, 1971.

11. Dahl, E.: Craniofacial morphology in congenital clefts of the lip and palate. Acta Odont. Scand., (Suppl. 57), Vol. 28, Copenhagen, 1970.

12. Graber, T. M.: A study of cranio-facial growth and development in the cleft palate child from birth to six years of age in Hotz, R. (ed.): Early treatment of cleft lip and palate. Berne, Han Huber, 1964.

13. Aduss, H.: Craniofacial growth in complete unilateral cleft lip and palate. Angle Orthodont., 41:202–213, 1971.

14. Monroe, C. W., and Rosenstein, S. W. in Grabb, W. C., Rosenstein, S. W., and Bzoch, K. R. (eds.): Cleft Lip and Palate, Boston, Little, Brown, pp. 573–584, 1971.

15. Trausch, E. S.: A study of the morphologic changes in the oral cavity induced by eccentric muscular activity in cerebral palsy children. Master's thesis, Northwestern University, 1954.

16. Sollar, E. M.: Torticollis and its relationship to facial asymmetry. Master's thesis, Northwestern University, 1947.

17. Weinmann, J. P., and Sicher, H.: Bone and Bones. 2nd ed. St. Louis, C. V. Mosby Co., 1955.

18. Todd, T. W.: Facial growth and mandibular adjustment. Am. J. Orthodont. & Oral Surg., 16:1243–1267, 1930.

19. Chapple, C. C., and Davidson, D. T.: A study of the relationship between fetal position and certain congenital anomalies. J. Pediat., 18:483–493, 1941.

20. Spiegel, R. N., Sather, A. H., and Hayles, A. B.: Cephalometric study of children with various endocrine diseases. Am. J. Orthodont., 59:362–375, 1971.

21. Rosenstein, S. W.: New concept in early orthopedic treatment of cleft lip and palate. Am. J. Orthodont., 55:765–774, 1969.

22. Kamin, S.: Dysgnathic abnormalities in mental retardation and associated disorders. Bull. N. Y. Soc. Dent. Child., 22:11–23, 1971.

23. Tulley, W. J.: Methods of recording patterns of behavior of the oro-facial muscles using the electro-myograph. D. Record, 73:741, 1953

24. Lear, C. S. C., Moorrees, C. F. A.: Bucco-lingual muscle force and dental arch form. Am. J. Orthodont., 56:379–393, 1969.

25. Gould, M. S. E., and Picton, D. C. A.: A study of the pressures exerted by the lips and cheeks on the teeth of subjects with Angle Class II, Division 1, Class II, Division 2, and Class III malocclusions, compared with those of subjects with normal occlusion. Arch. Oral Biol., 13:527–541, 1968.

26. Doty, R. W., Richmond, W. H., and Storey, A. T.: Effect of medullary lesions on coordination of deglutition. Exp. Neurol., 17:91–106, 1967.

27. Doty, R. W., and Bosma, J. F.: An electromyographic analysis of reflex deglutition. J. Neurophysiol., 19:44–60, 1956.

28. Bosma, J. F.: Human infant oral function in Symposium on Oral Sensation and Perception. Springfield, Ill., Charles C Thomas, 1969.

29. Garrett, F. A., Angelone, L., and Allen, W. L.: The effect of bite opening, bite pressure, and malocclusion on the electrical response of the masseter muscles. Am. J. Orthodont., 50:435–444, 1964.

30. Luffingham, J. K.: Lip and cheek pressures exerted upon teeth in three adult groups with different occlusions. Arch. Oral Biol., 14:337–350, 1969.

31. Jacobs, R. M.: Muscle equilibrium: fact or fancy. Angle Orthodont., 39:11–21, 1969.

32. Powell, R. N.: Tooth contact during sleep; association with other events. J. Dent. Res., 44:959–967, 1965.

33. Moyers, R. E.: Temporomandibular muscle contraction patterns in Angle Class II, Division 1 malocclusions: an electromyographic analysis. Am. J. Orthodont., 35:837, 1949.

34. Perry, H. T., Jr.: Kinesiology of the temporal and masseter muscles in chewing a homologous bolus. Doctoral thesis, Northwestern University, 1961.

35. Carlsöö, S.: Nervous coordination and mechanical function of the mandibular elevators. Acta Odont. Scand. (Suppl. 11), 10:9–126, 1952.

36. Ahlgren, J.: Mechanisms of Mastication; a quantitative cinematographic study of masticatory movements. Acta Odont. Scand. (Suppl. 44), 1966.

37. Simon, P.: Fundamental Principles of a Systematic Diagnosis of Dental Anomalies. Translated by B. E. Lischer. Boston, Stratford Co., 1926.

38. Rogers, A. P., Dinham, W. R., and Logan, H. L.: Symposium on muscle function. Internat. J. Orthodont. Oral Surg., 16:254–276, 1930.

39. Cleall, J. F.: Deglutition: A study of form and function. Am. J. Orthodont., 51:566–594, 1965.

40. Ballard, C. F.: A consideration of the physiological background of mandibular posture and movement. D. Practitioner & D. Record, 6:80, 1955.

41. Speidel, T. M., Isaacson, R. J., and Worms, F. W.: Tongue thrust therapy and anterior dental open-bite. Am. J. Orthodont., 62:287–295, 1972.

42. Kawamura, Y.: Dental significance of four oral physiological mechanisms. J. Canad. Dent. Ass., 34:582–590, 1968.

43. Cleall, J. F., Alexander, W. J., and McIntyre, H. M.: Head posture and its relationship to degluti-
    tion. Angle Orthodont., 36:335–350, 1966.
44. Tulley, W. J.: A critical appraisal of tongue thrusting. Am. J. Orthodont., 55:640–650, 1969.
45. Proffit, W. R., and Norton, L. A.: The tongue and oral morphology: influences of tongue activity
    during speech and swallowing. ASHA Reports, no. 5, 106–115, 1970.
46. Lear, C. S. C., Flanagan, J. B., and Moorrees, C. F. A.: The frequency of deglutition in man.
    Arch. Oral Biol., 10:83–99, 1965.
47. Winders, R. V.: An electronic technique to measure the forces exerted on the dentition by the
    peri-oral and lingual musculature. Am. J. Orthodont., 42:645, 1956.
48. Milne, I. M., and Cleall, J. F.: Cinefluorographic study of functional adaptation of the oropha-
    ryngeal structures. Angle Orthodont., 40:267–283, 1970.
49. Fletcher, S. G.: Processes and maturation of deglutition. ASHA Reports, no. 5, 92–105, 1970.
50. Yip, A. S. G., and Cleall, J. F.: Cinefluorographic study of velopharyngeal function before and
    after removal of tonsils and adenoids. Angle Orthodont., 41:251–263, 1971.
51. James, W.: Psychology. New York, Henry Holt & Co., 1923.
52. Haryett, R. D., Hansen, F. C., Davidson, P. O., and Sandilands, M. L.: Chronic thumbsucking:
    the psychologic effects and the relative effectiveness of various methods of treatment.
    Am. J. Orthodont., 53:569–585, 1967.
53. Davidson, P. O., Haryett, R. D., Sandilands, M. L., and Hansen, F. C.: Thumbsucking: habit
    or symptom? J. Dent. Child., 33:252–259, 1967.
54. Barton, E. A.: Septicity in thumbsucking. Lancet, Feb. 15, pp. 348–349, 1930.
55. Freud, S.: Three Contributions to the Theory of Sex. 3rd ed. New York, Nervous and Mental
    Diseases Publishing Company, 1918.
56. Kaplan, M. J.: Note on psychological implications of thumbsucking. J. Pediat., 37:555–560,
    1950.
57. Henry, R. G.: The effect of thumbsucking on the dentition. D. Practitioner & D. Record, 8:300–
    304, 1958.
58. Reider, N., and Korner, A. F.: Psychological effect of device to correct thumbsucking. J.A.D.A.,
    45:114, 1952.
59. Kjellgren, B.: Fingersugningsvana hos barn fran dentalortopedisk synpunkt. Nord. Med.,
    3:918–924, 1939.
60. Popovich, F.: The incidence of sucking habits and its relationship to occlusion in 3-year old
    children, Burlington Orthodontic Research Center, Progress Report Series no. 1, University
    of Toronto, 1956.
61. Davis, A., et al.: Effects of cup, bottle and breast feeding on oral activities of new-born infants.
    Pediatrics, 2:549–558, 1948.
62. Muller, A.: Nursing nipples. Zahnartzliche Welt, 6:109, December, 1951.
63. Gesell, A., and Ilg, F.: Infant and Child in the Culture of Today. 2nd ed. Philadelphia, Harper
    & Brothers, 1943.
64. Graber, T. M.: The fingersucking habit and associated problems. J. Dent. Children, 25:145–151,
    1958.
65. Baril, C., and Moyers, R. E.: An electromyographic analysis of the temporalis muscles and
    certain facial muscles in thumb and fingersucking patients. Int. J. Dent. Res., 39:536–553,
    1960.
66. Graber, T. M.: Thumb and fingersucking. Am. J. Orthodont., 45:258–264, 1959.
67. Moore, G. J., McNeill, R. W., and D'Anna, J. A.: The effects of digit sucking on facial growth.
    J.A.D.A., 84:592–599, 1972.
68. Graber, T. M.: The "three M's": muscles, malformation, and malocclusion. Am. J. Orthodont.,
    49:418–450, 1963.
69. Najera, A.: A critical evaluation of early feeding procedures and their implications on oro-facial
    morphology and related factors. Master's thesis, St. Louis University, 1963.
70. Anderson, W. S.: The relationship of the tongue-thrust syndrome to maturation and other
    factors. Am. J. Orthodont., 49:264–275, 1963.
71. Eysenck, H. J.: Learning theory and behavior therapy. J. Ment. Sci., 105:6175, 1959.
72. Moyers, R. E.: Postnatal development of the orofacial musculature. A.S.H.A. Reports, no. 6,
    38–47, 1971.
73. Graf, H.: Bruxism. D. Clin. North America, 13:659–666, 1969.
74. Palermo, D. S.: Thumbsucking: a learned response. Pediatrics, 17:392–399, 1956.
75. Linder-Aronson, S.: Adenoids: their effect on mode of breathing and nasal airflow and their
    relationship to characteristics of the facial skeleton and the dentition. Acta Oto-Laryng.
    (Suppl. 265), Uppsala, 1970.
76. Huddart, A. G., North, J. F., and Davis, M. E. H.: Observations on the treatment of cleft lip and
    palate. Dent. Pract., 16:265–274, 1966.
77. Huddart, A. G.: The application of computers to the study of maxillary arch dimensions. Brit. D.
    Jour., 130:397–404, 1971.
78. Wiemann, C.: Behandlungsbedürftigkeit von Dysgnathien im Milchgebiss. Deutsche Stomat.,
    20:272–279, 1970.
79. Rosenstein, S. W., Jacobson, B. N., Monroe, C., Griffith, H., and McKinney, P.: Cleft lip and
    palate children five years after undergoing orthopedic and bone-grafting procedures.
    Angle Orthodont., 42:1–8, 1972.

chapter 7

ETIOLOGY OF MALOCCLUSION: LOCAL FACTORS

ANOMALIES IN NUMBER OF TEETH

With the advent of general use of dental radiographs, it became apparent that variations in number of teeth are frequent. Several theories have been advanced to explain supernumerary or congenitally absent teeth. Heredity plays a strong part in many cases.[1] Why this is so is still unknown. Some authorities feel that the appearance of extra teeth is merely a leftover from the primitive anthropoids who had a dozen more teeth than *Homo sapiens.* There is a relatively high frequency of extra or missing teeth associated with congenital deformities such as cleft lip and cleft palate. Generalized pathoses, such as ectodermal dysplasia, cleidocranial dysostosis, and others, may also affect the number of teeth in the dental arches.

SUPERNUMERARY TEETH

There is no definite time when supernumerary teeth may develop. They may form prior to birth or as late as 10 to 12 years of age[2] (Figs. 7–1 to 7–5). It is usually a supernumerary tooth which erupts at an advanced age that is responsible for what the newspapers dub "a third set of teeth." Supernumerary teeth occur most commonly in the maxilla although they may erupt in any area of the mouth (Figs. 7–6 to 7–14). At times these teeth are so well-formed that it is difficult to determine which ones are the "extras" (Figs. 7–5, 7–16 to 7–19).

A frequently seen supernumerary tooth is the mesiodens, which occurs near the midline, palatal to the maxillary incisors. It is usually conical in shape and occurs most often singly although it may be present in pairs. Occasionally it is fused to the right or left maxillary central incisor. As is true for all supernumerary teeth, the mesiodens may point in any direction. Not infrequently a supernumerary tooth may erupt toward the floor of the nose instead of toward the palate (Fig. 7–4).

(Text continued on page 336)

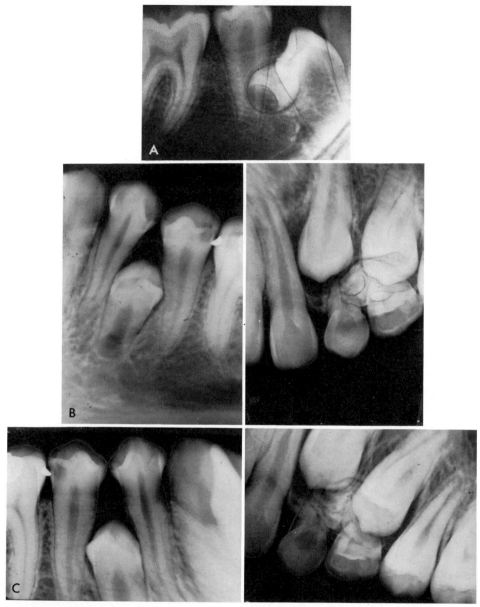

Figure 7–1   A, Developing supernumerary premolar. B, Supernumerary premolars attempting to erupt between first and second premolars. C, Dentigerous cyst interfering with normal eruption of canine and premolar.

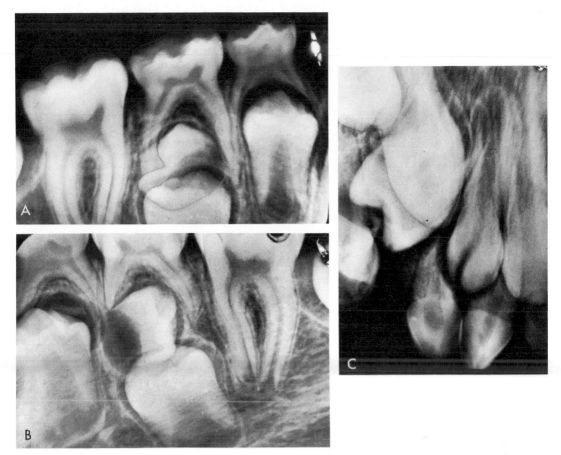

Figure 7-2 A and B, Supernumerary right and left second premolars interposed between developing lower second premolars and second deciduous molars. C, Supernumerary lateral incisor and first premolar, with conically shaped deciduous right lateral incisor. These are all in the same mouth.

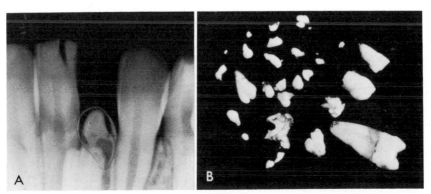

Figure 7-3 A, Dentigerous cyst preventing eruption of mandibular incisor. B, Cystic elements removed from maxillary premolar region.

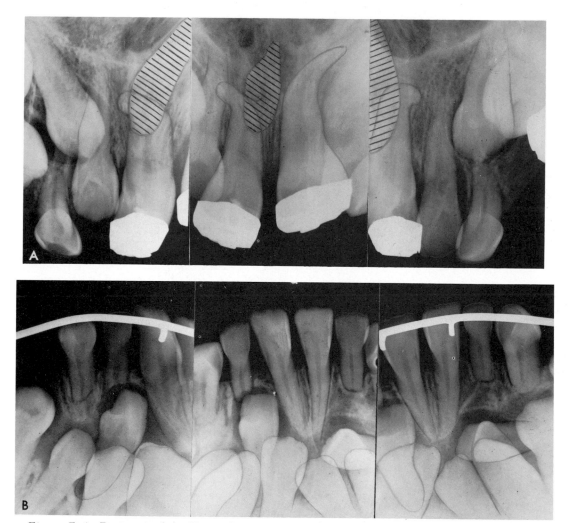

Figure 7-4   Patient with malformed permanent teeth and a number of supernumerary incisors. A, Mesiodens is present between malformed apical portions of maxillary central incisors. B, Three supernumerary teeth are preventing the eruption of permanent lateral incisors and canines.

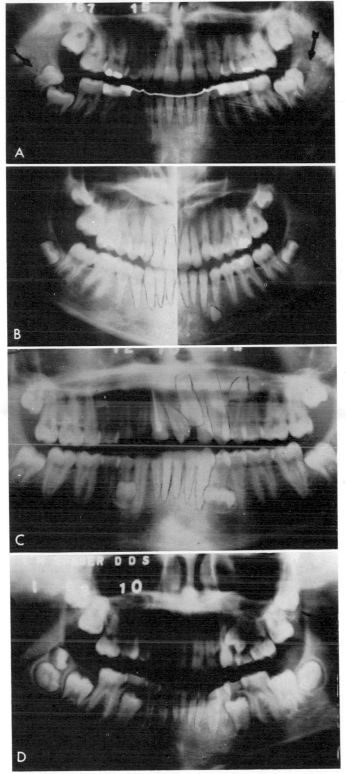

Figure 7–5 A, Fourth molars interfering with eruption of third molars after removal of first premolars and orthodontic treatment. B, Supernumerary in canine area, not interfering with dentition; it should probably be left alone. C, Mesiodens and premolar supernumeraries that were being "watched" for four years by the dentist. D, Lower fourth molar. Like the mesiodens, the fourth molar is not infrequently seen. Laminagraphic radiography shows many more supernumerary teeth than had been expected, using intraoral radiographs alone.

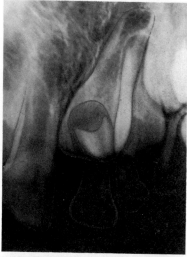

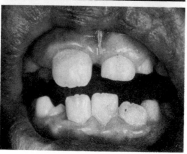

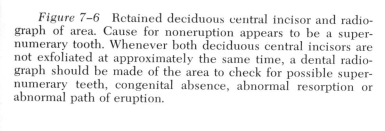

Figure 7–6 Retained deciduous central incisor and radiograph of area. Cause for noneruption appears to be a supernumerary tooth. Whenever both deciduous central incisors are not exfoliated at approximately the same time, a dental radiograph should be made of the area to check for possible supernumerary teeth, congenital absence, abnormal resorption or abnormal path of eruption.

Some authorities believe that unerupted supernumerary teeth have a tendency to become cystic if allowed to remain. Others contend that if such teeth are completely out of line of occlusion and have no effect on the dental arches they should be left alone. Sometimes the removal endangers the apical regions of contiguous permanent teeth. Multiple radiographic examination and a careful diagnosis must be made.

Of major concern to the dentist is the frequency of deflection or noneruption of the maxillary permanent central incisors as a result of supernumerary teeth (Fig. 7–7). In many cases a supernumerary tooth does not have to be in contact with the permanent incisor to prevent it from erupting normally. The careful removal of a supernumerary tooth usually allows the permanent tooth to erupt, though it may be malposed. However, this is not always true; surgical and orthodontic intervention may be necessary. *In any patient who shows a marked difference in times of eruption of permanent maxillary central incisors, this condition should be considered suspect and investigated radiographically.* Early detection and treatment, if necessary, is preventive orthodontics. This is true whether the cause is a supernumerary tooth, congenital absence or merely a mucosal barrier that is preventing the tooth from erupting. It hardly seems necessary to admonish a dentist to "count teeth," but more than one man has been embarrassed to find five lower incisors or two maxillary lateral incisors on the same side after he has been working on the patient for two or three visits (Figs. 7–16 to 7–18).

(Text continued on page 348)

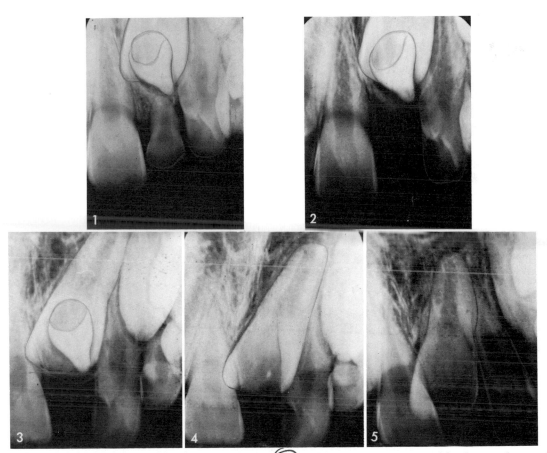

Figure 7-7   Similar problem to Figure 7-6. 1, Patient was nine years old when radiograph revealed supernumerary tooth as probable cause for noneruption of central incisor. 2, Deciduous central incisor was removed to try to stimulate some eruption. 3, Very little occurred in a year's time, and supernumerary was removed. 4, Six months later some eruption had occurred. 5, Orthodontic procedures were required to complete proper positioning after another six months.

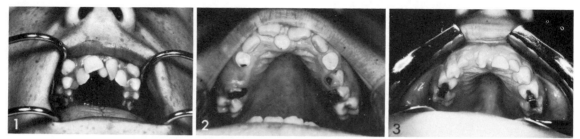

Figure 7–8   "Mesiodens" type supernumerary teeth that have erupted. (Views 2 and 3, courtesy W. R. Mayne.)

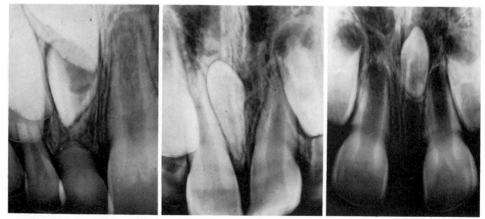

Figure 7–9 Supernumerary teeth in maxillary incisor region. (Courtesy J. R. Jarabak.)

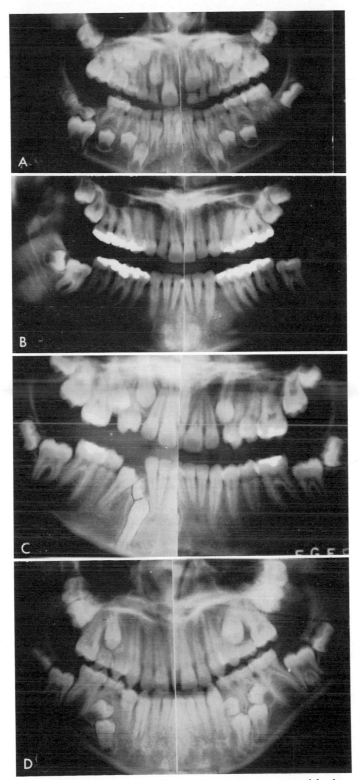

Figure 7–10 Supernumerary teeth. A, Dentigerous cyst blocking eruption of lower first molar. B, Fourth molars developing in a 21-year-old female, where first premolars had been removed previously for orthodontic reasons. C, Noneruption of canine because of supernumerary. D, Abnormal eruption and noneruption, due to premolar supernumerary.

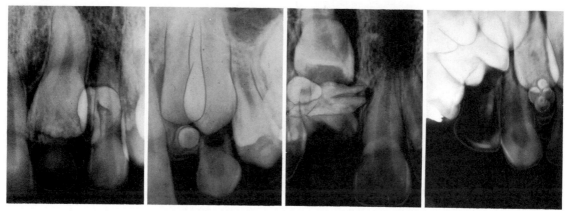

Figure 7–11   Dentigerous cysts and odontomas in maxillary incisor region. (Courtesy J. R. Jarabak.)

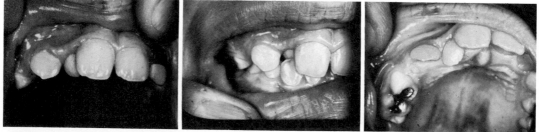

Figure 7–12   Supernumerary right lateral incisor in lingual cross-bite. Permanent lateral incisor has been deflected distally, causing premature loss of the right maxillary deciduous canine.

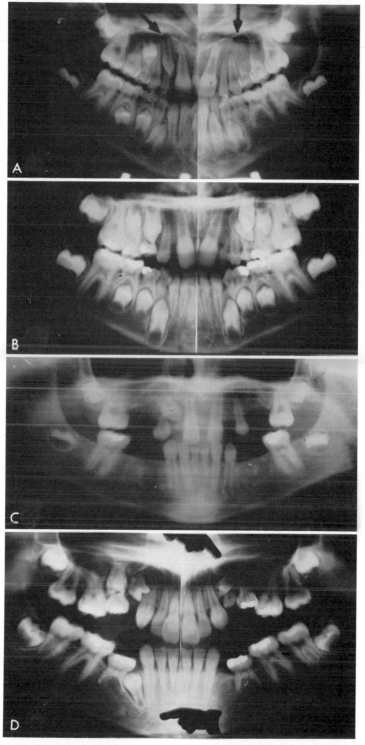

Figure 7–13 Congenital absence. A, Missing lateral incisor and premolar. Note canine erupting into incisor position. B, Missing lateral incisor, but canine erupting distally. C, Multiple congenital absence. D, Congenital absence, ankylosis and abnormal eruptive paths. Panoral radiograph shows such conditions well.

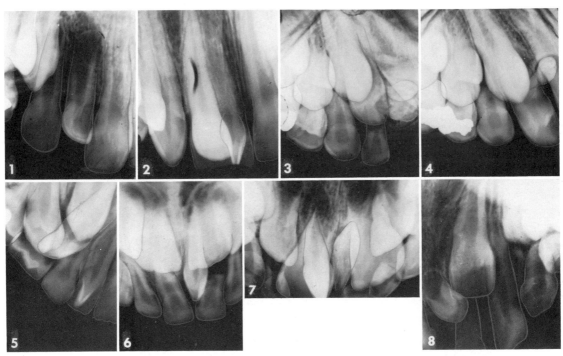

Figure 7–14 Dental radiographs of more supernumerary teeth in maxillary incisor region. 1, Dental radiograph of Figure 7–12. 2, Supernumerary combined with twinned central incisor and malposed lateral incisor superimposed over central incisor. 3, Dentigerous cyst, incisor area. 4, Same case as 3, but surgeon did not remove all cystic elements. 5, Two supernumerary lateral incisors are present. 6, Mesiodens is about to erupt before permanent central incisors. 7, Two supernumerary teeth are present in central incisor region and are deflecting the permanent teeth. 8, Supernumerary responsible for noneruption of central incisor. (View 2, courtesy S. Signorino; Views 5 and 7, courtesy J. R. Jarabak.)

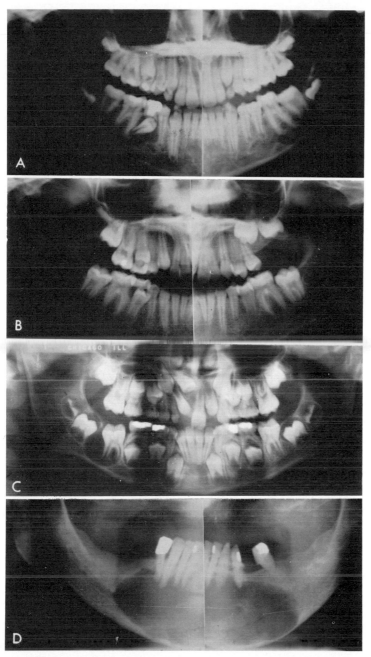

Figure 7–15 (A.) Infected cyst from deciduous molar which involves lower second premolar. (B) Despite removal of cyst in upper right first molar region, upper right first molar has not erupted. Early removal would have allowed the first molar to erupt normally. Note overeruption of opposing lower first molar. (C) Noneruption of upper central incisor that is blocked by contiguous lateral incisor, plus eruption cyst around lower first molar. Remaining first molars have erupted. (D) Large cystic involvement at symphysis. Pain was diagnosed by dentist, without radiograph, as being due to calculus.

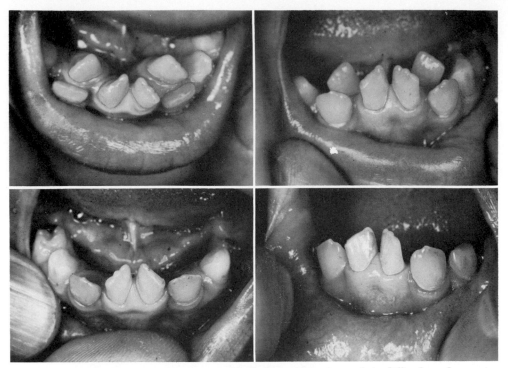

Figure 7–16   Supernumerary mandibular lateral incisors. It is difficult to determine which incisors are supernumerary. The lingually malposed teeth were removed (lower figures), however, since the remaining lateral incisors were in more nearly normal position.

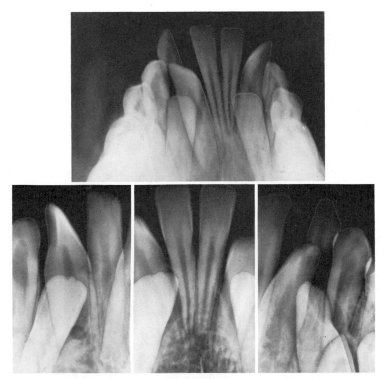

Figure 7–17   Occlusal and periapical radiographs of supernumerary mandibular lateral incisors; similar to problem in Figure 7–16.

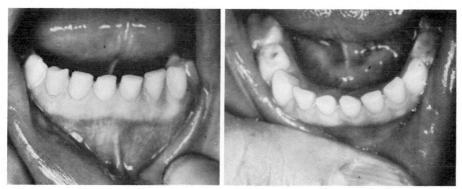

Figure 7–18 Patient with five deciduous mandibular incisors. He is a younger brother of patient in Figures 7–15, 7–16. As with congenital absence, there is a strong hereditary component with supernumerary teeth.

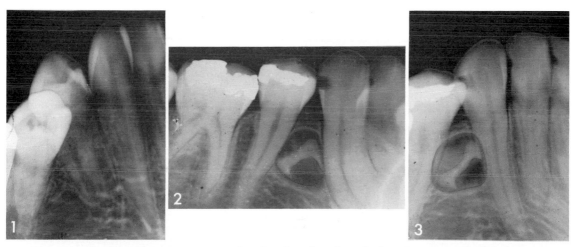

Figure 7–19 Supernumerary premolar that has developed after the removal of four first premolars and complete orthodontic therapy. 1, At the beginning of orthodontic treatment, radiograph shows only a slightly rarified area between first and second premolars. 2 and 3, At the end of the retention period, a well-defined supernumerary has formed. Note how this developing tooth has forced the root of the second premolar distally.

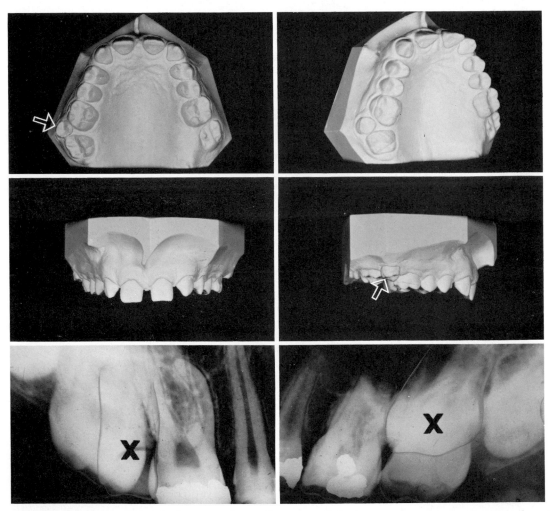

Figure 7-20 Congenital absence of maxillary lateral incisors and supernumerary molars in the same mouth. There is a familial history of missing incisors, but none of supernumerary teeth.

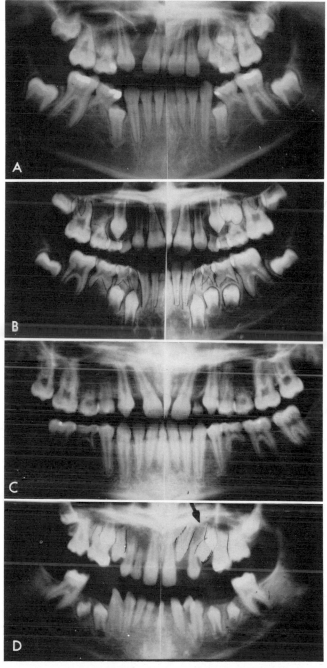

Figure 7-21 A, Congenital absence. Consolidation of spaces and prosthetic replacement are indicated. B, Maxillary canines erupting distally into missing premolar space. Some plan must be made for future rehabilitation. C, Multiple congenital absence. Mandibular second deciduous molars are often retained until the fourth decade of life. D, Abnormal eruption and congenital absence. All possible permanent teeth should be guided into place by removal of interfering deciduous teeth. Orthodontic therapy should place teeth in best positions for reception of prosthesis.

MISSING TEETH

Congenitally missing teeth are many times more frequently found than supernumerary teeth. Whereas supernumerary teeth are usually found in the maxilla, missing teeth are frequent in both jaws, though some writers believe that they are actually absent more often in the maxilla. The order of frequency of absence is: (1) maxillary and mandibular third molars, (2) maxillary lateral incisors, (3) mandibular second premolar, (4) mandibular incisors, (5) maxillary second premolars.[1] In patients with congenitally missing teeth, deformities in tooth size and shape (such as peg laterals) are more frequent. It is possible for supernumerary teeth to appear in the same mouth where there are congenitally missing teeth (Fig. 7–20). Congenital absence problems are more likely to be bilateral than are supernumerary teeth. Occasionally, a second premolar may be missing on one side while the tooth on the opposite side is quite atypical and forms only partially with no eruptive force (Fig. 7–21). Partial or total anodontia is seen more rarely (Fig. 7–22), but the patient should be carefully checked if there is any history of missing teeth in the family.[3] Heredity seems to play a more significant role for missing teeth than supernumerary teeth. Congenital absence is more frequent in the permanent than in the deciduous dentition (Figs. 7–23 to 7–25). Where permanent teeth are missing, the roots of these deciduous predecessors may not resorb. This cannot be predicted in advance and must be checked at periodic intervals. Where maxillary lateral incisors are congenitally missing, the permanent canines may often erupt mesial to the deciduous canines, into the space of the missing teeth (Figs. 7–26 to 7–29). It seems to be a matter of chance whether or not the roots of the deciduous canines resorb. Usually it is sound procedure to attempt to maintain the deciduous tooth, unless it is creating irregularities in the dental arch because of its larger mesiodistal dimension (Fig. 7–30). Even then the tooth may be reduced in size by disking. This is discussed in greater detail in Chapter 14.

Teeth may also be lost as the result of accidents. Many an incisor has been

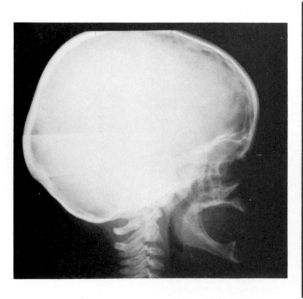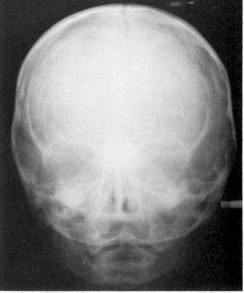

Figure 7–22   Child with complete anodontia. No teeth will develop later.

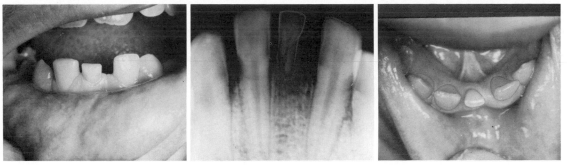

Figure 7–23 Congenital absence of permanent mandibular incisors; retention of deciduous incisor.

lost through contact with a playmate's head, a drinking fountain or the sidewalk (Figs. 7–31 to 7–33). If the lost anterior tooth is deciduous, space maintenance is usually unnecessary unless there is a tendency toward crowding already or unless the space serves as the inciting factor for a tongue thrust habit. If it is a permanent central or lateral incisor the picture is different. Even the slightest crowding tendency will result in drifting of the contiguous teeth into the edentulous area (Fig. 7–33). If considerable crowding is present it is wise to seek the counsel of an orthodontist before maintaining space; one phase of orthodontic therapy may be tooth removal, and a planned program of serial extraction may be necessary. (See Chap. 15.) Frequently incisor teeth are lost because of their undue prominence. In most instances this protrusion is only a

(Text continued on page 356)

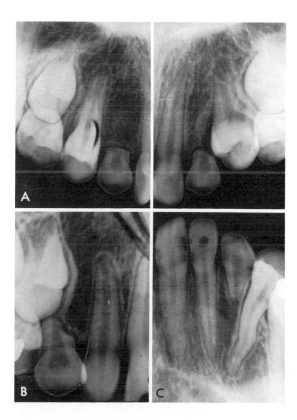

Figure 7–24 Congenital absence of canines. A, Bilateral absence of maxillary canines in same patient. B, Unilateral absence of right maxillary canine with atypical right lateral incisor. C, Unilateral absence of mandibular left canine.

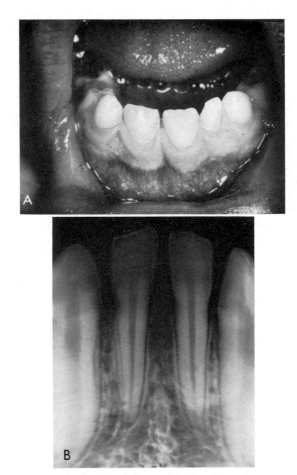

Figure 7-25   Congenital absence of mandibular lateral incisors. A, With retained deciduous lateral incisor. B, Radiograph showing generalized spacing usually present when deciduous lateral incisors are not retained.

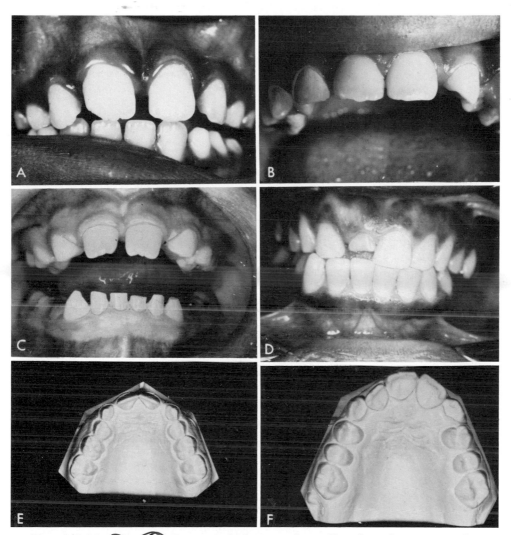

Figure 7–26 (A and C,) Congenital absence of maxillary lateral incisors with generalized spacing. *B,* Maxillary centrals in contact despite absence of lateral incisors. *D,* Congenital absence of maxillary central incisor, with deciduous right central incisor retained. *E,* Bilateral absence of lateral incisors; canine—first deciduous molar and central incisor contact tight but space inadequate to replace missing lateral incisors. *F,* Congenital absence of maxillary left lateral incisor. Space has closed autonomously and contact is established from canine to canine.

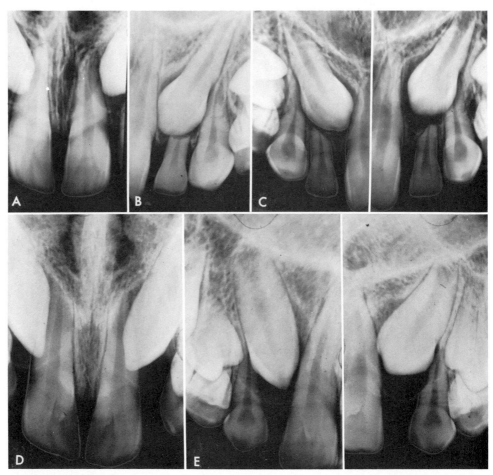

Figure 7–27 Congenital absence, maxillary lateral incisors. Deciduous lateral incisors already lost in A, D and E. Little resorption is observed on the root of the deciduous canine in B and C. Permanent canines are mesial to normal position because of congenital absence of the lateral incisors.

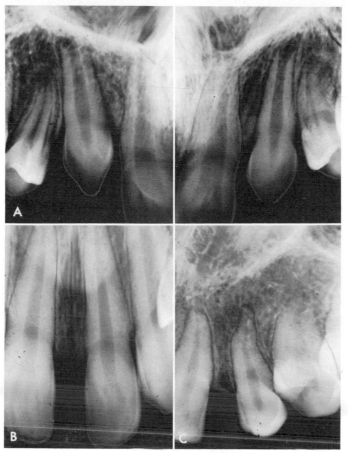

Figure 7–28 Varying positions of permanent canines in cases of congenital absence of lateral incisors. A, Right and left sides, with canines between first premolar and central incisor. B, Canine in contact with central incisor; diastema between incisors. C, Canine has erupted in contact with first premolar; diastema in missing lateral incisor area. There is little predictability regarding path of canine eruption when the lateral incisors are missing.

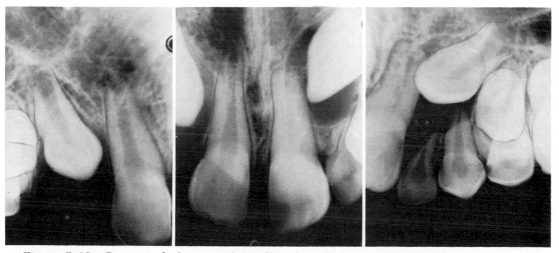

Figure 7–29 Congenital absence of maxillary lateral incisors. Both canines were cystic, but cyst was removed on right to allow canine to erupt. Cyst still present on left. Note beginning damage to left maxillary central incisor apical portion. Cysts appear to occur more frequently in congenital absence problems.

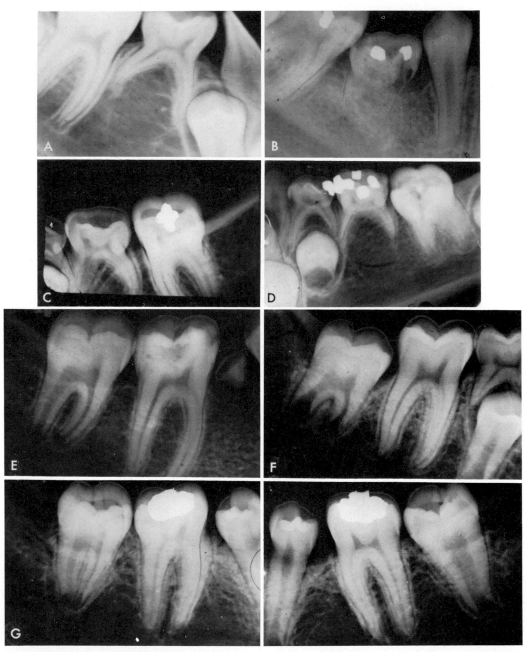

Figure 7–30 Congenital absence of premolar and molar teeth. Despite absence of premolar in A, note crowding of first premolar and rotation and distal tipping of canine. In B, retained second deciduous molar is ankylosed and should be removed. In C, D and E, second premolars are absent; second permanent molar also absent in C; third molar absent in E. Third molar probably is missing in F but a lateral jaw or lateral cephalometric headplate should be made to confirm diagnosis and a new examination made a year or two later. In G, first permanent molars are missing bilaterally.

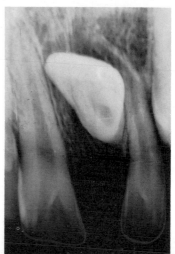

Figure 7–31 Maxillary left central incisor malposed as a result of an accident. The deciduous central incisor was driven up into the alveolar process, deflecting the permanent successor from its normal eruptive path. Intraoral view shows lack of space to accommodate incisors.

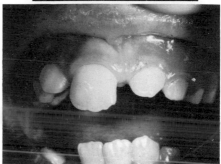

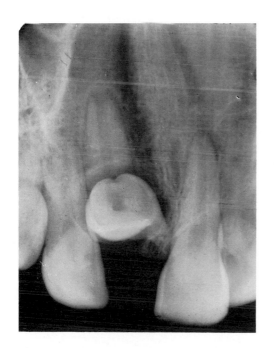

Figure 7–32 Di-lacerated maxillary right permanent central incisor. Early blow injured developing tooth bud, creating the malformation seen. (Courtesy Warren Wayne.)

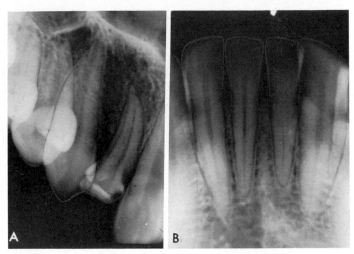

Figure 7–33   A, Accident has reduced mesiodistal width of incisor crown, allowing drift of contiguous teeth. B, Left central incisor completely knocked out 13 years previously. Prompt action by dentist sterilizing and replacing tooth has prevented a malocclusion. Note complete calcification of root canal. (View A, courtesy, J. R. Jarabak.)

symptom of a Class II, Division 1 malocclusion. Again, orthodontic consultation is indicated before placing a space maintainer that might interfere with orthodontic therapy.[11]

ANOMALIES OF TOOTH SIZE

The size of teeth is largely determined by heredity. Like all other structures in the body, there is great variation, both from individual to individual and even within the same individual. Since crowding is one of the major characteristics of dental malocclusion, it might be assumed that there is a greater tendency in this direction with the large teeth than with the smaller teeth. From various research studies, this does not seem to follow.[4]

In *The Dentition of the Growing Child* by Moorrees, several observations were made on the size of teeth and malocclusion.[5] (Children between 3 and 18 years of age were the subjects of this study.) The tables (Tables 2–3 to 2–6) show the mesiodistal crown diameters of deciduous and permanent teeth for male and female. Table 2–6 shows mesiodistal crown diameters of deciduous teeth expressed as a percentage of those of their permanent successors. As can be seen, width increments are greater in males than females, with the sex difference being more pronounced in the permanent than in the deciduous teeth. The canine shows the greatest difference. There does not seem to be any correlation between tooth size and arch size, and between spacing and crowding of teeth. Quite frequently, however, there is a variation in tooth size within the same individual (Figs. 7–34, 7–35). Often one maxillary lateral incisor will be of normal size and configuration while the other is diminutive. Anomalies of size are relatively frequent in the mandibular premolar area. Sometimes a tooth size discrepancy can be noted when comparing maxillary and mandibular dental arches. Occasionally, developmental aberrations occur with one or more teeth

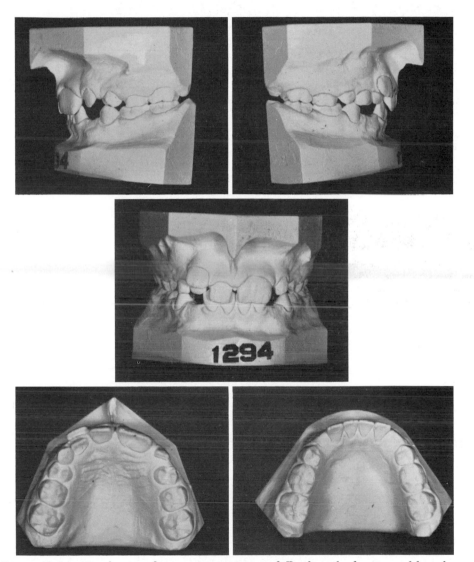

Figure 7-34 Tooth size discrepancy poses a difficult orthodontic problem here.

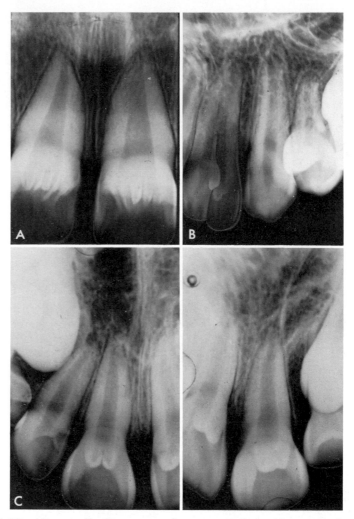

Figure 7–35   Abnormally large central incisors A have abnormal shape. In B, left lateral incisor is geminated. Shovel-shaped incisors C have heavy marginal ridges that are characteristic of the Japanese. (Views A and B, courtesy J. R. Jarabak.)

being anomalous in shape or fused with a neighboring tooth. The significant increase in arch length cannot be tolerated and a malocclusion results (Figs. 7–36, 7–37).

ANOMALIES OF TOOTH SHAPE

Intimately related to tooth size is tooth shape. The most frequent departure from normal is the "peg lateral." Because of its diminutive size, excessive spacing will often occur in the maxillary anterior segment. Maxillary central incisors vary a great deal in shape. Like lateral incisors, they may be deformed owing to a congenital cleft (Fig. 7–38). Occasionally the cingulum is quite pronounced and, particularly with the Japanese, the marginal ridges can be sharp and well defined, bounding the lingual fossa (Figs. 7–35, 7–37). The presence of an exaggerated cingulum or heavy marginal ridges can force the involved teeth labially

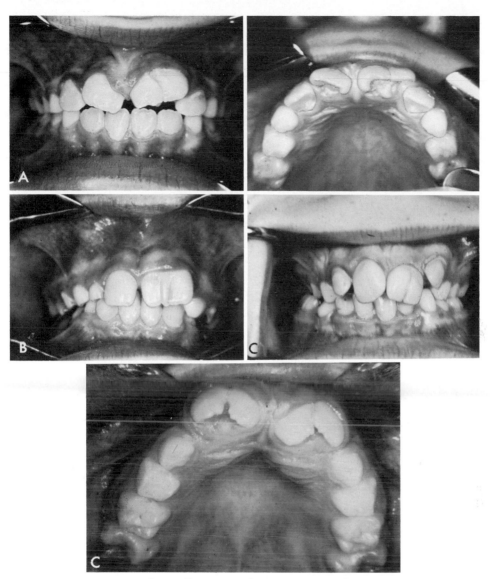

Figure 7–36 Twinned maxillary central incisors. Lateral incisors present in A and C, but left lateral incisor congenitally missing in B. History of missing teeth in C in family. (Views A and B, courtesy J. R. Jarabak.)

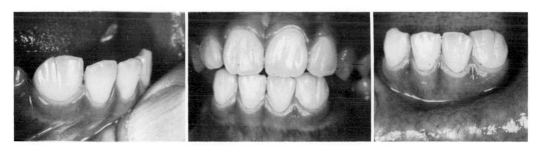

Figure 7–37 Twinned canines and lateral incisors.

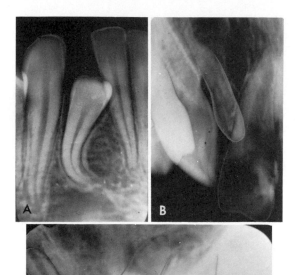

Figure 7–38 A, Abnormally shaped lateral incisor in cleft palate child. B and C, Abnormal root formations that can cause a malocclusion.

and prevent the establishment of a normal overbite-overjet relationship. The mandibular second premolar also shows great variation in shape and size. It may have an extra lingual cusp, which usually serves to increase the mesiodistal dimension. Such a variation reduces the autonomous adjustment space that the loss of the second deciduous molar usually gives.

Other anomalies of shape occasionally occur as a result of developmental defects, such as amelogenesis imperfecta, hypoplasia, gemination, dens in dente, odontomas, fusions and congenital syphilitic aberrations such as Hutchinson's incisors and mulberry molars.

ABNORMAL LABIAL FRENUM

A controversial subject in orthodontics has been the connection between the labial frenum and the diastema that occurs between the maxillary incisors. Most of this controversy is due to an incomplete understanding of the role of heredity, tooth size, local habits and the processes of growth and development, with attendant changes in tooth position. Spacing between the maxillary central incisors and the presence of the fibrous tissue attachment such as the labial frenum provide an excellent "chicken and egg" routine for controversy. Which came first? (Figure 7–39.) In the past, thousands of labial frena have been "clipped" needlessly to allow the space to close. In a large percentage of these cases it is likely that closure would have occurred autonomously with the eruption of the permanent canines. In many other instances, because of the lack of recognition of habit problems, tooth size discrepancy, congenitally missing teeth or midline supernumerary teeth, the clipping of the frenum has done little to close the space. A thorough examination and a differential diagnosis are imperative before the dentist sets out to clip the frenum. At birth the frenum is attached to the alveolar ridge, with fibers actually running into the lingual interdental papilla. As the teeth erupt and as alveolar bone is deposited, the frenum attachment migrates superiorly with respect to the alveolar ridge. Fibers may persist between the maxillary central incisors and in the V-shaped intermaxillary suture (Fig. 7–40), attaching to the outer layer of the periosteum and connective tissue of the suture.

As Faustin Weber has noted, the diastema may be due to other factors, and any and all of the following list should be eliminated as possible causative factors: microdontia, macrognathia, supernumerary teeth (especially a mesiodens), peg laterals, missing lateral incisors, heavy occlusion against the lingual surfaces of the maxillary incisors, habits such as thumb sucking, tongue thrust, lip biting or lip sucking, and midline cysts.[6] That the interincisor spacing will close in most cases without any interference is confirmed by Taylor[7] who noted the following figures:

Age	Incidence of Diastema
6	97%
6– 7	88%
10–11	48%
12–18	7%

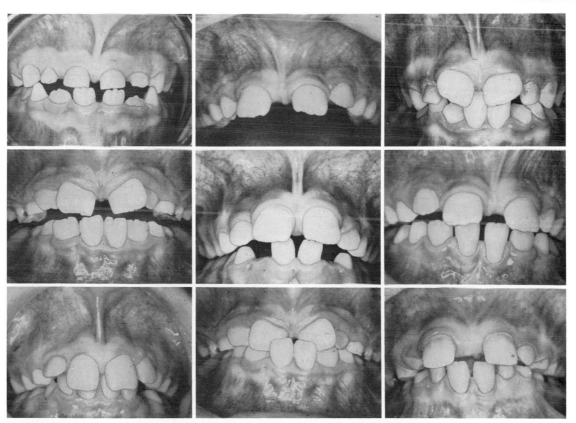

Figure 7–39 Anterior diastemas associated with various shapes and sizes of labial frena. The frenum is not necessarily the cause of the spacing. (Courtesy W. R. Mayne.)

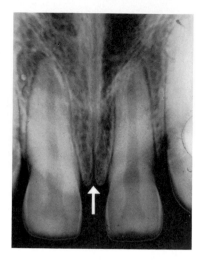

Figure 7–40 Notching of intermaxillary suture often seen in conjunction with heavy and fibrous labial frenum and a diastema between the maxillary central incisors. A successful frenectomy usually requires dissecting out frenum fibers in the notch.

Existence of a heavy fibrous frenum does not always mean that spacing is present (Fig. 7–41). Frequently during the course of orthodontic therapy the interposed fibers will atrophy, making a frenectomy unnecessary.[8] One diagnostic adjunct that helps to determine the role of the frenum is the "blanche test." Ordinarily, the frenum has migrated sufficiently superiorly by 10 to 12 years of age that a tug on the upper lip causes no demonstrable change at the maxillary central inderdental papilla. Where there is a heavy fibrous frenum that may be contributory, however, a "blanching" of the tissue just lingual to the maxillary central incisors can be noted. This usually means that the fibrous attachment still remains in this area. This attachment may well interfere with the normal developmental closure of the spacing, as Broadbent has outlined in his explanation of the "ugly duckling" stage (see Chap. 2). The difficulty lies in establishing whether this fibrous attachment is "causative" or "resultant" or whether it is primary or secondary to such problems as excessive overbite, local habits, tooth size discrepancy. The hereditary component is a major factor in persistent diastemas. Therefore, a check of parents and siblings is advisable whenever a diastema is observed. (The spacing of maxillary incisors is discussed from a treatment point of view in Chap. 13). It is sufficient to say here that the mere clipping of the frenum attachment will not solve the diastema problem.

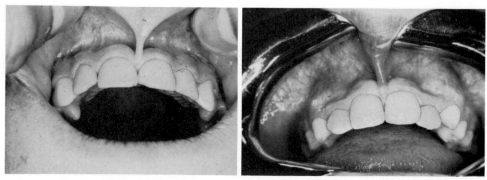

Figure 7–41 Heavy fibrous frenum, but no diastema present. (Courtesy W. R. Mayne.)

PREMATURE LOSS OF DECIDUOUS TEETH

In Chapter 2 it was pointed out that the deciduous teeth serve not only as organs of mastication, but as "space savers" for the permanent teeth. They also assist in maintaining the opposing teeth at the proper occlusal level. While it is probable that early writers in the field overstressed the importance of premature *loss* of deciduous teeth, the importance of recognizing the possibilities of alleviating a malocclusion by premature *extraction* of deciduous teeth cannot be overemphasized. Where there is a generalized lack of arch length in both maxillary and mandibular dental arches, the deciduous cuspids are frequently shed prematurely, and nature attempts to provide more space to align the permanent incisor teeth that have already erupted (Fig. 7–42). This type of premature loss is often a clue for further guided extraction of deciduous teeth and possible removal of first premolars later. (See Chap. 15.) To maintain space in these cases may render a disservice to the patient. By contrast, where there is a normal occlusion to start with, and radiographic examination shows that there is no arch length deficiency, the premature removal of posterior deciduous teeth because of caries means a probable malocclusion unless space maintainers are placed. (See Chap. 13.) With as many as 48 teeth in the alveolar process at the same time, the struggle for space in the expanding and growing medium of bone is at times critical. The unscheduled loss of one or more dental units may throw off the delicate timetable and prevent nature from achieving a normal healthy occlusion.

In the maxillary or mandibular anterior areas, space maintenance for deciduous teeth is seldom necessary in a normal occlusion. Growth and developmental processes are such that mesial drifting of contiguous teeth is minimal. It is a different story with an arch length deficiency or overjet problem, however. Spaces can close rapidly (Fig. 7–43).

The loss of the first or second deciduous molar, however, is almost always a matter of concern, even when the occlusion is normal. In the mandibular arch the combined width of the deciduous canine, first deciduous molar and second deciduous molar is on the average of 1.7 mm. greater on each side than the permanent successors. In the maxillary arch this "leeway" space averages only 0.9 mm. because of the greater size of the permanent canine and first and second premolar teeth. (See Chap. 2.) This space differential is necessary to allow for the occlusal adjustment and final alignment of the incisors and a "settling in" of the occlusion as the terminal plane relationship is corrected. Premature extraction of a deciduous second molar will very likely lead to mesial drift of the first permanent molar and blocking of the erupting second premolars (Fig. 7–44). Even when the premolar erupts, it is deflected buccally or lingually into a position of malocclusion. As the maxillary molar drifts mesially it often rotates with the mesiobuccal cusp moving lingually, and the tooth tends to tip (Fig. 7–45). In the mandibular arch the first permanent molar may show less rotation but more frequently tips over the unerupted second premolar (Fig. 7–46). The mesial drifting and tipping of first permanent molars does not always occur. If the occlusion is "locked" and if there is quite adequate space for erupting succedaneous teeth, the tendency for space closure in the prematurely extracted deciduous molar region is less. A differential diagnosis is essential. (See Chap. 13.)

With respect to premature extraction of deciduous teeth, it is wise for the dentist to keep in mind that it does not take very much to throw off the delicate timetable of dental development. It is up to him to do all he can to maintain this

(Text continued on page 367)

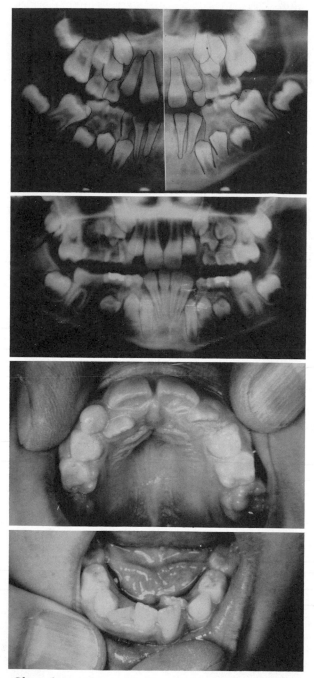

Figure 7–42   Clues for guided extraction. Premature loss, ectopic eruption, lingual malposition of lateral incisors, arch length deficiency, flaring of lateral incisors—just a few of the danger signs an observant dentist should see and have checked for possible serial extraction guidance.

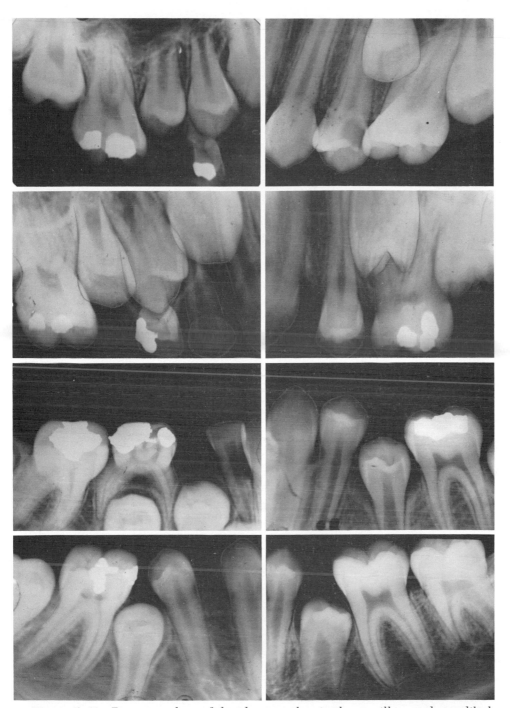

Figure 7–43 Premature loss of deciduous molars in the maxillary and mandibular arch. Encroachment on space for erupting premolar is usually mesial as well as distal.

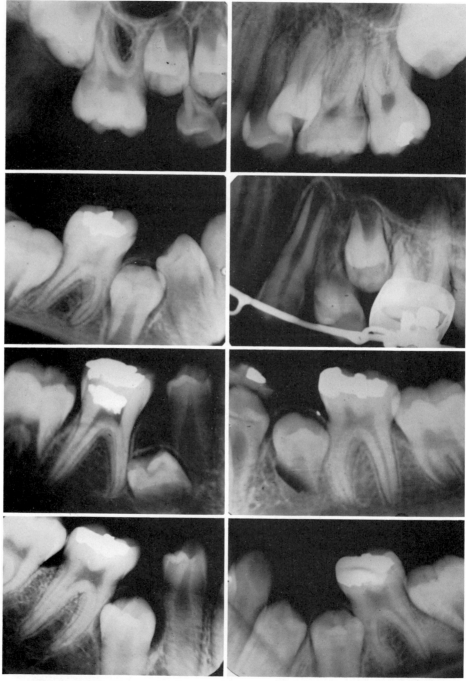

Figure 7–44 Premature loss problems require orthodontic assistance.

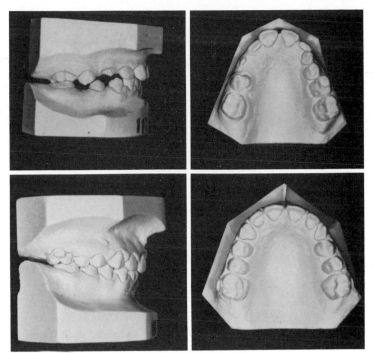

Figure 7-45 Premature loss, upper right second deciduous molar, with no space maintainer to prevent mesial drift of first molar (upper pictures). Orthodontic therapy was necessary to restore integrity of the dental arch (lower pictures).

timetable on schedule by anatomically correct restoration of deciduous teeth and maintenance of the integrity of the dental arch in harmony with the developmental pattern. If there is any question as to what procedure to follow, he should seek the advice of an orthodontist. It cannot be emphasized too strongly that a consultative relationship should be set up with an orthodontist and used frequently. When in doubt—check!

The early loss of permanent teeth should be considered just as severe a "malocclusion maker" as the loss of deciduous teeth. Too many children lose their first permanent molars to the onslaught of caries and dental neglect. If the

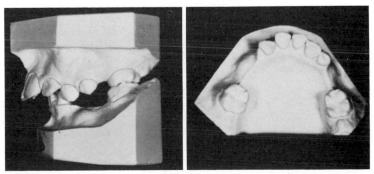

Figure 7-46 Premature loss, lower first and second deciduous molars and left deciduous canine. First permanent molars have tipped and rotated mesially. Space now inadequate for succedaneous teeth.

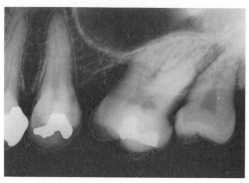

Figure 7–47 Early loss of a maxillary first permanent molar. The health and longevity of the entire dentition is endangered by the ever-increasing malocclusion development.

loss occurs before the dentition is complete, the disturbance is likely to be particularly marked (Fig. 7–47). The resultant shortening of arch length on the side of the loss, tipping of the contiguous teeth, overeruption of opposing teeth and the future periodontal implications are not calculated to enhance the longevity of the dental mechanism. At the risk of seeming repetitious, because of the great importance of this dynamic concept, it is pointed out again that morphogenetic, anatomic and functional forces maintain a dynamic balance of the occlusion. The loss of a tooth can upset this balance. It is the duty of the dentist to restore the occlusal harmony. Not to do so invites widespread damage to the dentition (Fig. 7–48).

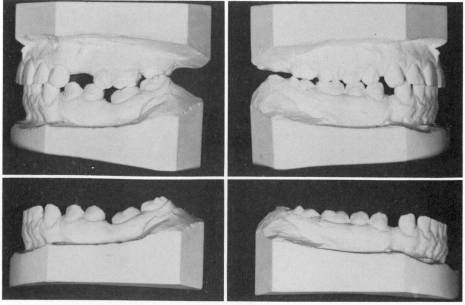

Figure 7–48 Unilateral malocclusion with arch length deficiency, teeth receiving stress in an abnormal manner, functional prematurities, overeruption of the opposing teeth, etc. Compare the occlusal plane on the mutilated side (left) with that on the normal side (right). Proper dental care would have prevented this problem.

PROLONGED RETENTION AND ABNORMAL RESORPTION
OF DECIDUOUS TEETH

In the child's constantly changing, shifting, growing dento-alveolar complex, timing is a critical matter. This has been emphasized in the discussion of what can happen because of the premature loss of deciduous teeth and of the effect that premature loss may have on eruption schedule and availability of space for permanent teeth. No less an upset in the developmental pattern is the prolonged retention of deciduous teeth. Mechanical interference can deflect an erupting permanent tooth into a position of malocclusion. If the roots of the deciduous teeth are not resorbed properly, uniformly or on schedule, the permanent successors may be either withheld from eruption at a time when the same teeth are erupting in other segments, or they may be deflected into malposition (Figs. 7–49 to 7–52).

One basic rule to follow is that *the dentist should maintain the tooth-shedding timetable at about the same level for each of the four buccal segments*. If the canine, first premolars or second premolars are clinically present in one or more segments while the deciduous counterparts are still firmly anchored in one or more of the remaining segments, an immediate radiographic examination is essential. The dentist should be sure that good periapical or laminagraphic views of the retained deciduous tooth are obtained (Fig. 7–53). It is tragic to remove a deciduous tooth only to find that the permanent tooth is congenitally missing. More frequently, however, one root or part of a root does not resorb along with the rest of the roots (Fig. 7–54). Then it is the duty of the dentist to remove the deciduous tooth. This is truly preventive orthodontics. Many pa-

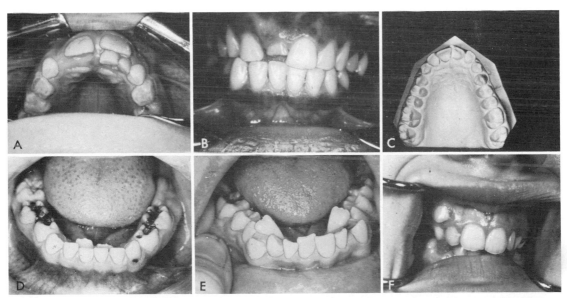

Figure 7–49 Prolonged retention. A, Permanent central incisor has erupted labially because of retained deciduous central and lateral incisors. B, Blow devitalized the upper right deciduous central incisor, and it has not resorbed. The permanent successor is in contact with the nonresorbing root. C, Retention of deciduous canines deflected the permanent canines mesially. The increased arch length comes primarily from an excessive overjet. D, Retained deciduous central incisors; permanent centrals erupting lingually. E, Retained deciduous lateral incisors; mandibular permanent lateral incisors deflected into transposed coronal positions. F, Retained deciduous canine.

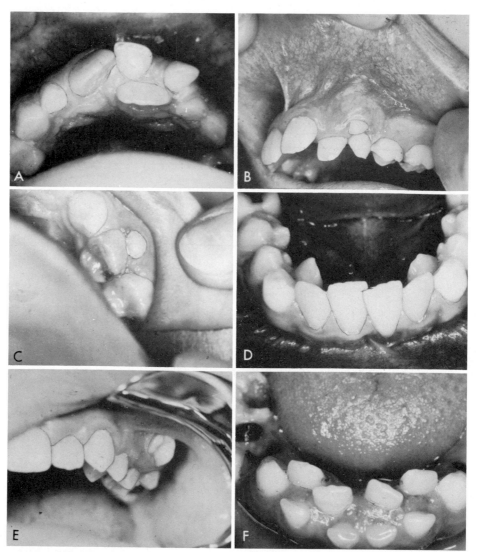

Figure 7–50 Prolonged retention. A, Maxillary incisor in lingual cross-bite. B, Maxillary canine being deflected buccally—a frequent occurrence. C, First premolar erupting into buccal malposition. D, Mandibular canines being forced lingually. E, Maxillary second molar erupting buccally. F, Mandibular incisors crowded lingually by prolonged retention of deciduous counterparts.

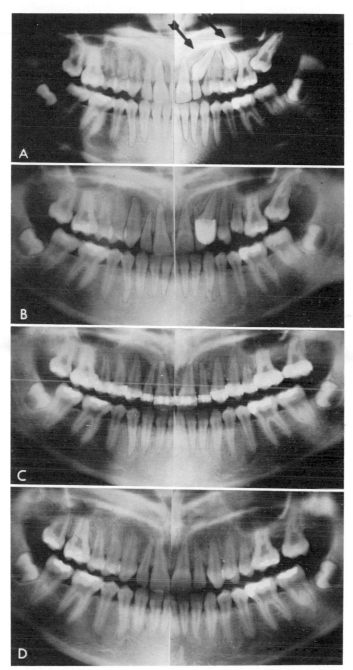

Figure 7–51 Fifteen-year-old girl under routine dental care. A, Note impacted maxillary canine and second molar, prolonged retention of second deciduous molar, noneruption of second premolars and congenital absence of maxillary third molars. B, Six months later after surgical uncovering of canine and crown placement, removal of deciduous molar and surgical tipping of second molar. C, Orthodontic appliances placed to complete tooth movement. Note pocket between first and second molar on right of picture. D, After appliance removal, two years after A, with bone still rarified between upper first and second molars on right. Surgical intervention three years earlier would have improved prognosis.

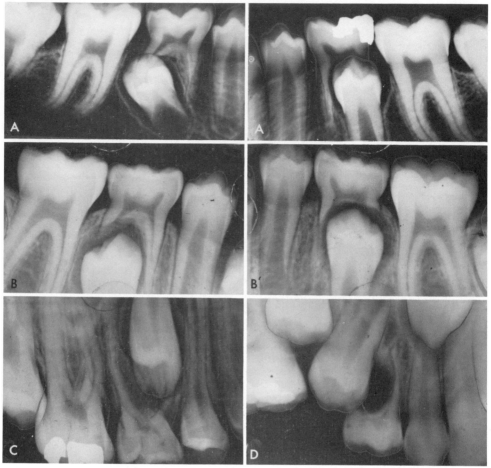

Figure 7–52   A, Abnormal resorption of second deciduous molars, with deflection of lower right second premolar. B, Resorption is normal in lower left second premolar area, but abnormal in the lower right second deciduous molar area. C and D, Abnormal resorption is deflecting maxillary permanent successors, with the maxillary right second premolar completely impacted.

tients would not have needed orthodontic treatment had adequate guidance been given to the critical exchange of the teeth.

The subject of prolonged tooth retention versus abnormal eruption has "chicken and egg" overtones. Which came first? Which is primary? Is the permanent successor being deflected by the abnormal resorption, or is there abnormal resorption of the deciduous tooth because of the abnormal path of eruption of the permanent tooth? Is is not always possible to make a firm differential diagnosis, as indicated in the sections on *Delayed Eruption of Permanent Teeth* and *Abnormal Eruptive Path*, which immediately follow this discussion. The important thing is to recognize departure from the normal. Regardless of the primary or secondary status of deciduous versus permanent tooth, the method of control is usually the same—removal of the deciduous tooth according to the timetable established by the same tooth in the remaining quadrants of the mouth, and creating a tract, if need be, for the permanent tooth to erupt toward its normal position in the mouth. If the dentist looks for them, he will be

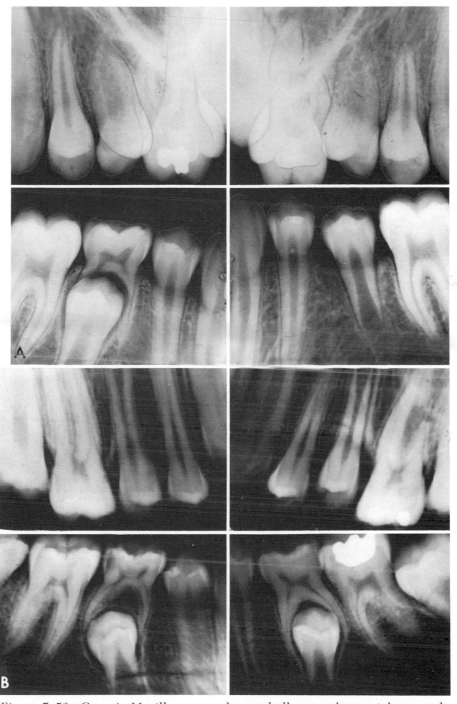

Figure 7-53 Case A. Maxillary premolars and all except lower right second premolar have erupted. Abnormal resorption of mesial root of deciduous molar is preventing its loss. This tooth should be removed. Case B. Maxillary second deciduous molars were lost on schedule but mandibular counterparts were still retained, with no resorption of roots. These teeth should be removed and the crowns of the second premolars uncovered to enhance their eruption.

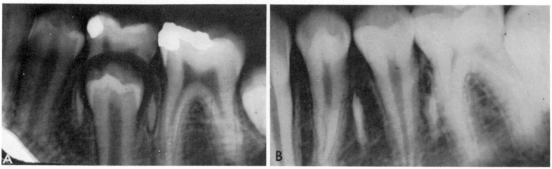

Figure 7–54   A, Second deciduous molar roots resorbing abnormally. B, These root fragments are often retained and incorporated if not caught in time. They may prevent proper autonomous adjustment of the occlusion and occasionally act as a focus for a cyst. Careful periodic radiographic examination can prevent most of these problems.

amazed at how frequently he will spot abnormal resorption phenomena, particularly in the mandibular second deciduous molar area. Procrastination can only lead to dental disaster.

There is a broad range of normalcy for loss of deciduous teeth. Some children are precocious and lose their teeth early; others are quite slow. Both patterns may be normal. Thus, the dentist must maintain the exchange of teeth schedule for the *individual* patient, and not attempt to follow a "norm table" compiled from thousands of youngsters. One clue to the pattern for a particular patient is the eruption time of the deciduous dentition. Another is the loss of the deciduous incisors and their replacement by the permanent teeth. Usually a child that completes his deciduous dentition early is likely to follow the same trend in the permanent dentition. Hereditary pattern is a factor here and the parents should be questioned about their own dental development and that of siblings. A full radiographic examination assists the dentist in determining the relation of the dental developmental age to the chronologic age. Uniformity is the watchword for guidance during the critical tooth exchange period.

If the dental developmental age is either abnormally advanced or retarded, a check into the endocrine history should be made. Hypothyroidism is a relatively frequent occurrence in our society, and the tendency can be inherited. If there is a history of hypothyroidism, a delayed developmental pattern is common. Frequently prolonged retention of deciduous teeth is one of the characteristic signs. With precocious gonadotrophic hormonal development, the dental developmental pattern is markedly accelerated. Since maturation occurs early, crowding is more likely. It is quite possible for any hormonal or endocrine disturbance to upset the timetable of dental development. It is not infrequent that an alert dentist is the first to pick up signs of this systemic disturbance. Medicine makes more frequent use of cortisone and other steroids in treatment of a variety of general diseases today. These substances affect the metabolic climate and endocrine balance. In turn, the dental developmental pattern may become abnormal. Thus, medication may be the ultimate *cause* of a malocclusion, and not the cure. A few simple questions asked early in the game may save the dentist considerable embarrassment later.

Even when the deciduous teeth appear to be lost on time, the patient should be observed until the permanent teeth erupt. Frequently fragments of deciduous roots are retained in the alveolar process (Fig. 7–54). These fragments, if not resorbed, may deflect the permanent tooth in its eruptive path and most certainly may prevent the closure of contacts of permanent teeth. Whenever root fragments are found, periodic radiographic examination is necessary to check their status. These fragments are usually incorporated in the alveolar process and remain asymptomatic. Retained root fragments can and occasionally do serve as foci for cysts. Such fragments should be removed, if this is possible without endangering the adjoining teeth. (The management of retained roots and prolonged retention of deciduous teeth is discussed in more detail in Chap. 13.) Another possible factor in prolonged retention of deciduous teeth will be discussed under Ankylosis—rupture of periodontal membrane at one or more points and establishment of a bony bridge between the tooth and lamina dura, preventing normal eruption.

DELAYED ERUPTION OF PERMANENT TEETH

There are times during the exchange-of-teeth period that deciduous teeth are lost, but it seems to both parent and patient that the permanent successors will *never* erupt. In addition to the possibility of an endocrine disorder (such as hypothyroidism), the possibility of congenital absence of the permanent tooth, and the presence of a supernumerary tooth or deciduous root ("road block"), there is the relatively common chance of a "mucosal barrier." The heavy mucosa usually deteriorates before the advancing tooth—but not always. If the eruptive force is not vigorous, the mucosa can effectively stop the erupting tooth for a considerable period of time. Since root formation and eruption go hand-in-hand, the delay in all probability further reduces the eruptive force. It is good preventive dentistry to excise the mucosa when the unerupted tooth appears ready to "pop" but does not. A check of the relative state of eruption of the same tooth in the other segments of the mouth will help the dentist decide whether to excise or not. (See Chap. 13.)

The premature loss of a deciduous tooth may require more careful observation of the eruption of the permanent successor, whether or not a space maintainer is placed. Frequently early loss of the deciduous tooth means early eruption of the permanent tooth, but occasionally a bony crypt forms in the line of eruption of the permanent tooth. Like the mucosal barrier, it effectively bars the eruption of the tooth (Figs. 7–55 to 7–57). Careful radiographic examination

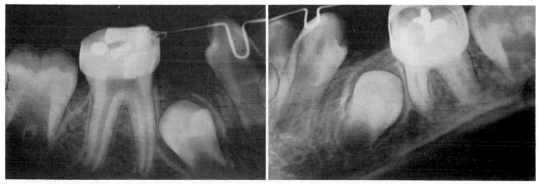

Figure 7–55 Bony barrier apparently preventing mandibular second premolars from erupting, despite orthodontic assistance in creating space. Surgical uncovering of crowns from occlusal is now indicated.

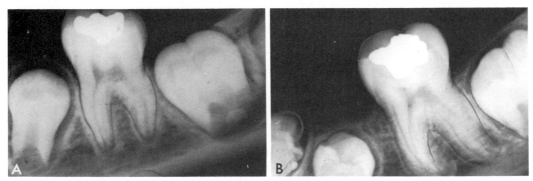

Figure 7–56   Second deciduous molars lost prematurely in A and B. Premolars appear to be erupting normally but should be watched carefully, particularly B.

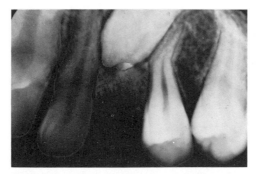

Figure 7–57   Maxillary left canine being prevented from erupting, apparently by a sclerotic bone concentration. This should be removed and coronal portion of tooth exposed partially.

and a check of the timetable in the other segments should be made before making a decision to curette the bony barrier. (See Chap. 13.)

ABNORMAL ERUPTIVE PATH

In listing all possible causes of dental malocclusions, the possibility of an abnormal eruptive path should not be overlooked. This is usually a secondary manifestation of a primary disturbance. Thus, with a hereditary pattern of severe crowding and totally inadequate space to accommodate all the teeth, deflection of the erupting tooth may be merely an adaptive response to the conditions present (Figs. 7–58, 7–59). Furthermore, because of the presence of a super-numerary tooth, retained deciduous tooth or root fragment, or possible bony barrier, a physical barrier often influences the direction of eruption, setting up an abnormal path as a result. There are cases, however, where no space problem exists and where no visible barrier is recognized, but where teeth are erupting obviously in an abnormal direction (Figs. 7–60 to 7–74). A blow is a possible cause of such eruption. In this manner a deciduous incisor may be driven into the alveolar process, and though it erupts later, it may turn the developing successor in an abnormal direction (Figs. 7–31 to 7–33). Mechanical interference by orthodontic treatment also can cause a change in eruptive path. Early Class II therapy against the maxillary arch to "move" the maxillary dentition posteriorly can cause the maxillary second molar teeth to erupt into cross-bite or can impact the developing third molars more deeply.

Coronal cysts can also cause abnormal eruptive paths (Figs. 7–29, 7–65). Such cysts occur with relative frequency and require prompt surgical elimination. If caught in time, tooth sacrifice is not usually necessary.

Some abnormal eruptive paths are of idiopathic (unknown) origin (Fig.

(Text continued on page 388)

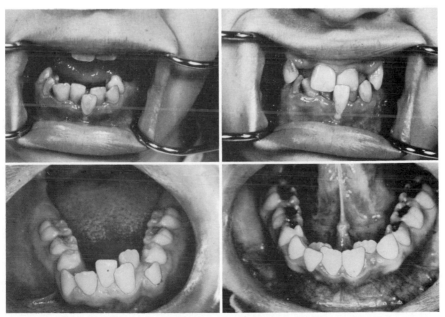

Figure 7–58 Crowding as a result of generalized arch length deficiency. Malocclusion is a likely result of nature's adaptation to the tooth size-basal bone discrepancy.

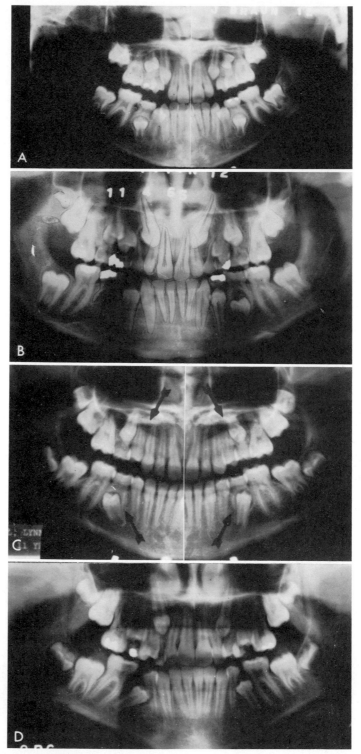

Figure 7–59   Abnormal eruptive path. A, Inadequate space, maxillary canines, upper right second premolar erupting distally. B, Upper canines erupting mesially; lower left second premolar and third molars congenitally missing. C, Abnormal path of eruption of all second premolars; ankylosis, lower right second deciduous molar. D, Abnormal path of eruption, lower left second deciduous molar; caries, lower left first molar, arch length deficiency.

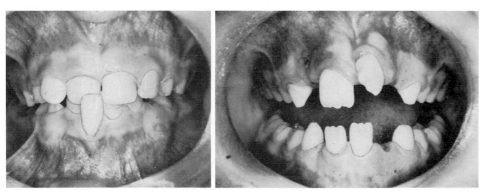

Figure 7–60 Malposition of maxillary central incisors with no known cause for abnormal eruptive path. (Courtesy W. R. Mayne.)

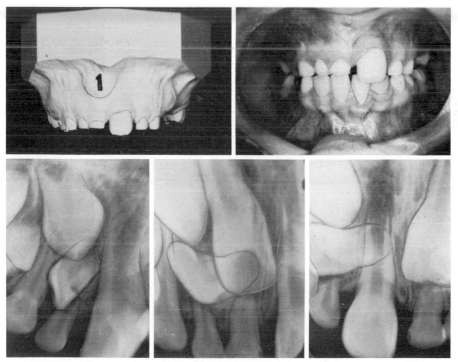

Figure 7–61 Noneruption of maxillary central incisor because of abnormal eruptive path of maxillary lateral incisors. (Courtesy W. R. Mayne.)

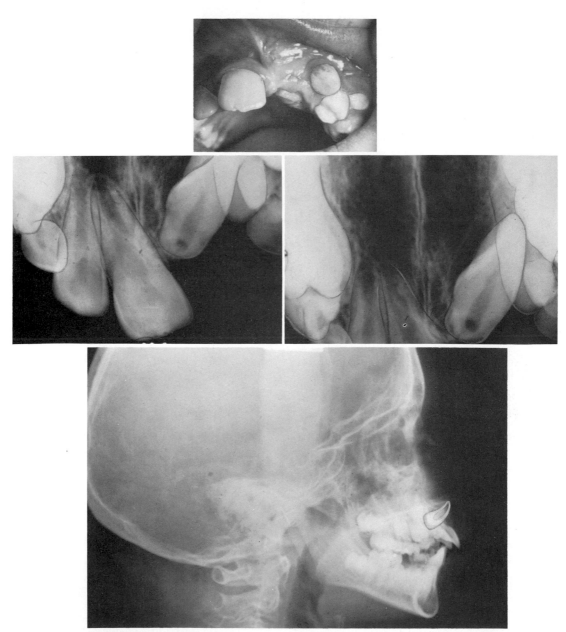

Figure 7–62   Noneruption, left central incisor. No history of supernumerary; earlier radiograph showed left central incisor crown in apparently normal position. (See Fig. 8–25.)

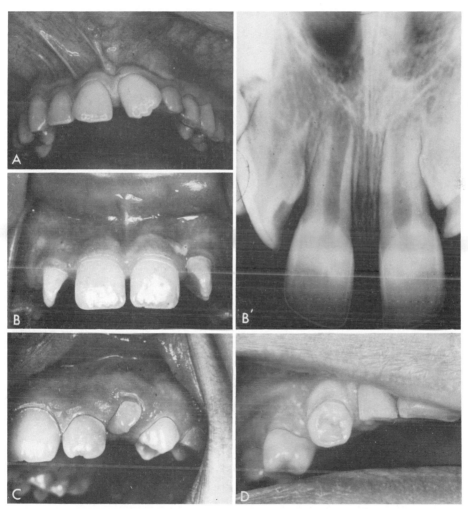

Figure 7–63   A, Left central incisor malposed because of canine transposition and resultant pressure against distal root surface. B, Malposed maxillary lateral incisors. Canines are erupting mesial to normal and have influenced the incisor position. C, Canine rotated, mesial angle lingually. D, Marked canine rotation with lingual surface to the labial.

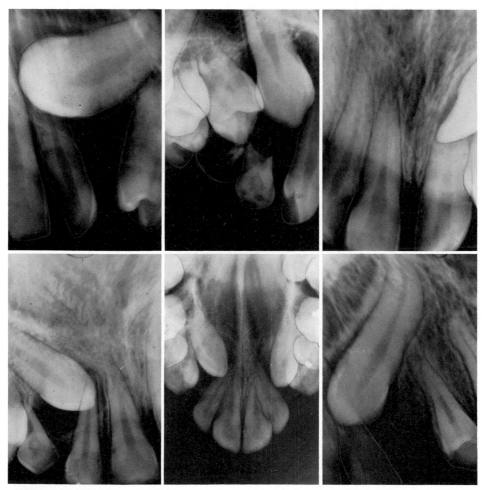

Figure 7–64   The maxillary canine may assume a number of abnormal eruptive paths. Most of the time the direction is mesial to normal, but the canine may lie lingually or labially.

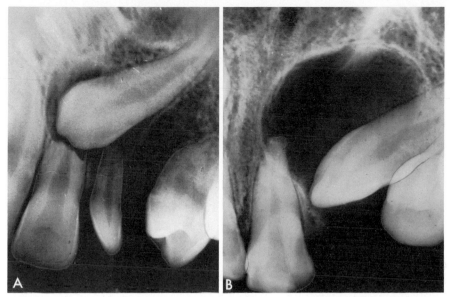

Figure 7–65 Destructiveness of abnormal canine eruption path. A, Resorption of central incisor root. B, Coronal cyst (dentigerous cyst); lateral incisor already lost. (From Fastlicht, S.: Treatment of impacted canines. Am. J. Orthodont., 40:891–905, 1954.)

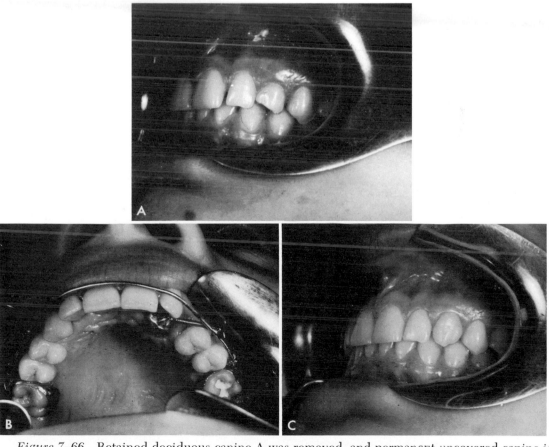

Figure 7–66 Retained deciduous canine A was removed, and permanent uncovered canine is being moved B into normal position C. (From Fastlicht, S.: Treatment of impacted canines. Am. J. Orthodont., 40:891–905, 1954.)

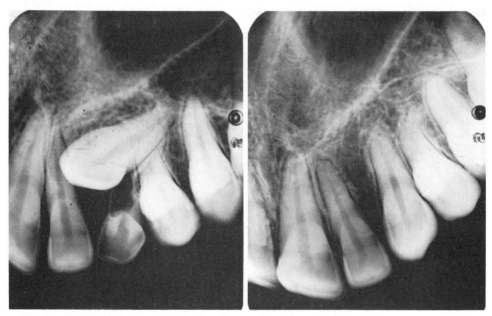

Figure 7–67   Before and after radiographs of Figure 7–66. (From Fastlicht, S.: Treatment of impacted canines. Am. J. Orthodont., 40:891–905, 1954.)

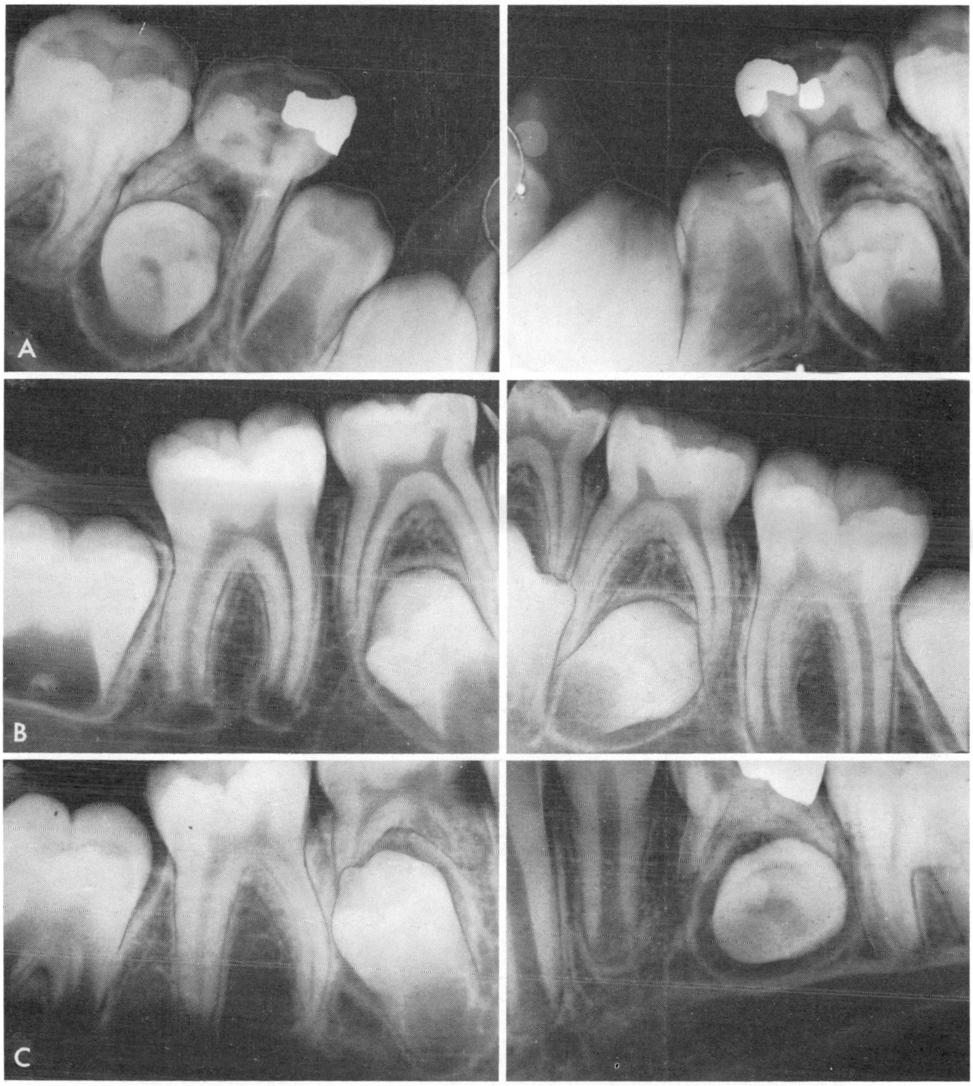

Figure 7–68   A, Right premolar erupting in an abnormal direction, left second premolar erupting normally. B, Both second premolars erupting in a distal direction. This is usually seen in arch length deficiency cases. C, Left and right second premolars both erupting abnormally but in different directions. Periodic examination is necessary, and the deciduous second molars should be removed at the proper time. Crowns of the second premolars may also need uncovering.

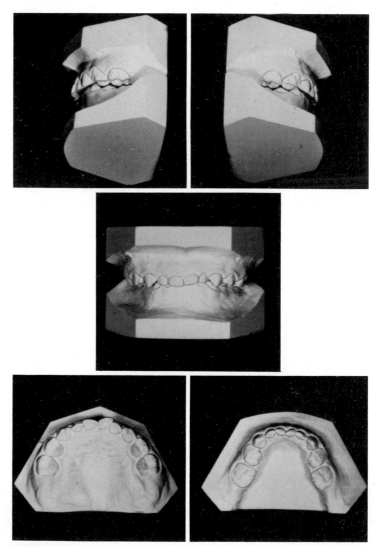

Figure 7–69   Abnormal eruption of maxillary and mandibular buccal segments resulting in a total maxillary cross-bite (scissors-bite) in the deciduous dentition.

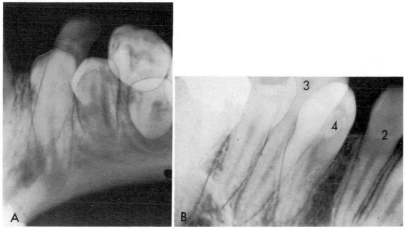

Figure 7-70 A, Transposed mandibular left lateral incisor. B, Transposed mandibular right canine and first premolar teeth.

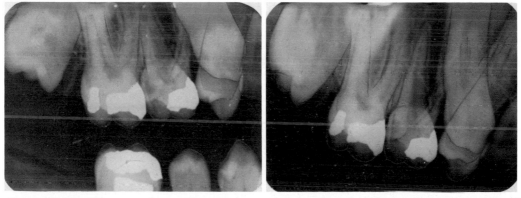

Figure 7-71 Transposed maxillary right canine combined with congenital absence of the maxillary right second premolar; picked up on a routine bite-wing radiograph (left) and seen more clearly on a periapical view (right).

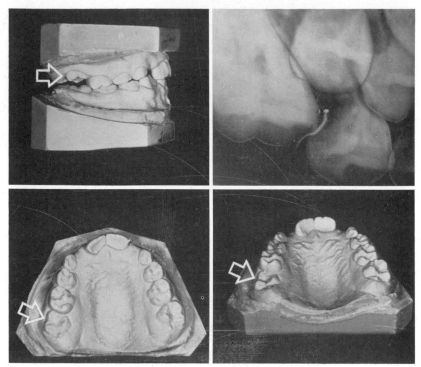

Figure 7–72   Ectopic eruption, upper right first molar. Radiograph (upper right) shows attempt by dentist to "unlock" impacted molar by using brass wire wrapped tightly around contact. There is a generalized arch length deficiency in this case, and guided extraction procedures may be necessary.

7–60). A canine or premolar will erupt buccally, lingually or transposed, with no apparent cause (Figs. 7–70, 7–71). Careful radiographic examination permits the detection of this aberration, and preventive orthodontic procedures are possible. (Chap. 13.)

First and second permanent molars are occasionally impacted; third molars are frequently impacted by an abnormal path of eruption. This is not always due to lack of space and often poses a difficult problem of correction for the orthodontist. More often than not, however, such problems are finally solved by the oral surgeon. Early referral to the oral surgeon is strongly recommended because of the developmental timing factor in surgical uprighting. A differential diagnosis—removal versus uprighting—should be made early. (See Chap. 15.)

Another form of abnormal eruption is referred to as ectopic eruption. In its most common form, a permanent tooth erupting through the alveolar process causes resorption on a contiguous deciduous tooth or permanent tooth, rather than its predecessor (Figs. 7–72 to 7–73). Frequently the maxillary first permanent molar is the offending tooth, causing abnormal resorption of the maxillary second deciduous molar as it erupts beneath the distal convexity of this tooth. Ectopic eruption may generally be considered a manifestation of arch length deficiency; it is a good clue to future sacrifice of dental units, if a harmonious relationship between tooth material and basal bone is to be maintained. It may also indicate immediate study and possible institution of a planned program of serial or guided extraction. (See Chap. 15.)

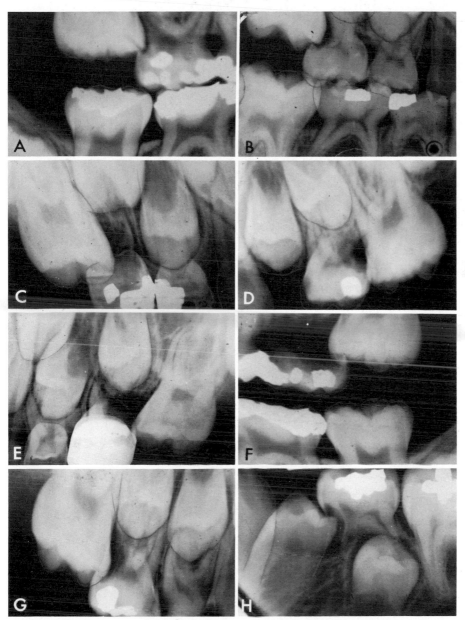

Figure 7-73 Various stages of ectopic eruption. These are all associated with arch length problems in the particular case. In D, the first permanent molar has finally passed the distal convexity of the second deciduous molar, but this is at least partly due to mesial drift of the deciduous tooth, which is now encroaching on the first premolar space. The second premolar is imminently impacted in E, F and G. In H, the first premolar will probably erupt into the arch, but the lower second premolar will be locked by the contiguous teeth. Complete orthodontic diagnostic records should be made to determine the advisability of "watchful waiting," or there should be selected removal of deciduous teeth early to allow autonomous adjustment (see Chap. 15). (Views A, F, G and H, courtesy J. R. Jarabak.)

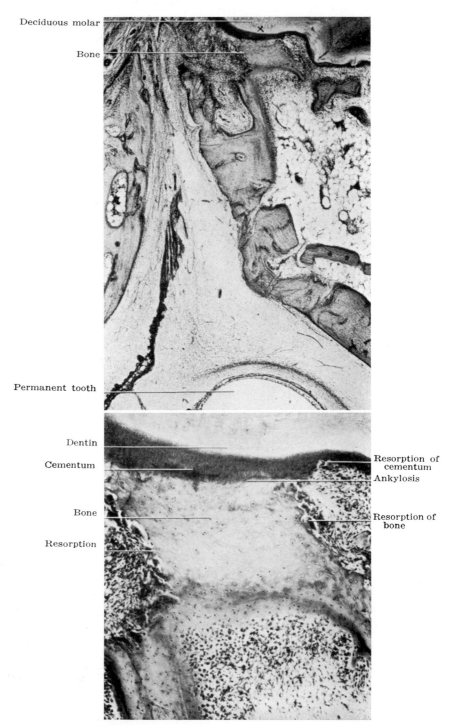

Figure 7–74   Histologic section of ankylosis of deciduous tooth. A, General view.
B, High magnification of area marked X. (From Sicher, H.: Orban's Oral Histology and
Embryology. 7th ed. C. V. Mosby Co., 1972.)

ANKYLOSIS

Ankylosis or partial ankylosis is encountered relatively frequently during the 6- to 12-year age period. It is a phenomenon overlooked by entirely too many dentists.[9] The results of lack of recognition and failure to institute preventive orthodontic procedures can be quite dramatic (Chap. 13). Much remains to be learned about this phenomenon in which a tooth is fixed in its surrounding bone (Fig. 7–74) while the contiguous teeth continue to erupt and shift with growth and development.

Ankylosis is probably due to an injury of some sort, as a result of which a part of the periodontal membrane is perforated and a bony "bridge" forms, joining the lamina dura and cementum. This "bridge" need not be very large to stop the normal eruptive force of a tooth.[5] It may occur on the buccal and lingual aspects, and thus be totally unrecognizable in a dental radiograph. Clinically, the observant dentist sees what appears to be a "submerging" of the offending tooth (Figs. 7–75, 7–76). In actuality, the other teeth are erupting and the ankylosed tooth is not. If left alone, ankylosed teeth can actually be covered over again by the ever-growing mucosa (Figs. 7–76, 7–77), and the contiguous teeth often migrate into the space, effectively locking the tooth in the process. Surgical removal then is possible only through the buccal plate. The effects of ankylosed deciduous teeth on the erupting permanent successors, as well as the alveolar

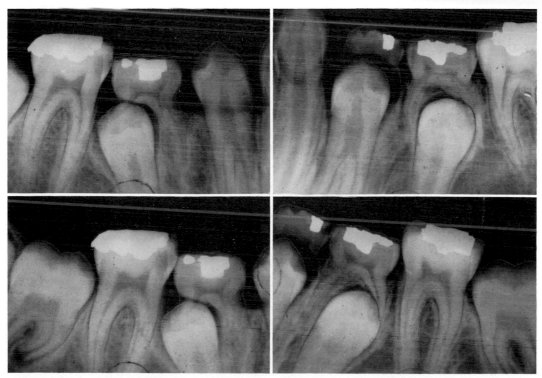

Figure 7–75 Patient with bilaterally ankylosed deciduous second molars. Lower right second premolar obviously deflected to distal. Mesial root on lower left second deciduous molar appears to be incorporated in the alveolar process. It is unlikely that either deciduous tooth will be lost naturally for some time. The dentist should be prepared to remove both left and right deciduous second molars, being careful not to break off the roots and being sure to uncover the crowns of the erupting successors.

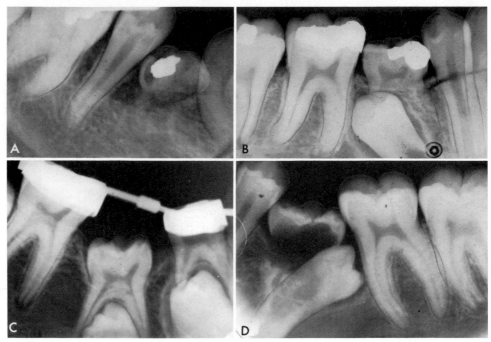

Figure 7–76   A, Ankylosed deciduous molar, no successor. B, Second premolar crown is in contact with the mesial root of the first permanent molar in a 16-year-old patient. Second deciduous molar is firm, with no signs of resorbing any further. C, Badly ankylosed second deciduous molar with second premolar beneath it, as dentist attempts to open space for the premolar, totally unaware of the ankylosis disclosed by a radiograph. D, Ankylosed molar has finally resorbed in this case after deflecting second premolar, but the first premolar and first molar teeth have tipped into the second deciduous molar area, locking the deciduous tooth in place. It is now necessary to remove the deciduous molar from the buccal, to uncover the crown of the second premolar and to open space orthodontically.

bone level, are obvious. Early recognition of such problems is of paramount importance. Criteria for removal or building up of or surgically subluxating ankylosed deciduous teeth along with problems of space maintenance are discussed in Chapter 13. Permanent teeth may also be ankylosed (Fig. 7–77). Accidents or trauma, certain endocrine conditions and congenital diseases like cleidocranial dysostosis predispose an indivdual to ankylosis (see Chap. 6). Often, however, ankylosis occurs with no apparent cause.

DENTAL CARIES

Dental caries may be considered among the many local causes of malocclusion. Thus, caries, which leads to the premature loss of a deciduous or permanent tooth, subsequent drifting of contiguous teeth, abnormal axial inclination, overeruption, bone loss and so on, is the proverbial straw that breaks the camel's back. It is basic that carious lesions should be repaired not only to prevent infection and loss of teeth but to maintain the integrity of the dental arches. More insidious and less dramatic than the actual loss of teeth is the loss of arch length due to a series of proximal carious lesions that are unrepaired (Figs. 7–78, 7–79). Immediate and correct anatomic restoration should be made of all teeth as a preventive orthodontic procedure.

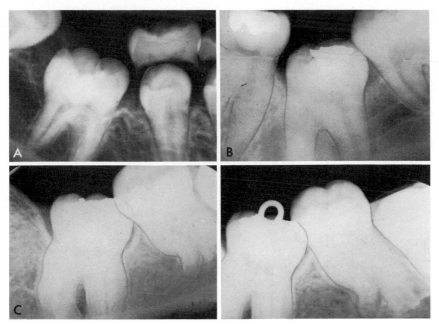

Figure 7–77   Ankylosis of lower right first molar (A) and lower left second molar (B). In C, lower left first molar is ankylosed; second premolar is absent. Hook has been placed in occlusal (right) to attempt to elevate molar into occlusion by intermaxillary elastics. (Views A and B, courtesy J. R. Jarabak; View C, courtesy S. P. Signorino.)

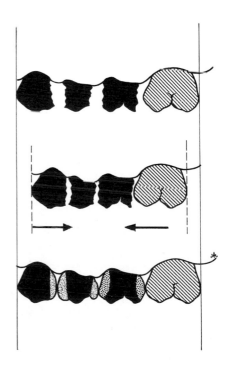

Figure 7–78   Effect of proximal caries on arch length. Great care must be exercised in maintaining the mesiodistal dimension through proper restoration of tooth contours and the contact relationship.

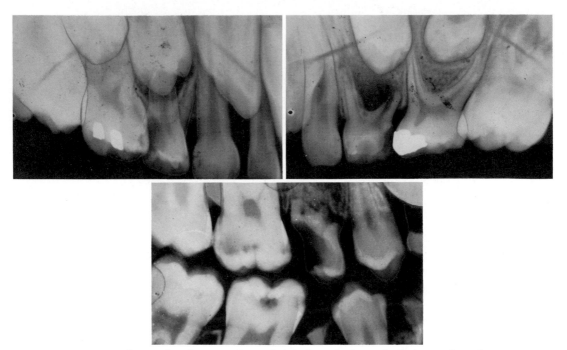

Figure 7–79   Radiographs showing loss of arch length through drifting of teeth contiguous to carious deciduous molars that have been reduced in mesiodistal dimension through caries.

IMPROPER DENTAL RESTORATIONS

In our zeal to restore carious teeth, we have been guilty too frequently of creating dental malocclusions. As noted in the discussion on eruption and growth and development, arch length is critical in the establishment of a normal occlusion. Even the prolonged retention of a mandibular second deciduous molar can cause a break in contacts and subsequent rotations. It is not unreasonable to assume that overextended proximal restorations can create the same effect — irregular mandibular incisors. Too many dental students have been taught a snap-ligature concept (super-tight mesial and distal contacts at all costs) without being told of the possible unfavorable sequelae. A proximal contact that requires the dentist to drive an inlay to place, forcing the contiguous tooth to give way, is just as harmful as one that is too loose and thus permits packing of food. Too tight a contact causes elongation of either the tooth being restored or approximating teeth, creates functional prematurities and severely strains the canine-lateral contact (Fig. 7–80). With more than one restoration in a segment placed with "snap-ligature" precision, the arch length is increased to the point that a break in the continuity of the arch is only a matter of time.

If gutta-percha or temporary stopping is used as a temporary filling material before placing the permanent restoration, the approximating teeth may be moved apart by the plunger-like action of the rubberoid mass, even before the permanent restoration is placed. The restoration only serves to perpetuate the arch length increase. No gutta-percha filling should be left in occlusion or the slightest bit "high." Teeth have actually been moved into a cross-bite relationship by a poorly placed temporary restoration. Mechanical separation also encourages increase of arch length as the dentist strives for a tight contact in an area that has been wedged and restored abnormally apart, much like a jackscrew

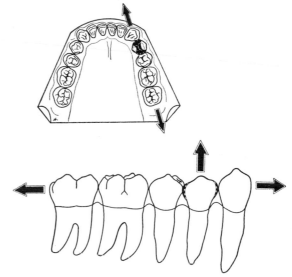

Figure 7–80 An increase in arch length through improper restoration of one or more carious proximal surfaces may result in the creation of broken contacts, rotations, crossbite conditions and functional prematurities.

OVER EXTENDED PROXIMAL RESTORATION
---- ORIGINAL MESIODISTAL DIMENSION
—— RESTORED MESIODISTAL DIMENSION

moves teeth in an orthodontic appliance. Silver-mercury alloy restorations have a tendency to "flow" under pressure. Large proximal restorations change gradually under the assaults of occlusal forces, and arch length is increased. The net result is a break in contact in the immediate area, the creation of functional prematurities or a contact break or rotation in the anterior segment or at the critical canine-lateral region. Remember, as we saw in Chapter 3, the opposing teeth are in contact only 2 to 6 per cent of the time, at most. And the time in habitual occlusion or centric occlusion is only a fraction of that. Thus, it is not wise to rely solely on the "locking" of the occlusion to maintain stability and to prevent drifting, prematurities and other unfavorable adaptations. A routine check with articulating paper to determine prematurities, glides, etc., plus a set of study models to serve as a "base line" for future changes, is part of the preventive orthodontic service. (See Chap. 13.)

The dentist must not forget that the individual teeth are preformed building blocks in a plastic medium. A change in size of the block will cause other blocks to adapt to the change. The adaptation is almost always unfavorable. The need for anatomic restorations is not limited to the mesiodistal dimension. Poor contacts, even with correct restoration of actual mesiodistal dimension, encourage tooth shift. With loose contacts and food packing, teeth also tend to move apart. Bone loss makes this easier. Lack of anatomic detail in restoration of cuspal areas of a tooth can permit elongation of opposing teeth or, at the very least, create functional prematurities and possible tooth guidance foci for mandibular shifts. This subject is discussed further in Chapter 13, Preventive Orthodontics.

REFERENCES

1. Muller, T. P., Hill, I. N., Petersen, A. C., and Blayney, J. R.: A survey of congenitally missing permanent teeth. J.A.D.A., 81:101–107, 1970.
2. Gupta, L. D., and Vacher, B. R.: Supernumerary teeth and malocclusion. J. Indiana Dent. Ass., 42:123–126, 1970.

3. Adler-Hradecky, C., and Adler, P.: Partial anodontia as an orthodontic problem. Oest. Z. Stomat., 66:294–297, 1969.

4. Dickson, G. C.: The natural history of malocclusion. Dent. Pract., 20:216–232, 1970.

5. Moorrees, C. F. A.: The Dentition of the Growing Child. Cambridge, Harvard University Press, 1959.

6. Weber, F. N.: Personal communication, January 23, 1972.

7. Taylor, J. E.: Clinical observations relating to the normal and abnormal frenum labii superioris. Am. J. Orth. & Oral Surg., 25:646–660, 1939.

8. Van der Veen, J. A., and Woldringh, S. J.: The central diastema. Nederl. T. Tandheelk., 77:60–64, 1970.

9. Biederman, W.: Etiology and treatment of tooth ankylosis. Am. J. Orthodont., 48:670–684, 1962.

10. Hemley, S.: A text on orthodontics, showing its relationship to every phase of dentistry. Washington, D.C., Coiner Publications, 1971.

11. Siersbaek-Nielsen, S.: Rate of eruption of central incisors at puberty: an implant study on eight boys. Tandlaegebladet, 75:1288–1295, 1971.

12. Garn, S. M., and Burdi, A. R.: Prenatal ordering and postnatal sequence in dental development. J. Dent. Res., 50:1407–1414, 1971.

DIAGNOSTIC PROCEDURES, AIDS AND THEIR INTERPRETATION

It is important to know the various types of malocclusions and to be able to classify them. Thorough knowledge of the possible etiologic factors is essential to the dental student in the development of a total concept of the field of orthodontics. However, it is only through a proper diagnostic routine that he can gain and *utilize* such information. Proper diagnostic procedures and an intelligent analytical interpretation of pertinent diagnostic aids are the basis of a comprehensive plan of orthodontic therapy. Modern technical advances and efficient armamentaria provide the dentist with excellent therapeutic tools that he can learn to use in a relatively short time. But it may take years of study and careful analysis of the information available from many sources before he can develop a "diagnostic sense."

The clinician already starts to interpret his findings as they are collected and may unconsciously make a tentative diagnosis or diagnoses. As more information is obtained and "weighed" in the light of previous evidence and conscious and unconscious opinions and as previous experience on similar cases is recalled, a firm diagnosis is finally established, and a treatment plan developed (Fig. 8–1). Yet, the development of the treatment plan may not be a direct consequence of a diagnosis, for, as Moorrees and Grøn[1] observe, "seemingly similar types of malocclusion often require different timing and different planning of treatment." The Ackerman-Proffit diagnostic classification (Chap. 5) is a step toward differentiating malocclusion characteristics and preventing "shotgun" therapeutic decisions, aimed at broad classes of malocclusions.[2] Many diagnostic facets must be analyzed, a different diagnosis must be made, and in the light of clinical experience, the indications and contraindications of "therapeutic modifiability" must be weighed. The question may be *whether* to treat, after all information is sorted and sifted, not *how* to treat. Even if therapy is indicated, the successful clinician knows that any treat-

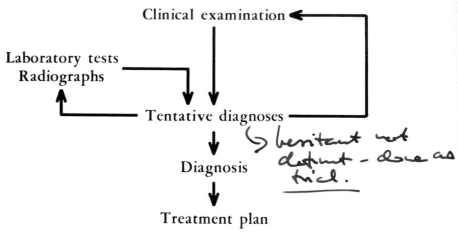

Figure 8–1   Diagnostic, prognostic and therapeutic interrelations. (From Moorrees, C. F. A., and Grøn, A. M.: Principles of orthodontic diagnosis. Angle Orthodont., 36:258–262, 1966.)

ment plan must be regarded as tentative and must be open to modification or even abandonment, depending on tissue response, patient cooperation, growth and development and other factors not amenable to accurate assessment at the time that therapy was instituted (Fig. 8–2).

It is incumbent upon the dentist to know where to turn for specific information; he must know how to wield a deft brush as he blends each contribution into the total diagnostic picture. It is no exaggeration to say that the success or failure of all subsequent efforts may well rest on his acrostic ability to complete the mosaic of diagnosis and case analysis.

It cannot be overemphasized that diagnosis is a *tentative* and continuing process. Therapeutic response to decisions made at the beginning of treatment constantly alters treatment plans for the most experienced and expert diagnostician. There is no pat formula, no magic combination of cephalometric creations or study cast measurements. For a fuller discussion of diagnostic procedures,

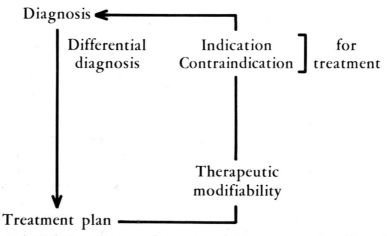

Figure 8–2   Relations between diagnosis and the treatment plan. (From Moorrees, C. F. A., and Grøn, A. M.: Principles of orthodontic diagnosis. Angle Orthodont., 36:258–262, 1966.)

reference is made to Chapter 1 of *Current Orthodontic Concepts and Techniques* by the author.[3]

ESSENTIAL DIAGNOSTIC CRITERIA.   Whether the dentist limits his practice to orthodontics or not, the following diagnostic criteria are essential:

1. Case history
2. Clinical examination
3. Plaster study casts
4. Radiographs — periapical, bite-wing and panoramic
5. Facial photographs

SUPPLEMENTAL DIAGNOSTIC CRITERIA.   Other diagnostic criteria that provide valuable information at one time or another but require equipment that the average dentist does not have are:

1. Special x-ray views
   a. Cephalometric headplates — skeletal (teeth in occlusion) and function patterns
      (1) Lateral projection with teeth in occlusion
      (2) Lateral projection, postural resting position
      (3) Frontal projection
      (4) Functional records
         (a) Incision — end-to-end "bite"
         (b) Phonation
         (c) Wide-open mouth
         (d) Views with radiopaque media
      (5) 45 degree lateral projections, right and left
   b. Occlusal intraoral films
   c. Selected lateral jaw views
2. Electromyographic examination — muscle activity
3. Wrist x-rays — bone age, maturation age
4. Basal metabolic rate and other endocrine tests

ESSENTIAL DIAGNOSTIC CRITERIA

CASE HISTORY

This should be a written record. Usually it is made up of a medical history and a dental history. A medical history may occasionally yield information of value to the orthodontist. It is a good idea to record the various childhood diseases, allergies, operations, congenital deformities or unusual diseases in the immediate family. A record of medications which have been taken, past and present, may be quite valuable, particularly if it includes corticosteroids and other endocrine extracts. If possible, a dental examination should be made of the parents and a record kept. Because of the significant role of heredity, valuable information can be gained from such an examination. Dental abnormalities in members of the family certainly should be recorded. Since the manner of feeding during infancy may be relevant it should be noted. Also, a history of abnormal oral habits such as finger sucking, nail or lip biting, tongue thrust, etc., should be included.

Many elaborate case history record forms are available commercially. These may be adapted to individual use. However, if a check list of the criteria just listed is made on a 4 × 6 inch or 5 × 8 inch card, and then made part of the patient's record file, it may prove more practical and may be used more conscientiously. Much of the case history data can and should be obtained by a good dental assistant even before the dentist has made his examination, saving valuable chair time. A call to the family pediatrician may be in order and may provide needed case history background. In addition, a favorable professional rapport is established.

CLINICAL EXAMINATION

A large part of the information needed to guide the patient's orthodontic management can be seen and recorded by the dentist at the first visit. It is then that the development of the "diagnostic sense" comes to the fore. The use of other definitive diagnostic criteria such as dental radiographs and panoramic films has not made examination of the patient himself any less important. In fact, the vitally important information that is gained from the examination helps to interpret and enhance the value of other diagnostic criteria.

It cannot be stressed too much that the dentist can render significant service without any special tools merely by using his fund of knowledge and excellent powers of observation. He can determine the growth and developmental pattern of the patient, the health of the teeth and investing tissues, facial type, esthetic balance, dental age, posture and function of the lips and mandible, tongue function, type of malocclusion, premature loss or prolonged retention of teeth. As we know from our study of the etiology of malocclusion, this may well be the bulk of information needed. Other diagnostic criteria may be substantiative or correlative.

For the initial examination the dentist needs a mouth mirror or tongue blade, a No. 17 explorer (or equivalent), a Boley gauge, a pair of dividers, thin articulating paper, a sensitive set of finger tips and a clear mental picture of just what should be normal for that particular patient (Fig. 8–3). The last

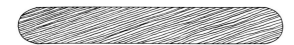

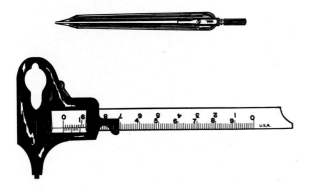

Figure 8–3 Essential armamentaria for initial clinical examination of the patient.

requisite is indeed the most important. It is not possible to recognize and describe the abnormal without a thorough understanding of individualized normality. Some system is necessary in recording the clinical observations. The following routine is suggested.

1. General health, body type and posture
2. Facial features
   a. Morphologic
      (1) Facial type (dolichocephalic, brachycephalic, mesocephalic)
      (2) Profile analysis (anteroposterior and vertical relationships)
         (a) Protruded or retruded mandible
         (b) Protruded or retruded maxilla
         (c) Relation of maxilla and mandible to cranial structures
      (3) Lip posture at rest (size, color, mentolabial sulcus, etc.)
      (4) Relative symmetry of facial structures
         (a) Size and shape of nose (This may mitigate against treatment results and the possibility of a rhinoplasty may be mentioned to the parent, diplomatically.)
         (b) Chin button size and contour (As with the nose, there are limits imposed on profile improvement of "chinless wonders." Surgical assistance — genioplasty — with alloplastic and cartilage or bone implants is highly successful, and may be indicated.)
   b. Physiologic
      (1) Muscle activity during:
         (a) Mastication
         (b) Deglutition
         (c) Respiration
         (d) Speech
      (2) Abnormal habits or mannerisms (mouth breathing, tics, etc.)
3. Examination of the mouth (initial or preliminary clinical exam)
   a. Classification of malocclusion with teeth in occlusion (Class I, Class II, Class III [Angle], etc.)
      (1) Anteroposterior relationship (overjet, procumbency of maxillary and mandibular incisors, etc.)
      (2) Vertical relationship (over-bite)
      (3) Lateral relationship (cross-bite)
   b. Open mouth examination of teeth
      (1) Number of teeth present and absent
      (2) Identity of teeth present
      (3) Record of any abnormality of size, shape and position
      (4) Restorative status (caries, fillings, etc.)
      (5) Tooth to bone ratio (adequacy of space for eruption of permanent teeth)
         (a) If mixed dentition, either measure deciduous teeth present with calipers and record space available for successors or merely make a general notation of space adequacy and defer to a careful mixed dentition analysis, using the study models and dental radiographs.
      (6) Oral hygiene
   c. Soft tissue appraisal
      (1) Gingivae (color and texture, hypertrophy, etc.)
      (2) Labial frenum, upper and lower
      (3) Tongue size, shape, posture
      (4) Palate, tonsils and adenoids
      (5) Vestibular mucosa
      (6) Lip morphology, color, texture and character of tissue
         (a) Hypotonic, flaccid, hypertonic, functionless, redundant, short, long, etc.

d. Functional analysis
   (1) Postural resting position and interocclusal clearance
   (2) Path of closure from resting position to occlusion
   (3) Prematurities, point of initial contact, etc.
   (4) Displacement or tooth guidance, if any
   (5) Range of mandibular motion—protrusive, retrusive, lateral excursions
   (6) Clicking, crepitus or "popping" of the temporomandibular joint during the function range
   (7) Excessive mobility of individual teeth when palpated by finger tips during closure
   (8) Position of upper and lower lips with respect to maxillary and mandibular incisors during mastication, deglutition, respiration and speech
   (9) Tongue position and pressures exerted during functional movements

To illustrate the use of this diagnostic "check list," a sample case report is given at the end of this chapter.

At first glance the above outline for the clinical examination seems complicated. Experience will show that this is not true. All the above information can be obtained by a competent dentist in five minutes or less, but it is five minutes well spent. Utmost care and keenness of the "diagnostic sense" at this time will save hours later and perhaps enable the dentist to prevent the development of a severe orthodontic problem. It is at this point that the preventive and interceptive phases of orthodontics are initiated. Use of a small chair-side tape recorder for dictating clinical observations from the check list is an excellent means of obtaining information. This may be typed later and incorporated into the patient's record.

As serious as the information gained may or may not be, levity with the child as he is being seated has a beneficial disarming effect. Apprehension can be reduced or dispelled if it is made clear that this first appointment is a hunting or exploring expedition. The mother's presence is usually desirable at this time. Hand holding or other overprotective activities should be avoided, however. Gentle but precise palpation with the finger tips and checking thickness of lips, character of tissue, nodes, temporomandibular joint activity, mucobuccal vestibule and interdental papillae provide considerable information without creating apprehension on the part of the patient.

Facial form and balance are important. Frequently it is the facial appearance that has made the patient come in for an examination. Record all asymmetries, evidences of imbalance, nasal and chin contours, etc. Lip contours, symmetry or lack of same are of concern to the patient and the parents. It is here that the greatest motivation for treatment may lie. Some treatment is conducted for facial disfigurement. One of the best ways to learn an orthodontic examination routine is to predict the malocclusion from the facial examination, and then to thoroughly check it afterward. A little practice makes a dentist quite adept. If the dentist adheres to his diagnostic outline, much as the pilot does to his preflight check list, uniformly good records should result. A brief summary should then be given to the parent in terms that both she and the child will understand.

In most instances the clinical examination only "whets the appetite" for further diagnostic information. This means that a full set of dental radiographs or bite-wings and a panoramic view are essential to interpret "the part of the iceberg that is under water."

It is a good routine during the initial clinical examination to tell the parent that guidance of the dental development of the child requires that the dentist have all relevant information available at his finger tips to permit him to project future guidance with a minimum of actual treatment. This is more than good relations propaganda. Truly significant service without appliances may be rendered to many children, with a minimum of chair time. To do this the clinical examination must be correlated with information taken from dental radiographs, plaster casts, facial photographs and possibly other specific information gleaned from cephalometric x-ray pictures. Since the general dentist seldom has equipment in his office for cephalometric or panoramic radiographs, this record can be made by an x-ray laboratory if needed.

Adequate guidance during the delicate and complex formative years from 6 to 12 requires a thorough clinical examination, radiographs and plaster casts at periodic intervals. If it is possible, impressions should be taken for the study casts at the first visit, along with full mouth radiographs and facial and intraoral photographs. An appointment can then be made with the parent to go over the recorded and transcribed clinical examination observations and further details obtained from the study casts and dental, panoramic or cephalometric radiographs.

PLASTER STUDY CASTS

Plaster casts provide a "reasonable facsimile" of the occlusion of the patient (Fig. 8–4). Despite a comprehensive clinical examination, it is still better to have a set of plaster casts to correlate additional information from intraoral and cephalometric radiographs. The dentist should not depend on his memory and notes as he recalls the exact status of the occlusion of the child. Even more important, study casts taken at a particular time in the development of the child provide a permanent record of the time-linked situation. Together with subsequent similar records, they constitute a continuing record of the accomplishment or lack of accomplishment of a normal developmental pattern. If such records have been made previously by another dentist they should be obtained, if possible. Although the classification and individual malpositions, arch relationship, overbite, overjet and so forth have been recorded in the

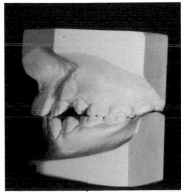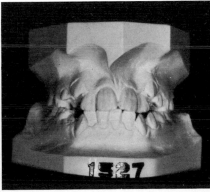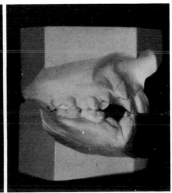

Figure 8–4 A symmetrically and smoothly finished set of study casts. The art portions of the casts are so trimmed that when resting on their back surfaces, upper and lower casts may be moved together into full occlusal contact. To maintain uniformity, top and bottom surfaces are perpendicular to the back surface. The occlusal plane is maintained roughly parallel with the top and the bottom surfaces.

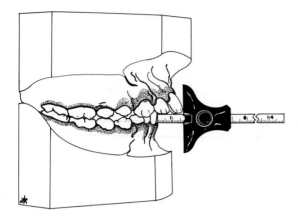

Figure 8–5 Measurement of overbite, overjet, arch width, available space for erupting teeth, etc., is done more easily and accurately on the study models than directly in the mouth.

clinical examination, these can be corroborated by careful analysis of the study casts. Measurement of arch length or lack of arch length, tooth size discrepancies, available space, total arch length, etc., is usually more precise when taken from the study casts than from the patient's mouth directly (Fig. 8–5).

THE IMPRESSION TECHNIQUE

Care must be exercised to obtain as nearly perfect a reproduction of teeth and investing tissues as possible. Alginate impression materials are ideally suited for this purpose. It is recommended that a quick-setting type be used. The time which elapses from mixing to completion of the set should not exceed 90 seconds, or longer than 45 to 60 seconds in the mouth. Accelerating additives do not reduce the accuracy of the alginate, but they do make patient management much easier and the whole procedure more pleasant for the patient. Trays first should be fitted carefully. Strips of soft utility wax or mortite are then adapted to the tray periphery to hold in the alginate impression material and to assist in reproducing the details of the vestibular fornix (mucobuccal fold) (Figs. 8–6, 8–7). The wax has the added advantage of reducing the pressure of the impression tray metal rim on the displaced tissue during the impression-taking procedure. The child's fears and tensions during the tray-fitting procedure can be greatly alleviated in most instances if this is approached as a game. By likening each object to something the child already knows, the dentist will find less apprehension. Thus, the tray becomes a spoon or cup, the utility wax which rims the tray becomes a red licorice and the alginate becomes ice cream or even tooth paste or chewing gum.

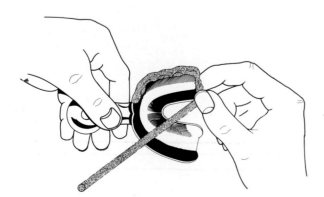

Figure 8–6 Adapting the wax beading to impression tray periphery.

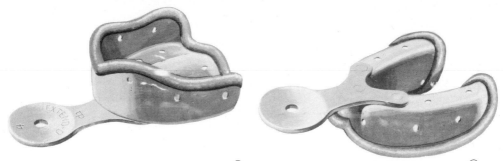

Figure 8–7 Upper and lower Extend-O® impression trays rimmed with Mortite® (a single strip of wax can also be used) for patient comfort and to aid in retention of impression material. Special extra-deep trays ensure adequate reproduction of alveolar processes—an important factor for beautiful, accurate orthodontic casts. (Courtesy of T. P. Laboratories.)

A pre-impression "mouthwash cocktail" of a colored, pleasant-tasting astringent commercial mouthwash serves a dual purpose. It is a pleasant experience for the apprehensive child, often reducing his fears, and it leaves the mouth with a clean, pleasant feeling. Equally important, the wash removes debris and reduces the surface tension of the teeth and tissues, cutting down on bubble formation during the impression-taking procedure.

If the tray is fitted properly, a minimum of material is needed. The lower impression is usually easy to take and a good means of getting the child's confidence. As the tray is seated, one should be careful to pull the lip away from the periphery of the tray and allow the alginate to squeeze down into the mucobuccal fold in order to record the muscle attachments. As part of the game, daubing a bit of the alginate on the tip of the nose distracts the child and serves to indicate when the chemical reaction is completed. Eye-to-eye contact is most desirable during the impression-taking procedure. On the upper impression, because of the greater chance of gagging, it is important that the posterior periphery of the tray be adequately dammed with a roll of utility wax. It is often a good idea to wipe the teeth first with a cotton roll. This reduces the bubbles that sometimes appear around the gingival margin. Wiping the impression material on the tray with a wet finger before insertion will also produce a smoother surface. The greatest concentration of impression material should be in the anterior portion of the tray, at least level with the wax-beaded periphery. A blob of impression material may be placed in the palatal vault of the patient just behind the incisors before inserting the tray, if the operator desires, to ensure the elimination of trapped air and to ensure a faithful reproduction of palatal tissues.

The upper tray should be inserted so that the anterior periphery of the tray first fits under the upper lip. The tray is then pushed upward to force the alginate out into the mucobuccal fold to record muscle attachments. At the same time, the tray is gradually rotated upward and backward until the operator can see the alginate starting to squeeze past the utility wax dam (Fig. 8–8). The impression should be stabilized at this point. The upper lip is pulled up and away from the tray periphery to observe whether the impression material has reproduced the muscle attachments. If not, the pressure on the anterior part of the tray is increased to squeeze out more material, and then the operator pulls down on the upper lip to "muscle trim" the periphery. A little experience will make the impression taking procedure practically effortless and uneventful. The rotation of the tray upward and backward in a smooth continuous motion during the

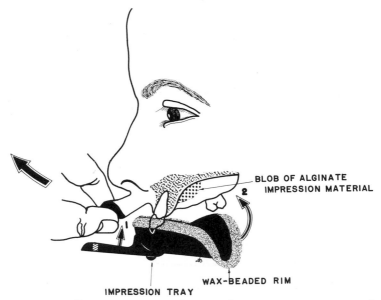

Figure 8–8   Maxillary impression-taking technique. Insert tray gently in incisor region (1) after pulling away upper lip with thumb and forefinger; blob of impression material has already been placed in palate to prevent trapping air. Then rotate tray upward and backward (2) until impression material starts to extrude past palatal wax post dam. Exert a slight but constant pressure to keep tray seated and pull cheeks and lips out and down to muscle trim impression periphery.

impression taking prevents the trapping of air or saliva in the palate. Careful observation prevents material from squeezing back into the throat and inciting the gag reflex. (Throughout the whole procedure it is important that the operator maintain an easy, relaxed and confident manner mixed with humor or firmness when needed. The child quickly recognizes a nervous dentist, which only increases apprehension.) A good maxillary and mandibular impression will show a "peripheral roll" and will record muscle attachments. Both the retromolar pad in the lower jaw and the tuberosity in the upper should be included, if possible (Fig. 8–9).

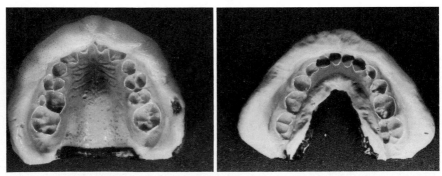

Figure 8–9   Maxillary and mandibular impressions with adequate peripheral roll. Wax may show through impression material as it is molded by impression-taking procedure. If desired, a sheet of baseplate wax may be attached on the lower impression between the flanges before pouring in plaster. This will eliminate the need for heavy cutting away of plaster to provide a flat "floor" for the tongue area of the lower model. (Figs. 8–22, 8–23)

WAX BITE RECORDS

A wax bite record is valuable, permitting the dentist to relate the upper and lower casts correctly in full occlusion. Two layers of a soft baseplate wax, roughly shaped to arch form and warmed in water, may be used to make a satisfactory record (Fig. 8–10). Care must be exercised in obtaining the "bite" because, like prosthetic patients, children are prone to give a protrusive mandibular relationship or not close completely. For this reason many orthodontists do not take "bites" routinely, but rely on careful observation of the patient's occlusion and the "fit" of the casts when articulated. A little experience will make the observational approach uniformly successful. A wax bite should always be taken in patients where there are open bite problems, where many teeth are missing or where there is any question whether the casts will articulate properly when placed together. The wax bite may also assist in holding the maxillary and mandibular casts in proper relationship when the back surfaces of the casts are trimmed flush with each other. The wax reduces the chance of fracturing the anterior teeth on the casts, also.

THE STUDY CAST

One of the things that impress a parent most in a dental office is a cabinet of gleaming white study casts, carefully trimmed, precisely angled and well polished. But parental reaction is not the reason why orthodontists try to make such records. It *is* true that uniformly trimmed casts look good, appear neat and impel a favorable psychological reaction in parents and patients (as do precise workmanship and a neat, clean dentist, competent and careful about all dental procedures). More important, these casts provide a precise record of a particular condition at a particular time. The measurements so often necessary for arch length problems can be taken accurately from the casts. They serve as valuable adjuncts in discussion of the problem with the patient, parent or other patients with similar problems. Unlike "rough" casts full of bubbles from "snap" impressions, they require no apology from the dentist. They are trimmed so that the correct articulation is apparent, and they are easily reproduced. Cast

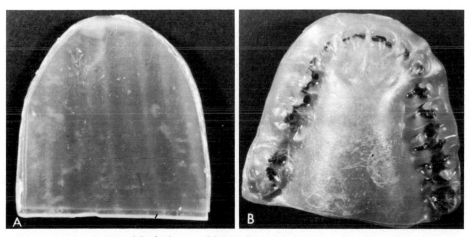

Figure 8–10 A, Doubled sheet of baseplate wax trimmed and ready to warm and insert for wax bite. B, Maxillary side of completed wax bite shows how thin wax should be in occlusal area if correct occlusal relationship has been obtained.

pouring and trimming can be entrusted to a good dental assistant or technician. The assistant does this in most orthodontic offices.

POURING THE IMPRESSION. If the following admonitions are observed, uniformly good records can be obtained.

A good grade of white model plaster is usually satisfactory to "pour up" the impressions. Many orthodontists use white stone for the anatomic portion of the cast and model plaster for the art portion. This reduces the likelihood of breakage of the important tooth portion and yet allows easy trimming of the base. But this method leaves a definite line between the two materials which is considered objectionable by some men. Another way is to mix white dental stone and model plaster in equal parts and to use this mixture to pour up both anatomic and art portions at the same time. At present this is the most popular method. Addition of stone lengthens the setting time, so the operator is not rushed.

The impression is rinsed and excess water shaken out. This removes mucin and debris that might reduce the quality of the surface reproduction. A diluted solution of one of the popular detergents makes an excellent rinse and has the added advantage of reducing surface tension on the impression surface, ensuring a freer flow of the plaster. Commercial "de-bubble-izers" are also available for this purpose.

By the time that a dental student reaches his senior year or is in practice, it might be taken for granted that he knows how to mix plaster. Unfortunately, this is not true in many cases. The urge to follow the "flour and water" technique is great. But guessing at the amount of plaster needed, pouring in the approximate amount of water required for a mix of the desired consistency and then whirling away with the spatula with great gusto is not calculated to produce a proper result. About all one can be sure of is that a chemical set will take place and that a good job of incorporating as *much* air as possible has been done. Air means bubbles, and bubbles mean poor study casts. It is strongly urged that a mechanical spatulator or vacuum mixer be used. If one is not available, the plaster, or plaster and stone, may be mixed according to predetermined proportions on a mechanical vibrator as the spatulating is done, to bring the bubbles to the surface. The rewards in a stronger, superior cast and reduced trimming and polishing time will be obvious.

In the actual pouring up, a mechanical vibrator is essential. This not only eliminates bubbles from the important tooth depressions in the impression but permits the use of a heavier "mix." A heavier "mix" is much easier to handle in pouring up the anatomic and art portions and produces a stronger cast. Most dentists introduce the plaster at one end of the impression and carefully and slowly vibrate it around to the opposite side, adding small amounts of material at the initial point of insertion. If the impression has been rinsed in a detergent

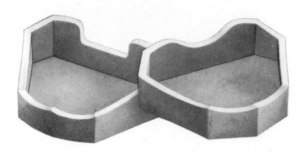

Figure 8–11 Rubber study model bases provide neat and uniform art portions for study models with a minimum of effort. (Courtesy Columbia Dentoform Corp.)

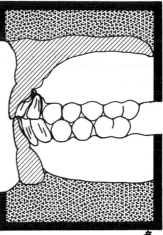

Figure 8–12 Cross section of plaster casts in rubber mold base formers. Occlusal plane should be parallel with top and bottom cast surfaces. The back surfaces of the casts should be related in exactly the same plane, perpendicular to top and bottom cast surfaces.

solution and the excess rinse eliminated, if the actual mixing of the plaster has been done to keep bubble incorporation to a minimum and if the mix is mechanically vibrated into the impression, bubbles just will not occur. The technique is not difficult and can be learned readily by a dental assistant.

FORMING THE BASE   The art portion, or base, is then poured. Most orthodontists have learned a technique of "pouring" cast bases that does not require a boxing medium, or form. It is easier for the neophyte or technician, however, to use rubber base molds that are readily available (Fig. 8–11). They serve to confine the plaster and are fabricated to shape the base in artistically pleasing contours. They allow the operator to orient the tray and anatomic portion in the center of the mold, with the occlusal plane parallel with the cast base and table top, and are easy to clean and re-use (Fig. 8–12).

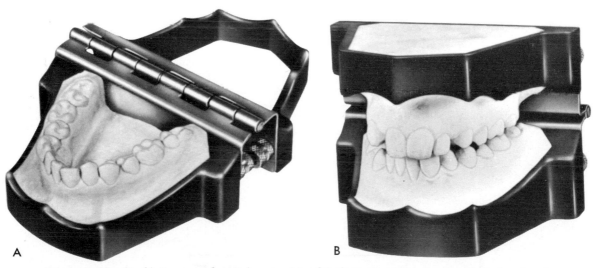

A   B

Figure 8–13 (Left) Broussard cast former. Mandibular cast oriented properly in bottom former with occlusal plane parallel with bottom surface. (Right) Maxillary and mandibular casts have now been poured. Cast former may now be removed or allowed to remain and serve as a hinge type articulator. (Courtesy Rocky Mountain Dental Products Co.)

The Broussard cast former may be used to establish symmetrical cast shape. It may be removed and re-used or left on and allowed to serve as a hinge type articulator (Fig. 8–13). Where just the anterior maxillary and mandibular tooth relationship is desired, this may be obtained by one impression with the teeth in occlusion and the use of a rubber base former (Fig. 8–14). This type of study cast is particularly useful where there is an anteroposterior discrepancy or open bite. A minimum of chair and laboratory time is needed to obtain routinely excellent plaster reproductions.

With all the cast base formers, the most frequent mistake is to use too thin a plaster mix and to invert the impression portion that has already been poured, onto the base portion before the plaster starts to set. The impression starts to "sink." The operator helplessly lifts it, traps air or resigns himself to heavy trimming after the set of the plaster has been completed. If a heavy mix is used and if the operator waits until he has definitely detected a marked thickening of the consistency due to the setting, he can then invert the impression with no danger

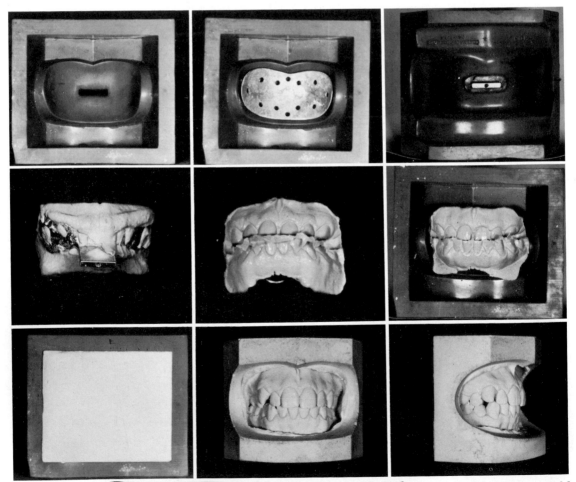

Figure 8–14 Columbia anterior segment single unit study cast. Top row shows rubber mold inside, empty tray inserted and outside of mold with tray handle extending through slot. Middle row shows outside of impression, inside of alginate impression and impression inserted in rubber mold, ready to pour in plaster. In bottom row, plaster has been poured in mold and is setting; front and side cast views show cast after separating from mold.

of the material running out and can carefully position the tray in the center of the mold, with the base of the tray parallel with the base of the mold. If his timing is correct—a little experience will soon determine this—some pressure will actually be needed to "seat" the plaster-filled impression properly on the plaster-filled mold. The periphery of the tray can then be wiped with a wet finger to smooth the plaster and reduce the amount of trimming needed. After half an hour the impression and rubber base are carefully peeled away. If the impression is separated within two hours after pouring up, the chance of breaking teeth is reduced.

CAST FINISHING

BUBBLE REMOVAL. Bubbles that appear at the gingival margin can be removed nicely with a small universal scaler. Bubbles reproduced from the impression in the mucobuccal fold area can be removed with a Kingsley type scraper. After the bubbles have been removed the anatomic portion can be made symmetrical by carving an even periphery where it joins the art portion of the base. Final finishing can be done with fine waterproof sandpaper where the knife or scraper has been used and with an Arkansas stone and water on the base, or art portion.

INDIVIDUALIZATIONS OF CASTS. Although preformed base casts appear uniform and neat, most orthodontists "individualize" each set of casts because of the additional information that can be gained and the more accurate orientation with the occlusal plane parallel with the cast base. Even the most careful positioning of the inverted tray during the pouring up procedure permits only an approximation of the occlusal plane relationship. With a few additional refinements, both top and bottom cast bases can be made to parallel the occlusal plane, and the casts can be trimmed so that the midline is perpendicular to the back surface. By so doing, they can be articulated correctly merely by placing them together on the back surfaces. These modifications require a cast trimmer or a set of plaster files. If a cast trimmer is not available, a jig-saw can be used for the rough shaping.

STEPS IN BASE FABRICATION. With a study cast trimmer a minimum amount of time is needed, and accurate angles can be made readily by a relatively inexperienced assistant. The assistant should be instructed to take the following steps:

1. Start with a maxillary cast and remove enough plaster from the base top so that the occlusal plane of the cast and the base are parallel. A good proportion for the thickness of the cast is tooth portion, one third; soft tissue, one third; and art portion, one third. (See Fig. 8–15.)

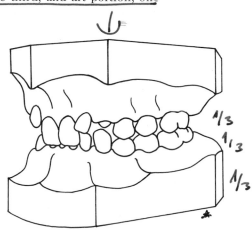

Figure 8–15 The approximate proportions of a well-trimmed set of study casts. Tooth portion should be one third, soft tissue portion one third, and art portion one third.

2. With a fine line pencil, carefully draw a line down the median raphe of the maxillary cast. The posterior surface should then be finished down with a cast trimmer or with a plaster file so that it is exactly perpendicular to the median raphe and to the base top. This step will permit easy visualization of arch asymmetries. Care must be exercised not to trim the posterior surface too closely, cutting off the tuberosity or portions of the last tooth.

3. Placing the maxillary cast on the base, the sides should be trimmed so that they are parallel with the buccal segments and perpendicular to the base top. They should form approximately the same angle with the posterior surface of the cast. Be careful not to duplicate a mistake made by many beginners—cutting the base too close to the anatomic portion and destroying the impression of muscle attachments.

4. Placing the maxillary cast on the case, carefully trim the front portion so that the two flat surfaces meet as an expanded "V" at the midline of the cast. (See Fig. 8–16.)

5. The mandibular cast is then carefully articulated with the trimmed maxillary cast and the casts are inverted so that the mandibular cast is on top with the teeth in occlusion. If a wax bite has been taken, this will orient the casts properly and serve to protect the anterior teeth from breakage during the trimming procedure. Placing the articulated casts on the maxillary base, the posterior surface of the mandibular cast is gently brought into contact with the grinding wheel of the cast trimmer. It is trimmed down so that it is exactly parallel with the posterior surface of the maxillary cast, with both posterior surfaces just contacting the grinding wheel. This can be checked by setting both the upper and lower casts together on the back surfaces. If they remain nicely in occlusion, this step has been performed correctly. It is important here that tuberosity and retromolar detail be allowed to remain.

6. Placing the mandibular cast on its posterior surface, the mandibular base is then trimmed so that it is perpendicular to the posterior surface and the thickness of the art portion is approximately one third; the anatomic portion, one third; and the tooth portion, one third. This may be checked by articulating the maxillary and mandibular casts in a correct occlusal relationship to make sure that the bases and occlusal plane parallel each other and the table top.

7. Placing the mandibular cast on its base, the sides are finished down so that they parallel the buccal segments. The surfaces should be perpendicular to the mandibular base. As with the maxillary cast, the two sides should form approximately the same acute angle with the posterior surface. Be careful not to remove too much of the tissue "roll."

8. The most commonly used design for the trimming of the front of the cast is an ellipse or curved surface from canine to canine (Fig. 8–16). This is done roughly with the cast trimmer so that the curve should approximate the curvature of the dental arch in this area.

9. The maxillary and mandibular casts are occluded, and the angles formed by the posterior surfaces and right and left sides are trimmed off. Two more surfaces, one half to three quarters of an inch wide, are created, forming approximately equal obtuse angles with the posterior surface and the respective sides of the casts. (See Fig. 8–16.)

10. The lingual portion of the mandibular cast, which is normally occupied by the tongue, is then trimmed with an office knife so that the floor parallels the mandibular base, and the sides are a continuation of the lingual tissue contour. The art portion is smoothed with water proof sandpaper together with an Arkansas stone and water, to remove any marks left by the plaster cast trimmer. Fine sandpaper can then be used on the remaining art portion surfaces.

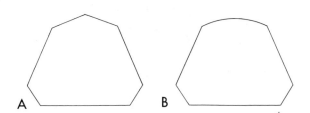

A   B

Figure 8–16 Maxillary (A) and mandibular (B) base shapes for art portion of study casts.

After the cast has thoroughly dried, application of ordinary talc and polishing with a chamois will leave a pleasing semigloss finish. Some operators soak the dried and polished casts in a soap solution and finish the polishing with a chamois. Commercial plaster cast gloss soap preparations have less tendency to turn yellow with age, but ordinary soap flakes in solution will work.

CAST TRIMMING TO INDICATE OCCLUSAL PLANE RELATIONSHIPS. While mounting the occlusal plane parallel with the table top is the most popular method, the gnathostatic technique reproduces the inclination of the occlusal plane with reference to the eye-ear (Frankfort) plane (Fig. 4–9). Trimmed in this fashion, the casts show the approximate inclination of the occlusal plane in the face of the patient. This information is valuable, but can be gained more accurately with the use of a cephalometric headplate. It is also important to relate the inclination of the occlusal plane to the mandibular plane, and this cannot be done very well with plaster casts (Fig. 8–40).

INFORMATION OBTAINABLE FROM STUDY CASTS

After the clinical examination, there is no single more important diagnostic and prognostic criterion than the plaster casts that have been properly taken and prepared of the patient's teeth and investing tissues. Most of the information obtained by a careful study of the plaster casts serves to delineate more sharply and to corroborate the observations made during the oral examination.[4–12]

Problems of premature loss, prolonged retention, inadequate space, rotations, individual tooth malpositions, frenum diastemas, muscle attachments, and morphology of interdental papillae are immediately apparent. You, as the dentist, are in a position to directly appraise anomalies of size, shape and position. The questions of arch shape and symmetry, tooth symmetry, tooth size and shape discrepancies with the same jaw and from one jaw to the other may be answered if only the time is taken to look, to measure and to appraise. The thickness of the alveolar bone over the teeth, the depth of the inward curvature of the basal bone as it drops away from the gingival margin, the apical base relationship of the teeth within each jaw and the apical base relationships of the upper and lower dental arches to each other, both anteroposteriorly and from left to right, are important facets of diagnostic information that must be gleaned from some source if a complete diagnosis and treatment plan are to be made. Those sensitive finger tips we discussed earlier, as they wander over the teeth, the gingival tissue, the palatal vault, along the superior and inferior vestibules and over the buccal mucosa, can gather much of this information in the initial clinical examination, but the objectivity of a plaster cast analysis is greater, and permits mensuration of what was formerly only a clinical impression. Problems of drifting, tipping, overeruption, undereruption, abnormal curve of Spee and prematurities may be carefully noted and correlated with the functional analysis and with radiographic evidence. Even the palatal breadth, depth and configuration are important to note, as in Class II, Division 1 cases, for example.

The importance of making a detailed study of the plaster casts cannot be overemphasized.[12] This is one of the reasons why we have devoted so much space in the first part of this chapter to the proper methods of impression taking and cast pouring, trimming and polishing. No matter how astute you are, no matter how carefully you look into your dental mirror, no matter how you bend your head to get a better view of the patient's mouth as he sits in the dental chair with his jaws spread apart, you cannot achieve the degree of accuracy and attain the completeness that an analysis of study casts will permit—no, will actually demand. An additional "plus" is that you have a time-linked record, a longitudinal, three-dimensional record that establishes the status of the teeth and investing tissues at that particular time. As you render treatment and return to these records again and again, you will realize the value of such records for *every* patient, not only for those on which you are performing minor orthodontic services. In Chapter 9 are study casts of dental "cripples" (Figs. 9–6, 9–11). These situations did not develop overnight. Armed with a set of adequate diagnostic records, the dentist is well prepared to follow the developing pattern of use, disuse, tooth loss, drifting and shifting and he has the opportunity to show this to the patient in complete detail. He may intercept these changing and deteriorating disturbances that often occur so slowly and insidiously that they are *faits accomplis* before they have been observed and recorded on the patient's chart during the once or twice a year routine visits.

A modified Schwarz analysis is an effective method of organizing the cast information outlined (Table 8–1). Figure 8–17 shows a Class II, Division 1 mal-

TABLE 8–1   STUDY MODEL AND PLASTER CAST ANALYSIS

1. Classification of malocclusion

2. Overjet

3. Overbite

4. Upper to lower arch midline

5. Palatal contour
   (a) Sagittal
   (b) Transverse

6. Teeth clinically present   R ——————————————————— L

7. Tooth measurements   R ——————————————————— L

	Upper jaw	Lower jaw
8. Arch form and symmetry (a) Mesial displacement of buccal teeth		
9. Incisor midline to jaw midline		
10. Vertical tooth malpositions		
11. Horizontal tooth malpositions (including rotations)		
12. Abnormal tooth morphology		
13. Arch length determination (a) Canine to canine distance (b) First permanent molar to first permanent molar distance (c) Bolton, Rees, Howes, or Moyers Mixed Dentition Analysis (see Table 8–2) (d) Liability (incisors) (e) Leeway		
14. Axial inclination of teeth (a) Incisors (b) Canines (c) Buccal segments (buccolingual and mesiodistal)		
15. Facets of wear		
16. Muscle attachments (frenum, etc.)		
17. Diagnostic set-up needed? (a) If so, what is conclusion?		
18. Extraction necessary? (a) Which teeth?		

(From Graber, T. M. (ed.): Current Orthodontic Concepts and Techniques. vol. 1, p. 36, W. B. Saunders Co., 1969.)

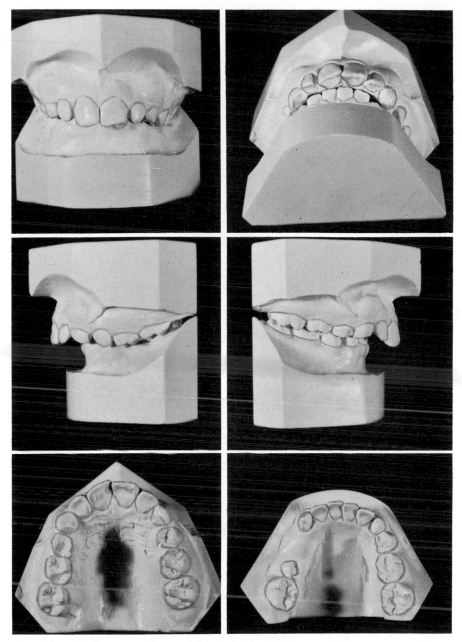

Figure 8–17   Plaster study models, patient S.C. (From Graber, T. M. (ed.): Current Orthodontic Concepts and Techniques. W. B. Saunders Co., 1969.)

occlusion study cast series. Table 8–2 shows how the cast analysis chart is completed with meaningful information gleaned from the casts, directly. This is coordinated with other criteria. Reference is made again to Chapter 1 of *Current Orthodontic Concepts and Techniques*, for a more detailed cast analysis discussion.[3] Refer to the tables in Chapter 2 on mesiodistal crown diameters of teeth (Moorrees) for differences between deciduous and permanent teeth. Remember, for the incisors, 11.6 mm. may be needed in the maxilla for boys, while for the posterior teeth, as much as 8.4 mm. may become available as leeway space. Conversely, very little space may be available, depending on the

TABLE 8–2   STUDY MODEL AND PLASTER CAST ANALYSIS CASE S. C.

1. Classification of malocclusion—*Class II, Division 1*

2. Overjet—*excessive*

3. Overbite—*deep*

4. Upper to lower arch midline—*Lower midline ½ tooth off to right*

5. Palatal contour
   (a) Sagittal—*normal*
   (b) Transverse—*normal*

6. Teeth clinically present

R $\dfrac{6 \quad V \quad 4 \quad III \quad 2 \quad 1}{6 \quad V \quad 4 \quad 3 \quad 2 \quad 1}$ $\Big|$ $\dfrac{1 \quad 2 \quad III \quad IV \quad V \quad 6}{1 \quad 2 \quad 3 \qquad \quad 5 \quad 6}$ L

7. Tooth measurements

R $\dfrac{12 \mid 10 \mid 9 \mid 8 \mid 7.5 \mid 10}{12 \mid 11 \mid 8.5 \mid 8.5 \mid 6.0 \mid 5.5}$ $\dfrac{10 \mid 7.5 \mid 8 \mid 8 \mid 10 \mid 12}{5.5 \mid 6 \mid 8.5 \mid \quad \mid 8 \mid 12.5}$ L

	Upper jaw	Lower jaw
8. Arch form and symmetry		
(a) Mesial displacement of buccal teeth—	*yes 6|6*	*yes, both buccal segments*
9. Incisor midline to jaw midline—	*to right, 2 mm*	*to right, 3 mm*
10. Vertical tooth malpositions—	*reverse curve of Spee*	*excessive eruption $\overline{2\ 1 \mid 1\ 2}$*
11. Horizontal tooth malpositions (Including rotations)	———	*$\overline{3\|3}$, primarily*
12. Abnormal tooth morphology	———	———
13. Arch length determination		
(a) Canine to canine distance	*35 mm*	*26 mm*
(b) First permanent molar to first permanent molar distance	*91 mm*	*71 mm*
(c) Bolton, Rees, Howes or Moyers Mixed Dentition analysis (see separate sheet)		
(d) Liability (incisors)	*None*	*None*
(e) Leeway	*2.5 mm*	*3 mm (leeway)*
14. Axial inclination of teeth		
(a) Incisors	*Normal*	*Normal*
(b) Canines	*Normal*	*Normal*
(c) Buccal segments (buccolingual and mesiodistal)	*Normal*	*Slight lingual inclination*
15. Facets of wear	*III|III*	
16. Muscle attachments (frenum, etc.)	*Normal*	*Normal*
17. Diagnostic set-up needed? (a) If so, what is conclusion?	*No*	*No*
18. Extraction necessary? (a) Which teeth?	*Probably not*	*Probably not*

(From Graber, T. M. (ed.): Current Orthodontic Concepts and Techniques. vol. 1, p. 53, W. B. Saunders Co., 1969.)

individual patient. So a careful cast analysis, together with measurement of long cone radiographs, is essential for each case.[14]

Take study casts of every patient; learn to look for the variations of the normal and the departures from that normal listed above. Make a check list so that you don't miss anything. On each subsequent visit, take out the study casts and compare the present status of the mouth with that of the study casts taken earlier. What changes have occurred? Are they favorable or unfavorable? Is there any drifting, overeruption, prematurities, abnormal facets of wear, overbite problems? Catch these before they develop. This is dentistry at its best—a preventive and interceptive service.

MIXED DENTITION ANALYSIS.   Considerable detail has been given on the development of the dentition in Chapter 2. The importance of adequate space at specific times was emphasized and the critical nature of this problem, even in normal occlusions.[15, 16] "To treat or not to treat" or "to extract" are important questions for patients between 8 and 11 years of age. The answers come from careful study of diagnostic criteria—the patient first, together with radiographs, photographs and plaster casts. It is important to know the size of the deciduous teeth and their successors.[15, 16] Direct measurements in the mouth are possible and measurements of properly taken intraoral radiographs give an idea of the size of unerupted permanent teeth. Properly taken long cone technique intraoral radiographs or occlusal radiographs may be measured fairly accurately, and this exercise is to be encouraged, using fine-line dividers and a millimetric scale. Direct measurements are preferable for the most accurate appraisal. Of course, it should be remembered that rotations are difficult to measure on the two-dimensional x-ray image; distortion and magnification are continual problems. Carefully taken supplemental occlusal views can actually give even better appreciation of tooth position and size, but because of the short target film distance, some slight allowance for the magnification should be made (Fig. 8–18). Measurement on the study casts is more accurate than measurements taken directly in the mouth. Also, the perimeter measurement of arch length available, the mesial side of the first permanent molar, around to the mesial side of the opposite first permanent molar, is more accurately determined on the plaster cast (Fig. 8–19). A number of mixed dentition analyses, based on a combination of

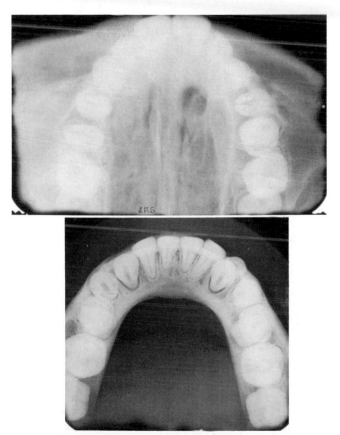

Figure 8–18 Maxillary (top) and mandibular occlusal films, illustrating use for measuring mesiodistal dimensions of unerupted teeth. Less distortion is likely than with conventional periapical films. (Courtesy W. S. Brandhorst.)

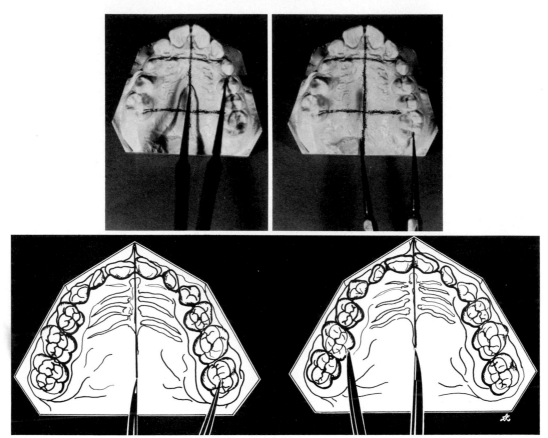

Figure 8–19 (Top) Marked mesial drift of upper left first molar, impacting second premolar, shows well when a perpendicular is drawn to the median raphe. Casts should be routinely analyzed in this manner. Both anteroposterior and bilateral asymmetries can be discerned readily after drawing the midsagittal plane. Fine line dividers (Fig. 8–3) help in this analysis. (Bottom) In addition to drawing a line down the median raphe and constructing perpendiculars to it to determine symmetry of the arch, precise measurements may be made with fine line dividers and recorded on the patient's record. Subsequent measurements may be taken directly in the mouth and compared with pretreatment figures. Caliper or fine line measurements are particularly valuable in space-opening problems, giving a precise indication of changes obtained by orthodontic therapy.

study cast and radiograph measurements, are available. The Bolton analysis is widely used. Arch length and tooth size discrepancies are discussed in greater detail in Chapter 15, together with the Mayne analysis for potential serial extraction cases. Owen has developed a comprehensive cast analysis, which is described briefly. Properly used, it provides precise three-dimensional assessment of malrelationships seen on the study casts[14] (Fig. 8–20).

What is the information you desire most during the period of mixed dentition? Obviously, it is whether there will be enough room to accommodate the unerupted canines and the first and second premolars. When the demands are not too critical and the dentist wants a "ball-park" impression of space adequacy, then the mixed dentition analysis developed by Moyers provides this quickly, without a full-mouth, long cone survey that can be difficult to obtain where there are apprehensive young children or parents who are opposed to radiation[17] (Fig. 8–21). It has the following advantages:

1. It has minimal error and the range of possible error is precisely known.
2. It can be done with equal reliability by the beginner and by the expert.

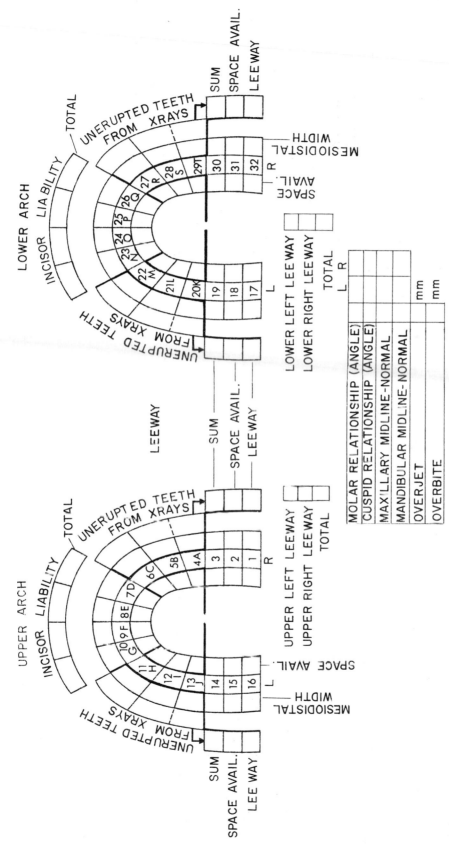

Figure 8-20 University of Chicago Cast Analysis. New numbering system, with 1 to 32 for permanent teeth and A to K to designate deciduous teeth in both arches. (Courtesy D. G. Owen.)

MIXED DENTITION ANALYSIS

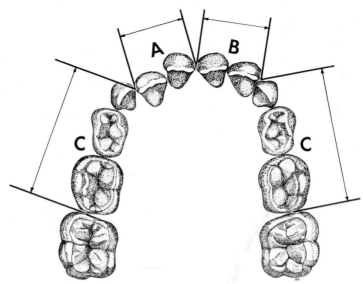

Figure 8–21   A and B, Measurement on arch perimeter of the combined widths of the central and lateral incisors on each side. Distal mark will actually lie on canine crown—if arch length is deficient—and is seldom short of canine contact. C, Distance from mesial aspect of first permanent molar to mark made on arch perimeter after exact widths of central and lateral incisors have been marked off on arch circumference. Predicted width taken from table is then subtracted from this figure to give actual arch length left over. (From R. E. Moyers.)

3. It is not time-consuming.
4. It requires no special equipment.
5. It can be done in the mouth as well as on the casts.
6. It may be used for both arches.

The basis for the Moyers mixed dentition analysis is that there is a high correlation among groups of teeth. Thus, by measuring one group of teeth—the mandibular incisors, for example—it is possible to make a prediction on the size of other groups of teeth with a fair degree of accuracy (Fig. 8–21). Mandibular incisors erupt first and offer the earliest opportunity of measurement and they are also less variable and more reliable than the maxillary incisors. Probability charts have been developed for predicting the sum of canine and premolar widths from the sum of mandibular incisor width for both arches. These are given at different confidence levels, and the technique is described in detail in the Moyers text.

Since the maxillary arch is not the contained arch, space deficiency is regarded as less critical, as downward and outward growth to a larger perimeter is to be expected to some degree with maxillary alveolar growth. The unpredictability of this growth assist in both amount and timing militates against any "sure fire" space availability prognostication. A M.D.A. should serve as a guide and must be correlated with other diagnostic information.

Because of the lack of correlation between size of deciduous teeth and their permanent successors, and even the variability between segments of the permanent dentition, it is still recommended that measurements be made on accurate, properly taken long cone technique intraoral radiographs, whenever possible, even though a mixed dentition analysis has been done.[15, 16, 18]

FUNCTIONAL ANALYSIS AND EQUILIBRATION OF OCCLUSION

Equally important is a functional analysis, a study of the patterns of attrition and the facets of wear. Many a functional mandibular displacement has been discovered by looking at the inclined planes and cusps of the teeth on the casts. Armed with this information, a sheet of baseplate wax and thin articulating paper strips, the dentist may return to the mouth to check for prematurities, tooth guidance, cuspal interference and possible trauma. The problem may be just overeruption of the mandibular third molar; it may be a premolar in buccal or lingual cross-bite; it may be improper restoration of a contact relationship. It may be that very frequent and largely unrecognized habit of bruxism so often associated with deeper than normal overbite and high nervous irritability. In this case occlusal equilibration may not be the therapy of choice, but rather a bite-plate. Study casts enable the dentist to see these things much more clearly and to correct them before the patient himself becomes aware of them through pain, looseness of teeth, inflamed or bleeding gingival tissues or loss of supporting bone.

One of the most valuable services a dentist can render is the equilibration of his patient's occlusion. Without a set of study casts this is a hazardous procedure. For this service it is advisable that the casts be mounted on an anatomic articulator to better reproduce the normal functional movements. This will be discussed in greater detail in Chapter 14.

CLASSIFICATION OF MALOCCLUSION. Classification of malocclusion is made easier by occluding the maxillary and mandibular casts. The basal relationship is more readily apparent than from an oral examination alone. A view of the lingual cusps and surfaces during function may be just as important as the labial and buccal surfaces. It is possible, of course, only with the study casts. It is emphasized here again as it was in Chapter 5 that classification of the malocclusion is just one diagnostic facet that creates arbitrary categories based on morphologic, spatial and functional variances. Its purpose is to organize the thinking of the dentist, not to regiment it.[2] As Brader[71] observes, "The test of time and accumulated clinical experience leads . . . toward the inevitable conclusion that the Angle classification of dental malocclusion is inadequate for the diagnostic evaluation of complex dentofacial problems." Thus, it would be a mistake to rely solely on categorizing as a basis for therapeutic decisions. As a clue to treatment—yes; as a crutch—no. Individual variability makes a differential diagnosis a paramount consideration for each patient, with the tentative treatment plan based on the entire battery of diagnostic criteria: clinical examination, radiographic evidence, laboratory tests where indicated, case history, plaster casts and photographs.

Plaster casts provide a record of a particular condition at a specific time. Because bone is plastic; because there a variety of forces exerted on the dentition by the musculature, food, etc.; because teeth become carious and must be repaired; because teeth may be lost, leaving spaces that are to be restored; because there is mesial drift and actual wear at the contacts, it is vitally important that a set of study casts be made for each patient if the dentist wants to render optimal service. With study casts and dental radiographs, truly interceptive orthodontics and interceptive dentistry are possible throughout life. Without them the dentist is usually confronted with a *fait accompli* and must then resort to corrective or reparative procedures.

POST-TREATMENT STABILITY. When a patient undergoes orthodontic treatment, original casts are valuable to demonstrate the progress to the patient and

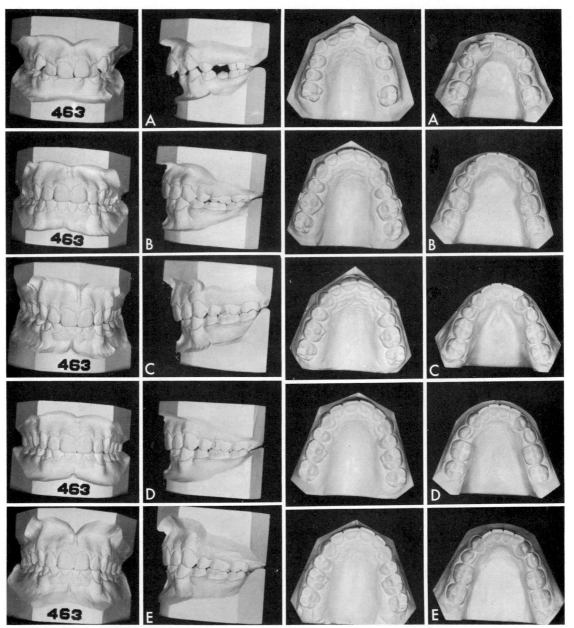

Figure 8–22   (Left) Frontal and lateral views of plaster study casts before orthodontic treatment (A), after appliances were removed (B), after retention (C), one year later (D) and two years later (E). (Right) Occlusal views of maxillary and mandibular study casts at same time intervals. Changes that have occurred over a 7-year span of orthodontic and postorthodontic management may be precisely analyzed. The result appears stable.

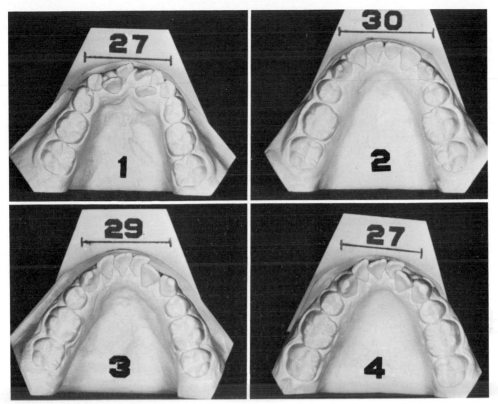

Figure 8–23 Occlusal view of mandibular plaster study cast. Before treatment (1), after orthodontic treatment (2), two years later (3) and four years later (4). Note change in intercanine dimension with return to original measurement of 27 mm. despite the removal of premolars during orthodontic therapy.

parents. There is no better check on post-treatment stability (Figs. 8–22, 8–23). If treatment objectives are not being accomplished, if unwanted tooth movement occurs or there are unwanted post-treatment changes, this can be seen more readily with the original casts at hand. Finally, a case history and record of oral conditions is no less important to the patient than similar records of other parts of the body. Knowing how important longitudinal or continued records are to the dentist in helping him render a better professional service, the dentist can fully appreciate that these records would be of equal importance to another practitioner in the event that the patient moves to a different locality. How often has the dentist said as he saw a patient for the first time, "How did this patient get this way?" Or he may ask himself, "Is this a stable occlusion or a changing one?" The patient may talk of shifting teeth, of increasing irregularity of incisors, of spaces opening or closing, conditions which may or may not exist. The plaster cast provides an accurate time-linked record of any such changes. The dentist is thus protecting the patient and himself with these records. (See Chap. 9.)

INTRAORAL AND PANORAMIC RADIOGRAPHS

As with an iceberg, hidden factors may be of greater importance than those which are readily apparent. An astute dentist with sensitive fingers and a sharp eye may palpate canine bulges high in the mucobuccal fold, or he may note a suspicious bulge in the palate; he may see an edentulous area and suspect that a tooth is either missing or erupting abnormally; he may see an ankylosed deciduous first molar dropping below the level of occlusion. Indeed, he may see a number of things clinically, but he must turn to the intraoral radiograph or panoramic radiograph for confirmatory evidence of his clinical observations (Fig. 8–24). Frequently the information obtained from the radiographic examination may not have been suspected clinically. But dental radiographs by themselves, like study casts alone, are incomplete. The dentist must not be lulled into relying on any one criterion. There should be a "team" or "total diagnostic"

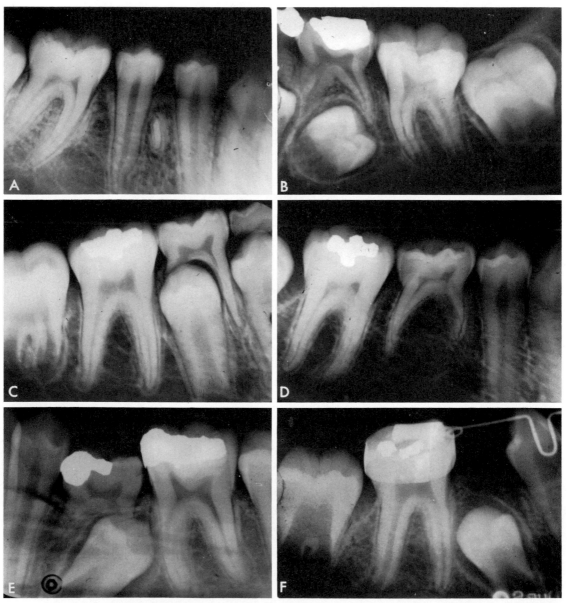

Figure 8–24 Some conditions in which dental radiographs provide significant information. A, Retained deciduous root fragment. B, Abnormal path of eruption. C, Abnormal resorption. D, Congenital absence. E, Ankylosis. F, Noneruption and orthodontic treatment.

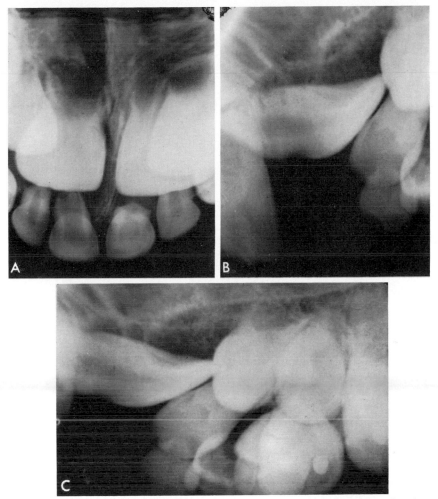

Figure 8-25 Three views of same patient showing value of longitudinal periodic radiographic examination. A, Apparently normal pattern at 6 years of age. B and C, Markedly rotated and malposed left central incisor that has greatly changed position in the two years since A was taken. (See Fig. 7–62.) Interrogation of the patient disclosed that there had been a heavy blow against the incisor region from a baseball when he was 6½ years of age.

approach, with information gained from a number of sources—information that is corroborated or correlated by more than one diagnostic criterion, if possible.

Chapters 6 and 7 on etiology of malocclusion show that the delicate timetable of growth and development and accomplishment of a normal occlusion is vulnerable to many attacks. To ward off these attacks and keep the progress of the developing dentition on schedule, the dental radiograph is invaluable. The average dentist is aware of this, because he is well trained in interpretation of the dental radiograph and he recognizes the importance of routine radiographic examinations (Fig. 8–25).

To enumerate just a few of the conditions requiring radiographic observation and confirmation: (1) pattern and amount of resorption of roots of deciduous teeth; (2) presence or absence of permanent teeth; their size, shape, position and relative state of development; (3) congenital absence of teeth or presence of supernumerary teeth; (4) character of alveolar bone and immediate lamina

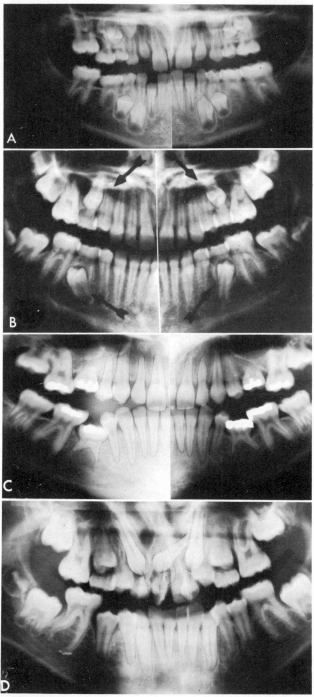

Figure 8–26 A, Congenital absence of one upper first permanent molar and ectopic eruption of the other, congenital absence of lower second premolars, all second molars and probably third molars. Lower second deciduous molar is probably ankylosed. B, Abnormal eruptive path of all second premolars with possible beginning ankylosis of lower second deciduous molars. C, Congenital absence and advanced ankylosis. D, Malpositions, abnormal eruptive path and arch length deficiency. This type of information is seen better and correlated more effectively on laminagraphic radiographs.

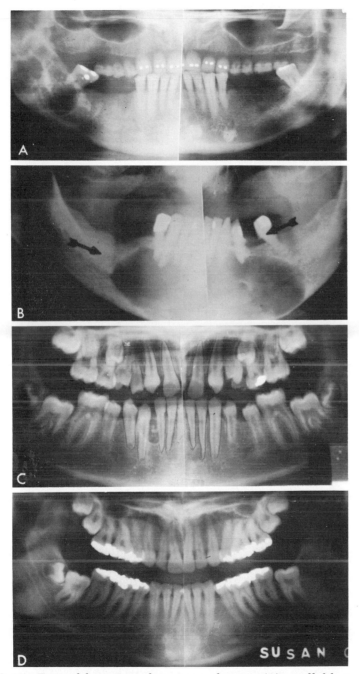

Figure 8–27   Panoral laminagraphic views, showing (A) amelloblastoma, unrecognized by prosthodontist who made denture. B, Large cyst, also not discovered in routine dental check-ups. C, Developing cyst in lower incisor area, with congenital absence of maxillary lateral incisors. D, Four first premolars removed for orthodontic purposes earlier, but fourth molars are developing in three quadrants.

dura and periodontal membrane; (5) morphology and inclination of roots of permanent teeth; (6) pathologic oral conditions such as caries, thickened periodontal membrane, apical infections, root fractures, retained deciduous roots, cysts, etc.

Special consideration must be given to panoramic radiography. With more than 3500 units now in action and many laboratories providing panoramic radiography service for dentists, the real value of this diagnostic tool must be stressed. By virtue of its ability to take a single picture of the entire stomatognathic system—teeth, jaws, temporomandibular joints, sinuses, etc.—important information may be obtained routinely with a fraction of the radiation needed for a full mouth intraoral examination and without even placing the film in the mouth. The entire picture taking procedure takes less than 90 seconds, and developing is limited to one film.[19–22, 75]

In guiding the developing occlusion, yearly panoramic radiographs would be invaluable. The status of the dental timetable is easily determined by noting the following: deciduous root resorption, permanent root development, path of eruption, premature loss, prolonged retention, ankylosis, supernumerary teeth, congenital absence and malformed teeth, impactions, cysts, fractures, caries, apical involvement—and this is only a partial list (Figs. 8–26, 8–27). For serial extraction procedures, invaluable information is obtained (see Chap. 15). As a "correlator" of other diagnostic criteria, the panoramic view assists in the synthesis of the diagnostic and therapeutic phases of patient management.

FACIAL PHOTOGRAPHS

Even as plaster casts serve as a record of the teeth and investing tissues at a specific time, so does the photograph. The photograph assumes even greater importance when the dentist does not have equipment permitting him to take cephalometric headplates.

Facial harmony and balance are considered important therapeutic objectives by the orthodontist. With favorable growth and development, elimination of muscular perversions and proper appliance therapy, the facial changes in certain cases can be most rewarding and quite dramatic (see Chap. 1). A permanent record of the original profile and full face appearance as compared with similar post-treatment records is a graphic example for both patient and parent of what can be accomplished by orthodontics (Fig. 8–28). While all favorable facial changes are not wrought solely by orthodontic therapy, therapy in conjunction with growth and maturation often produces a significant change. Photographs, like intraoral radiographs, plaster casts and the case history, are only one part of the total picture. Interpretations made on the photographs should be correlated with other records and should be weighted by data gathered from other diagnostic criteria. Thus, a short, hypotonic upper lip, a lower lip that cushions to the lingual aspect of the upper incisors and an excessive overjet should be recorded in the initial clinical examination and corroborated by an analysis of the articulated plaster study casts. A mandibular retrusion apparent from a study of the articulated plaster casts will usually show up on the profile photograph. The dentist can then decide whether this is purely a dental mandibular retrusion, a total retrusion or a combination of both.

Not all these features can be changed by orthodontics alone. "Team effort," with surgical assistance in the form of rhinoplasties, chin implants, and even lip-lengthening procedures, will result in a better total service to the patient.

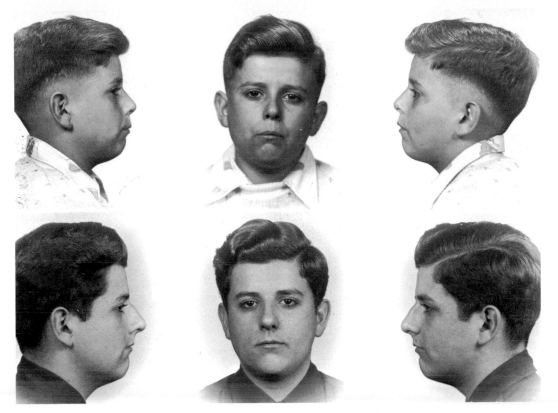

Figure 8-28   The type of facial change that can be wrought by orthodontic procedures. Note restoration of normal muscle function.

Parents should be made aware of the dominance of morphogenetic pattern, the influence of soft tissues over the skeletal structures (the functional matrix) and of the possible need later to alter nose, lip or chin contour.

Forehead slant affects facial balance. Even hair style is important. The "beatle," "natural" or "Afro" look can change the impressions of effective facial length and width. Hair style may thus add or detract from facial appearance, depending on the problem.

Facial type is important to the orthodontist (Fig. 8-29). He has learned by bitter experience through the years that he cannot change facial type but must work with it. A long narrow face, for instance, requires a certain arch form to fit that face. Arch form is just one of many characteristics reflecting facial type. Many orthodontists show beautiful "Hollywood" straight face profiles, attributing this to their orthodontic endeavors. In actuality, the facial type was there already, as a study of hereditary pattern and cephalometric radiographs would show. If the patient and the photograph show a convex facial profile and if the parents and siblings mirror this facial convexity, the dentist would do well to build his orthodontic result around this facial type. Many an orthodontist has encountered serious trouble by ignoring facial type and arch form that depend so strongly on hereditary and functional forces. Recent orthodontic literature has stressed the importance of axial inclination of the upper and lower incisors. Some authors categorically state that the lower incisors should be set as close to 90 degrees with the mandibular plane as possible, or an equally empiric and unrealistic 65 degrees to the Frankfort horizontal plane. (See discussion of cephalometrics later in this chapter.)

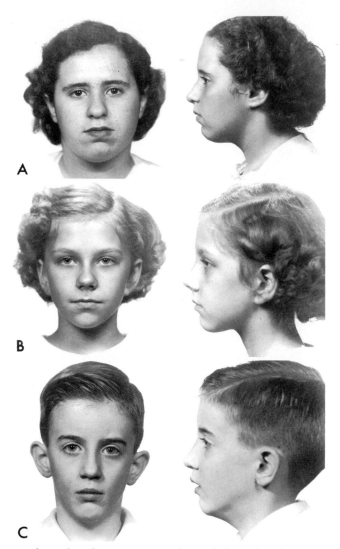

Figure 8–29   Three facial types. A, Brachycephalic is likely to have a broad dental arch to go with the board facial structure. B, Mesocephalic will probably have an average dental arch form. C, Dolichocephalic is most likely to have a long and narrow dental arch form to harmonize with the long and narrow face. Mixture of hereditary components, however, produces significant exceptions to the general rule.

Pont's index or similar measurements of tooth size are used to determine arch width, with no regard for basal bone and muscle system limitations.[23] They are of little value. Extraction or nonextraction is too often determined by a single angular measurement of the lower incisor. Racial and facial types, sex, age, apical base differences, etc., are blandly ignored.[24–28] How tragically arbitrary and unthinking such an approach is! This sort of advice ignores individual differences, functional forces and the limitations of mechanotherapy. What is normal for one individual and one facial or racial type may be abnormal for another. Even malocclusion is a state of balance for a particular patient at a particular time. In a convex face, for example, the upper and lower incisors are likely to be more procumbent or tipped further forward. This is perfectly normal for this facial type. A concave facial type usually has more erect upper and lower incisors (Fig. 8–36). Worship of any arbitrary tooth-oriented, standard is unphysiologic and bound to disillusion the dentist. Even if he is able to achieve the arbitrary axial inclination by virtue of his appliance manipulation, as soon as these appliances are removed, slowly, inexorably, insidiously, the axial inclination returns to the position determined by hereditary pattern, by bone relationships and by functional forces. Photographs are an important clue for facial type. Do not ignore this clue.

SUPPLEMENTAL DIAGNOSTIC CRITERIA

Thus far we have discussed diagnostic criteria that are considered essential. In addition to these there are a number of other criteria that on occasion are valuable and give additional information that assists the dentist in making the all-important diagnostic decisions. The dentist is usually not equipped to utilize these criteria, however, and must turn to the orthodontic specialist, the laboratory or the radiologist for assistance. If he suspects that such information will aid him in diagnosis, he should not hesitate to get it by referring the patient to the proper agency. Some of these records and the information they impart are discussed in the following pages. If he carries any number of active orthodontic patients in his practice, some of these supplemental diagnositc criteria must be transferred to the "Required" list. Reference is again made to the chapter on diagnosis in the two-volume specialty-oriented text, *Current Orthodontic Principles and Techniques.*[3] Cephalometrics is discussed at length because of the importance it has in routine orthodontic practice. There is no question that much of the information gained can find use in general dental practice as more dentists learn to use this tool.

SPECIAL X-RAY VIEWS

CEPHALOMETRIC RADIOGRAPHS

Photographs are an excellent aid in appraising facial balance, facial type and harmony of external features, but they leave much to be desired in an analysis of relationship of bony parts. Soft tissue frequently masks hard tissue configuration. The teeth are an integral part of the craniofacial complex, as any dentist soon finds out by manipulating tooth-moving appliances. The discussion in Chapter 3 of bony architecture and stress trajectories and of the physiology of the stomatognathic system in general, emphasizes the interdependence of cranial, facial and dental building blocks. This concept is not new. Ever since Camper investigated prognathism craniometrically in 1791, anthropologists have been interested in the ethnographic determination of facial form and pattern. Anthropometrics, or "the measurement of man," found the human head a fertile source of information because of the relatively little change in the bony parts as a result of death. By studying different ethnic groups, different age groups, male and female, and by measuring the size of the various parts and recording variations in position and shape of cranial and facial structures, it became possible to devise certain broad standards that were descriptive of the human head. As a specialized part of anthropometrics, study of the head became known as craniometrics or cephalometrics. Certain landmarks and measure points were developed to assist the anthropologist in interpreting craniofacial relations. The limitations of "dead-house diagnosis" soon became obvious to investigators attempting to analyze the problems of living phenomena. Skeletal material was often of unknown ethnic origin, the age only an approximation, and the cause of death unknown. The effects of the environment after death served as an added variable. To establish a "norm" meant lumping assorted groups of skulls together and making a cross-sectional analysis. Despite these limitations, anthropologists did make significant contributions. Much of what we know today about facial types and growth and developmental changes was first described in anthropologic literature.[29]

Because of the drawbacks of a cross-sectional analysis, obviating study of the individual pattern, Simon developed gnathostatics as a diagnostic medium relating the teeth and their bases to each other and to craniofacial structures. Gnathostatics played an important role in making the orthodontist more conscious of basal relationships, of facial balance and harmony, of the cant of the occlusal plane, inclination of the mandibular plane, of arch asymmetries, etc. But much of the diagnosis was based on the facial photograph, and the underlying bony structures often did not duplicate the apparent soft tissue contours. (See Chaps. 1, 4, 5.) Yet, it was obviously important to ascertain the true relationship of the tooth, bone and neuromuscular systems.

From Simon and gnathostatics to Todd, Broadbent and Hofrath and roentgenographic cephalometrics was a short step.[30–32] Here was a method which combined the face-conscious longitudinal approach of Simon with the anthropologic mensuration of the underlying bony structures of the living individual through the medium of carefully oriented sagittal and anteroposterior headplates. Even as the conventional intraoral radiographic examination and panoramic views augment the clinical examination, verifying the clinical impressions and providing new information, so also does the oriented craniofacial x-ray picture add to the image of the teeth, jaws and cranium (Figs. 8–30, 8–31).

CEPHALOMETRIC LANDMARKS.   Roentgenographic cephalometrics has taken over many anthropometric landmarks. Most of these are for the lateral (sagittal) headplate which is used most commonly for orthodontic diagnosis (Figs. 8–31, 8–32). Some of the important landmarks are listed below.

A   *Subspinale.*   The deepest midline point on the premaxilla between the anterior nasal spine and prosthion (Downs).

ANS   *Anterior nasal spine.*   This point is the tip of the anterior nasal spine seen on the x-ray film from norma lateralis.

Ar   *Articulare.*   The point of intersection of the dorsal contours of process articularis mandibulae and os temporale (Björk).

B   *Supramentale.*   The most posterior point in the concavity between infradentale and pogonion (Downs).

Ba   *Basion.*   The lowermost point on the anterior margin of the foramen magnum in the midsagittal plane.

Bo   *Bolton point.*   The highest point in the upward curvature of the retrocondylar fossa (Broadbent).

Gn   *Gnathion.*   The most inferior point in the contour of the chin.

Go   *Gonion.*   The point which on the jaw angle is the most inferiorly, posteriorly, and outwardly directed.

Me   *Menton.*   The lowermost point on the symphysial shadow as seen in norma lateralis.

Na   *Nasion.*   The intersection of the internasal suture with the nasofrontal suture in the midsagittal plane.

Or   *Orbitale.*   The lowest point on the lower margin of the bony orbit.

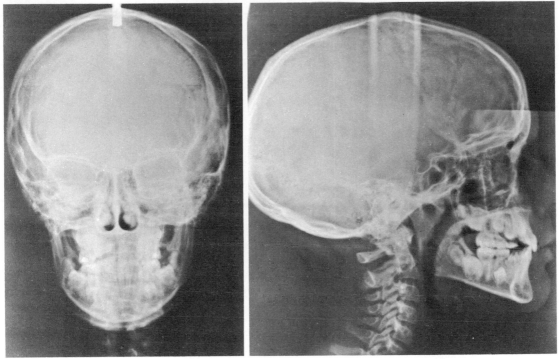

Figure 8–30   Lateral and frontal radiographs, with teeth in habitual occlusion. (From A. Björk.)

PNS *Posterior-nasal spine.*   The tip of the posterior spine of the palatine bone in the hard palate.

 Po *Porion.*   The midpoint on the upper edge of the porus acusticus externus located by means of the metal rods on the cephalometer (Björk).

Pog *Pogonion.*   Most anterior point in the contour of the chin.

Ptm *Pterygomaxillary fissure.*   The projected contour of the fissure; the anterior wall represents closely the retromolar tuberosity of the maxilla, and the posterior wall represents the anterior curve of the pterygoid process of the sphenoid bone.

 "R" *Broadbent registration point.*   The midpoint of the perpendicular from the center of sella turcica to the Bolton plane.

  S *Sella turcica.*   The midpoint of sella turcica, determined by inspection.

 SO *Spheno-occipital synchondrosis.*   The uppermost point of the suture.

Naturally, not all these landmarks are used in routine cephalometric analysis. A sizable number are more difficult to discern accurately from patient to patient. The more variable landmarks, such as porion, orbitale, gonion, Bolton point, basion, anterior and posterior nasal spines and point A (Fig. 8–33), can produce significant differences in interpretation in cephalometric criteria from observer to observer.[33, 73] As Johnston shows, experimental error is likely to be more variable than the biometric analysis of the data itself, even when using a computer and taking X-Y Coordinate information directly from the film.[34, 35]

Using combinations of dimensional and angular criteria which employ the various measure points and landmarks, cephalometrics offers the dentist valuable information in the following categories.

1. Growth and development
2. Craniofacial abnormalities
3. Facial type

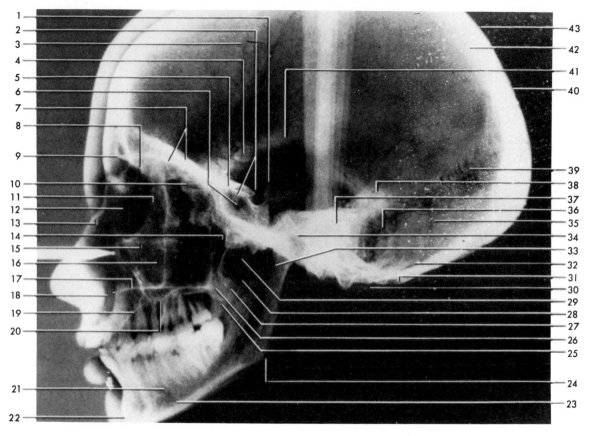

1. POSTERIOR CLINOID PROCESS AND DORSUM SELLAE
2. ANTERIOR CLINOID PROCESS
3. CORONAL SUTURE
4. GREATER WING OF SPHENOID BONE
5. FLOOR OF ANTERIOR CRANIAL FOSSA IN THE MIDLINE
6. SPHENOID SINUS
7. ROOF OF ORBIT AND FLOOR OF ANTERIOR CRANIAL FOSSA LATERAL TO MIDLINE
8. SUPRAORBITAL MARGIN
9. FRONTAL SINUS
10. ETHMOID SINUS
11. LATERAL BORDER OF ORBIT
12. ORBIT (MEDIAL WALL)
13. NASAL BONES
14. PTERYGOMAXILLARY FISSURE
15. ZYGOMA
16. MAXILLARY SINUS
17. FLOOR OF NOSE AND ROOF OF PALATE (MIDLINE)
18. ANTERIOR NASAL SPINE
19. ROOF OF THE PALATE (MIDLINE)
20. FLOOR OF THE MAXILLARY SINUS

21. MENTAL FORAMEN
22. MENTUM
23. BODY OF MANDIBLE
24. GONION
25. MAXILLARY TUBEROSITY
26. CORONOID PROCESS
27. HAMULAR PROCESS
28. MANDIBULAR NOTCH
29. LATERAL PTERYGOID PLATE
30. MASTOID PROCESS OF TEMPORAL BONE
31. POSTERIOR BORDER OF FORAMEN MAGNUM
32. FLOOR OF POSTERIOR CRANIAL FOSSA
33. NECK OF CONDYLE
34. TEMPOROMANDIBULAR JOINT
35. OCCIPITOMASTOID SUTURES
36. MASTOID CELLS
37. PETROUS PORTION OF TEMPORAL BONE
38. PARIETOMASTOID SUTURE
39. LAMBDOID SUTURE
40. LAMBDA
41. SQUAMOPARIETAL SUTURE
42. INNER TABLE
43. OUTER TABLE

(Courtesy David Marshall.)

Figure 8–31 Cephalometric and anthropometric landmarks, as seen on the lateral head film directly.

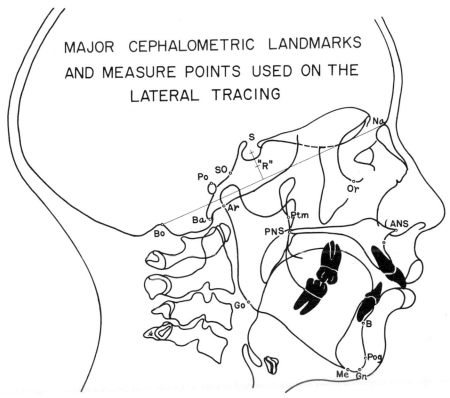

Figure 8–32 Landmarks and measure points approved for use by the First and Second Cephalometric Workshop. *S*, Sella turcica; *SO*, spheno-occipital synchondrosis; *Ba*, basion; *Bo*, Bolton point; *Na*, nasion; *Po*, porion; *"R,"* registration point; *Or*, orbitale; *Ptm*, pterygomaxillary fissure; *Ar*, articulare; *PNS*, posterior nasal spine; *ANS*, anterior nasal spine; *A*, Point A, or subspinale; *B*, Point B, or supramentale; *Pog*, pogonion; *Gn*, gnathion; *Me*, menton; *Go*, gonion.

4. Case analysis and diagnosis
5. Progress reports
6. Functional analysis

GROWTH AND DEVELOPMENT. The first and major use of cephalometrics is to appraise the growth and developmental pattern. Since Class II and Class III malocclusion correction particularly must rely on growth contributions if the dentist is to cope successfully with the problem of jaw malrelationship, a knowledge of what is "normal" is vital. Broadbent compiled over 20,000 records in his study of 5000 Cleveland school children.[31] Krogman,[36] Savara,[13] Meredith,[37] Popovitch,[38] Woodside,[39] Björk,[45–47] and others have made similar longitudinal studies, using cephalometric radiographs.[40–44]

As a result of these and similar studies by many investigators, much is known about growth increments, growth direction, differential growth and growth of component parts of the craniofacial complex (Figs. 8–34, 8–35). Clinically, the orthodontist is better able to time his mechanical procedures to coincide with pubertal growth spurts and to predict with some degree of accuracy what the end-result will be, based on interpretation of the cephalometric headplate. (See Chap. 2.)

CRANIOFACIAL ABNORMALITIES. The oriented lateral headplate is an excellent check on dental radiographs, not only for what they may miss—and many dental radiographs are technically deficient—but for areas that are beyond their scope. In addition to picking up impactions, congenital absence of teeth, cysts and supernumerary teeth, the headplate, by virtue of the constant direction of the central ray perpendicular to the midsagittal plane, gives a truer picture of the inclination of unerupted teeth. Tonsillar and adenoid tissue is easily detected in the lateral headplate, and its role in obstructing the nasal and oral airways can be assessed. Structural deformities imposed by less frequent conditions such as birth injuries, cleft lip and palate, macroglossia, fractures and mandibular prognathism are readily apparent. (See illustrations in Chaps. 6 and 7, Figs. 6–29 to 6–32.)

FACIAL TYPE. The relations of facial components vary broadly, depending on the facial type—whether the face is concave or convex—whether the face is forward divergent or backward divergent. The relationships of the jaws and the positions of teeth are intimately tied up with facial type.[10] The orthodontist who chooses to ignore typal implications is likely to be called upon by anxious parents to explain the major post-treatment "adjustments" that occur in tooth position after the removal of restraining appliances. The diagnostic decision, therapeutic accomplishment and ultimate stability reflect the limitations imposed by the morphogenetic pattern (Figs. 8–36, 8–37). There are two major considerations: the position of the maxilla anteroposteriorly in the face (with reference to the cranium) and the relation of the mandible to the maxilla, which is responsible for the convex, straight or concave profile line.

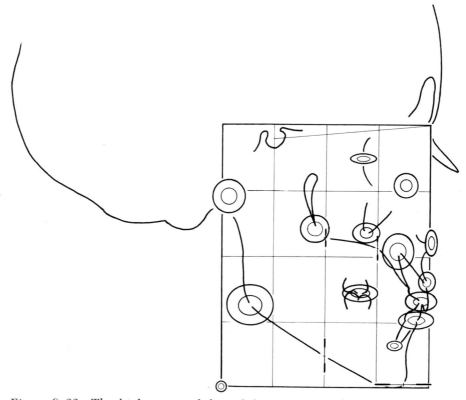

Figure 8–33 The biologic variability of the various landmarks is shown by concentric circles, indicating one and two standard deviations from the mean values for picking up cephalometric criteria. (Courtesy C. F. A. Moorrees.)

Case:T. C. age :	4	5	6	7	8	9	10	11	12	13	14
SNaA	85.5	83.5	84.0	82.0	80.0	80.0	79.5	80.0	79.0	79.5	79.5
A B Diff.	10.5	8.0	9.5	8.5	6.0	5.0	5.5	5.0	3.5	4.0	4.0
NaS—GoGn	33.0	34.0	35.0	35.0	35.0	34.0	36.0	33.5	32.5	33.5	32.0
U1—NaS	98.0°	86.0°	84.5°	88.0	89.5	95.0	93.0	93.0	93.0	93.0	97.0
L1—GoGn	80.5°	83.0	89.5	92.0	92.5	93.0	88.0	93.0	92.0	91.0	97.0
U1—NaPog(mm)	11.5°	7.5°	7.0°	6.0	6.5	7.5	7.5	7.5	7.0	7.0	7.5

• deciduous teeth

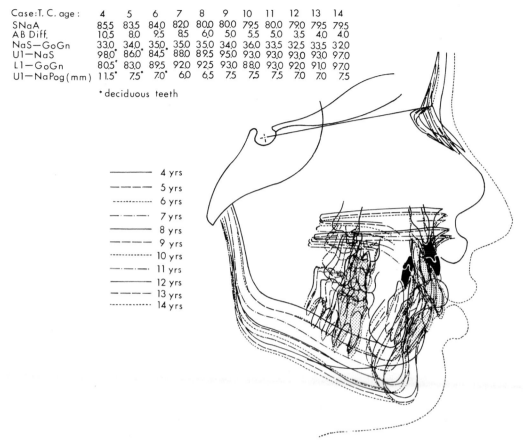

———— 4 yrs
– – – – 5 yrs
·········· 6 yrs
– · – · 7 yrs
———— 8 yrs
– – – – 9 yrs
·········· 10 yrs
– · – · 11 yrs
———— 12 yrs
– – – – 13 yrs
·········· 14 yrs

Figure 8–34 Severe Class II, Division 1 malocclusion. Note primary vertical direction of growth until pubertal spurt. Then there is a horizontal swing. Although radiographs are taken yearly, increments vary in amount as cephalometric tracings indicate.

If the maxilla is protracted in its relationship to the cranium, the profile is more likely to be convex. If the maxilla is retracted, the profile is more likely to be concave. However, with a maxillary protraction the face can be convex, straight or concave. The same profile variations hold true in a face where the maxilla is retracted in relation to the cranium. This is further complicated by an appraisal of general facial type, whether it is dolichocephalic (long and narrow) or brachycephalic (short and broad) (Fig. 8–29). Observations of large groups would seem to indicate that the dolichocephalic individual (or so-called Nordic type) is more likely to have a straight facial profile. The brachycephalic type (Slavs, eastern European groups, etc.) is more prone to profile convexity. Drummond, in research at Baylor University, did a study of 40 Negroes from 8 to 23 years of age to determine differences from the Caucasian race. The maxilla is more anteriorly placed with respect to the cranial base, the maxillomandibular basal difference is greater, the upper incisor more procumbent, and the lower incisor even more procumbent. Negroes also have a steeper mandibular plane.[26] Racial admixtures make any clear-cut correlation impossible. Nevertheless, incisor tooth inclinations vary depending on the maxillary protraction or retraction and the relative facial convexity.

The skeletal morphology strongly affects the tooth position and inclination. From our studies of clinically excellent occlusions, it appears that the apical base difference (maxilla to mandible) is routinely greater when the maxilla is

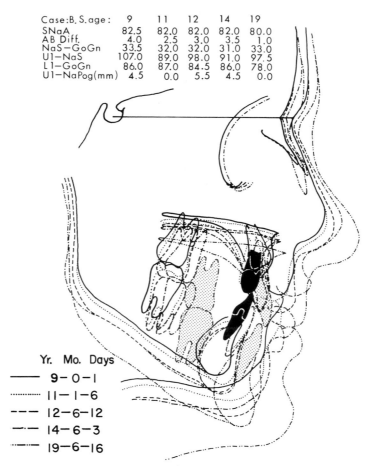

Case:B, S, age:	9	11	12	14	19
SNaA	82.5	82.0	82.0	82.0	80.0
AB Diff.	4.0	2.5	3.0	3.5	1.0
NaS—GoGn	33.5	32.0	32.0	31.0	33.0
U1—NaS	107.0	89.0	98.0	91.0	97.5
L1—GoGn	86.0	87.0	84.5	86.0	78.0
U1—NaPog(mm)	4.5	0.0	5.5	4.5	0.0

Yr. Mo. Days
——— 9— 0 — 1
·········· 11— 1 — 6
— — — 12— 6 —12
—·— 14— 6 — 3
—··— 19— 6 —16

Figure 8–35 Class III problem from 9 to 19 years, under orthopedic guidance, from 9 to 14 years. Observe changing direction of growth to a more dominant horizontal vector after termination of retrusive force against the mandible.

protracted in relation to the cranium. In such cases, there is a markedly greater tendency toward facial convexity and incisor procumbency. In patients with maxillary retraction, the incisor teeth seem to be more upright over basal structures. The anteroposterior apical base discrepancy is consistently less. For example, Figure 8–38 shows profile pictures of two patients with clinically excellent occlusions. An examination of the cephalometric tracings will show a broad difference in the relation of facial and dental components. In the straight face, with a maxillary retraction the upper incisors are 98 degrees to the S-Na plane, the lower incisors 85 degrees to the mandibular plane and the anteroposterior apical base difference is 1 degree. In the convex face, with maxillary protraction the upper incisors are relatively procumbent at 113 degrees; the lower incisors are 99 degrees; the apical base difference is 5 degrees.

The Frankfort-mandibular plane angle in both patients is 26 degrees. Both dentures are in balance and are healthy, functioning units. This is not a sporadic example, for in the study of a large group of individuals with clinically excellent occlusions it has been shown that the balance of parts obtained by nature varies as the relative maxillary protraction or retraction and the degree of convexity vary. There is a positive correlation between the anteroposterior

PROTRACTED   MAXILLA

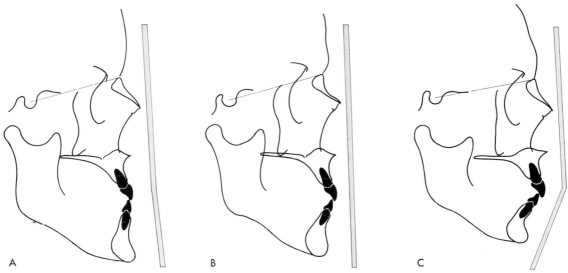

A   B   C

Figure 8–36   Protracted maxilla, foward with respect to cranium. Facial type may be concave (A), straight (B) or convex (C). When the maxilla is forward in the face, facial type is most frequently convex, anteroposterior apical base difference is greater, and maxillary and mandibular incisors are more procumbent.

RETRACTED   MAXILLA

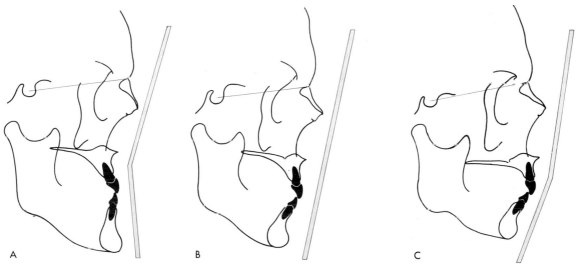

A   B   C

Figure 8–37   Retracted maxilla, retruded with respect to cranium. Facial type may be concave (A), straight (B) or convex (C). With the maxilla retruded in the face, the profile is most frequently straight, anteroposterior apical base difference is small, and maxillary and mandibular incisors are more upright.

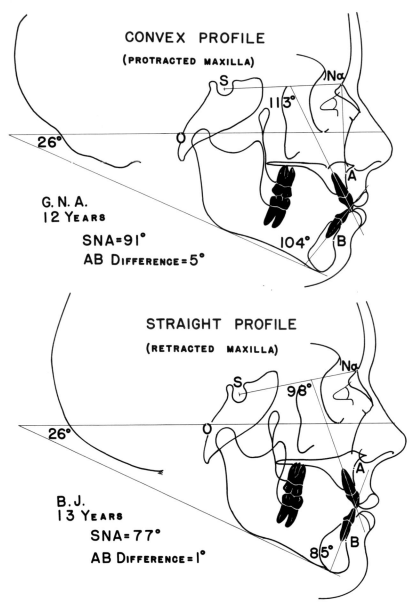

Figure 8–38   Convex and straight profiles associated with normal occlusion. Note particularly the difference in apical base relationship and the variability in incisor procumbency.

apical base difference and the amount of incisor procumbency. Corollary to this is the observation that there are larger maxillomandibular basal differences in individuals whose maxillary apical bases are protracted in relation to the cranium.

CASE ANALYSIS AND DIAGNOSIS.   A number of so-called "analyses" have been developed by orthodontists to assist in evaluating the original malocclusion and in projecting what the measurements should be at the end of orthodontic treatment. These analyses are usually confined to the lateral headplate with the teeth in occlusion. The validation for these analyses and for the use of lateral headplates taken at frequent intervals during treatment is the pattern of differential growth. Not all parts of the head grow at the same rate. The brain and brain case grow rapidly and are completed relatively early, while the face, which follows the general bodily growth curve, takes much longer to reach maturity and reflects pubertal growth spurts (Fig. 2–24). Thus, a relatively complete cranial base changes little while appreciable change is seen in the orofacial region.

Since there are a number of analyses (groups of cephalometric criteria) that actually duplicate each other in one or more areas, the First and Second Cephalometric Workshops, consisting of leaders in the fields of anthropology, anatomy, growth and development and cephalometric radiography, developed a series of measurements, based on the landmarks previously described.[48, 49]

Downs has shown diagrammatically the division of the face into parts which grow at different rates and are variable in their response to orthodontic therapy (Fig. 8–39).

Because of the differential growth rate, it is possible to use the relatively complete and stable cranial base from which to measure changing facial and dental dimensions.

CEPHALOMETRIC PLANES. There are two commonly used planes in the cranium (Fig. 8–40): Bolton plane (Bolton point-nasion) and the sella-nasion plane. Both perform essentially the same function, serving as a relatively stable base from which to appraise dynamic changes in the dentofacial complex. Nearer the face, but also used by some orthodontists as a base plane, is the time-honored Frankfort plane, a horizontal construction that joins the landmarks

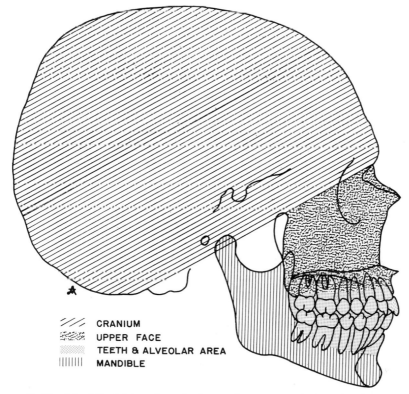

CRANIUM
UPPER FACE
TEETH & ALVEOLAR AREA
MANDIBLE

Figure 8–39 Modified lateral cephalometric tracing showing cranium, maxillary and mandibular bases, and teeth and supporting bone where the greatest reactions of orthodontic therapy are observed. (After Downs.)

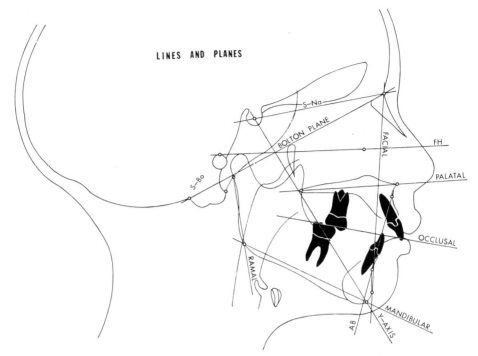

Figure 8–40   Base planes: *S-Na*, sella-nasion; *Bo-Na*, Bolton plane; *Po-Or*, Frankfort horizontal. *S-Bo* joins Bolton point and sella turcica to complete Bolton triangle. Facial planes: palatal, occlusal and mandibular planes; also facial plane, Y-axis, orbital plane and ramal plane.

porion (earhole axis) and orbitale (lowest point on the inferior margin of the orbit). The sella-nasion plane is easiest to establish, with minimum error between observers. However, as Moorrees and his co-workers show, sella may be high or low, with respect to a vertical profile line. This affects angular criteria, using the SN plane as a base (Fig. 8–41). In the face, three planes are used most commonly in cephalometric studies: the palatal plane paralleling the floor of the nose (or joining ANS and PNS); the occlusal plane, which bisects the first molar and incisor overbite; and the mandibular plane. The mandibular plane may be constructed as a tangent to the lower border (a) as a plane joining gonion and gnathion or (b) as a plane joining gonion and menton. Any one method chosen must be used consistently, of course.

The Y-axis (sella-gnathion) is used by a number of orthodontists to indicate the position of the chin-point in the face, the direction of mandibular growth, or the relative retraction or protraction of the mandible.

The lack of reliability in the use of intracranial and intrafacial reference planes should be recognized in the light of normal biologic variation.[50–52] We cannot expect nasion, sella, orbitale or porion to remain unaffected by racial, sex, age and individual differences. The marked difference in cranial base is shown in tracings of two females with close similarity of profile (Fig. 8–41). Because of the endochondral dominance of the anterior cranial base, its early completion and relative stability would seem comparatively more reliable. Use of nasion, an ectocranial landmark, militates somewhat against the sella-nasion plane. Clinically, however, for the astute observer, the use of nasion is tempered by the use of other criteria.

CEPHALOMETRIC CRITERIA.   Angular criteria are the most used of cephalometric analyses. They help compare qualitative similarity or difference within the total facial pattern or components with that pattern, making the dentist better able to evolve a concept of harmony or disharmony for the patient. Because of technical errors inherent in reducing a three-dimensional object (the head) to a two-dimensional projection (the film), and problems of magnification, distortion, etc., angular assessment is usually preferable to linear measurement.

There are three basic components of a representative cephalometric analysis: a *skeletal* analysis (Fig. 8–42), a *profile* analysis (Fig. 8–43) and a *denture* analysis (Fig. 8–44).

The *skeletal analysis* has as its major purpose an appreciation of facial type and an appraisal of anteroposterior apical basal bone relationship, particularly for Class II and Class III malocclusions. Facial type and basal relationships markedly influence the therapeutic objectives and accomplishments of the dentist. Two thirds of the malocclusions treated by the average orthodontist involve abnormal jaw relationships, with the teeth reflecting the anteroposterior dysplasia. In other words, the position of the teeth in Class II and Class III problems is caused by the position of the jaws (modified, of course, by the adaptive and deforming musculature).

For the purpose of analysis, malocclusions can be divided into three groups:

1. *Skeletal dysplasias:* malrelationship of the maxillary and mandibular

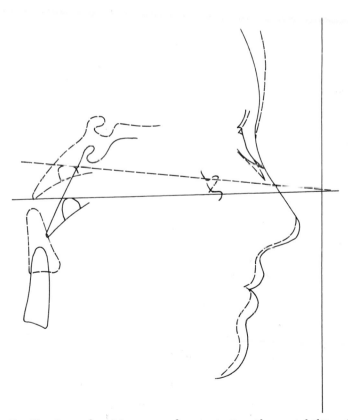

Figure 8–41 Tracing, after Moorrees, demonstrating the variability of sella turcica (high or low), with respect to a vertical profile line. Angular measurements may thus vary as much as 13 degrees, depending on the position of sella in the cranial base. (Courtesy C. F. A. Moorrees.)

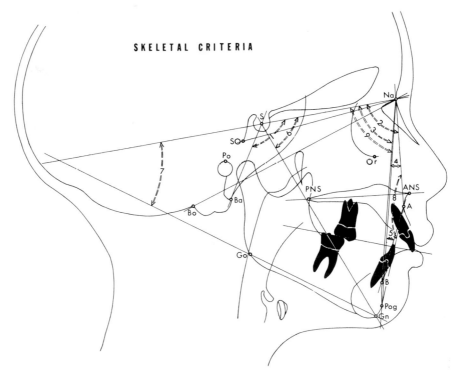

Figure 8–42 1, *Ba-S-Na*, cranial base flexure. 2, *S-Na-A*, maxillary base prognathism. 3, *S-Na-B*, mandibular base prognathism. 4, *A-Na-B*, apical base difference. 5, *AB-Na-Pog*, apical base-profile angle. 6, *Na-S-Gn*, Y axis angle. 7, *S-Na-Go-Gn*, mandibular-cranial base inclination. 8, *Na-A-Pog*, angle of facial convexity. 9, *S-Na-Pog*, relative mandibular prognathism. (University of Chicago Analysis.)

bases, with the teeth reflecting this malrelation but perhaps in fairly good position when compared with their basal bone alone.

2. *Dental dysplasias:* good skeletal pattern, with the malocclusion manifest only in tooth areas.

3. *Skeletodental dysplasias:* combination of basal and local malrelationships of varying degrees. This involves the four tissue systems—bone, muscle, nerve and tooth.

There are several methods to measure the apical base relationship—relation of maxilla to mandible and of both to the cranial base. One of the simplest is to make angular measurements of point "A" on the maxilla and point "B" on the mandible, to a reference cranial base line (S-Na-A and S-Na-B). The difference between the two angles determines the maxillomandibular difference. Measurement of the angle A-Na-B will give the same information. As Hasund and Sivertsen show, the greater the degree of facial prognathism (as indicated by anteroposterior positions of points A (subspinale) and B (supramentale) on maxilla and mandible, respectively), in relation to the Na-S line at nasion, the more procumbent the lower incisors. AB relationship affects incisor inclination.[50]

In addition to the facial typing just outlined on the previous pages, one may measure the angle formed by the facial plane and Frankfort horizontal plane, and by an angle connecting nasion, point "A," and pogonion (angle Na-A-Pog), to help in assessing the anteroposterior position of the mandible. The latter criterion records the convexity or concavity of the facial profile. A large anteroposterior basal discrepancy in a patient with a Class II or Class III malocclusion makes basal (maxillomandibular) adjustment imperative as the primary therapeutic goal. It is here that the orthodontist must utilize the patient's dentofacial growth potential if he is to achieve a reasonably stable and permanent correction.

Of the three planes in the facial portion—palatal, occlusal and mandibular—the inclination of the latter seems most significant clinically. A steep mandibular plane may be seen with Class II or Class III malocclusions and is considered by most orthodontists as an unfavorable condition. The steeper the plane, the more difficult both overbite and open bite are to correct.

The *profile analysis* is primarily an appraisal of the soft tissue adaptation to the bony profile; of lip size, shape and posture; of soft tissue thickness over the symphysis; of nasal structure contour and relationship to the lower face, etc. (Fig. 8–43). However, it is recognized that certain skeletal angular criteria influence the profile. In addition to the facial angle (Na-P with Frankfort horizontal) and Na-A-Pog already pointed out by Downs, there are such criteria as angles S-Na-A, S-Na-B, S-Na-Pog, Na-S-Gn, the inclination of the mandibular plane with a cranial base plane and AB-Na-Pog.

The *denture analysis* consists primarily of those descriptive elements that appraise tooth relationships with each other and with their respective bony bases (Fig. 8–44). This refers primarily to maxillary and mandibular incisors. The information desired usually is the degree of inclination of the incisors to their respective bases, to the occlusal plane and to each other. A linear measurement from the maxillary central incisal margin perpendicular to the Na-Pog line, helps to assess the anteroposterior position of the maxillary incisors with respect to the facial profile.

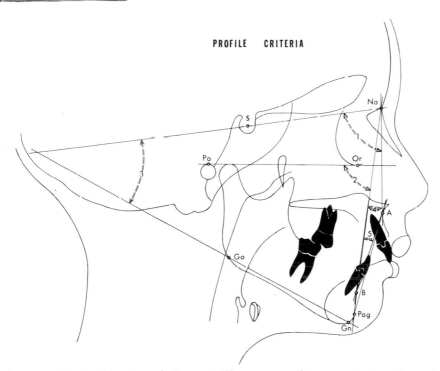

PROFILE   CRITERIA

Figure 8–43 1, *S-Na-A*, relative maxillary prognathism. 2, *FH-Na-Pog*, Downs' facial angle. 3, *S-Na-Go-Gn*, steepness of mandibular plane. 4, *A-Na-B*, apical base difference. 5, *AB-Na-Pog*, apical base-profile angle. Size and shape of nose, forehead slant, thickness, length and posture of lips and thickness of soft tissue over symphysis are essential profile criteria that require value judgments without mensuration. (University of Chicago Analysis.)

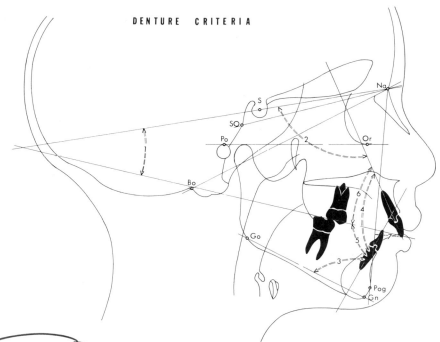

DENTURE CRITERIA

Figure 8–44 1, *S-Na-Occlusal Plane.* 2, *Upper incisor-S-Na.* 3, *Lower incisor-Go-Gn.* 4, *Inter-incisal.* 5, *Lower incisor-occlusal plane.* 6, *Upper incisor-occlusal plane.* 7, *Upper incisor incisal tip to Na-Pog plane.* These angles establish relationships of teeth to base planes, occlusal plane and to each other. A millimetric measurement of the upper incisor to the facial plane establishes relative prominence. Steepness of occlusal plane, related to cranial base, conditions procumbency of lower incisors to basal and occlusal plane. (University of Chicago Analysis.)

It is unwise to attach too much importance to any single criterion, such as the axial inclination of the lower incisors. The arbitrary 90 degree angulation has no place in physiology. Kobayashi and Takano showed a range from 84 to 105 degrees in Japanese with clinically excellent occlusions.[54, 55] The mean lower incisor inclination in their group was 96.6 degrees. In a like group, the range was 87.3 to 116.3 degrees, with a mean of 95.3 degrees.[56] Another study of 100 Japanese arrived at a mean of 95.5 degrees.[53] Miura[57] shows similar values for denture analysis, but a greater Class II tendency among pure Japanese than shown in the studies of Japanese-Americans by Takano, Kobayashi, Chang and Uesato.[25, 58] In a Chinese sample, the range was 90 to 108 degrees, with a mean of almost 98 degrees.[54] In a comparable Negro sample, the range was from 86 to 112 degrees, with a mean of 96.6 degrees.[54] Another Negro study showed a mean FMIA (Frankfort plane-mandibular incisor angle) of 49.4 degrees, while various studies on Caucasians show mean values ranging from 56.4 to 65 degrees.[26]

This substantiates the Hasund group research. Increasing prognathism means increasing incisor procumbency as a normal consequence of facial type.[59] Lundström, in his study of supposedly straight-faced Swedes, found that the mean lower incisor inclination was 95.9 degrees, with a standard deviation of 5.4 degrees.[60] Normalcy is obviously a broad range for all cephalometric criteria. For this reason current orthodontic "philosophies" which build their treatment objectives and make extraction decisions around single cephalometric criteria are merely "using" cephalometrics as ex post facto justification for a prior decision to remove teeth and treat according to the "bible."

In the cephalometric synthesis, none of the three analyses—skeletal, profile and denture—can stand alone. Integration with one another is essential, and then the conclusions require conditioning by other equally important clinical diagnostic aids, such as plaster casts, intraoral and panoramic radiographs, photographs and visual and digital examination of the patient.

PROGRESS REPORTS. The value of progress evaluation—an analysis of what has been accomplished during orthodontic treatment or full mouth reconstruction—cannot be overestimated. Our greatest lessons seem to come from such studies. There is all too little of this objective cephalometric approach in the analysis of "finished" cases today. Serial tracings offer much more information on developmental changes and on stability of orthodontic accomplishment than isolated head films taken prior to orthodontic therapy. Progress information can be gained without even measuring the various angles that make up a static cephalometric analysis such as has just been described (Figs. 8–45, 8–46).

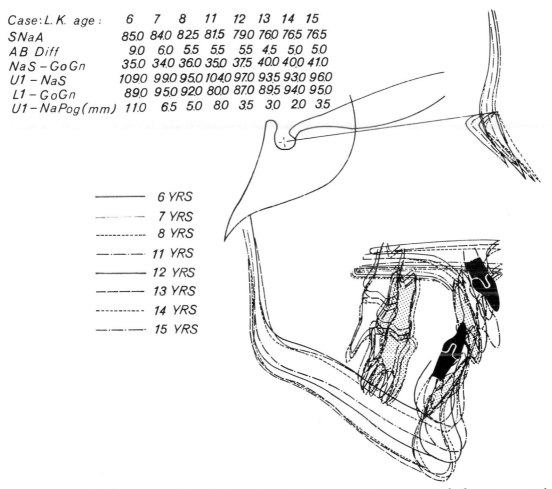

Case: L. K. age:	6	7	8	11	12	13	14	15
SNaA	85.0	84.0	82.5	81.5	79.0	76.0	76.5	76.5
AB Diff	9.0	6.0	5.5	5.5	5.5	4.5	5.0	5.0
NaS – GoGn	35.0	34.0	36.0	35.0	37.5	40.0	40.0	41.0
U1 – NaS	109.0	99.0	95.0	104.0	97.0	93.5	93.0	96.0
L1 – GoGn	89.0	95.0	92.0	80.0	87.0	89.5	94.0	95.0
U1 – NaPog (mm)	11.0	6.5	5.0	8.0	3.5	3.0	2.0	3.5

——— 6 YRS
— - — - 7 YRS
---------- 8 YRS
— - — - 11 YRS
——— 12 YRS
— — — 13 YRS
---------- 14 YRS
— - — - 15 YRS

Figure 8–45 This series of cephalometric tracings, over a ten-year period, demonstrates the major therapeutic challenge with an unfavorable direction of mandibular growth. A severe Class II malocclusion, growth was downward and backward, making continuing orthopedic guidance against the maxilla necessary to reduce the apical base difference. S-Na-A angle was reduced from 85 degrees to 76.5 degrees. The effective apical base dysplasia reduction was only 4 degrees, however. Stringent torque was required and was rather successful. The upper incisors were moved back almost 8 mm. with respect to the facial plane.

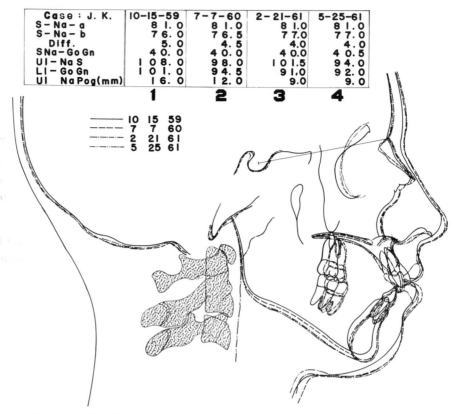

Case : J. K.	10-15-59	7-7-60	2-21-61	5-25-61
S – Na – a	81.0	81.0	81.0	81.0
S – Na – b	76.0	76.5	77.0	77.0
Diff.	5.0	4.5	4.0	4.0
SNa – Go Gn	40.0	40.0	40.0	40.0
UI – Na S	108.0	98.0	101.5	94.0
LI – Go Gn	101.0	94.5	91.0	92.0
UI Na Pog (mm)	16.0	12.0	9.0	9.0

1   2   3   4

———— 10 15 59
----- 7 7 60
–·–·– 2 21 61
–··–·· 5 25 61

Figure 8–46 Cephalometric tracings made (1) before placing appliances, (2) during treatment, (3) after removal of appliances, (4) three months later. Progress report (2) shows need for lingual root torque of maxillary incisors, and it has been largely achieved in (3). A tendency to reversion of labial position of the maxillary incisor apices is evident in (4). (From Graber, T. M.: Clinical cephalometric analysis *in* Kraus, B. S., and Reidel, R. A. [eds.]: Vistas in Orthodontics. Lea & Febiger, 1962.)

With radiographs and tracings made before treatment has started, it is a simple matter to take pictures during treatment to measure the progress or lack of progress (Figs. 8–46, 8–47). A more objective position on the extraction of teeth as a therapeutic adjunct becomes possible. Therapeutic modifiability is the hallmark of a competent clinician, where diagnosis, even with the best of criteria, is tentative. During treatment, cephalograms and panoramic radiographic surveys are a must. The reward of a higher level of accomplishment is augmented by less potential iatrogenic damage.[61] Certainly, there is some truth to the admittedly facetious observation of the prosthodontist who gave a talk on "The Recovery of the Human Denture from the Pathologic Manipulations of Orthodontics." The prognosis of treatment and retention of the finished result can be predicted to a large extent by study of cephalometric headplates taken before, during and after therapy.[75]

Where growth is a significant factor — and this includes the majority of cases under orthodontic treatment — annual records are not frequent enough. Neither the amount of growth nor the direction of growth is constant (Fig. 8–47). Yet this is vital information for the orthodontist who would correct Class II and Class III malocclusions. Since he is unable as yet to predict accurately just when he may expect an "assist" from vital growth processes, the prudent orthodontist takes cephalometric headplates every three to four months during orthodontic treatment. He may alter his plan of treatment, postpone certain steps, accelerate others or rely on future orthodontic mechanotherapy to achieve the therapeutic goal, depending on what he sees in serial cephalometric appraisals. Danger from radiation is practically nil, especially with the newer high speed equipment and faster film emulsions. Growth changes can occur in a short period of time; tooth movement is often quite rapid. Too long an interval between progress headplates masks the more detailed changes, levels out the pattern of accomplishment and may allow deleterious effects of appliance therapy to occur.

FUNCTIONAL ANALYSIS. In the discussion on Physiology of the Stomatognathic System (Chap. 3), it was pointed out that when an infant is born the gum pads are not clamped together, as pictured in many anatomy texts. Rather, the jaws are apart, the mandible being suspended by the facial, masticatory and skeletal muscles (Figs. 3–16, 3–26).

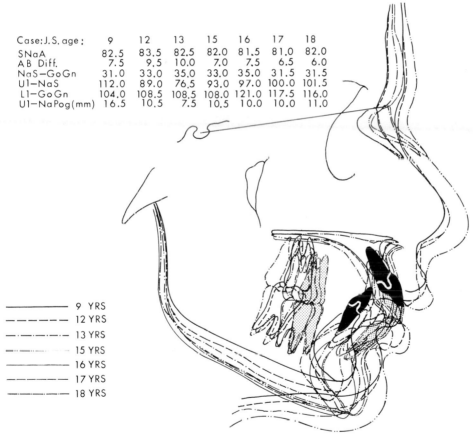

Case: J.S. age:	9	12	13	15	16	17	18
SNaA	82.5	83.5	82.5	82.0	81.5	81.0	82.0
AB Diff.	7.5	9.5	10.0	7.0	7.5	6.5	6.0
NaS−GoGn	31.0	33.0	35.0	33.0	35.0	31.5	31.5
Ul−NaS	112.0	89.0	76.5	93.0	97.0	100.0	101.5
Ll−GoGn	104.0	108.5	108.5	108.0	121.0	117.5	116.0
Ul−NaPog(mm)	16.5	10.5	7.5	10.5	10.0	10.0	11.0

——————— 9 YRS
— — — — — 12 YRS
—·—·—·—· 13 YRS
—··—··—·· 15 YRS
——————— 16 YRS
— — — — — 17 YRS
—··—··—·· 18 YRS

Figure 8–47 An example of poor therapeutic achievement, and lack of maxillary incisor torque when badly needed. Maxillary incisors were tipped lingually from 112 degrees to 76 degrees in an effort to reduce the large overjet (16.5 mm. incisor to facial plane measurement). During this time the mandible grew downward and backward, and was probably rocked down and back by the lingual tipping. Mandibular incisors, already procumbent at 104 degrees, moved to 108 degrees. Pubertal growth and release of teeth from appliances (except a retainer) resulted in a horizontal vector of mandibular growth and labial movement of maxillary incisors. Inexplicably, despite strong horizontal growth, mandibular incisors have moved further labially to 116 degrees. The maxillary incisors have returned to 101.5 degrees. Mandibular plane inclination is the same as it was at the beginning of therapy.

IMPORTANCE OF POSTURAL RESTING POSITION. A number of cephalometric studies have elaborated on this concept and have demonstrated that the physiologic resting position, or postural resting position, of the mandible is the most stable dental relationship throughout life and is least affected by growth disturbances and environmental influences.[62-64] This positioning of the mandible by the functional matrix is made possible by the maintenance of a predeterminable resting length of component muscle fibers under tonal contraction. Thus, the occlusal relationships (i.e., with the plaster casts related in occlusion) are frequently not true records of skeletal and dental dysplasia. These occlusal relationships may indicate an apparent malocclusion that is of entirely different proportions when seen with the mandible in a postural resting position. Occlusal aberrations are reflected in varying interocclusal clearances (space between the occlusal surfaces of the posterior teeth with the mandible at postural resting position). This emphasizes the three-dimensional nature of the orthodontic problem. Vertical growth increments are the greatest, and thus subject to the most potential abnormality. Vertical dysplasias affect anteroposterior occlusal relationships that simply cannot be seen from casts clamped in habitual occlusion.[65]

The vertical discrepancies in malocclusions are seldom due to derangement of muscular positioning of the mandible; almost always they are attributable to basal or alveolar bone dysplasia or lack of eruption (or overeruption in open-bite problems) of the teeth themselves. Such dysplasias lead to functional problems (as illustrated by Fig. 8–48). Without postural position cephalometric lateral

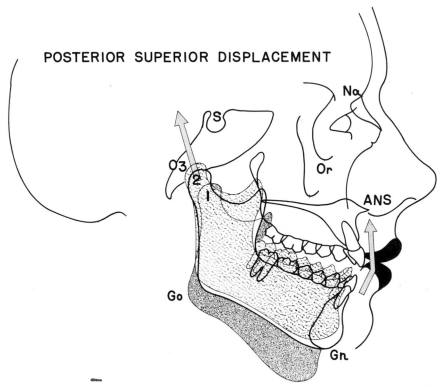

POSTERIOR SUPERIOR DISPLACEMENT

Figure 8–48 Lateral cephalometric tracing showing functional displacement. 1, Mandibular condyle position at open mouth. 2, Condyle and mandible at postural resting position. 3, Posterior superior displacement of condyle as a result of premature incisal guidance before habitual occlusion has been reached. Normally, condylar movement should be primarily rotary from 2 to 3, instead of translatory.

headplates, functional problems may be easily missed. For this reason, when a functional problem is suspected, a lateral headplate with the teeth in occlusion is inadequate. (See Chap. 3, discussion of vertical dimension.)

TECHNIQUE OF FUNCTIONAL ANALYSIS. First of all, a lateral projection with the mandible at postural resting position is required (Fig. 8–49). It is one thing to understand the importance of postural resting position and another thing to obtain it clinically. Nevertheless, with some experience the dentist can develop a fairly accurate technique of registering postural resting position. The patient is accurately placed in the cephalometric head positioner with the ear rod loosely inserted and then asked to repeat certain consonants. The letters "M" and "C" are quite satisfactory. Constant repetition of these letters over a 6- to 10-second interval tends to relax the mandible. With the letter "M" particularly, the lips are in gentle unstrained contact at the terminal phase of the sound. If the patient is instructed not to move immediately after the phonation of the consonant, exposure can usually be made with a fair degree of accuracy. Another method is to have the patient swallow and immediately instruct him not to move and then make the exposure 3 to 4 seconds after completion of the deglutitional act. The mandible habitually returns to postural resting position at the terminus of the deglutition cycle.

After the films are developed, tracings can be made (OVD and PVD) and superimposed on one another. The amount of interocclusal clearance can be recorded and the path of closure is indicated by joining the incisal margins of the lower incisors in postural resting position and occlusion and by drawing a straight line between these two points extending superiorly (Fig. 8–48). Normally, this line shows an upward and forward path of closure from postural resting position to occlusion. If the line is vertical or upward and backward, this may indicate a functional problem with probable tooth guidance and condylar displacement. (See Chap. 3.) Additional cephalometric records should then be made to confirm this functional abnormality. A wide open mouth cephalogram shows the outline of the condyle clearly. A template can be made of the condyle and transferred to the resting and occlusal headplates, where the condyle is often obscured by bony superimposition. This permits a clearer picture of the direction and amount of condylar displacement from postural resting position to occlusion. Normally, as was pointed out in Chapter 3, condylar movement should be rotary with little or no translatory movement from rest to occlusion (Fig. 3–37).

If clinical examination indicates that initial contact is in reality premature contact and that continued closing of the mandible is under aberrant tooth guidance, it is probable that habitual occlusion is not harmonious with centric relation. Lateral headplates taken with the teeth at initial contact help to define the path of closure more clearly. If a tracing is then made of the initial contact headplate and superimposed on the postural resting position and occlusal posi- tion headplate tracing, a functional problem becomes immediately apparent. The mandible closes upward and forward to the point of initial contact. Thereafter, a marked change in the path of closure occurs, usually changing to an upward and backward direction for the remainder of closure to full occlusion, with dominant posterior temporalis muscle activity. This clinical picture often indicates an excessive interocclusal clearance and incisal guidance. The correction of the vertical discrepancy may eliminate this abnormality. How this may be done is discussed in Chapter 16 in the section on excessive overbite.

Additional cephalometric records that are occasionally of value are the end-to-end "bite," or incision; a lateral projection taken during the phonation of

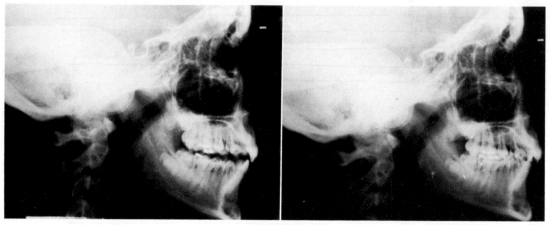

Figure 8–49   Lateral cephalograms in postural resting and habitual occlusal positions. This patient has a functional retrusion as a result of lingually inclined maxillary central incisors. The path of closure is thus upward and forward to point of initial contact, then upward and backward from the remaining closure into occlusion, under the influence of tooth guidance. (From Graber, T. M.: The "three M's": muscles, malformation, and malocclusion. Am. J. Orthodont., 49:418–450, 1963.)

the sound "ooo"; or special views taken with barium, iodochloral or other radiopaque media to determine soft tissue function. The incision headplate helps analyze the curve of Spee and the amount of space between the posterior segments with the incisors in contact. A phonation headplate shows tongue and soft palate position and may assist the speech therapist. Views with radiopaque media are particularly useful in cleft lip and cleft palate patients, helping to analyze velopharyngeal function. Such a headplate is indispensable to the prosthodontist who would fabricate a cleft palate prosthesis. (See Fig. 3–46.) Radiopaquing paste over the profile will assist in visualizing the soft tissue outline. This aids in the cephalometric profile analysis.

OTHER SPECIAL X-RAY VIEWS

THE 45 DEGREE LATERAL PROJECTION.   Since the two lateral aspects of the body of the mandible proceed from the symphysis backward on an expanding "V," the lateral cephalometric headplate, with the central ray perpendicular to the midsagittal plane, does not present a true picture of the contact relationship of the posterior teeth. Intraoral radiographs of the molar teeth often distort second and third molar images, too. The 45 degree lateral headplate, or lateral jaw projection, gives a more accurate recording of actual tooth position in either the left or right buccal segment, depending on which side is approximately perpendicular to the central ray (Fig. 8–50). These projections are of value in following the progress of serial extraction cases (Chaps. 11, 15) and third molar eruption. Panoramic laminagraphic views, if available, obviate the need for projections.[19, 20]

OCCLUSAL INTRAORAL FILMS.   Because of the limitations of size of the conventional intraoral periapical film and because both left and right sides are superimposed on the lateral headplate, the use of the larger intraoral occlusal film will permit the dentist to check for supernumerary or congenitally missing teeth more carefully and to observe abnormal eruption patterns, particularly of the canines (Fig. 8–51). Special occlusal film cassettes with intensifying

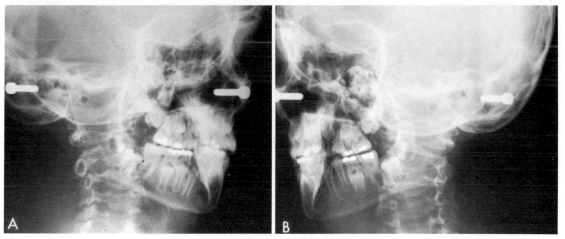

Figure 8–50 (A) Left and (B) right 45 degree cephalograms of case similar to that shown in conventional lateral and frontal cephalograms in Figure 8–30. This type of oriented headfilm gives a more accurate picture of the relationship of erupted and nonerupted teeth than conventional lateral jaw films. It may be used to advantage for serial extraction cases and as a record of longitudinal changes because of precise and reproducible orientation factors. (Courtesy W. S. Hunter, University of Western Ontario.)

Figure 8–51 A, Mesiodens supernumerary as seen in occlusal projection. B, Occlusal films show patient under orthodontic treatment, with maxillary canines blocked lingually. C, Occlusal view shows second premolar and canine position clearly.

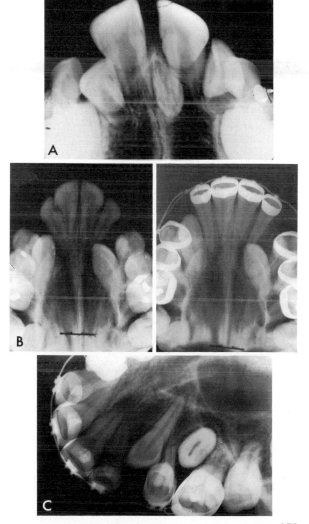

screens reduce the exposure time considerably. Whenever an impacted canine is to be uncovered in the palate, an occlusal view of this area is mandatory. Occlusal views are also of value in an arch length analysis, instead of long cone technique intraoral films. Although magnification is greater, individual tooth malpositions are seen, and the error is minimal.[11]

ELECTROMYOGRAPHIC EXAMINATION

The dentist seldom has access to and rarely needs equipment which provides electromyographic records. But, knowing the importance of muscle activity and the effect of abnormal muscle function on the dentition, there are times when such records are of value. In a severe Class II, Division 1 malocclusion, it can be seen clinically that the mentalis muscle is hyperactive and the upper lip is hypofunctional, while the lower lip strongly extends upward and forward during swallowing to force the maxillary incisors labially. Electromyographic studies verify this clinical observation (Fig. 6–55). In addition, they indicate that the buccinator may contract excessively. In Class II, Division 1 malocclusion the posterior fibers of the temporalis seem to exert greater influence than with a normal occlusion.

Vertical dimension problems are also amenable to electromyographic study.[66, 67] Overclosure, with concomitant retrusive posterior temporalis and deep masseter activity, can create anteroposterior discrepancies, accentuating the Class II malocclusion, for example. It is a simple matter to check muscle fiber group contraction. Space age telemetry provides monitoring equipment that is now available in a number of medical laboratories. The dentist should develop a connection with the laboratory, as does the physician, to obtain information not available from equipment in his own office.

With further progress in electromyography it is quite possible that more definitive studies may be made on pterygoid muscle activity. This may give us a clue to the solution of some of our temporomandibular joint problems. Analysis of tongue function is essential, and this may be possible with improved techniques. If the patient has had poliomyelitis, and there is an asymmetrical arch form, electromyographic examination may show that the selective attack of polio has "knocked out" certain muscle components, accounting for the asymmetry. For the same reason, an electromyographic examination may also be of value in children with cerebral palsy. Paralysis or hyperkinetic activity of muscles associated with the stomatognathic system undoubtedly leave their mark.

HAND-WRIST RADIOGRAPH

Since the orthodontist works with growth, it helps to have as much information as possible on the growth pattern and the degree of accomplishment of that pattern for each patient. Development of the Todd maturation series has shown that the hand-wrist radiographic examination can give an accurate bone age picture. Frequently the chronologic age is advanced or retarded when compared with the bone age. Because the orthodontist works primarily with teeth and bone, the bone age can give him information that may not be obtainable from other diagnostic criteria. Such information may help him coordinate treat-

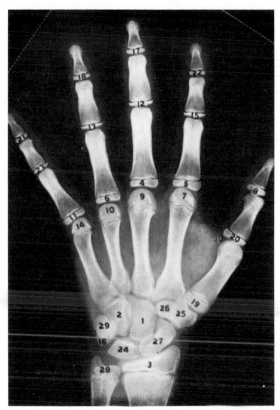

Figure 8–52   The individual carpals and epiphyses in the numbered hand above are numbered approximately in the order in which their ossification begins: 1, capitate; 2, hamate; 3, distal epiphysis of the radius; 4,° epiphysis of proximal phalanx of the third digit; 5,° epiphysis of proximal phalanx of the second digit; 6,° epiphysis of proximal phalanx of the fourth digit; 7, epiphysis of the second metacarpal; 8, epiphysis of distal phalanx of the first digit; 9, epiphysis of the third metacarpal; 10, epiphysis of the fourth metacarpal; 11, epiphysis of proximal phalanx of the fifth digit; 12, epiphysis of middle phalanx of the third digit; 13, epiphysis of middle phalanx of the fourth digit; 14, epiphysis of the fifth metacarpal; 15, epiphysis of middle phalanx of the second digit; 16, triquetral; 17, epiphysis of distal phalanx of the third digit, 18, epiphysis of distal phalanx of the fourth digit; 19, epiphysis of the first metacarpal; 20,° epiphysis of proximal phalanx of the first digit; 21, epiphysis of the distal phalanx of the fifth digit; 22, epiphysis of distal phalanx of the second digit; 23,° epiphysis of middle phalanx of the fifth digit; 24,° lunate; 25,° trapezium; 26,° trapezoid; 27,° scaphoid; 28, distal epiphysis of the ulna; 29, pisiform; 30, sesamoid of adductor pollicis (the sesamoid of flexor pollicis brevis is visible through the head of the first metacarpal, just below the numeral 2 on the epiphysis of the proximal phalanx of the thumb).

°Irregularities in the order of appearance are most apt to occur in those centers indicated by asterisks. (Courtesy Greulich, W. W., and Pyle, S. I.: Radiographic Atlas of Skeletal Development of the Hand and Wrist. 2nd ed. Stanford University Press, 1959.)

ment procedures with vital growth processes. While these records are not in widespread use and while the average dentist is not able to interpret hand-wrist radiographs properly, if taken and correctly interpreted by a qualified radiologist they may also assist the orthodontist in outlining his treatment plan as well as his treatment timing.[30, 68] The carpals and distal ends of the radius and ulna are most practical to use in assessing skeletal or bone age, showing a rather good correlation with downward and forward lower face growth. Growth spurts during puberty and at other times are reflected in the dentofacial complex as well as in other parts of the body. The condyle cannot be used as an area of maturational assessment, however, since it is not a true epiphysis. Qualifying any bone age assessment are the sex differences, familial maturational patterns and metabolic and nutritional factors. Figure 8–52 shows the approximate order of ossification. Figure 8–55 indicates average ages of ossification of various centers for boys and girls. Figure 8–53 gives average age of appearance and fusion of ossification centers for boys and girls. From these and standards developed for all ages, a good clue to growth accomplishment and amounts of growth yet to be accomplished may be seen. There is a wide range of normal, however, and it is recommended that the dentist emulate the physician and send his patients directly to the laboratory for a bone age assessment and for expertise in picture quality, detail and accuracy in age projection, based on visualization of the hand-wrist radiograph. It should be emphasized that the interpretation may give a general idea of *amounts* of growth but not *direction* of growth, which is of clinical im-

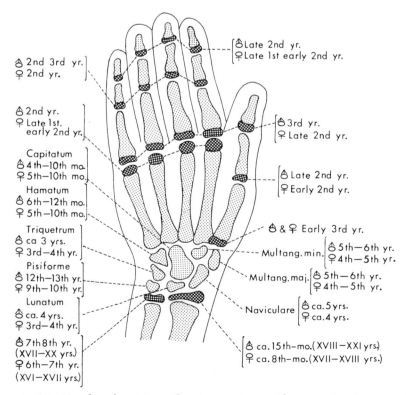

Figure 8–53   Hand and wrist ossification centers with approximate time of appearance and fusion for both male and female. (After Scammon.)

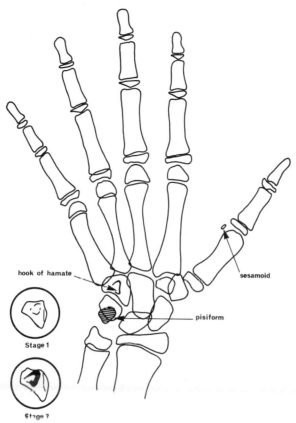

hook of hamate

sesamoid

pisiform

Stage 1

Stage 2

Figure 8–54 Ossification events inspected in final analysis. (Courtesy K. C. Grave.)

portance in treating basal malrelationships of teeth and jaws. Great amounts of downward and backward growth in a Class II, Division 1 malocclusion require entirely different therapeutic objectives and similar amounts of downward and forward lower face growth. Familial patterns and serial cephalometric radiographs provide a good source of information here.

Certain centers in the hand-wrist radiograph seem to have more significance than others. Absence of a sesamoid bone at the average age of onset of puberty in a female means likely retardation of pubertal development. Björk uses the ulna-sesamoid center as an indicator of growth completion, but Krogman attributes more variability to this center. Nevertheless, it is a good clue.[46, 69, 83]

Grave has demonstrated that the developmental status of a child is better measured in relationship to specified stages of maturation—in other words, against a scale of events rather than chronologically.[70] The maturational events he uses are shown in Figure 8–54. In his study, using the pisiform, hamate and sesamoid bones, Grave assessed the relations between timing of maturation events, maximum growth in body height and maximum facial growth during the circumpuberal period. Results showed that the initial ossification of the pisiform and the hook of the hamate preceded peak growth in most boys and girls. While initial ossification of the sesamoid of the thumb and advanced ossification of the hook of the hamate coincided with peak growth in most boys, this was true in only about half of the girls (Fig. 8–55).[70, 82]

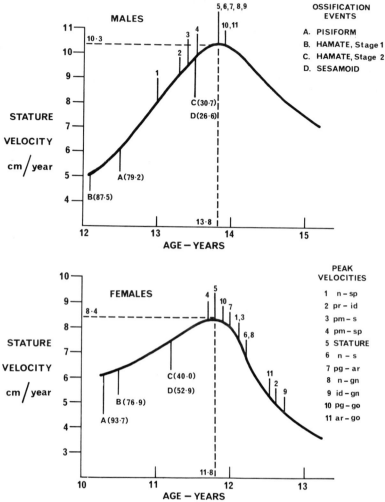

Figure 8–55   Mean time interval between ossification events and peak velocity in stature and facial dimensions. Percentage of subjects in which ossification events occurred before peak velocity in stature shown in brackets. (Courtesy K. C. Grave.)

BASAL METABOLIC RATE AND OTHER ENDOCRINE TESTS

It was pointed out in Chapter 6 on the Etiology of Malocclusion that endocrine upsets may produce, or at least be partly responsible for, dental malocclusions. One of the characteristic sequelae of hypothyroidism, for example, is the delayed eruption pattern. Whenever the dentist suspects endocrine problems, he should refer the patient to the family physician or to an endocrinologist for further testing. Of special value are the T-3 – T-4 (thyroid profile examination), PBI, B.M.R., etc. A negative B.M.R. may be the first indication of a thyroid disturbance. The dentist must not only recognize and intercept dental problems; it is equally his responsibility to see that the patient receives general medical care for any disturbance that may originate outside the stomatognathic system, with secondary oral manifestations.

BIOSTATISTICS

Here is a final word on dentistry and statistics in this chapter on diagnosis. It is not within the purview of this text to delve into the intricacies of biometric analysis. Yet in many fields besides dentistry and in most dental specialties, a knowledge of the fundamental principles of statistics is essential, if for no other reason than to be able to appraise the current literature and the increasingly computerized existence we lead. Brader, Solow and others have already pointed out the possibilities of the computer in diagnostic procedures.[4, 35, 71]

Ricketts has developed a computerized cephalometric analysis that is claimed to have a high degree of accuracy on growth prediction.[72, 76] Walker has a similar computerized cephalometric approach. This service is now available commercially and should improve as the data bank continues to enlarge. Using the coordinate system, headfilms may be analyzed directly on the viewer, and the information is fed directly into the computer for storage, analysis and retrieval. The experimental error inherent in making a pencil tracing is eliminated and the stochastic error in general is reduced.[74, 77–80]

As other diagnostic criteria are programmed for computer handling and information from multiple sources is stored, objective diagnosis becomes a reality. Therapy will be based less and less on teleology and selected clinical responses to a particular type of appliance, and more on the biomechanical foundation of orthodontics, transcending all so-called treatment philosophies.[81]

CASE ANALYSIS

J. L., age 13 years, Caucasian, male

1. General health is good; physique and posture normal.

2. Face is mesocephalic, profile convex, with familial pattern (mother) of mandibular retrusion. Two previous siblings were treated who had similar malocclusion. Premaxillary segment seems protrusive with respect to mandible and cranial structures. Lower face height gives impression of vertical deficiency.

Lip posture shows hypotonic, flaccid and hypofunctional upper lip, with lips habitually parted. Lower lip is curled, somewhat redundant, with marked mentolabial sulcus.

Face is symmetrical, nose of average shape and size; chin button adequate.

Muscle activity during deglutition, respiration and speech is abnormal, with excessive mentalis activity and with lower lip cushioning to the lingual aspect of maxillary incisors. Sibilant speech defect noted. Mouth breathing is chronic, but mother says that child also has a history of allergy.

3. Examination of mouth reveals a Class I malocclusion showing Class II, Division 1 characteristics, with usual sequelae of excessive overjet and deep overbite. Upper arch is narrow but no cross-bite is present.

All permanent teeth are present except upper right canine, lower right first premolar, lower left second premolar, lower left canine, upper second molars and all four third molars. The upper left and lower left deciduous second molars are still retained. Upper left canine just erupting and upper right canine appears about to erupt. Maxillary central incisors appear overly large. Dental caries is seen clinically, at buccal, lower left first molar.

Arch length is deficient, with some crowding in lower anterior segment; lower left canine and right first premolar spaces are inadequate. This makes tooth-to-bone ratio questionable and dependent on teeth present and yet unerupted, on cephalometric analysis, etc.

Oral hygiene appears adequate.

The soft tissue appraisal shows normal texture and color of gingival and mucosal tissue, except on labial side of lower anterior teeth, where there is hemorrhage. Labial

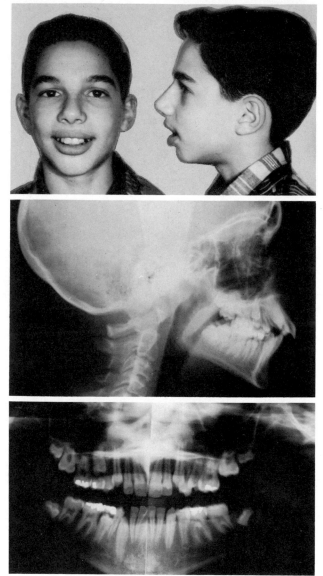

Figure 8–56 Photographs, headplate and panoramic view of J. L. Muscle imbalance, protrusion and congenital absence are immediately apparent.

frenum, lingual frenum, tongue size and shape appear normal. Palate, tonsils and adenoids are negative; vestibular mucosa normal. No nodes are palpated. Lip morphology appears adaptive to malocclusion with short, functionless upper lip, redundant lower lip, habitually parted. Some cracking of lower lip is present and may be attributed to mouth breathing.

A functional analysis indicates an easily attainable postural resting position, excessive interocclusal clearance and normal path of closure from rest to habitual occlusion with no apparent prematurities or tooth guidance or posterior mandibular displacement. No clicking, crepitus or abnormality noted in temporomandibular joints. Normal range of mandibular movement in protrusive, lateral excursive and retrusive maneuvers. Lower lip cushions to the lingual side of upper incisors during function; upper lip has relatively little activity. No excessive mobility of teeth is found on tapping in habitual occlusion. Tongue tends to thrust slightly, but pressures appear within normal limits on deglutition.

CAST ANALYSIS

Cast analysis is made in conjection with panoramic and cephalometric radiographic records. Lower right first premolar is missing; lower left canine present but with inadequate space to erupt. There is a 3 mm. discrepancy of tooth size, with maxillary central incisors overly large. Both maxillary first molars are rotated, indicating slight mesial drift. Right side shows more drift and this results in a slight asymmetry. Mesial drift is more apparent at lower right buccal segment because of absence of first premolar. Deciduous molars are about to be shed. Individual tooth malpositions are already noted in clinical examination. No signs of abnormal attrition or facets indicating tooth guidance.

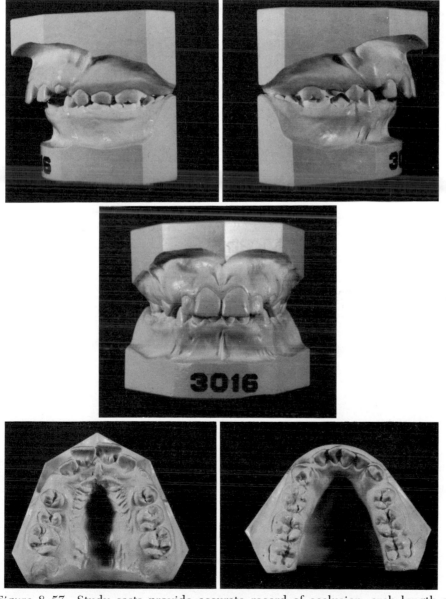

Figure 8–57 Study casts provide accurate record of occlusion, arch length adequacy, etc.

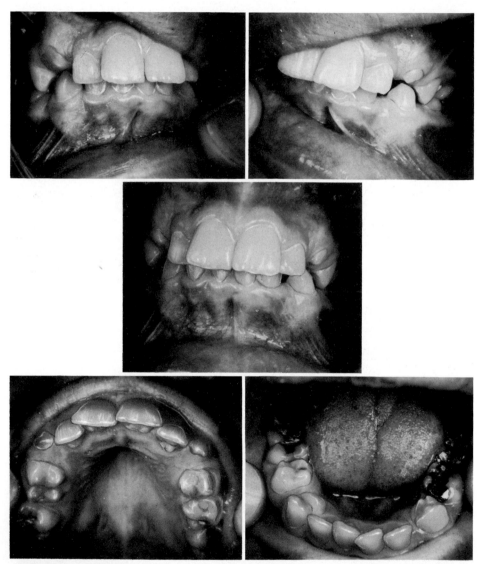

Figure 8–58 Intraoral views which are permanent records of tooth arrangement and soft tissue configuration at the beginning of treatment.

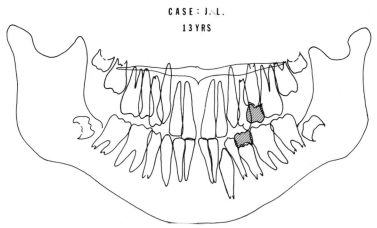

Figure 8–59 Tracing of panoramic radiograph shown in Figure 8–56. Congenital absence of the lower right first premolar has allowed eruption of permanent canine; lack of arch length on lower right as well as in maxillary arch is illustrated.

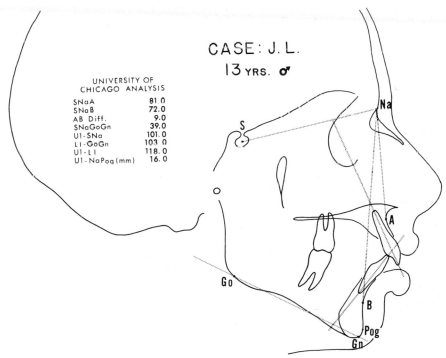

Figure 8–60 Cephalometric tracing of headplate on 8–56. Excessive basal difference, steeper than normal mandibular plane, labial inclination of lower incisors, more acute angle of facial convexity and excessive prominence of the upper incisors with regard to the facial plane are the obvious observations.

RADIOGRAPHIC ANALYSIS

Since the oral examination indicates clinical absence of upper right canine, lower right first premolar, lower left second premolar, lower left canine, upper second molars and all third molars, perusal of the panoramic radiograph is indicated to check out the clinical observations. The clinically missing teeth are all found to be present, except the lower right first premolar. The remaining deciduous teeth show imminent exfoliation. Arch length deficiency is corroborated in the lower left canine and upper left second premolar regions, as well as the upper right canine area. Teeth show a good state of caries repair, except for cavity previously noted. An interesting observation which supports the original impression of mesial drift of the lower right buccal segment is the distance between the developing lower right third molar and the distal aspect of the second molar which has already erupted. On the left side, where there are no missing teeth, there is less space. Yet the direction of eruption of the third molar on the left is better than the mesially inclined third molar on the lower right. The upper left second premolar appears rotated in the alveolar process. Condylar morphology and relationships appear within normal limits.

The cephalometric analysis indicates an excessive anteroposterior dysplasia, with an apical base difference of 9 degrees. This is a familial pattern, and probably unrelated to the missing tooth in the lower arch. The mandibular plane is also steeper than normal, and the facial profile decidedly convex. Lips are parted, with the upper lip short and hypotonic and the lower lip heavy and redundant. This correlates with clinical and photographic evidence. The inclination of the maxillary incisors is within normal limits, but they appear protrusive because of the mandibular retrusion. Actually, the position with respect to the cranium is close to the mean values for the maxillary apical base. The mandibular incisors show some procumbency, but with a convex face this is not necessarily abnormal. But the intersection of the long axes of the upper and lower incisors shows a more acute angle than normal, and this, together with the higher reading of the lower incisor (101.0 degrees) to mandibular plane, could be interpreted as labial inclination of the lower incisors. The fact that the upper incisors are as much as 16 mm. ahead of the facial plane (NaPog) is clinically and esthetically significant. All signs point to the mandibular retrusion as a major factor. With one tooth more in the maxillary arch than in the mandibular arch, elimination of the discrepancy without tooth removal would seem unlikely. Yet it will be difficult to maintain correct maxillary incisor inclination, preventing excessive lingual inclination and return of a deeper than normal overbite after therapy.

PHOTOGRAPHIC ANALYSIS

Facial and intraoral photographs corroborate clinical and cephalometric evidence of a convex profile, deep overbite, short hypotonic upper lip, heavy, redundant lower lip, normal size and shape of nose and reasonably adequate chin button. Early tetracycline administration during tooth formation lends a grayish cast to the incisors.

TREATMENT OBJECTIVES

Obviously, as much as possible should be done to establish normal facial balance and to position the teeth in harmony with this naturally convex profile. Elimination of abnormal muscle habits and establishment of proper lip position and activity are of high priority.

The correction of the dental malocclusion, the arch length deficiency, the imbalance of tooth material in one arch as opposed to the other — not only in number, but in size of teeth — and the establishment of proper interdigitation must be attempted.

Since the patient is a boy, and just beginning his pubertal growth spurt, it is hoped that there will be an "assist" because of this, but the steeper than normal mandibular plane, the excessive apical base difference and the familial Class II pattern militate against any appreciable help or optimism. The growth may occur, but the direction may be largely vertical, rather than downward and forward.

Any appreciable correction in profile and muscle patterns must come from retropositioning the maxillary and mandibular incisors, without increasing the overbite. The third molars are developing normally and should erupt if there is adequate space. Therefore, the removal of the three remaining first premolars (the lower right first premolar is missing) is indicated.

The real challenge will be to move the maxillary anterior segment bodily posteriorly without tipping the maxillary incisors excessively lingually. This means constant application of lingual tipping forces to the apical portions of the incisors (i.e., torque). The steeper than normal mandibular plane and the excessive apical base difference make establishment and maintenance of a normal overbite difficult. Prognosis is poor in this respect. "Control" is the appliance watchword; objectives require a fixed multibanded appliance that will achieve maximum torque, root control for uprighting of teeth over basal bone and for closing extraction space by paralleling contiguous teeth. Such appliances must exert a depressing force on anterior teeth, to eliminate excessive overbite. Lower incisors may still have to remain somewhat procumbent to correct the overjet, to compensate for apical base dysplasia and to reduce the tendency to tip the maxillary incisors lingually.

Retention will be demanded of the type that prevents reoccurrence of excessive overbite and overjet. Individual tooth malpositions should be no problem.

REFERENCES

1. Moorrees, C. F. A., and Grøn, A. M.: Principles of orthodontic diagnosis. Angle Orthodont., 36:258–262, 1966.
2. Ackerman, J. L., and Proffit, W. R.: The characteristics of malocclusion: a modern approach to classification and diagnosis. Am. J. Orthodont., 56:443–454, 1969.
3. Graber, T. M. (ed.): Current Orthodontic Concepts and Techniques. Philadelphia, W. B. Saunders Co., 1969.
4. Biggerstaff, R. H.: Computerized diagnostic setups and simulations. Angle Orthodont., 4:28–36, 1970.
5. Boersma, H.: The set-up. Nederl. T. Tandheelk., 76:459–469, 1969.
6. Boersma, H.: Disharmony of mesiodistal measurements of the maxillary teeth in relation to those of the mandibular teeth., Nederl. T. Tandheelk., 75:836–854, 1968.
7. Sanin, C., Savara, B. S., Clarkson, Q. C., and Thomas, D. R.: Prediction of occlusion by measurements of the deciduous dentition. Am. J. Orthodont., 57:561–572, 1970.
8. Bowden, D.: A clinical assessment of mixed dentition crowding. Aust. Dent. J., 14:90–98, 1969.
9. Bolton, W. A.: The clinical application of a tooth size analysis. Am. J. Orthodont., 48:504–529, 1962.
10. Hasund, A., and Sivertsen, R.: Dental arch space and facial type. Angle Orthodont., 11:140–145, 1971.
11. Shepard, E. E.: Orthodontic undergraduate clinical procedure (manual), St. Louis, Washington University, 1971.
12. Riedel, R. A.: Diagnosis and treatment planning on orthodontics. D. Clin. North America, 12:175–187, 1969.
13. Sanin, C., and Savara, B. S.: An analysis of permanent mesiodistal crown size. Am. J. Orthodont., 59:488–500, 1971.
14. Owen, D. G.: Plaster cast analysis. Unpublished data, University of Chicago, 1972.
15. Moorrees, C. F. A., and Reed, R. B.: Correlations among crown diameters of human teeth. Arch. Oral Biol., 9:685–697, 1964.
16. Moorrees, C. F. A., and Chadha, J. M.: Crown diameters of corresponding tooth groups in deciduous and permanent dentition. J. Dent. Res., 41:466–470, 1962.
17. Moyers, R. E.: Handbook of Orthodontics. 3rd ed., Chicago, Yearbook Medical Publishers, 1972.
18. Garn, S. M., Lewis, A. B., and Kerewsky, R. S.: Size inter-relationships of the mesial and distal teeth. J. Dent. Res., 44:350–353, 1965.
19. Graber, T. M.: Panoramic radiography in dentistry. J. Canad. Dent. Ass., 31:158–173, 1965.

20. Graber, T. M.: Diagnosis and panoramic radiography. Am. J. Orthodont., 53:799–821, 1967.
21. Hauck, R. M.: Documentation of tooth movement by means of panoral radiography. Am. J. Orthodont., 57:386–392, 1970.
22. Zach, G. A., Langland, O. E., and Sippy, E. H.: The use of the orthopantomograph in longitudinal studies. Angle Orthodont., 39:42–50, 1969.
23. Joondeph, D. R., Riedel, R. A., and Moore, A. W.: Pont's Index: a clinical evaluation. Angle Orthodont., 40:112–118, 1970.
24. Hunter, W. S., and Garn, S. M.: Evidence of a secular trend in face size. Angle Orthodont., 39:320–323, 1969.
25. Uesato, G.: Esthetic facial balance of American-Japanese. Am. J. Orthodont., 54:601–611, 1968.
26. Drummond, R. A.: Determination of cephalometric norms for the Negro race. Am. J. Orthodont., 54:670–682, 1968.
27. Choy, O. W. C.: Cephalometric study of the Hawaiian. Angle Orthodont., 39:93–108, 1969.
28. Bang, G., and Hasund, A.: Morphologic characteristics of the Alaskan Eskimo dentition. Am. J. Phys. Anthrop., 35:43–47, 1971.
29. Hellman, M.: An introduction to growth of the human face from infancy to adulthood. Int. J. Orth. Oral Surg. Radiol., 18:777–798, 1932.
30. Todd, T. W.: Atlas of Skeletal Maturation. St. Louis, C. V. Mosby, 1937.
31. Broadbent, B. H.: Ontogenetic development of occlusion. Angle Orthodont., 11:223–241, 1941.
32. Hofrath, H.: Die Bedeutung der Röntgenfern- und Abstandsaufnahme für die Diagnostik der Kieferanomalien. Fortschr. Orthodont., 1:34–41, 1931.
33. Van der Linden, F. P. G. M.: A study of roentgenocephalometric bony landmarks. Am. J. Orthodont., 59:111–125, 1971.
34. Johnston, L. E.: Statistical evaluation of cephalometric prediction. Angle Orthodont., 38:284–304, 1968.
35. Solow, B.: Computers in cephalometric research. Comput. Biol. Med., 1:41–49, 1970.
36. Krogman, W. M.: Biological timing and the dento-facial complex. J. Dent. Child., 35:377–381, 1968.
37. Meredith, H. V.: Serial study of change in a mandibular dimension during childhood and adolescence. Growth, 25:229–242, 1961.
38. Popovitch, F.: Prevalence of the sucking habit and its relationship to malocclusion. Oral Health, 57:498–499, 1967.
39. Woodside, D. G.: Distance, velocity and relative growth rate standards for mandibular growth for Canadian males and females age 3 to 20 years. American Board of Orthodontics thesis, 1969.
40. Leighton, B. C.: The value of prophecy in orthodontics. Dent. Pract., 21:359–372, 1971.
41. Leighton, B. C.: Some observations on vertical development and the dentition. Proc. Roy. Soc. Med., 61:1273–1277, 1968.
42. Susami, R.: A cephalometric evaluation of dentofacial growth in mandibular protrusion subjects. J. Osaka Univ. Dent. Sch., 9:25–35, 1969.
43. Subtelny, J. D.: Cephalometric diagnosis, growth and treatment: something old, something new? Am. J. Orthodont., 57:262–286, 1970.
44. Abraham, R. A.: A cephalometric investigation of craniofacial growth based on an occlusal reference system. Angle Orthodont., 39:198–208, 1969.
45. Björk, A.: Prediction of mandibular growth rotation. Am. J. Orthodont., 55:585–599, 1969.
46. Björk, A.: The use of metallic implants in the study of facial growth in children: method and application. Am. J. Phys. Anthrop. 29:243–254, 1968.
47. Björk, A., and Helm, S.: Prediction of age at maximum puberal growth in body height. Angle Orthodont., 37:134–151, 1967.
48. Graber, T. M.: Implementation of the roentgenographic cephalometric technique. Am. J. Orthodont., 44:906–932, 1958.
49. Krogman, W. M.: Validation of the roentgenographic cephalometric technique. Am. J. Orthodont., 44:933–939, 1958.
50. Hasund, A., and Sivertsen, R.: An evaluation of the diagnostic triangle in relation to the facial type, the inclination of the horizontal facial planes and the degree of facial prognathism. Acta Universit. Bergensis, Medisinske Avhandl., 4, 1969.
51. Myklebust, S., Hasund, A., and Bøe, O.: The use of the nasion-pogonion line as a reference line to the position of the upper incisors. Fasett, no. 2, 113–122, 1970.
52. Myklebust, S., Hasund, A., and Bøe, O.: The use of the nasion-pogonion line as a reference line to the position of the lower incisors. Fasett, no. 3, 165–174, 1970.
53. Iijuka, T., and Ishikawa, F.: Normal standards for various cephalometric analyses in Japanese adults. J. Jap. Orth. Soc., 16:4–12, 1957.
54. Cotton, W. N., Takano, W. S., and Wong, W. W.: The Downs analysis applied to three other ethnic groups. Angle Orthodont., 21:213–224, 1951.
55. Kobayashi, F.: A study of cephalometric characteristics of Japanese-American in Orange County, California. American Board of Orthodontics thesis, 1961.
56. Kayukawa, H.: Roentgenographic-cephalometric cranio-facial morphology of Japanese. J. Jap. Orth. Soc., 13:6–17, 1954, 14:6–12, 1955.
57. Miura, F., Inoue, N., and Suzuki, K.: The standards of Steiner's analysis for Japanese. Bull. Tokyo Med. Dent. Univ., 10:387–395, 1963.

58. Chang, T. G. M.: An evaluation of the "norm" in the Oriental face and its comparison to Downs and Steiner standards. Master's thesis, University of Southern California, 1964.
59. Hasund, A., and Ulstein, G.: The position of the incisors in relation to the lines NA and NB in different facial types. Am. J. Orthodont., 57:1–14, 1970.
60. Lundström, A.: Introduction to Orthodontics. New York, Blakiston, 1965.
61. Ackerman, J., and Proffit, W.: Treatment response as an aid in diagnosis and treatment planning. Am. J. Orthodont., 57:490–496, 1970.
62. Bosma, J. F.: Evaluation of oral function for the orthodontic patient. Am. J. Orthodont., 55:578–584, 1969.
63. McDowell, C. S.: A reappraisal of cephalometrics, I & II, J. Clin. Orth., 4:82–92, 134–145, 1970.
64. Schwindling, R., and Stark, W.: An electronic investigation of rest position of the mandible. Stoma, 21:15–24, 1968.
65. Graber, T. M.: Overbite—the dentist's challenge. J.A.D.A., 79:1135–1145, 1969.
66. Proctor, A. D., and DeVincenzo, J. P.: Masseter muscle position relative to dentofacial form. Angle Orthodont., 40:37–44, 1970.
67. Nagy, L., and Denes, J.: Electromyographic analysis of temporal and masseter muscle activity in persons with normal occlusion and deep bite. Fogorv. Szemle, 61:235–238, 1968.
68. Greulich, W. W., and Pyle, S. I.: Radiographic atlas of skeletal development of the hand and wrist. Palo Alto, Stanford University Press, 1959.
69. Krogman, W. M.: Personal communication, October 26, 1971.
70. Grave, K. C.: Timing of facial growth in Australian aborigines. Adelaide, University of Adelaide, 1971.
71. Brader, A. C.: Differential orthodontic diagnosis and treatment planning. Am. J. Orthodont., 51:806–815, 1965.
72. Ricketts, R. M.: The evolution of diagnosis to computerized cephalometrics. Am. J. Orthodont., 55:796–803, 1969.
73. Baumrind, S., and Frantz, R.: The reliability of head film measurements. 1. landmark identification. Am. J. Orthodont., 60:111–127, 1971.
74. Huddart, A. G., Clarke, J., and Thacker, T.: The application of computers to the study of maxillary arch dimensions. Brit. Dent. J., 130:397–404, 1971.
75. Brown, C. E., Christen, A. C., and Jerman, A. C.: Dimensions of the focal trough in panoramic radiography. J.A.D.A., 84:843–847, 1972.
76. Ricketts, R. M., Bench, R. W., Hilgers, J. J., and Schulhof, R.: An overview of computerized cephalometrics. Am. J. Orthodont., 61:1–28, 1972.
77. Krogman, W. M.: Use of computers in orthodontic analysis and diagnosis: Introduction. Am. J. Orthodont., 61:219–220, 1972.
78. Walker, G. F.: A new approach to the analysis of craniofacial morphology and growth. Am. J. Orthodont., 61:221–230, 1972.
79. Savara, B. S.: The role of computers in dentofacial research and the development of diagnostic aids. Am. J. Orthodont., 61:231–244, 1972.
80. Biggerstaff, R. H.: Computerized analysis of occlusion in the postcanine dentition. Am. J. Orthodont., 61:245–254, 1972.
81. Grewe, J. M., and Hagan, D. V.: Malocclusion indices: A comparative evaluation. Am. J. Orthodont., 286–294, 1972.
82. Brown, T., Barrett, M. J., and Grave, K. C.: Facial growth and skeletal maturation at adolescence. Tandlaegebladet, 75:1211–1222, 1971.
83. Helm, S., Siersbaek-Nielsen, S., Skieller, V., and Björk, A.: Skeletal maturation of the hand in relation to maximum puberal growth in body height. Tandlaegebladet, 75:1233–1234, 1971.
84. Hixon, E.: Simplified mechanics: a means of treatment based on available scientific information Am. J. Orthodont., 62:113–141, 1972.

chapter 9

UNFAVORABLE SEQUELAE OF MALOCCLUSION

To most people, orthodontics is purely for "looks." While this is one benefit that may accrue from the correction of a dental malocclusion, it is only a small part of the total picture. As the following list shows, facial esthetics is just one of 14 possible sequelae. Yet, as Moorrees and Grøn write, "Esthetics takes a special place among the indications for treatment because it is the foremost reason for patients, or their parents, to seek orthodontic consultation. Both orthodontists and plastic surgeons deal, therefore, with the important relation between esthetics, self image and psychologic adjustment. Both use the same approach to therapy, namely a change in morphology to improve well-being."[1]

It is not fair, however, to create the incorrect impression that orthodontists or, for that matter, dentists who place porcelain jackets on anterior teeth, are little more than glorified cosmeticians. As the following list indicates, a majority of the items concerns dental health, function of the stomatognathic system, longevity of the teeth and investing tissues and psychosocial sequelae, already alluded to in the previous quotation.

1. Unfavorable psychological and social sequelae
   a. Introversion, self-consciousness
   b. Response to uncomplimentary or derisive nicknames like "Bugs Bunny," "buck teeth" or "Bucky Beaver."
2. Poor appearance
3. Interference with normal growth and development and accomplishment of pattern
   a. Cross-bites causing facial asymmetries; effect on condylar growth of mandible
   b. Overbite and overjet influence on maxillary and mandibular anterior segments; possible retardation of normal pattern accomplishment
4. Improper or abnormal muscle function
   a. Compensatory muscle activities such as hyperactive mentalis muscle activity, hypoactive upper lip, increased buccinator pressures and tongue thrust that occur as a result of spatial relationships of teeth and jaws. These activities are unfavorable and serve to increase the departure from the normal.
   b. Associated muscle habits
      (1) Lip biting
      (2) Nail biting
      (3) Finger sucking

  (4) Tongue sucking
  (5) Temporomandibular joint disturbances
  (6) Bruxism
5. Improper deglutition
 a. Changed function as a result of adaptive demands of hard tissue structures on the musculature regularly associated with swallowing, and recruitment of musculature not ordinarily a part of the swallowing act
6. Mouth breathing
 a. Increased respiratory involvement (ear, nose, throat disorders)
 b. Enlarged tonsils and adenoids
 c. Enlarged turbinates
7. Improper mastication
 a. Abnormal function may increase malocclusion, as with abnormal swallowing.
 b. Possible nutritional deficiency
 c. Increased work load on digestive tract
8. Speech defects (sibilants, fricatives, plosives, anterior escapage, tongue position, etc.)
9. Increased caries incidence (result of less self-cleansing areas, poor contact surface apposition, packing of food, more difficult hygiene, etc.)
10. Predilection to periodontal disease
 a. Sequelae of poor hygiene ("Vincents," hypertrophic gingival tissue, etc.)
 b. Poor contacts, spaces and tipped teeth permit wedging of food and debris in gingival crevice.
 c. Lack of normal exercise
 d. Abnormal axial inclination, abnormal stresses, jiggling of teeth due to functional prematurities
 e. Earlier loss of teeth
11. Temporomandibular joint disorders; functional problems
 a. Tooth guidance, abnormal muscle function, overclosure or bruxism may cause clicking, crepitus, pain, limited motion and trismus.
12. Predilection to accidents
 a. Fractured teeth, devitalized or lost incisors
13. Impacted and unerupted teeth, possible follicular cysts, damage to other teeth
14. Prosthetic rehabilitation complications
 a. Space problems, poor contacts, teeth tipped and receiving abnormal stress

MALOCCLUSION AND UNFAVORABLE PSYCHOLOGICAL AND SOCIAL BEHAVIOR

One has only to see a few of the shy, self-conscious, withdrawn or overly demonstrative youngsters with protruding upper incisors and a typical "adenoidal facies" to realize the profound psychological impact that a malocclusion can have (Fig. 9–1). For many of these children who desperately want to look like other children, one glance in the mirror convinces them that they do not. And if this is not enough, the constant jibes of "Bugs Bunny," "bird beak," "Bucky Beaver" and similar epithets are not calculated to increase self confidence and feelings of acceptance.

The youngster who sucks his finger beyond the time that it is normal to do so frequently faces a psychological problem. He knows that his parents in particular and society in general frown on his behavior. He often sees that he is causing a facial abnormality and unpleasant appearance and is frustrated because he wants to stop and cannot. Many of these children and their parents are totally unaware that simple orthodontic procedures can help them to eliminate the habit and can restore normal appearance. Often these children become

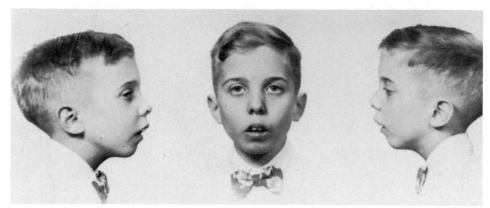

Figure 9–1 Adenoidal facies of a mouth breather whose dental malocclusion prevents him from closing his lips properly.

exceedingly introvertive or overassertive, and their social behavior is quite immature. Unfavorable psychological effects tend to accompany speech defects that are attributable to dental malocclusions. Certainly it is within the sphere of the dentist to remove these roadblocks to a normal, balanced psyche and a mature social attitude. Reasons of mental health are no less impelling than reasons of physical health of the teeth and investing tissues.

POOR APPEARANCE

Corollary to the psychological implications of malocclusion is the question of appearance. In our face-conscious society it seems that any departure from the usual or the "normal" attracts attention[2] (Fig. 9–1). For children this often means derision and ridicule. Obviously, because the child wants to be like his playmates and because facial disharmony is predisposing to psychological aberrations just mentioned, the dentist should do all he can either to intercept the malocclusion or to refer the child to an orthodontist for specialty care as indicated. Too often it is the parent who asks the dentist, "Doctor, don't you think we really ought to see an orthodontist about Susan? Her teeth stick out badly. She bumped them with a skate board the other day and nearly broke one tooth off."

Therapy may not be indicated at this time, but the orthodontist should make the decision, based on clinical experience and knowledge of the broad ramifications of dental malocclusion, concerning just what should be done at the earliest possible time. We cannot laugh off the child's or the parent's concern about unsightly teeth. One recent survey indicates that only 5 per cent of general dental practitioners make routine orthodontic referrals. This surely does not reflect their knowledge or seeming interest in their patients' welfare.

INTERFERENCE WITH NORMAL GROWTH
AND DEVELOPMENT

In the chapters on etiology of malocclusion it was stressed that abnormal growth and developmental patterns are apt to be a major basis for malocclusions. Such patterns are largely hereditary. But a normal developmental pattern may still be side-tracked by obstacles along the road toward the maturity of the

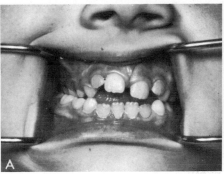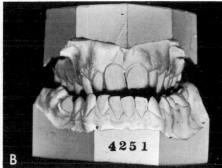

Figure 9–2 A, Right unilateral posterior cross-bite forces the mandible to shift to the right on occlusion. Compensatory tongue activity maintains the anterior open bite. B, Adult cross-bite, open bite and facial asymmetry resulting from uncorrected malocclusion during childhood.

stomatognathic system. Abnormal finger sucking habits, perverted perioral muscle function, premature loss and similar factors may upset the timetable and cause morphologic and functional changes detrimental to the dentition. A frequent result of a prolonged thumb sucking habit, with associated perioral muscle malfunction, is a posterior crossbite (Fig. 9–2). (See Fig. 6–63.)

Even though the narrowing of the maxillary arch is usually bilateral, the "convenience swing" is habitually to one side. Prolongation of this abnormal relationship can cause permanent changes in tooth position, in the bony support and possibly in the temporomandibular joint growth center. In many adults, facial asymmetry is traceable to a childhood unilateral crossbite that was not corrected.

Excessive overbite and an abnormal lower lip habit both exert strong lingual pressures on the mandibular anterior segment (Fig. 6–50). A break in contacts, rotations or a flattening of the mandibular anterior segment may ensue. If the malocclusion is intercepted, the integrity of the mandibular arch is often maintained, without the unfavorable dental and alveolar response.

In Class III malocclusions the maxillary anterior segment may suffer the same fate that the mandibular anterior segment does in Class II, Division 1 malocclusions. Particularly in a pseudo Class III malocclusion, where the condyle actually comes downward and forward in closure from postural resting position to occlusion, there is a constant retracting vector on the premaxillary region. The "flattened" alveolar process is mute testimony to the restrictive forces (Fig. 6–51).

IMPROPER OR ABNORMAL MUSCLE FUNCTION

ADAPTATION

Even as abnormal muscle function may be causative, or at least contributory, in the formation of a dental malocclusion it may also be resultant. In our analysis of etiology of malocclusions, we have not yet reached the point at which we may be sure which is cause and which is effect. In a number of instances a single factor may operate as both. It is likely that muscle activity is in this category. A hereditary basal malrelationship type of Class II, Division 1 malocclusion, for example, requires certain adaptive or compensatory muscle responses (Figs. 9–3 and 9–4). To swallow, the lower lip cushions behind the maxillary incisors; the tongue thrusts forward to "close off" or create an anterior seal required by deglutition. Thus, as was pointed out in Chapter 6, the lips no longer restrain the forward translation of the dental arches. The lower lip actually assists maxillary protrusion while exerting an abnormal lingual pressure on the mandibular anterior segment. The deformity is made worse by this compensatory activity. The idiomatic "vicious circle" is a most appropriate description (Figs. 6–76, 6–78).

Correction of the malocclusion in most instances eliminates the abnormal lip, tongue and buccal muscle activity. The hypoactive upper lip associated with Class II, Division 1 malocclusion, and the redundant and hypofunctional lower lip seen with Class III malocclusions, leave the "slackers' club" and join "the team."[6]

Even where the jaw relationship is normal and no compensatory muscle activity is required for mastication and deglutition (as in Class I malocclusions, for example), individuals may elicit an asynchronous contraction pattern of the masticatory muscles.[7] According to Moyers, motor impulses initiate occlusal movements, but are modified by disorganized proprioceptor responses in the PDM or TMJ, triggered at initial contact. Adaptive activity may induce aberrant patterns of occlusal activity as a result, enhancing the original malocclusion.

Furthermore, these adaptive responses may alter the degree of the tonal contraction under peripheral and central nervous system stimuli. Usually the

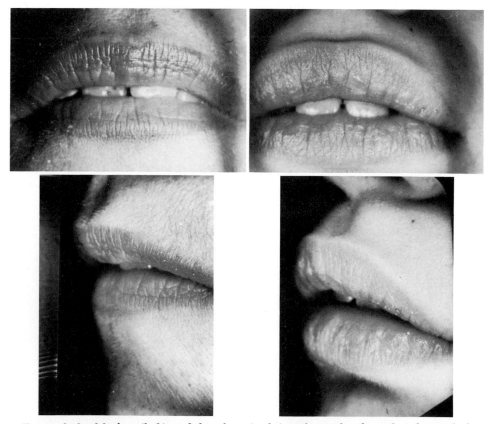

Figure 9–3   Mother (left) and daughter (right) with similar dentofacial morphology. It is likely that this is a hereditary type Class II, Division 1 malocclusion.

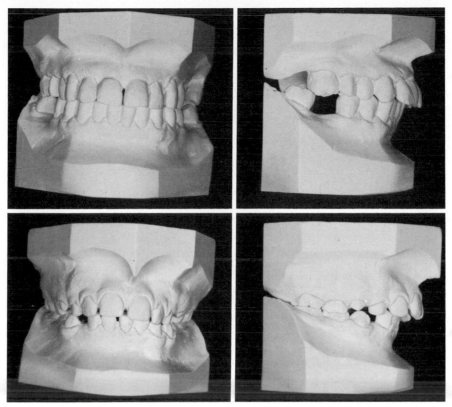

Figure 9–4   Plaster casts of Figure 9–3, mother (above) and daughter (below). Abnormal function and occlusal aberrations are main reasons for tooth loss and advanced periodontal involvement for mother. Note tooth guidance in right molar area. Mother complains of "tired jaw."

alteration is in the nature of a hypertonic response. Such a reaction is thus due to a combined occlusal disharmony and increased nervous excitability. Thus, even as perverted function of the perioral musculature in Class II, Division 1 malocclusions tends to increase the severity of the overbite and overjet, so hypertonicity that has developed in response to the occlusal disharmony and adaptive reaction in turn enhances the occlusal abnormalities. Injury to the supporting structures, fatigue and discomfort may lead to outright pain and trismus as the cycle develops under the guidance of the "feedback" mechanism. Temporomandibular joint disturbances are a logical result of the deteriorating situation, and may become the predominant clinical entity originating from an obscure occlusal disharmony or malocclusion.[8, 9]

ASSOCIATED MUSCLE HABITS

Associated with Class II malocclusions particularly are certain abnormal habits. Tongue thrust and sucking occur with greater frequency in children that have a Class II, Division 1 malocclusion (Fig. 6–79). In these cases, is the habit etiologic, symbiotic or resultant? Very probably the answer differs from individual to individual, and combinations of factors vary. It is likely that in a large number of children the tongue habit is at least partly the result of the inherent morphogenetic pattern of malocclusion. Lip biting and nail biting are also in the same category. A recent study by the author showed that a significantly larger percentage of children with basal or true maxillomandibular Class II, Division 1 malocclusions sucked their fingers than children with normal occlusions. The impression is correct that there is a higher percentage of retained infantile mechanisms such as tongue thrust and finger sucking. The longer period of transitional swallowing activity, from the infantile to the mature swallowing pattern, is evident. Here again, while the finger habit and tongue habit are partly causative, they also may be partly the result of the inability of abnormal perioral muscle function to satisfy the kinesthetic-neuromuscular and delicate sensory demands of the growing child. This important avenue of establishing a feeling of well-being (euphoria), is discussed in detail in Chapter 6.

BRUXISM

The picture of bruxism is equally clear. There is a strong correlation seen clinically between malocclusion and the incidence of "night grinding," clenching or bruxism.[10] (Chaps. 4 and 6). Occlusal disharmonies and excessive overbite are associated most frequently with these functional aberrations. Although the exact cause of clenching and bruxism is unknown, it is recognized that certain sensory and proprioceptive impulses are involved, as with the temporomandibular joint disturbances. Thus, a malocclusion with premature contacts or a deep overbite is apparently able to "trigger" the habit. Anyone who has heard the grating, cracking and rending noise associated with bruxism can appreciate the forces involved and the need for the elimination of the habit, if possible. Other factors are involved, nervous tension and the individual's psychic superstructure being the most important. But a "high" filling, a malposed tooth or deep overbite is frequently contributory. Orthodontic and equilibrative procedures are indicated. If nothing is done, periodontal deterioration may well be the result (Fig. 9–5). (See Chaps. 16 and 17.)

IMPROPER DEGLUTITION

Abnormal swallowing is usually corollary to abnormal muscle function. But additional muscle groups are involved, and the functional demands on the musculature of the stomatognathic system itself are different from those for mastication, respiration and speech. For example, an abnormal swallowing habit leads to increased hyoid bone movement in some individuals. In children with cleft palate the bolus of food is managed differently from that in other children. By inductive reasoning and an awareness of the effect of muscle pressures on bone, it is not too difficult to construct a picture of certain types of malocclusions that could be attributed at least partly to abnormal deglutition. Such a reconstructive or analytical approach is in complete harmony with basic physiologic principles (Fig. 3–42).

MOUTH BREATHING

Also intimately associated with abnormal muscle function is the mouth breathing habit (Fig. 9–1). Long considered a primary causative factor in the creation of dental malocclusion, this habit is now deemed as more of an associ-

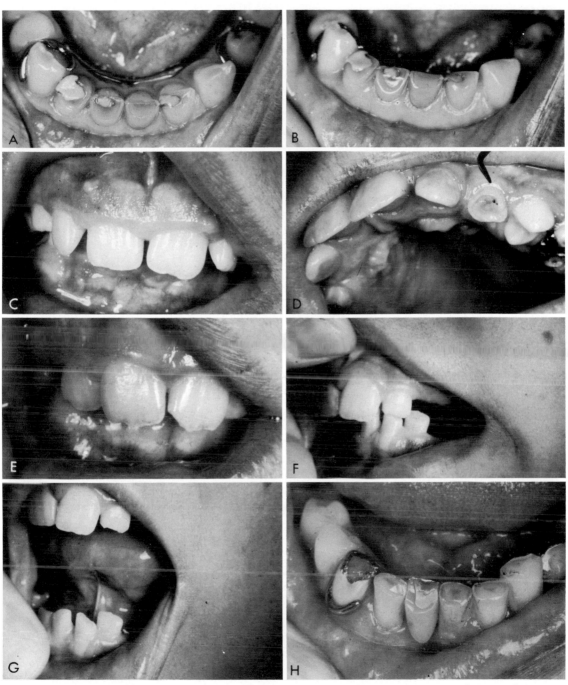

Figure 9–5 Examples of bruxism, associated with excessive overbite. A and B, Incisor wear, associated with partial denture and lack of harmonious occlusal vertical dimension. C and D, Deep bite and resultant wearing down of maxillary canine. E, F and G, Ten-year-old boy with compulsive grinding habit, day and night. Note wearing away of distal angle of lateral incisor in G. H again shows deficient occlusal vertical dimension and bruxism. Prosthetic restoration in these cases is difficult without eliminating deep bite. (See Figure 6–86.)

ated or symbiotic factor and, to a lesser degree, a result of the inherent mal-occlusion. As with other habits, any arbitrary assignment of cause, association and effect would be most precarious. It is apparent that the mouth breathing habit contributes to all three phases of the dynamics of malocclusion.

Ear, nose and throat specialists often note that respiratory ailments are more common in a habitual mouth breather. The filtering, warming effect of the nasal passages is lost and nasal obstructions such as enlarged turbinates occur more frequently. Enlarged tonsils and adenoids and frequent middle ear involvements may be associated. Such ill effects are not certainties; many other factors are involved, not the least being individual resistance. But it does make eminently good sense that if the danger to the child's health does exist and if the "adenoidal facies" is a detriment to the child's appearance, the orthodontist should assist where he can. In many cases elimination of excessive overjet and the establishment of normal perioral muscle function reactivates the upper lip, makes lip closure possible and stimulates normal nasal breathing.[6]

IMPROPER MASTICATION

The inability to chew properly is largely an associated factor or a result of malocclusion. Irregular or missing teeth often initiate a particular pattern of chewing. Most people favor one side more than the other and seldom distribute the bolus evenly. A "high" restoration or missing or malposed teeth on one side are quite sufficient reasons for the masticatory selectivity for the working side. The buccal segment that does not get adequate exercise and massage may show periodontal abnormalities more readily. Coupled with improper deglutition, the combined abnormal function may increase the severity of the malocclusion.

The importance of nutrition in a growing child need not be emphasized here. It is also easy to understand why a child who has difficulty chewing meat, or who must literally tear his food off by holding it in between the buccal segments, is less likely to eat the foods he should to satisfy the important nutritional needs. Since he does not chew his food properly the bolus is not mixed with saliva as it should be to prepare it for the digestive processes that follow; trituration is only partial. This throws an additional load on the digestive system. Since the human body is a wonderfully adaptive mechanism, it can usually take the load, but not always. Particularly when a child is sick, this is a "weak link" in the metabolic cycle.

SPEECH DEFECTS

The positions of teeth and the relationship of the supporting tissues are basic in speech physiology. It is through the relative positional changes of these hard and soft tissues as they inflect the outgoing air stream and vocal tone that normal or abnormal speech sounds are produced. It has been recognized by many speech authorities that dental malocclusions serve as a factor in speech pathology. In most instances adjustive, adaptive or compensatory activity largely overcomes the malocclusion handicap, but not always. The articulation of consonants and vowels may be attributed to a functional *maladaptation* to the dental malocclusion. Bloomer[11] notes that the effects on speech may be both direct and indirect: *direct* by virtue of the mechanical difficulties imposed as the person tries to obtain the proper position and movement of the articulators of speech; and *indirect* because of the influence which the deformities may have on the physical and mental health of the individual (Fig. 3–44).

EFFECTS OF MALOCCLUSIONS ON SPEECH

As an example of direct influence of malocclusion, a Class II, Division 1 malocclusion with a protruding premaxillary segment makes the normal production of bilabial consonants difficult. An anterior open bite permitting anterior escapage interferes with the normal production of sibilants. Since the teeth, supporting structures, tongue and lips are directly involved in the production of consonants requiring pneumatic control for fricative and plosive characteristics and since they modify the air column by blocking it (widening, narrowing or otherwise altering the passageway), most speech sounds can show the effects of malocclusion. The accurate formation of vowels and diphthongs may also suffer, though this is less critical than the enunciation of consonants.[11] Most of the defects are in the nature of dyslalic phenomena (defective articulation due to faulty learning or abnormalities of the external speech organs—not due to lesions of the central nervous system). The problem is not a simple cause-and-effect relationship. Some of the most severe malocclusions produce no discernible speech pathology because of the excellent adjustive mechanism. But certain types of malocclusion are more difficult to compensate for and more likely to cause speech abnormalities. These are Class I problems with anterior open bite or missing anterior teeth, Class II, Division 1 problems characterized by excessive overbite and overjet and abnormal perioral muscle function and Class III malocclusions with total absence of incisal contact, a redundant lower lip and perverted tongue function. (See Chaps. 5 and 6.) With an open bite deformity it is more difficult to produce acoustically acceptable sibilants. Bilabial consonants may suffer because of the habitual parting of the lips and the greater conscious effort required to effect closure. In Class II, Division 1 maxillary protraction problems, the same speech elements suffer. Lip incompetence is greater and anterior escapage combines with abnormal tongue position to produce a lisp-like sound. Correction of the malocclusion often eliminates the speech defects spontaneously. With Class III malocclusions, the mandibular prognathism, abnormally low tongue position and lethargic tongue function reduce the quality of sibilants. Fricatives and plosives may also suffer because of the retrognathic upper lip and redundant, hypofunctional lower lip.

EFFECTS OF CLEFT LIP OR PALATE

Obviously, speech problems are associated with cleft lip and cleft palate deformities. Phonation, resonation and articulation may be profoundly disturbed. Velopharyngeal incompetence, naso-oral communication, abnormal palatal morphology, severe dental malocclusion, abnormal tongue posture and function, and pathologic lip involvement mitigate strongly against production of normal speech sounds. Despite surgical assistance many of these patients are beyond the range of adjustment and they are limited regarding degree of improvement from speech therapy. Much depends on the type of cleft deformity, the technique and timing of surgical assistance, the growth and developmental pattern, hearing involvement and assistance from the other services, e.g., the prosthodontist and the speech therapist.

DENTAL CARIES AND MALOCCLUSION

Dental caries that leads to loss of arch length and ultimately the teeth themselves serves as a causative factor in dental malocclusions (Figs. 7–79, 1–1). But like many other sequelae of malocclusion discussed in this chapter, malocclusion can also affect caries control adversely. Dental irregularities make the self-cleansing action of the bolus of food, tongue and cheeks less effective. Oral hygiene is more difficult to perform, particularly for children. In susceptible mouths, food that lodges between malposed teeth is apt to decalcify the enamel; very likely, a carious lesion will be the end-result. Proper proximal contact relationship and normal tooth position and morphology make food packing between teeth almost impossible. Rotated and tipped teeth have no such defense mechanism. Scrupulous attention must be paid to oral hygiene if the incidence of caries is to be reduced. This is only a stopgap until the orthodontist can restore normal tooth relationships, eliminating those conditions which trap and impact food.

PERIODONTAL DISEASE AND MALOCCLUSION

Many orthodontists consider the periodontal implications of dental malocclusion the most important from a long-range point of view. It is the firm

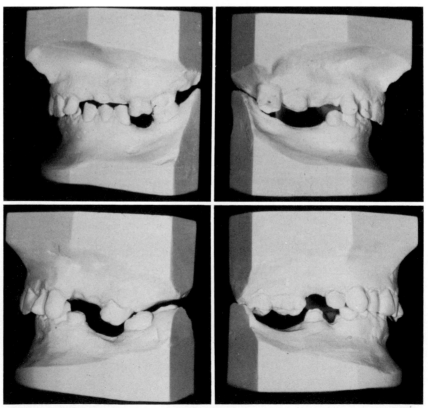

Figure 9–6 Malposed teeth, abnormal stresses, abnormal function and advanced periodontal involvement are the result of neglected malocclusions during childhood. Overeruption of teeth opposing edentulous areas makes restoration of the integrity of the dental arches most difficult.

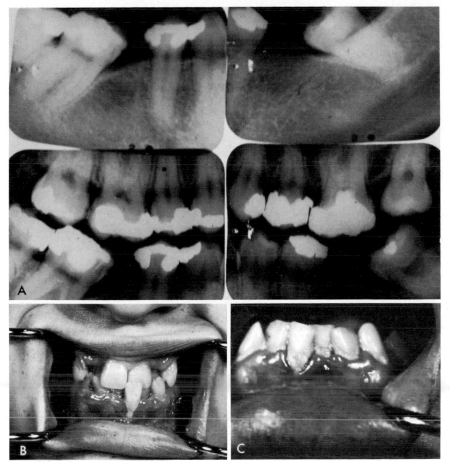

Figure 9–7   A, Pocket formation and bone loss beginning as a result of tipped teeth receiving abnormal stress. B, Damage to investing tissues as a result of anterior crossbite. C; Tissue breakdown in mandibular anterior segment in conjunction with deep overbite and poor prophylaxis.

conviction of some observers that periodontal disease and bone loss, drifting, spacing and ultimate loss of teeth in the geriatric period of dental service can be traced to malocclusions that were neglected during the pediatric phase of dental care (Figs. 9–5, 9–6). The same factors that increase the incidence of dental caries operate on the soft tissue.[12] Packing of food in interproximal areas is injurious to the mucosa and the gingival crevice. Pocket formation is but a step away. Lack of proper massage and natural stimulation, so important to maintain the integrity of the soft tissues, aggravates the hygiene problem. Hyperemic, edematous, puffy, interdental papillae become fibrous. Pockets deepen as abnormal proximal contact relations stimulate the pathologic process.

Abnormal axial inclinations and tipping of malposed teeth set up abnormal stresses. No longer are the functional stresses distributed evenly to all teeth primarily through the long axes. Lateral vectors of force cause jiggling and premature contacts; the alveolar crest succumbs to the onslaught (Fig. 9–7). Loss of bony support permits contacts to open and teeth to shift, and enhances abnormal axial inclination. All these factors react to accelerate bone loss and make the demise of the dentition merely a matter of time. Constitutional factors modify this sequence; hereditary predisposition may be important and certain idiopathic phenomena are contributory—but these do not alter the basic pattern. Malocclusion predisposes a patient to a certain degree of periodontal involvement, the extent of which depends on the type of malocclusion, the preventive or interceptive dental care and certain systemic factors.

With certain types of malocclusion, periodontal involvement is especially severe. Anterior cross-bite, for example, must be corrected immediately because tissue breakdown occurs quickly in the cross-bite area (Fig. 9–7). Overeruption may cause tooth guidance and a mandibular shift, setting up abnormal stresses on the dentition. Anterior open bite or a severe Class III malocclusion takes incisor segments out of masticatory function. The trabecular structure of the supporting bone becomes more rarified, and these teeth undergo a process akin to disuse atrophy, with a significant reduction in their longevity. (See Chaps. 5, 6 and 7.)

So important are the periodontal implications that malocclusions are frequently corrected in the adult; not to do so means temporizing by treating the symptoms and merely delaying the eventual loss of the teeth. Orthodontic procedures and appliances are more and more a part of every periodontist's armamentaria. The scope of service of the general dentist is being enlarged as he sees the value of uprighting teeth preparatory to placing fixed appliances, and as he sees bite plates and other removable appliances help patients with deep overbite, shifting incisors and similar problems. (See Chaps. 16 and 17.)

TEMPOROMANDIBULAR JOINT DISORDERS

Manhold has noted that temporomandibular joint dysfunction is being met by the physician with increasing frequency.[13] Certainly the orthopedic surgeon is receiving a larger number of complaints in this area. The dentist, too, as he learns more about the physiology of the stomatognathic system, has become aware that the influence of the teeth and of the functions of mastication, deglutition, respiration and speech extends well beyond the oral cavity. The alignment of stress trajectories and the pneumatization and buttressing of the upper face and cranium to resist functional oral stresses were discussed in Chapter 3. Pathologic ramifications of stomatognathic system function also occur outside the mouth proper. The physiology of the temporomandibular joint is a wonderful phenomenon to behold (Chap. 3). The unique fibrous condylar covering, and division into two separate joint cavities by the articular disk, qualifies the temporomandibular joint for the many stresses it receives. But malocclusion and resultant tooth guidance can cause pathology here. The synchrony of normal condylar and articular disk movement with relation to each other and the articular eminence can be destroyed. Most of the damage is done in the functional range from postural resting position to habitual occlusion. In the majority of cases, a vertical discrepancy—deeper than normal overbite—is an associated factor.[16]

ANALYSIS OF TYPICAL DISORDER

In analyzing a typical temporomandibular joint disorder, it will be noted that the movement of the condyle is essentially normal in the closure from postural resting position to point of initial contact, primarily a rotary motion of the condyle in the lower joint cavity. The disk is in retruded position with respect

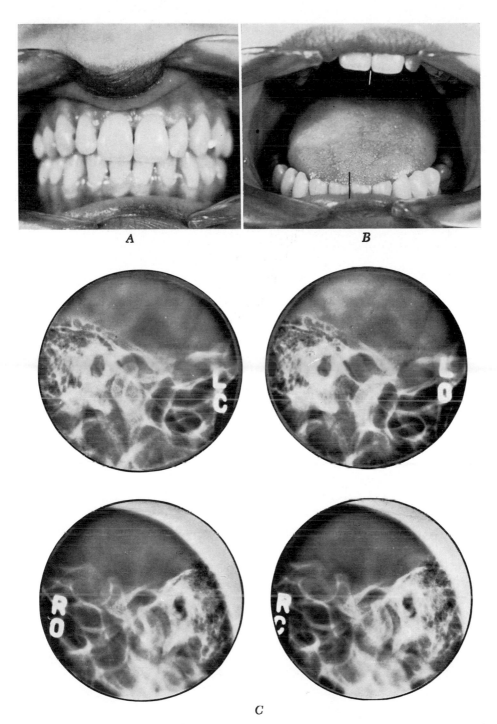

Figure 9–8 Limited mandibular opening with deviation of the midline to the right. Joint radiographs show marked forward movement of the left condyle (middle) but only slight translation of the right condyle from closed to open position. (From Schwartz, L., and Chayes, C. M.: Facial Pain and Mandibular Dysfunction. W. B. Saunders Co., 1968.)

to the articular eminence, and is held from going farther posteriorly by fibers of the external pterygoid muscle and the capsular ligament. At the point of initial contact—which is still centric relation—only certain teeth contact. Normally, initial contact should also be a centric occlusal relationship. But because of the malocclusion and vertical discrepancy, initial contact assumes the role of premature contact with respect to full habitual occlusal relationship. From this point on, tooth guidance through inclined plane relationship and facets of wear dictate the path of closure.

The upward and forward direction of closure from postural resting position to point of initial contact is abruptly changed. It can become a vertical vector, actually upward and backward, or a lateral shift, depending on the type of tooth guidance. Since the articular disk is already in its most retruded position and is held by the external pterygoid fibers from being retruded further, the condyle itself is forced upward and backward as the teeth are guided into habitual occlusion (Fig. 8–48). The condyle rides the posterior lip of the articular disk, and in some instances actually rides over the raised periphery to impinge on the postarticular connective tissue.

Initiation of the opening movement in this hypothetical temporomandibular joint disorder can (1) pull the disk forward first—sort of "pulling the rug" from under the condyle as the external pterygoid fibers contract and the condyle snaps over the disk periphery against the postarticular connective tissue; (2) pull the disk forward first, with the posteriorly displaced condyle starting late but moving forward more rapidly and riding over the posterior periphery of the disk into a more normal relationship or (3) cause the posteriorly displaced condyle to snap forward first, riding up over the posterior thickened disk periphery. In all instances, a "snap, crackle or pop" sensation is elicited—and described variously as crepitus, grinding or clicking. Pain or limitation of movement may or may not be present, depending on resistance factors and the type of condyle-disk-articular eminence disharmony during function (Fig. 9–8).

COMMON EFFECTS OF DISORDERS

The constant traumatic experience of the condyle compressing the delicate postarticular connective tissue and capsular membrane sooner or later elicits a sensory response. Pain can be quite severe, largely of a referred nature. The patient may complain of a radiating sharp sensation in the circumauricular region. He often wakes up in the morning to find his muscles tired and slightly sore to touch because of a clenching during the night; he may have to "unlock" his jaw by swinging it from side to side in the morning; or there may be actual trismus and real limitation of motion. Posselt[14] has graphed the distribution of various temporomandibular joint symptoms as described by a number of authors (Fig. 9–9) and has charted the frequency of complaints (Fig. 9–10). Any check list should include these, though not all of them will be present in any one patient. (See section on Bruxism, Chap. 7.) Many a patient has wandered from general practitioner to ear specialist to orthopedic surgeon to psychiatrist before he finally sees his dentist and finds out that his constantly recurring pain is in reality of dental origin. Unless the dentist can correct the malocclusion and eliminate the traumatic experience, the patient may be in for a very long siege of discomfort and disability.[17, 18]

In an alarming number of cases, the dentist sees the patient too late, i.e., after the patient has undergone long periods of cortisone injections into the joint or after actual extirpation of the disk and sometimes partial facial paralysis

DISTRIBUTION OF SYMPTOMS

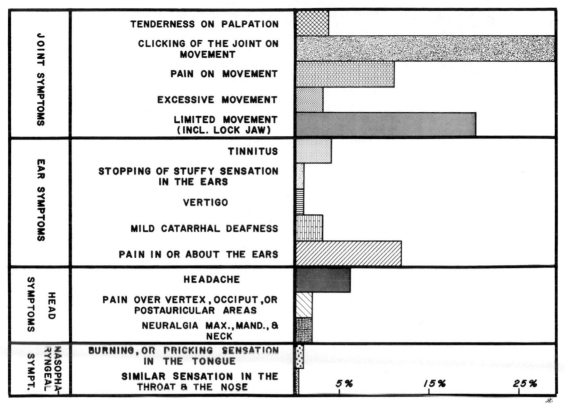

Figure 9–9   Distribution of temporomandibular joint symptoms, based on the research of a number of investigators, as compiled from a total group of 731 patients by Posselt. Clicking is included only in conjunction with other complaints and not when it is the sole symptom. (After Posselt, U.: The Physiology of Occlusion and Rehabilitation, F. A. Davis, 1968.)

after the surgery. It is tragic when the etiologic basis is of dental origin and the physician did not recognize this, or bother to find out.

Not all temporomandibular joint disturbances are of dental origin, of course. Arthritic changes can occur in this area as they do in any other joint in the body. Muscular dystrophy affects masticatory muscles; cerebral palsy and poliomyelitis can induce functional abnormalities similar to the pain-dysfunction syndrome so often seen with malocclusion. Even poor posture may be a factor.[15] A careful diagnosis must be made using all available criteria, and consultation must be had with the physician or psychiatrist, if necessary, before embarking on a plan of treatment. It should be obvious—but isn't always—that the dentist himself should not be guilty of creating or perpetuating a temporomandibular joint disturbance (Fig. 9–11). Nonphysiologic restorations damage the teeth and investing tissues; they create and accentuate TMJ disturbances. If a bridge is nothing more than a "space occupier" and splint between teeth that are tipped and ill prepared to receive the additional stress, the dentist is little more than a mechanic. The bridge might as well have been placed by the laboratory technician who probably did the actual fabrication of it in the first place.

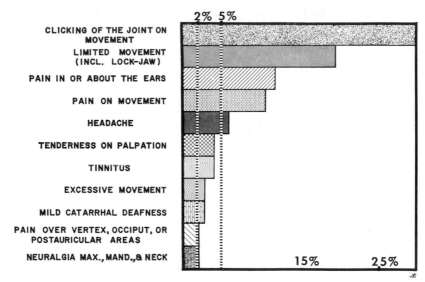

Figure 9–10   Frequency of symptoms listed in Figure 9–9. (From Posselt, U.: The Physiology of Occlusion and Rehabilitation. F. A. Davis, 1968.)

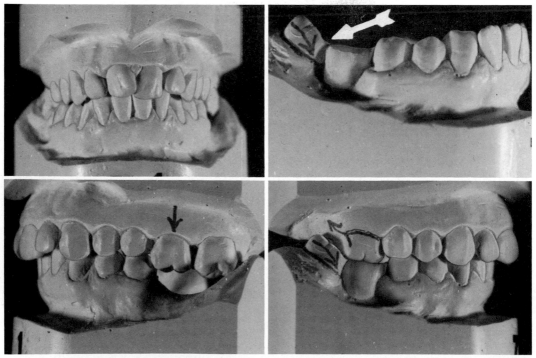

Figure 9–11   Severe temporomandibular joint disturbance with "built-in" predisposition. Innocuous anterior malposition is (upper left) hardly a problem; "the skid" in the upper right-hand view guides the condyle superiorly and posteriorly into a forced retrusion: Overeruption and non-restoration (lower left) accentuates the functional problem that is shown by the occluded maxillary and mandibular casts and arrows in the region of the skid where a so-called bridge has been placed, as seen in the lower right-hand illustration.

ACCIDENTS AND MALOCCLUSION

One of the unfortunate sequelae of a Class II, Division 1 malocclusion is the greater likelihood of damage to the maxillary incisors as a result of their protruded and relatively unprotected status. Falls, drinking fountain accidents, another child's head—and the child tearfully confronts his shocked parent with parts of one or more of the front teeth missing. If he is lucky the nerve is not exposed. If he is really fortunate, the tooth may not turn black as the pulp undergoes necrosis and dies, necessitating the removal of the pulp or the tooth. At the very least, he must wait until he is 16 or 17 years old before an adequate permanent restoration can be made (Fig. 9–12).

IMPACTED UNERUPTED TEETH

Premature loss and prolonged retention of deciduous teeth may interfere with the eruption of their permanent successors or neighbors (see Chap. 7). Some authorities believe that an impacted tooth that is retained within the alveolar process may at times initiate a dentigerous cyst. All too little is known about the cause-and-effect relationship between unerupted teeth and cystic formation. If the malocclusion can be corrected, thus permitting an unerupted tooth to emerge, a possible cystic focus is eliminated. Even when these malocclusion-impacted teeth do not become cystic, they can still pose a hazard to

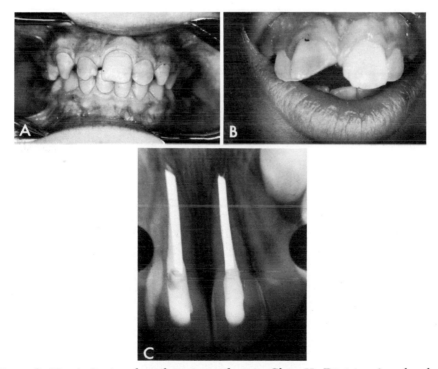

Figure 9–12   A, Incisor lost due to accident in Class II, Division 1 malocclusion. The space has closed autonomously. B, Fractured and nonvital right central incisor, a victim of a drinking fountain accident. C, Protruding incisors, a playmate's head, pulpal death and root canal fillings account for findings in this picture.

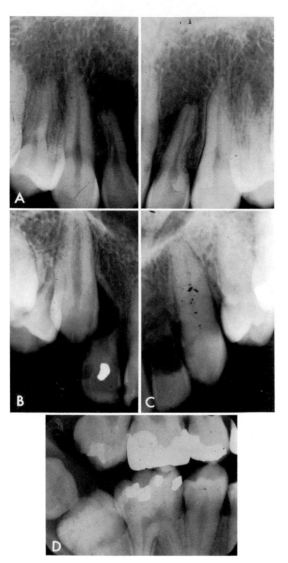

Figure 9–13 A, B and C, In malocclusions where crowding exists, impactions or partial impactions are common. Varying degrees of root resorption may result. The maxillary lateral incisor is particularly prone to damage from the erupting canine. D, The occlusion may be seriously jeopardized by third molar impaction. (Views A and B, courtesy J. R. Jarabak.)

geriatric dental service (partial and full denture rehabilitation). When partially impacted teeth do finally make the grade and erupt into the mouth, they may permanently damage contiguous teeth by resorbing part or all of their roots (Fig. 9–13). This is just another good reason for periodic full mouth dental radiographs.

COMPLICATIONS IN PROSTHETIC REHABILITATION

The instances are legion in which the dentist has looked at an adult mouth, shaken his head and said, "If only your remaining teeth were in normal position I could make you a good bridge." Malocclusion, with the usual characteristics of rotated or tipped teeth, poor contacts, elongation into opposing edentulous areas and space problems, can create insuperable obstacles for the dentist, anxious to render a satisfactory prosthetic service (Fig. 9–11). (See Uprighting

Molars and Opening and Closing Spaces in Preparation for Prostheses, Chap. 18.)

In addition to the physical impossibility of placing a proper restoration there is a problem of abnormal stress distribution. Tipped teeth no longer receive functional stresses primarily in the long axes (Figs. 9–6, 9–7). Normally, the stresses are absorbed largely by the periodontal ligament transmitting the force to the lateral walls of the alveolus mostly as tension. (See Figs. 18–13, 18–14.) Abnormal pressures result in lateral jiggling movements, with ultimate pocket formation and breakdown of the supporting crest structures. If this can happen before a fixed prosthesis is placed, it is not difficult to figure out that the additional stress on abnormally posed teeth, splinted in a position of mal-occlusion, will hurry the process. Much can be done to restore normal tooth position by preparing the remaining teeth to receive occlusal stresses in a physiologic manner before the placement of the fixed prosthesis.

REFERENCES

1. Moorrees, C. F. A., and Grøn, A. M.: Principles of orthodontic diagnosis. Angle Orthodont. 36:258–262, 1966.
2. Stricker, G.: Psychological issues pertaining to malocclusion. Am. J. Orthodont., 58:276–283, 1970.
3. Lewit, D. W., and Virolainen, K. M.: Conformity and independence in adolescents' motivation for orthodontic treatment. Child Develop., 39:1189–1200, 1968.
4. Baldwin, D. C., and Barnes, M. L.: Patterns of motivation in families seeking orthodontic treatment. J. Dent. Res., 45:412, 1966.
5. Hilzenrath, S. S., and Baldwin, D. C.: Achievement motivation – a factor in seeking orthodontic treatment. J. Dent. Res., 49:433, 1970.
6. Subtelny, J. D.: Malocclusions, orthodontic corrections and orofacial muscle adaptation. Angle Orthodont., 40:170–201, 1970.
7. Baril, C., and Moyers, R. E.: An electromyographic analysis of the temporalis muscle and certain facial muscles in thumb and finger sucking patients. J. Dent. Res., 39:536–553, 1960.
8. Perry, H. T.: Symptomatology of temporomandibular disturbance. J. Prosth. Dent., 19:288–298, 1968.
9. Bober, H.: Grundlagen der Therapie der Hauptformen des Zahneknirschens. Stomatol., 52:449, 1955.
10. Ramfjörd, S. P.: Bruxism, a clinical and electromyographic study. J.A.D.A., 66:21–44, 1961.
11. Bloomer, H. H.: in Travis, L. E. (ed.): Handbook of Speech Pathology. New York, Appleton-Century-Crofts, 1971.
12. Pearson, L. E.: Gingival height of the lower central incisors in orthodontically treated and untreated. Angle Orthodont., 38:337–339, 1968.
13. Manhold, J. H., Jr.: Temporomandibular joint dysfunction. Dent. Times, 8:7, 1965.
14. Posselt, U.: The Physiology of Occlusion and Rehabilitation. Philadelphia, F. A. Davis Co., 1966.
15. Crum, R. J., and Loiselle, R. J.: Temporomandibular joint symptoms and ankylosing spondylitis. J.A.D.A., 83:630–638, 1971.
16. Schwartz, L., and Chayes, C. M.: Facial Pain and Mandibular Dysfunction. Philadelphia, W. B. Saunders Co., 1968.
17. Laskin, D. M., and Greene, C. S.: Splint therapy for the myofascial pain-dysfunction (MPD) syndrome; a comparative study. J.A.D.A., 84:624–628, 1972.
18. Reitan, K.: Orthodontic treatment of patients with psychogenic, muscular and articulation disturbances. Tandlaegebladet, 75:1182–1197, 1971.

chapter 10

BIOMECHANICAL PRINCIPLES OF ORTHODONTIC TOOTH MOVEMENT

By the time the dental student or practicing dentist develops an interest in tooth movement, he knows fairly well what the various tissues look like under a microscope. He has undoubtedly been exposed to basic lectures on bone biology and is conversant with such terms as *osteoblast, osteoclast, fibroblast, Howship's lacuna* and *osteoid bone.* (Where bone is being built, osteoblasts are present; where bone is being destroyed, osteoclasts may be observed. Pressure seems to cause resorption; tension on bone seems to stimulate bone apposition.) If he has been an apt student in his histology courses and has done a little outside reading, he becomes aware of the tremendous amount of research that has been done on tooth movement, and also of the quite considerable controversy that has developed as various observers have attempted to analyze the experimental material. It is not the purpose of this text to add to the organized confusion. Rather, the aim is to outline briefly the changes that occur normally as the dentition develops—so-called "physiologic tooth movement"—and then to analyze what actually occurs with the use of orthodontic appliances as we know them today.

Some observers facetiously refer to orthodontic tooth movement as "a pathologic process from which the tissue recovers." In some instances the theme might be, "What price orthodontics?" The strong mechanical orientation of the dentist and the constant repetition of procedural tasks in routine practice sometimes obscure the importance of the biologic aspect of dentistry in the total service. This must not happen in the case of the man who would move teeth. "Tissue consciousness" is a vital prerequisite to mechanics. There are available today potent tooth-moving appliances that can accomplish almost any desired change, but if their use is not controlled by a profound respect for the biologic media in which they work, incalculable harm can be done. Resorbed roots, devitalized teeth, sheared alveolar crests, periodontal pockets, poor gingival health and failure to achieve the therapeutic objective await the man who ignores biologic principles (Fig. 10–1).

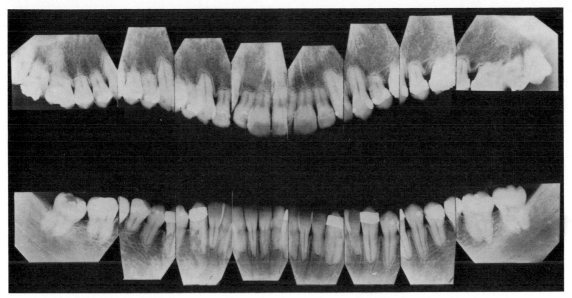

Figure 10–1   Root resorption as a result of previous orthodontic treatment. (Courtesy H. Becks.)

It is estimated that root resorption occurs in at least 12 per cent of all orthodontic patients presently being treated by competent orthodontists.[1] De Shields observed measurable resorption in 51 out of 52 cases of orthodontically treated Class II, Division 1 malocclusion.[2] Untoward sequelae are observed from time to time in the practices of the most careful operators. These sequelae must be kept to a minimum by a constant awareness of the response of living tissue to mechanical manipulations.

The tremendous increase in the amount of orthodontic treatment being done in general dental practice comes under the heading of iatrogenic or orthogenic malocclusions in too many cases. Specifically, this means that the attempts at orthodontic therapy created malocclusions and attendant unfavorable sequelae that would not have been present without appliance intervention. Wanton expansion with removable appliances under the guise of stimulating growth and development is contrary to most of what we know concerning growth and development. The collapse of the bulldozed dentition after the removal of appliances is not calculated to improve the dentist's public image, nor to enhance his own feeling of community service. Nor are the destroyed alveolar crests, the foreshortened apices, the gingival recessions or the pockets and periodontal lesions that comprise the residuum of misguided therapy going to increase the longevity and health of the teeth and investing tissues. Tissue consciousness is a *must* for every dentist. Just because he does not call himself an orthodontist as he moves teeth does not mean that he must not obey the same rules, heed the same admonitions and know the stringent limitations that are imposed on all who would change tooth positions with fixed or removable appliances.

PHYSIOLOGIC TOOTH MOVEMENT

To the layman, about the most rigid thing in his body is his set of teeth. The vitreous-like pegs of ivory are anchored in bone, like steel posts in concrete. He accepts the fact that they can wear down over the years, but if they move he expresses surprise, and even alarm. He knows nothing about the cushioning connective tissue, periodontal membrane, that is as vital as any tissue in the body, with its network of capillaries, nerves, lymph vessels and supporting fibers. There, as in the rest of the body, anabolic and catabolic processes are continuously active. He does not know that bone is a vital tissue and also undergoes constant reorganization; that teeth move — constantly, imperceptibly, but indubitably throughout life. With the wearing-away process, teeth continue to erupt. Contacts are worn, and contact points become contact surfaces. Mesial drift "takes up the slack" (Fig. 10-2). The loss of one or more teeth accelerates the process of drift or eruption; introduction of premature contacts or abnormal functional forces may cause further shifting. And as the teeth shift, the socket shifts with the tooth. Not all drifting of teeth is mesial, however. Zwarych and Quigley have observed distal physiologic drifting in mouse molars, and such activity is present in humans at one time or another — particularly where a tooth has been lost in the posterior segment.[3]

As Weinmann's illustration shows, bone is resorbed ahead of the drifting tooth and deposited behind it. Resorption is seen as an uneven scalloped margin, with the presence of osteoclasts — cells that are apparently phagocytic. Bone deposition appears histologically as concentric lamellae of bundle bone laid down in the presence and probably with the aid of the bone-building cells, the osteoblasts. As the alveolus or "socket" moves, maintaining space for tooth and periodontal membrane, bony reorganization outside the alveolus occurs. Ahead of the moving tooth, trabeculae show resorption on the side nearest the moving tooth, deposition of bone on the side farther away. Behind the moving tooth, bone is deposited on the side of the trabeculae nearest the tooth, while bone is resorbed on the side away from the tooth to maintain a constant length of the trabecular structure. The osteoblasts probably first lay down an organic matrix known as osteoid bone. This then becomes calcified as calcium salts are deposited in the matrix. Osteoid bone is more resistant to resorption. The growing surfaces of bone, as well as the entire root surface of the teeth, are protected by a layer of organic, uncalcified and acellular material.

The histologic picture seldom shows a clear mesial drift pattern or eruption

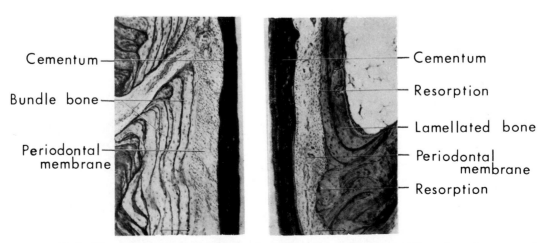

Cementum

Bundle bone

Periodontal membrane

Cementum

Resorption

Lamellated bone

Periodontal membrane

Resorption

Figure 10-2   Physiologic mesial drift. Tooth moving from left to right. There is active resorption on the mesial side as shown by the scalloped line of bone with osteoclasts. On the distal side, bundle bone has been built up by intermittent action. (Courtesy J. P. Weinmann.)

pattern. Even where drifting is the primary action at the moment, the tooth moves by imperceptible "wiggles" so that an entire surface will not show resorption on the side of drift, or pressure or bone deposition on either the side of tension or the side opposite the drift direction. Analysis of a series of slides taken from different regions up and down the length of the root surfaces will show both resorption and deposition taking place on the side in the direction of drift as well as on the remaining surfaces. DeAngelis likens regular orthodontic tooth movement to mesial drift, with a differential apposition-resorption pattern also induced by appliances. Possible regulatory action may come from alteration of the electric environment by stresses (piezo-electric effect).[4] Frost reaches the same conclusions in his studies.[5-7]

A tooth must be considered in three dimensions. A strain gauge or pressure gauge placed at various points along the root surfaces would show that force vectors are operative laterally, anteroposteriorly and vertically (and in infinite combinations of these three) on all root surfaces.[8] Bone, as a responsive tissue, reflects the manifold forces. Thus, while it is true that physiologic tooth movement occurs primarily in a mesio-occlusal direction, reorganization occurs on all surfaces. Time is an important fourth dimension. Somewhat analogous to the rings of a tree, like the neonatal line of Schour, are the resting and reversal lines observed in the alveolus.[9]

Brief rest periods occur at periodic intervals throughout life. During these rest periods it seems that the bundle bone is formed, and the reoriented periodontal membrane fibers are re-anchored in the bone to preserve the integrity of the attachment. After a certain amount of bundle bone has been deposited, reorganization from haversian systems in the bone already laid down takes place. Part of the bundle bone is converted into trabeculae. The cycle then begins all over again at this point and at countless other points. Resting and reversal lines are present on all surfaces and occur at different places at different times. The histologist unfortunately stops vital processes and obtains a picture of the situation at only one precise moment in time; but he is confident that if it were possible to take successive pictures of the same area he would observe the gamut of tissue changes without ever moving his "seeing eye." Actually, as Baer and Ackerman show, a two-color vital staining process can now be used most effectively to show longitudinal patterns of apposition.[10]

ORTHODONTIC TOOTH MOVEMENT

If bone is so biologically plastic and adaptive to developmental and functional forces, responding to pressure with *resorption* and to tension with *bone deposition*; if teeth move and reflect various environmental influences by positional modifications throughout life, why cannot the orthodontist channel these activities and move teeth? He can. Alveolar bone has been referred to as "the slave of the orthodontist." The essential processes are there and at work before he attempts guided tooth movement by mechanical appliances. These processes are attempting to perform their own job, laid out for them by nature, during the time that the orthodontist is interfering; and they will continue after he is finished. But before the orthodontist, emulating and enslaving nature, can guide teeth through bone to predetermined positions, he must search for the answers to a number of questions.

The last section of this chapter briefly discusses the means, the methods, the theoretical mechanics and engineering concepts of orthodontic appliances themselves. A glossary of terms is also given. The current biophysical and mathematical analysis of orthodontic therapy goes into greater depth and detail and is aimed primarily at the orthodontic specialist. Selected references are listed at the end of this chapter for the serious student. The 14 questions listed below have been answered on a nontechnical basis, with a primary tissue reaction orientation for the applied biologist. If mechanical background is desired first, then the reader should turn to the section on General Principles of Tooth Movement, later in this chapter.

1. When force is applied to the crown of a tooth, how do the tooth and surrounding tissues react?
2. How does a tooth react to a tipping force, a bodily force, a rotating force, an elongating force, a depressing force?
3. What is the tissue reaction to different amounts of force?
4. What is the role of the periodontal membrane?
5. Is there an optimal orthodontic force?
6. Should forces be continuous or intermittent? Through how great a distance should force be active?
7. What kind of force causes less root resorption?
8. Can forces be directed precisely?
9. What is the role of functional forces?
10. What is the soft tissue response?
11. What is the role of the supra-alveolar tissue?
12. Does tooth movement stimulate jaw growth, cause modeling changes in the bone itself or restrict jaw growth?
13. What is the age factor in tooth movement?
14. What are the changes during and after the retention period?

1. WHEN FORCE IS APPLIED BY PRESSURE TO THE CROWN OF A TOOTH, HOW DO THE TEETH AND SURROUNDING TISSUES REACT?

THE TOOTH ITSELF. The application of a constant pressure to the crown of a tooth will cause it to change position if the force applied is of sufficient duration and intensity and the path ahead is not blocked by the occlusion or another tooth. Sandstedt demonstrated this fact histologically for the first time, in 1901.[11] For example, lingual pressure on the labial surface of an incisor causes the incisor to move lingually if there is room and if the opposing tooth is not jammed against it on the lingual side (Fig. 10–3). But the movement is primarily a tipping or tilting of the tooth unless special appliances are used to effect bodily movement. Judging from histologic studies, this tipping, with an average orthodontic force, occurs with the axis of rotation at about one third of the root length from the apex.[12]

Variations in force intensity have been claimed to change the axis of rotation position. Oppenheim stated that if forces are light enough, the axis of rotation is at or close to the apex.[13] Excessive force moves the axis of rotation up the root toward the crown. If the application of force is near the incisal margin, the axis of rotation can, in some instances, actually approximate the lingual crest, swinging the apex to the labial.[14] Sicher points out that the pivotal axis is near the apex for functional movements, as evidenced by the entry of vessels and nerves at this point.[15]

Dijkman, in a purely mechanical appraisal of force delivery and magnitude on theoretical tooth models, found that the magnitude of force does not affect the pivotal axis, generally situated in the middle region of the root.[8] This does not take into account the biologic reaction to different magnitudes of force, the hydraulic effect, nature's attempt to protect the "umbilical cord" of structures at the apex, etc. He did point out, however, that single rooted teeth have less pressure exerted at the apex, owing to their surface area and configuration. It would seem then that there are two rotational axes: the mechanical axis, based on laws of physics, and the biologic axis, based on tissue reaction, fluid pressures, cellular activity, protective mechanisms, etc. The first is substantiated by precise physical experiments, using models; the second is validated by histologic surveys of actual osteoblastic and osteoclastic response to applied pressures (Fig. 10–3).

THE PULP.   Mild forces cause hyperemia of the pulp tissue.[61] Patients sometimes have a sensitivity to thermal changes in conjunction with a pulpitis after adjustments have been made in the orthodontic appliances. If the pressure is severe, partial or total pulpal degeneration is possible, and the tooth will turn dark as hemorrhage and necrosis occur. Experiments show that there is a reduced sensitivity to electric pulp testing methods during orthodontic treatment. The pulp reaction returns to normal after completion of orthodontic therapy.[16]

CEMENTUM.   The surface of the root normally has an acellular organic layer of cementoid over the cementum. When orthodontic pressures are applied, this protective cementoid layer may be perforated and semilunar areas of resorption appear in the cementum (Fig. 10–4). If the forces employed are intermittent or if treatment is completed, cementoblasts usually fill in the "punched out" areas, but the cementum is never quite the same in microscopic appearance as the original structure.[17]

DENTIN.   With severe pressures, a breakthrough of the cementoid layer and cementum resorption are followed by actual dentin resorption in some cases. While prolonged pressures seem to be a factor, and endocrine disturbances predispose patients to this type of resorption, the resorption phenomenon is not completely understood. The apices show a predilection for destruction, and once lost do not return. If the dentin damage is only a cupping out beneath cementum resorption, the cementoblasts invaginate into the depression and repair the dentin damage—with a cementumlike substance, of course (Fig. 10–4).

ENAMEL.   No tissue changes are observed in the enamel as a result of tooth movement, per se. Decalcification around bands as a result of debris that is not removed and an etching of the enamel rod's surface may be seen by the naked eye (or microscopically) in many cases.

THE SURROUNDING TISSUES.   THE ALVEOLAR BONE.   As the diagram

Figure 10–3   Simple pressure applied in a lingual direction against the crown of a maxillary incisor. Dotted cross in middle of root represents theoretical pivotal axis, based on mechanical principles. Solid cross shows actual axis of rotation, as shown by histologic survey of the tooth and its investing tissues. Scalloped outline indicates bone resorption or osteoclastic activity; concentric lines indicate bone deposition or osteoblastic activity. (Courtesy K. Reitan.)

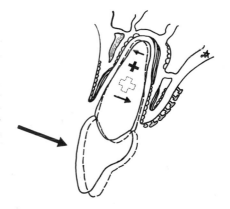

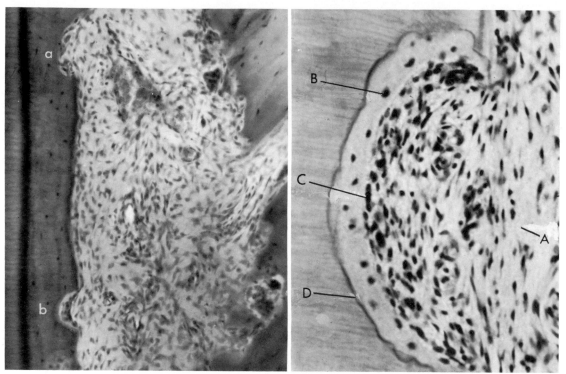

Figure 10–4 Compression and hyalinization has caused root resorption in two areas (a and b). This root resorption is incidental and not necessarily the result of excessive force. Picture on right is an enlargement of an area similar to b. Lettering indicates different structures. A is periodonta ligament, devoid of Mallasez' epithelial remnants as a result of earlier hyalinization. B is a cementoblast which is incorporated in new cementum. C indicates cementoblasts along cementoid layer. D is the demarcation line between dentin and cementum. (Courtesy K. Reitan.)

shows, the greatest resorption occurs at the lingual crest, reducing in degree as the proximity of the rotational axis is reached (Fig. 10–3). Proceeding apically past the axes of rotation, bone apposition may actually take place on the lingual apical third. On the labial surface, bone apposition occurs at the alveolar crest next to the tooth and diminishes in activity closer to the rotational axis. The labial apical third actually shows osteoclastic activity and bone resorption.

As the crown is tipped lingually, with resorption at the lingual crest area and deposition in the labial crest area, there is internal reorganization in the vicinity of the moving tooth. Resorption takes place on the external surface of the labial plate, with individual trabeculae mirroring this reaction (resorption on the side away from the labial surface of the tooth, deposition on the lingual aspect of the trabeculae). This helps maintain a constant thickness of the labial alveolar bone covering.

On the lingual aspect, modeling resorption and deposition of bone also take place, as individual trabeculae resorb on the side nearest the tooth and deposit on the side farther away. The greatest modification usually occurs at the crest because the majority of orthodontic patients undergo orthodontic therapy during a prolific growth period. Therapy is thus superimposed on normal eruptive processes. With or without orthodontic therapy, alveolar bone would be deposited at the crest. Tooth movement may alter the process and thus change the contours of this area. There is little evidence that orthodontic pressures can change the shape of the palatal bone that has already been laid down, but such pressure can influence bone being laid down in the proximity of the teeth being moved. Furstman and his co-workers note a differential response of maxillary to mandibular alveolar bone. Bone resiliency is greater in the maxilla and the maxillary teeth move further and more rapidly than mandibular teeth.[18]

PERIODONTAL MEMBRANE. Without the periodontal membrane the orthodontist could do very little. Serving as a source for proliferating cellular elements when stimulated by pressure or tension, the "builders" (osteoblasts) and the "wreckers" (osteoclasts) are pressed into service where needed. Using the same hypothetical example of a maxillary central incisor with lingual pressure applied to the crown, immediate physical changes would occur in the PDM. The most pronounced is the compression of the PDM at the lingual alveolar crest. The compression decreases closer to the rotational axis and is nonexistent at the rotational axis. The lingual apical third shows an increase in thickness with elongation of the periodontal membrane fibers, as this area is subjected to a tensional force. On the labial surface, the same tensional force, or increase in thickness of the PDM, is observed at the crest, reducing gradually as the observer approaches the rotational axis. The labial apical third shows the same compression phenomena as the lingual crest. PDM changes on the mesial and distal surfaces show both elongation and shortening of PDM fibers at the same time, depending on the area examined. For a given amount of force, there is some evidence that the periodontal ligament compresses more in the mandible.[18]

A critical factor here is the amount of force. Assuming the force to be optimal—not too much above the capillary pressure of 20 to 26 gm. per sq. cm.—the PDM will compress as much as one third its width at the lingual crest. There is an immediate increase in cell production and blood supply. The pressure on the lingual tissue stimulates osteoclastic activity on the approximating alveolar bone of the lamina dura, with the cells proliferating from the PDM at the site of pressure. On the labial surface, where the tooth movement force has been transmitted to the PDM as tension, osteoblastic cells proliferate (very probably both osteoclasts and osteoblasts differentiate from immature fibroblasts) and take up their job of depositing bone on the alveolar wall at the site of tension.

When a tooth is tipped with a conventional continuous force, the PDM is compressed in a circumscribed area situated close to the alveolar crest. This area becomes cell-free and blood vessels are occluded (Fig. 10–5). On the tension side the fibers are not usually torn and there is no hemorrhage. But the fibers will be stretched, which leads to the formation of new bone-building cells, the osteoblasts. Even with forces of the magnitude of 800 gm. fibers do not tear, according to Reitan.[19] However, necrosis may occur on the pressure side if the forces are as strong as 500 to 600 gm. and are acting over a long period. The compressed cell-free zone will then be much wider than with forces in the 100 gm. range, for example, and more time is required for the undermining bone resorption.

If the force greatly exceeds "physiologic" limits, the PDM is crushed at the lingual crest, blood vessels are mangled and occluded, and necrosis sets in. The PDM at the labial apical third is severely compressed and may show similar though less severe changes. At the labial-alveolar crest the PDM is stretched and some of the fibers may be torn partially at the intermediate zone or plexus of the periodontal membrane, with concomitant hemorrhage. With necrosis and stasis of fluids, activity at the immediate site of pressure is practically nil. On the labial surface both phagocytic and bone-building cells appear. Further up

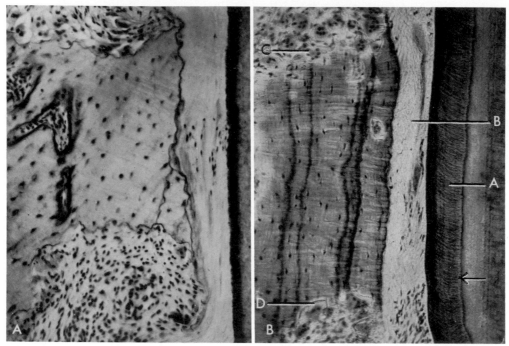

Figure 10–5   A, Undermining resorption in a 12-year-old person. This is a view from a short-rooted premolar tooth. Cementum covering of root surface has not been broken, though PDM is hyalinized at area of greatest pressure. Spicule of bone is being attacked from above and below, away from compressed PDM. B, Undermining resorption is again taking place in a 39-year-old person. No osteoclastic activity occurs in compressed PDM, but osteoclasts are at work on bundle bone that had been laid down previously from above and below area of greatest pressure. A, Thick cementum layer. B, Hyalinized periodontal ligament. C and D, Frontal undermining bone resorption on both sides of the cell-free area. (Courtesy K. Reitan.)

the root, away from the actual pressure site on the lingual side, blood supply is increased, osteoclasts proliferate and start to work on the alveolar bone in this area, literally tunnelling into the bone behind the necrotic pressure site to remove the bone and dead cells.[20] Tissue-building fibroblasts invade the area after phagocytic action to restore the continuity of the periodontal tissues. This phenomenon is known as "undermining resorption"[21] (Fig. 10–5).

It is likely that most tooth movement today, with multibanded techniques and heavy pressures, is accomplished by undermining resorption. Hence, the observation, "Orthodontics is a pathologic process from which the tissue recovers." But the tissue does not always recover, as will be discussed later in this chapter.[2]

With light, continuous forces, however, as prescribed in some differential light forces techniques, the tissue does indeed recover, and applied pathology is not the modus operandi. In tipping movements with fixed appliances, there need be no great concern over permanent damage as long as the forces remain in the 50 to 300 gm. range. Even with forces as light as 20 to 30 gm., there is formation of a pressure zone. But the duration of the undermining bone resorption will be fairly short. The duration of the cell-free zone is greatly influenced by the force factor. With a light tipping force (50 to 70 gm.), the cell-free area will be small and undermining resorption completed within a period of two weeks (Fig. 10–6).

An intriguing analysis of the periodontal membrane, or the "periodontal ligament," as he prefers to call it, has been made by Sicher. In 1923, in the histologic analysis of the eruption of teeth in a guinea pig, Sicher discovered what he called an intermediate zone or plexus in the periodontal membrane.[22, 23] Since the teeth of a rat or guinea pig erupt at a tremendously rapid rate — as much as one third of a millimeter per day — some adjustive process must take place within the periodontal membrane to allow for this change. Sicher showed that the principal bundle fibers are anchored in both the cementum of the tooth and the alveolar bone and run toward the center of the periodontal ligament. They are almost perpendicular at the crest, becoming more oblique farther down the root. These fibers meet in a network of fibers running in all directions at the center of the periodontal membrane, or ligament. He deduced that it was in this intermediate zone or plexus that the adjustive processes primarily take place (Fig. 10–7).

In animals with a much slower eruption rate, the intermediate zone or plexus would be much narrower. In man, whose eruption rates are quite slow, the intermediate plexus would be so thin that it could be overlooked entirely because of technical difficulties encountered during fixing and vital staining. Stretching and retraction of fibers during processing of the section could occur. Recently, in trying to explain some of the phenomena that occur with tooth movement, Sicher re-examined his sections and observed that the intermediate zone, narrow as it is, does exist in the human periodontal membrane.[24] If this is indeed true, the presence of this zone would explain a number of things.

First of all, at least part of the "give" during functional movements could be ascribed to the intermediate plexus' meshlike arrangement of individual fibers, stretching or widening somewhat under tension (Figs. 10–8, 10–9). As we know, the individual fibers are nonelastic. The existence of the intermediate plexus means that the growth of fibers would be at the free end and it would not be necessary for constant osteoblastic and cementoblastic activity to reanchor

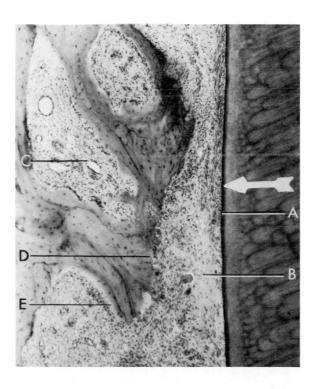

Figure 10–6   Tooth movement with light forces, pressure side. Period shortly after hyalinization. A, Root surface. B, Remnants of cell-free, formerly hyalinized tissue. C, Large marrow space in alveolar bone. D, Direct bone resorption. E, Compensatory bone formation in marrow space as a response to bone resorption on the side of the periodontal ligament. (Courtesy K. Reitan.)

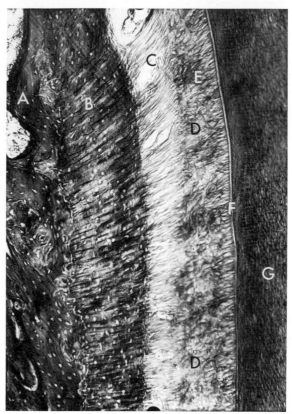

Figure 10–7   Intermediate plexus of a rat incisor. A, Haversian bone. B, Bundle bone. C, Alveolar fibers. D, Intermediate plexus. E, Dental fibers. F, Cementum. G, Dentin. (Courtesy H. Sicher.)

fibers literally torn from the bone under excessive pressures. Sicher thinks that the break occurs at the intermediate plexus, not at the alveolar bone or tooth surface. Under excessive pressures the intermediate zone unravels and the intertwining fibers are ripped apart, or unspliced, allowing the tooth to move in the direction of the force and exert intolerable pressures on the periodontal ligament on the opposing side. The necrotic changes in the pressure area, with its undermining resorption, are well known and previously described in this chapter (Fig. 10–5). Sicher prefers to emphasize the damage that occurs on the tension side as the greatest concern; to him, the resultant lack of protection of the PDM on the opposing side is secondary. With "normal" orthodontic forces (within the 50 to 300 gm. range), however, there need be no damage occurring on the tension side. Disengaged fibers will be reattached by the formation of

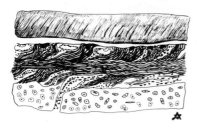

DENTINE
  ENAMEL
DENTAL FIBERS
  INTERMEDIATE
ALVEOLAR PLEXUS
  FIBER
BONE

Figure 10–8   Longitudinal section of the molar of a guinea pig to show intertwining of dental and alveolar fibers to form an intermediate plexus in the periodontal membrane. (After Sicher.)

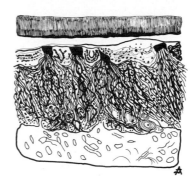

DENTINE
ENAMEL
DENTAL FIBERS

PLEXUS

ALVEOLAR FIBER
BONE

Figure 10–9   Cross section of guinea pig molar shows intermediate zone less clearly, but "splicing" of dental and alveolar fibers can be observed.

osteoid along the bone surface. Damage to fibers on the tension side occurs essentially as a result of a prolonged and traumatic occluding force.[25]

In this type of activity old fibers would not have to be replaced with new fibers on the traction side. On the pressure side only the alveolar fibers which become disengaged by resorption would have to be replaced, leaving the intermediary plexus and dental fibers still functioning. Sicher attributes the quick repair of the periodontal ligament to the presence of young argyrophilic-sensitive collagenous fibers and fibroblasts in the intermediary zone, which is, by its nature, a zone of growth and adjustment.

Zwarych and Quigley have not been able to demonstrate an intermediate plexus in their study of mouse molars.[3] Their research supported the concept of the continuity of the principal fibers across the periodontal space. The mesh-like arrangement is illustrated in Figure 10–10. This drawing shows where the fibers might become unspliced or broken in the center of the periodontal space, instead of ripping from the alveolar bone or the tooth. Actual sections are shown in Figures 10–11 and 10–12.

Sicher contends that the very narrow plexus is difficult to see in the mammal, but that it indubitably is present as a result of the evolutionary trend from reptilian ankylosis of teeth to mammalian syndesmosis, where the area of continual adjustment during growth and development is controlled in the alveolar

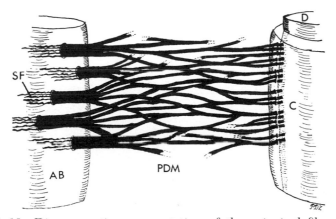

Figure 10–10   Diagrammatic representation of the principal fibers as they pass across the periodontal space. PDM, Principal fibers of the periodontal ligament. AB, Alveolar bone. C, Acellular cementum. D, Dentin. SF, Sharpey's fibers. (Courtesy Zwarych, P. D., and Quigley, M. B.: The intermediate plexus of the periodontal ligament; history and further observations. J. Dent. Res., 44:383–391, 1965.)

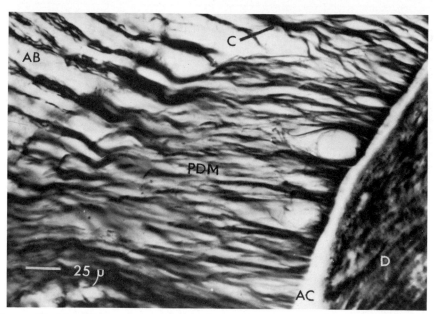

Figure 10–11 High power section showing continuity of principal fibers as they cross the periodontal space and the change in staining as the bundle becomes embedded in the alveolar bone. PDM, Periodontal ligament. AC, Acellular cementum. AB, Alveolar bone. C, Continuity of fibers from bone to tooth. D, Dentin. (Courtesy Zwarych, P. D., and Quigley, M. B.: The intermediate plexus of the periodontal ligament; history and further observations. J. Dent. Res., 44:383–391, 1965.)

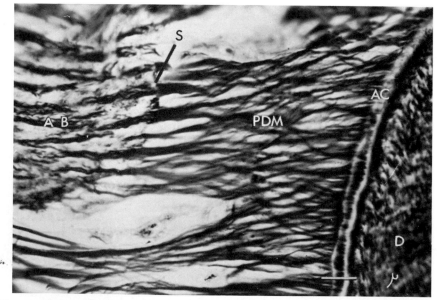

Figure 10–12 Higher power of Figure 10–11, again showing unbroken fibers and no intermediate plexus. PDM, Periodontal ligament. AC, Acellular cementum. AB, Alveolar bone. S, Abrupt change in staining of fibers as they become embedded in bone. D, Dentin. (Courtesy Zwarych, P. D., and Quigley, M. B.: The intermediate plexus of the periodontal ligament: history and further observations. J. Dent. Res., 44:383–391, 1965.)

socket and by ligamentous factors (the PDM).[26] In effect, all that is left of the number of bones that make up the mandible in the reptile is the dentary, which has become larger and larger in evolution. Therefore, the intermediary plexus is a natural consequence.

2. HOW DOES A TOOTH REACT TO A TIPPING FORCE, A BODILY FORCE, A ROTATING FORCE, AN ELONGATING FORCE, A DEPRESSING FORCE?

REACTION TO TIPPING FORCE.   The kind of movement, i.e. tipping or bodily, that a tooth undergoes can be more precisely evaluated by relating it to the location of the *center of rotation* for that specific movement. A tipping movement produced by application of a simple force to the crown will have a center of rotation approximately at a point one half the root length from the apex, while a pure moment or couple (torque) applied to the crown will result in a center of rotation at a point approximately 0.4 the root length measured from the alveolar crest. An increase or a decrease in the magnitude of the force or couple *when applied separately* can have very little effect upon the position of the instantaneous center of rotation.[8] Such changes in amount of force applied will only produce changes of intensity in the distribution pattern of the reactive stresses in the PDM.[27] It should be emphasized again that the physical and biologic centers of rotation may not coincide, because of reaction within the biologic continuum. A correlation of all factors is essential in arriving at an analysis of projected tooth movement.

The center of rotation of a tooth in movement *can* be shifted by the application of the proper *combination* of a force and a couple. In other words, the ratio of the magnitudes of force to couple determines the position of the instantaneous center of rotation of any tooth movement. This position can vary from anywhere on the root and crown portion in either direction out to infinity. Bodily movement means that the center of rotation is at infinity.

REACTION TO BODILY FORCE.   In the correction of many malocclusions, teeth must be moved bodily. Both the root and the crown must be changed in position to achieve proper axial inclination, overbite, overjet, etc. By use of "torque" force or by application of force at more than one point on the surface of a tooth, bodily tooth movement can be accomplished in most instances. As might be assumed, the histologic picture is similar to that for tipping. Bodily movement of a maxillary central incisor in a lingual direction would show resorption along the entire lingual surface and bone deposition along the labial surface. No axis of rotation should be expected (Fig. 10–13). Despite a clinical impression of bodily movement, however, there is some evidence that at least histologically, bodily movement is not quite that. A certain amount of "give" is present in all appliances—in brackets or wires. It is probable that a tooth moves bodily by "wiggling" or "jiggling" toward its new position. As Sicher has said, the tooth leads with its head, then its knee, then its elbow, then its foot. These are imperceptible tilts, but the histologist contends that he can demonstrate their presence. The "wiggling" allows both resorption and deposition to occur on the same surfaces to keep the tooth from becoming excessively mobile, to stabilize its position and to prevent traumatic injury to the delicate structures at the apex of the tooth and at the fundus of the alveolus.[4]

Clinically, with conventional fixed appliances, greater force is usually required for bodily movement. Evidences of root resorption are observed more frequently with this type of movement than with changes in tooth inclination.

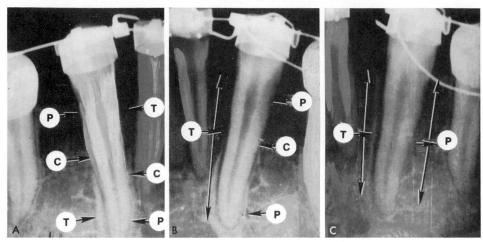

Figure 10–13   A, Lower right canine being moved distally by the tipping force of a sliding hook. B, Lower left canine, same mouth, three weeks later under an uprighting bodily force. C, Continued bodily movement of lower left canine. In A, note pressure P at alveolar crest on distal, at apex on mesial, with tension T at mesial alveolar crest and distal apex. Centroid C (rotational axis) is marked on both sides. In B, there is only tension on the mesial, only pressure on distal, but the rotational axis area has not yet disappeared. In C, the thickened periodontal membrane shows tension clearly on the mesial. Compare this with the pressure side. (Courtesy J. R. Jarabak.)

It should be emphasized that evidence of root resorption is highly correlated with force and time factors.[2] Experimental movement shows that bodily movement with light forces may be performed without the formation of pressure zones and with less root resorption than with a tipping movement conducted with the same force for the same duration.[28] Obviously, in the tipping movement, the force is concentrated in a smaller area, which accounts for this reaction.[29] Greater care must be exercised to produce the desired movement with a minimum of force. Excess force is damaging and may leave permanent scars such as root resorption, sheared crests or gingival detachment. Clinical evidence with differential light forces seems to indicate that bodily movement can be achieved rapidly with minimal force from high intensity spring wires of small gauge in many instances. The versatility of such continuous light force techniques is shown in Figure 10–13. Light wires produce (A) tipping, (B) beginning bodily movement and (C) continued upright and bodily movement. With the light wire technique, the tooth is frequently moved bodily in a slightly inclined position.

REACTION TO ROTATING FORCE.   The reaction of a tooth to a rotating force is somewhat more complex than tipping or bodily movement in one direction. Theoretically, it is bodily movement in one place; actually, it is usually a combined tipping and rotational action. A number of factors must be taken into consideration: tooth position, root size and form (most roots are ovoid in shape), arrangement of periodontal fibers, arrangement of free-gingival fibers and supra-alveolar tissue, degree, direction, distribution and duration of forces applied, and age of the patient. Because of the widespread effects of rotation forces, involving more than just bone and periodontal membrane, it is difficult to draw a concise picture. Since the root is seldom perfectly round, areas of pressure and tension will occur on various portions of the root, neighboring membrane and alveolar bone. Reaction should be similar to tipping or bodily stimulus. In addition, innumerable periodontal fiber bundles are stretched and realigned in the direction of pull (Fig. 10–14).

It has been noted that the reorganization of the principal periodontal fibers that run from the root surface to the bone surface proceeds fairly rapidly.[25] In this experiment on dogs, a retention period of 28 days seemed sufficient to prevent relapse. But the reaction of supra-alveolar fibers is an entirely different story. A retention period of 232 days was not enough to reorient supra-alveolar fibers.[30] Erikson, Kaplan and Aisenberg had noted the persistence of transseptal fibers.[31] The additional presence of a certain number of elastic fibers in the supra-alveolar tissues enhances the relapse tendency (Fig. 10–15). Relapse is thus caused by the contraction of the displaced gingival fibers and other supra-alveolar structures which, contrary to PDM fibers between root and alveolar

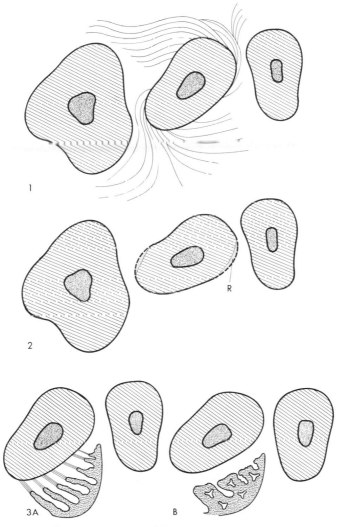

Figure 10–14   1, The arrangement of free gingival fibers following rotation of teeth. 2, R is the amount of resorption of the tooth root following extensive rotation. 3, A illustrates how bone spicules are formed along stretched fiber bundles; B shows the rearrangement of bone tissue following retention of the tooth moved. (After K. Reitan.)

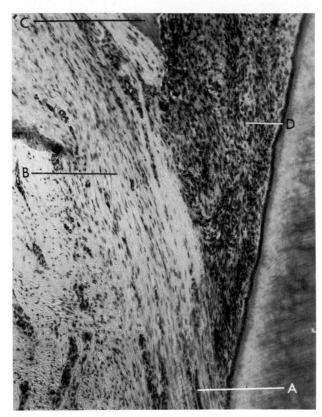

Figure 10–15   Twelve-year-old patient, marginal third of the root. A and B, supra-alveolar fibers. C, Alveolar bone undergoing direct resorption. D, Increase in the number of cells of the alveolar crest fibers. Note less increase in cellular elements of the supra-alveolar fibers. The tooth, previously moved toward the bone surface, had been left without appliances for four days. (Courtesy K. Reitan.)

bone, adapt very slowly to their new position. Reitan feels that over-rotation is advisable, transsection of stretched supra-alveolar fibers at the gingival margin might help, and — most certainly — rotation as early as possible is recommended.[60] This permits new fibers to form that will help maintain tooth position. Another factor in the persistent relapse tendency of orthodontically rotated teeth is the fact that this type of movement does not duplicate physiologic movement. More direct periodontal ligament adjustment is required on all surfaces than, for example, with a tipping movement.

REACTION TO ELONGATING FORCE.   Concerning the reaction of a tooth to an elongating force, one must take into consideration the fact that in most orthodontic cases this type of force is enhancing what would normally occur as a result of growth and development. It is difficult to assign any specific amount to natural causes or another equally arbitrary percentage of contribution to appliance manipulation. An elongating force tends to lift the tooth out of the socket. If unopposed by considerably greater functional forces and occlusal prematurities, the increased and continuous tension on the principal periodontal fibers causes deposition of bone on the walls of the alveolus — with little resorptive activity other than to realign and maintain trabeculae, replace bundle bone, and so on

(Fig. 10–16). A vitally important consideration is: What happens to the delicate structures that enter the apex of the tooth being elongated? Some clinicians have found the answer in darkened, nonvital teeth that were elongated. Apparently, of all orthodontic tooth movements, elongation is the one most likely to devitalize a tooth. Very light pressures and great caution are essential.

REACTION TO DEPRESSING FORCE. A depressing force against a tooth probably meets with less success in terms of absolute tooth movement than any other force applied (Fig. 10–16B). The oblique fibers of the periodontal membrane are so attached to the root surface and to the alveolar bone that a blow or pressure along the long axis of a tooth is strongly resisted by these fibers, as they cushion the fundus of the alveolus against damage. A depressing force in the long axis is transmitted as tension to both the tooth root and alveolar bone. The "give" of the oblique fibers is not enough under normal circumstances to create sufficient pressure at the apex for resorption, since the PDM is wider at this point. To actually depress a tooth, extremely strong force is required—a force sufficient to tear the fibers loose from their attachments, unsplice the intermediate plexus, rupture the delicate blood vessels of the periodontal membrane and then exert pressure on the alveolar walls and apex. Fortunately, the shape of the root as a reducing cone prevents the full force from being thrown against the apex, as the tooth "binds" on the converging lateral alveolar walls. Resorption is largely of an undermining nature in what is obviously a pathologic process.[32, 63]

Most clinical depression is not of this type. The pressures applied are not sufficient to rupture the periodontal fibers but serve to prevent the tooth being depressed from erupting normally as the remaining teeth not under this type of force will do. As with ankylosis of a deciduous molar, where the term "submerging molar" has often been used, there is no absolute depression. The other teeth merely erupt and elevate above the level of the tooth under depressing force; the net result is depression. Some adjustments that are placed in an arch wire are called "depressing adjustments." Since for every force applied there is an equal and opposite force, they could just as well be called "elevating or elongating" adjustments, with greater validity.

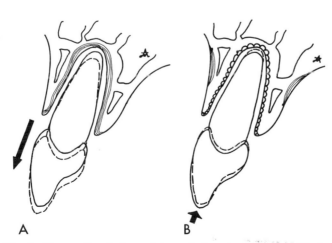

A   B

Figure 10–16 A, Generalized deposition of alveolar bone on the fundus of the alveolus during an elongating force. B, Diagram of the effect of a depressing force. Osteoclastic activity is generalized along surfaces of tooth socket. (Courtesy K. Reitan.)

3. WHAT IS THE TISSUE REACTION TO DIFFERENT AMOUNTS OF FORCE?

The reaction of the periodontal membrane and alveolar bone, as well as the cementum and dentin, varies with the degree of force applied. A light tipping force, as was discussed in the first question of this series, causes a compression of the PDM, but stimulates the formation of fibroblasts and osteoclasts on the side of pressure at hand in the vicinity of the site of pressure (Figs. 10–17, 10–18). PDM fibers are stretched in the areas under tension, unraveling partly in the intermediate zone, and osteoblasts form in the periodontal membrane. Using removable appliances and intermittent forces with rest periods during the day, Häupl actually observed an increase in bone-building cells on the side of pressure and a layer of osteoid bone at the lamina dura.[33] This substantiates the observation of Frost, an orthopedic surgeon and researcher, who observes the bone-building or osteoblastic reaction to certain types of pressure. Fränkel points out that a continuity of force application and force direction is needed to produce the classic reaction. Intermittent force is less likely than continuous force to produce resorption on the pressure side, if that force is not of sufficient duration or sufficiently oriented for a long enough time.[34]

With a gradually expanded fixed activator (see Chap. 11), worn at night over a short period of time, Reitan has shown that tissue changes are minimal on both pressure and tension side. In Figure 10–19, all the activator has done

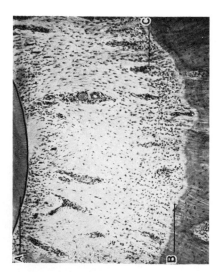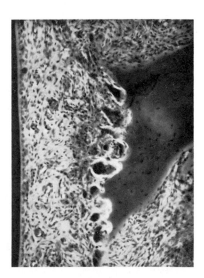

Figure 10–17   Histologic sections showing tooth reaction to a light force. (Left) The tooth (A) is being moved to the right. A definite osteoid layer of bone is seen at (B). There is an increase in cell number, considerably denser close to the bone and along the thickened fiber bundles extending from the osteoid layer (C). (Right) The tooth is also being moved to the right. Note the thin cementum line along the root and the large osteoclasts attacking a spicule of bone by direct frontal assault. (Courtesy K. Reitan.)

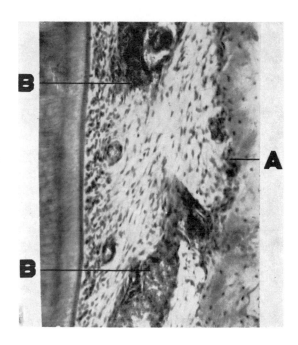

Figure 10–18 Reaction of pressure side to light force of short duration. The periodontal space is somewhat compressed. Cells with pycnotic nuclei are seen in the middle portion of this space, while there are normal cells along root surface. Direct bone resorption takes place along the bone surface at A. Note dilated capillaries at B. (Courtesy K. Reitan.)

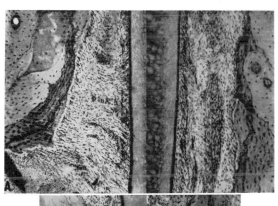

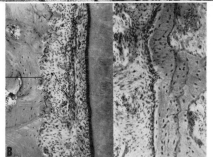

Figure 10–19 A, Tooth moved six nights with gradually expanded fixed activator. On tension side (left), formative changes prevail, but osteoid line is interrupted in several areas and there is no increase in cell number. On pressure side (right), no active bone resorption is seen; no capillary dilation has occurred, and osteoid lines are observed in some areas. Tooth was moved labially or to the right. This type of jiggling movement is seen with so-called Crozat appliances. B, The control tooth shows actual resorption on the lingual side (left) as the tooth migrates lingually. On the labial side of the control tooth (right), there is bone apposition along the inner bone surface as indicated by an osteoid line and chain of osteoblasts. Several resorbed areas are observed in closed marrow spaces. (Courtesy K. Reitan.)

is to interfere with a normal lingual migration, as seen in the control tooth. This can also be explained by the intermittent nature of the forces applied by the activator. Continuous light forces do not allow the pressure and tension sides to "recover," so few bone-building cells are seen on the pressure side during an adjustment period; no osteoid bone is observed on the bone surface being attacked by the osteoclasts. With light forces, the bone is resorbed directly by a frontal osteoclastic attack. Resorption of cementum and dentin appears less frequent, judging from clinical and radiographic evidence. The newer differential light force techniques of tooth movement claim to operate in this manner.[35]

Hixon notes that even though heavier forces produce more tooth movement than light forces, there is little evidence to support the "optimal" force theory. Because of the great variability from patient to patient, "It may be well to begin with light arches and gradually increase the diameter of the wire as the desired tooth movement is achieved."[36]

With forces well beyond the capillary pressure level, the periodontal membrane is compressed so severely at the site of pressure that hemorrhage, stasis and necrosis set in. Cells die instead of proliferating. The periodontal ligament suffers greatly on the tension side as fibers are parted in the intermediate zone. Adjacent to the pressure-necrosis area, circulation does increase and osteoclasts form. The osteoclasts infiltrate the alveolar wall in the compressed PDM sites above and below the point of greatest pressure. They move up to the alveolar bone to remove the bone from behind, in a flanking assault, or by "undermining resorption" (Fig. 10–5). After the clean-up of necrotic elements by phagocytosis, tissue reorganization recurs. With heavier pressures there is greater possibility of resorption of cementum and dentin of the tooth. Critical factors here are the degree of force, the distance through which the force is active and the length of force application. Strong continuous forces operating over a considerable distance are more likely to allow osteoclastic penetration of the resorption-resistant cementoid layer covering the root (Fig. 10–4). Continuous force prevents formation of both cementoid and osteoid bone at the site of greatest pressure.

4. WHAT IS THE ROLE OF THE PERIODONTAL MEMBRANE?

This has been particularized in the answers of the first three questions of this series. Specifically, however, it serves as:

A *protective cushion* against functional forces, protecting the delicate structures at the fundus of the alveolus. Because of the oblique position of the principal fibers, they literally suspend the tooth in a hammock-like sling, transmitting force applied in the long axis as tension to the alveolar wall.[14] Similarly, the PDM is a protective mechanism against accidental blows.

A *source of nutriment* for the periodontal tissues, bringing essential food and carrying off wastes through the periodontal circulatory apparatus.

A *storehouse of cells* (fibroblasts, osteoblasts, osteoclasts) for maintenance of physiologic activity, such as eruption and mesial drift. In addition, these cells serve nonphysiologic or pathologic demands (tooth movement).

A *sensory plexus* for proprioceptive demands.

5. IS THERE AN OPTIMAL ORTHODONTIC FORCE?

The most obvious answer would be the force that is required for such physiologic movement as eruption and mesial drift. It has been stated by

Oppenheim[17] and Schwarz,[21] as a result of their experiments, that this would be equivalent to the capillary pulse pressure—or 20 to 26 gm. per sq. cm. of root surface. With a force this light, tooth movement would be by direct osteoclastic activity in the area of greatest pressure; undermining resorption would not occur. In actual practice with current orthodontic appliances, few teeth are moved with such light forces. Furthermore, Reitan takes issue with this observation and points out that initially there is more tipping than bodily movement.[21, 25, 29] When a tooth is tipped, there is always formation of a cell-free zone on the pressure side, even with forces as light as 20 to 30 gm. If the tooth is moved bodily, there is still the formation of a small cell-free zone on the pressure side in most cases. He feels that this is caused by occlusal trauma created by the movement, together with the fact that the force may not be light enough. Experimentally, without the forces of occlusion acting, it has been proved that a bodily or torque movement may be performed with forces of 40 to 50 gm. without the formation of compressed hyalinized zones[37] (Fig. 10–20). Bodily movement with a force of 100 to 150 gm. causes undermining resorption for a fairly short period of 10 to 15 days. Schwarz did not detect the undermining resorption in his study because of the experimental design, with force being delivered unequally to several teeth in a quadrant.[40]

Whatever force is used, it would appear that the changes in rate of cell replication are the same on both pressure and tension sides. And the collagen synthesis decreases on both sides. Baumrind also noted that bone deflection can be caused by forces less than those required to decrease PDM width. "Bone deforms far more readily than PDM."[38, 39]

The measurement of forces employed is not accurate enough to tell magnitude at the cellular level at present. Tooth size, root shape, functional forces, point of application, type of force and hydraulic effect all influence the net amount of force reaching a particular area of root surface. Equally important are direction of force, duration of force, distance through which the force is

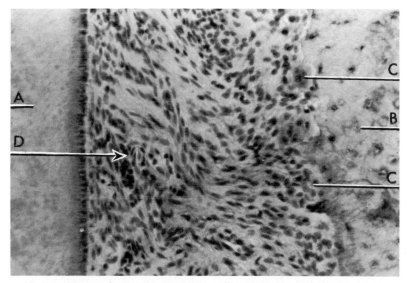

Figure 10–20 Direct bone resorption on the pressure side in a torque movement effected by light forces. A, Tooth; B, bone; C, osteoclasts in resorption lacunae; D, epithelial remnant of Malassez, indicating that there is a direct bone resorption. Arrow indicates direction of movement. (Courtesy K. Reitan.)

operating and continuity of the force. Very probably, patient age, individual tissue reaction and endocrine balance also make a difference.

Finally, in addition to the potent forces of occlusion, another force that has been ignored by many observers trying to arrive at a measure of optimal force to move teeth is the force exerted by the supra-alveolar structures. Particularly important are the elastic type transseptal fibers that "give" but do not change rapidly, and offer varying degrees of resistance to tooth movement — often recruiting additional teeth through their attachments, and actually moving these teeth as well as the tooth being moved primarily.[37]

To state categorically that capillary pressure is optimum is wrong. It might be better to say that the force should be one which moves the tooth most rapidly in the desired attitude and direction with the least tissue damage and the slightest amount of pain. The orthodontist must consider time an important practical factor. Patient convenience, increased possibility of decalcification around bands, chances of partial "washing out of cement," and soft tissue response must all be taken into account in arriving at a definition of an optimal force for orthodontic tooth movement. Recent advances in appliances employing differential light forces theoretically provide the answer. But usually, the force is considerably above capillary pressure. But it is well below the force stored in heavy gauge steel wires and released unchecked by some orthodontists employing multibanded techniques.

6. SHOULD THE FORCE BE INTERMITTENT (INTERRUPTED) OR CONTINUOUS? THROUGH HOW GREAT A DISTANCE SHOULD THE FORCE BE ACTIVE?

This is asked as a double-barreled question because clinical results indicate that these two factors are closely linked. Oppenheim, in his studies, recommended light, intermittent forces as best for tooth movement because the tissue had rest periods, allowing the bone and PDM to reorganize.[28] He felt that this resulted in less resorption. Schwarz, in his experience, has recommended light, continuous forces because this prevents the formation of resorption-resistant osteoid bone and certain reparative processes on the side toward which the tooth moves.[40] These processes actually slow down tooth movement. Stuteville has shown that fairly strong forces can be used, since the critical consideration is the *distance through which these forces act*.[14] Whether it is a light force or a heavy force, as long as this force is not active through a distance greater than the thickness of the periodontal membrane, the result is satisfactory, if not truly physiologic.[36]

USE OF HEAVY FORCES. Although, theoretically, Stuteville's statement is correct, it is not possible to apply the method in practice. The PDM is only 0.20 to 0.25 mm. wide, and heavy force application over as short a distance as this cannot be attained with orthodontic appliances. More to the point is the *interrupted force principle*,[41] whereby the force of considerable magnitude acts over a short distance, but the duration is limited. There is formation of a compressed hyalinized zone with undermining resorption of fairly short duration. During the resting period, the tissues are left ample time for reorganization. An example of interrupted force would be torque, as employed in many edgewise techniques.[7, 41] Heavy forces active through a short distance (forces that dissipate rapidly in intensity to a minimal level as the thickness of the PDM is reached, and then are followed by a rest period of some days to allow tissue reorganization and repair) produce relatively little tissue destruction or radiographically observable resorption. Heavy forces active through a much greater distance are more damaging to both the teeth and periodontal tissues and should not be used; damage may be irreparable. Even with heavy forces acting through a short distance, tooth movement is probably effected by undermining resorption in most instances.

USE OF LIGHT FORCES. An alternative to the relatively satisfactory use of heavy forces through very short distances by periodic intermittent applications that allow tissue repair between adjustments is the use of very light continuous forces. These forces move teeth primarily by frontal assault, with little necrosis of periodontal tissue at the point of greatest pressure. Because there is not the added load of removal of the necrotic remnants of the crushed, periodontal membrane, as with undermining resorption; because the periodontal tissue at the site of greatest pressure remains vital, with increased circulation serving as a source for phagocytic cells; and because osteoid bone does not form to retard resorption and tooth movement, many clinicians now prefer this type of force. They reason that with less tissue destruction during treatment (because of the light forces involved) there will be less permanent damage. With gentle, continuous forces, teeth appear to move more rapidly and with less pain to the patient.

PROBLEMS IN THEIR USE. There are problems, however, with the use of so-called light continuous forces. Because of the great range of individual differences, it is difficult to determine the optimal level of force application necessary for each individual patient.[36] Further, it is not easy to measure the exact force applied to each tooth after an arch wire has been tied into place. Such factors as reciprocal anchorage, functional forces during the period of force application and the mauling that a light wire appliance receives during mastication and cleansing of teeth, militate against maintenance of a continuous optimal force. With the knowledge that continuous forces beyond the optimal level can cause severe root resorption and great damage to the periodontal tissues, the dentist would do well to exercise caution in the use of these forces.

7. WHICH KIND OF FORCE CAUSES LESS ROOT RESORPTION?

As with the previous questions, the answer must be qualified. It has been shown histologically that the resorption-resistant layer of osteoid bone and the cementoid layer that covers the root of the tooth break down more slowly than alveolar bone.[24] For this reason, interrupted forces are less likely to produce root resorption than continuous forces of sufficient intensity to breach the protective cementoid barrier. It would seem that the question of intensity is the critical one. Light forces or forces approaching the level of so-called physiologic tooth movement probably produce little root resorption in most cases. It would seem with these light forces that the method of application — interrupted versus continuous — would make relatively little difference. Heavy forces that cause necrosis and undermining resorption can cause significant amounts of root resorption. If these heavy forces are of continuous duration and active over a distance well beyond the thickness of the PDM, chances of root resorption are increased appreciably. For heavy forces, particularly, *duration* as well as *intensity* must be considered. If appliances are left on the teeth for a long period of time, root resorption may occur as a result of repeated pressure. There is little tendency to root resorption within an 8- to 9-month period, provided that moderate forces have been used, and there are no endocrinologic predisposing factors. A prolonged tipping movement causes more apical root resorption than a bodily movement. Bodily tooth movement within the 50 to 200 gm. range does not ordinarily cause radiographically perceptible apical root resorption.[52, 54]

8. CAN FORCES BE DIRECTED PRECISELY?

If the dentist has the proper appliances, knows how to use them and understands the fundamental principles of biomechanics, he can usually move the tooth in the desired direction. He must be constantly aware, as discussed more fully later in this chapter, that for each force there is an equal and opposite force. He must make sure that he balances his reciprocal force in such a manner that the primary objective is accomplished—and not the movement of his "anchorage." The mere "tying in" with an arch wire often produces forces of which the dentist is unaware. Such forces may prevent the accomplishment of the primary objective or produce undesired tooth movement in other areas of the mouth. Even where forces can be directed precisely where desired, the response of the tooth or teeth to this force may not always be forthcoming. The lingual movement of the apices of the maxillary incisors and the distal movement of the mandibular molars may not be achieved in some cases, regardless of the force applied. Proper training, skill and experience are the best guarantors of the achievement of the therapeutic objective.

9. WHAT IS THE ROLE OF FUNCTIONAL FORCES?

In any analysis of the biomechanics of tooth movement, a thorough appreciation must be had of the effect of functional forces on the adjustments placed in tooth-moving appliances. Abnormal perioral muscle activity particularly can make it most difficult for the orthodontist to achieve his therapeutic objective. These forces are often acting in the opposite direction to which the orthodontist wants to move the teeth. With some types of appliances the orthodontist can utilize the potent functional forces to his advantage, but all too frequently these forces only serve to make the job more difficult. The inclined-plane relationship of the buccal segments may also serve as a roadblock to the desired changes in tooth position and inclination. As any dentist who has tried to correct posterior or anterior cross-bite problems knows, the antagonistic effect of function can be most frustrating.[42] Once the abnormal functional forces have been eliminated, however, and are no longer deforming the dental arch morphology, they "join the team" and serve as superb retaining adjuncts. After a tooth in cross-bite has "jumped the bite," the very same forces that interfered with the accomplishment of the orthodontic objective will now work on the side of the dentist. If abnormal muscle forces have not been eliminated and if the function in general is not supporting the result obtained by the correction of the malocclusion, the dentist can be sure of one thing—the subsequent remolding of the dental arches and the changes in individual tooth position necessary to achieve a dentition in balance with these forces. Changes in tooth position and arch form *must* be made in such a manner that a balance of *all* forces is obtained at the end of orthodontic treatment.

10. WHAT IS THE SOFT-TISSUE RESPONSE?

The orthodontist has often been accused of neglecting the gingival tissues when he moves teeth. While there may be validity to this accusation in some cases, there are certain extenuating circumstances. Orthodontic appliances usually interfere with the normal tissue exercise and massage that occurs during mastication, deglutition and speech.

With multibanded techniques the lip has a great deal of difficulty in cleaning the remnants of the bolus of food from the mucobuccal fold and from the gingivae because of the mechanical obstruction of the appliances. Food remains lodged in the gingival crevice and around the orthodontic appliances. Frequently the periphery of the orthodontic bands extends beneath the gingival margin, and the bands—together with the food debris—serve as constant irritating factors. With lack of proper exercise, with stasis of circulation and with irritation constantly present from the impinging appliances and collected decaying debris, it is no wonder that the gingival tissues become hyperemic, edematous and "puffy." The pink color is replaced by a reddish purple and these tissues bleed freely. If strong counter-measures are not taken, the proliferating interdental papillae become fibrous and will remain enlarged after the irritating influence of the appliances is removed.

Since most orthodontic therapy occurs at a time when the endocrine system is undergoing great changes and is most active, the patient may be unusually prone to an abnormal soft tissue response during orthodontic therapy. In severe cases there may be actual stripping of the labiogingival tissue or pocket formation. If the dentist realizes at the outset that he is robbing the tissue of its normal exercise and is introducing an irritant with orthodontic appliances and ensuing trapped debris, he can do much to maintain soft tissue health during the difficult treatment period (see Chap. 12). Constant massage and scrupulous hygiene are absolutely essential.

The elimination of bands and the attachment of brackets directly to the teeth, now becoming a practical technique, will reduce soft-tissue iatrogenic response, as well as decalcification of enamel in uncleansed interproximal areas.

11. WHAT IS THE ROLE OF THE SUPRA-ALVEOLAR TISSUE?

Reitan and others have emphasized the tensions in the supra-alveolar and subepithelial tissues during orthodontic tooth movement[18, 19, 20, 25, 28, 31, 43] (Figs. 10–14, 10–15). He shows conclusively in his experiments that the gingival fiber bundles are displaced by orthodontic tooth movement and that they remain displaced and stretched even after a retention period of 232 days.[19] This is in contrast with the periodontal fibers which run from the tooth to the bone surface and which rearrange themselves usually in less than 28 days.[37] Orthodontists who have moved individual teeth and watched contiguous teeth accompany them because of the influence of transseptal fibers know well the importance of the supra-alveolar tissue. It would appear from the latest work that rotated teeth must be retained for a long period of time to allow for the relatively slow reorganization of the supra-alveolar tissue.[59] Failure to do so means the relapse toward the original malposition. If the tooth movement is done quite early, just as the teeth erupt, and while the periodontal tissue is active from a growth standpoint, retention of rotated teeth may be more successful because of the formation of new fiber bundles formed in the apical region, which assist in maintaining the corrected position.

12. DOES TOOTH MOVEMENT STIMULATE GROWTH, CAUSE MODELING CHANGES IN THE BONE ITSELF OR RESTRICT JAW GROWTH?

TOOTH MOVEMENT AND GROWTH STIMULATION.   In the past, many claims have been made by orthodontists that their appliance manipulations stimulated jaw growth. Since most orthodontic patients are treated during an active growth period, it is difficult to determine how much growth is due to the inherent pattern and how much is due to orthodontic stimulation.

It is known that environmental influences can affect the total growth accomplishment. But the answer—at present—to the question whether orthodontic tooth movement, per se, makes the jaws grow any more than they would have under optimal conditions without orthodontic treatment must be that it probably does not. It is logical to assume that orthodontic procedures can remove the restricting influences of malocclusion and abnormal muscle function which, if left unattended, would prevent the full accomplishment of pattern. A good example of this is a Class II, Division 1 malocclusion with a severe overbite and active lip habit. The correction of the overbite and the elimination of the lip habit, which has flattened the mandibular anterior segment, may allow the mandible to come forward, seemingly because of growth, but actually because a functional retrusion is eliminated. The anterior arc of the mandibular denture is rounded successfully as a result of restoration of normal muscle function and continued unrestrained growth processes.

Claims have been made that the amount and direction of condylar growth can be changed by dentofacial orthopedic procedures. Experimental work on monkeys by Breitner and Baume indicates this possibility.[44, 45] There is considerable clinical substantiation for changing jaw growth direction and stimulating adaptive changes in the alveolar bone support of teeth, however. Heavy orthopedic force on the mandible in a Class III malocclusion can significantly reduce apical base discrepancy, as shown by this textbook author.[46–49, 62, 63]

Charlier, Petrovic and Linck showed positive experimental evidence of retardation of the prechondroblastic zone of the condyle, under chincap therapy. The resultant decrease in height of the chondroblastic zone demonstrates that mechanical appliances are capable of retarding mandibular condylar growth, although they are not able to inhibit epiphysial cartilage in long bones[46] (Fig. 10–21).

TOOTH MOVEMENT AND MODELING CHANGES.   While there is serious doubt that actual growth of the maxilla or mandible is enhanced by orthodontic therapy, there is much evidence that modeling changes in the alveolar bone nearest the teeth can be made. Most of these changes are accomplished in conjunction with the eruptive growth processes that occur during and following orthodontic therapy. For example, the retraction of the maxillary incisors in the correction of the Class II, Division 1 malocclusion significantly changes the contour of the contiguous labial plate. The lingual plate is also modified and assumes a more vertical inclination as alveolar bone continues to be deposited and the teeth erupt. Similar modeling changes can be observed routinely in the remaining segments of both the upper and lower dental arches. It is doubtful, however, that significant modeling changes can be routinely produced in basal bone that has already been laid down prior to orthodontic treatment. It is possible to torque maxillary incisor roots lingually *through* the palatal plate. It is questionable whether such torque forces, or any appliance manipulations, do much to change the contour of this area, at least at present.

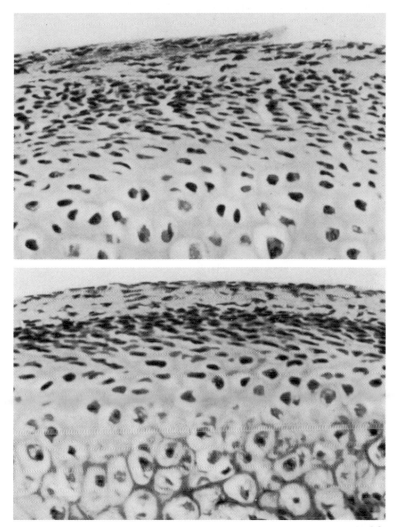

Figure 10–21 Top illustration shows chondroblastic and prechondroblastic zones without chincap pressure. Bottom illustration illustrates a reduced height of the prechondroblastic zone, after four weeks of chincap wear in the rat. The chondroblastic zone is also reduced in height as a result of the reduced proliferating activity of the prechondroblastic zone. The peculiar behavior of condylar cartilage may be explained by the fact that its growth is mainly appositional and only slightly interstitial. (From Charlier, J. P., Petrovic, A., and Linck, G.: La fronde mentionnière et son action sur la croissance mandibulaire. L'Orthodont. Franc., 40:100–113, 1969.)

Fränkel, with his functional corrector, which puts tension on buccal and labial periosteum, seems to show significant basal bone adaptation in the growing child.[34] Significant increases in width of the apical base are graphically demonstrated on oriented frontal headfilms and occlusal radiographs. Is this a growth response or adaptive response; is it harnessing the natural changes in a growing medium? Is it possibly a functional matrix type of response, as hypothesized by Moss (see Chap. 2)? We don't know—yet.

TOOTH MOVEMENT AND JAW GROWTH RESTRICTION. Another controversial question is whether orthodontic procedures can restrict jaw growth. Many clinicians today are firmly convinced that, particularly with the use of extraoral appliances, they can restrict or change direction of the growth processes that would occur normally during orthodontic treatment. After all, primitive tribes have caused bizarre changes in cranial and facial forms by crude bindings and constant pressures; the Chinese kept the size of women's feet at $4\frac{1}{2}$ inches for many centuries, so why cannot the orthodontist restrain jaw growth? The answer is that it can be done, but we must know more.

There is no question that the orthodontist can hold back the teeth and immediate alveolar supporting bone. When extraoral force is applied against a maxillary protrusion the maxillary incisors and bone around them quite obviously move downward and backward, instead of downward and forward as they would have if left alone. Under the same force, the maxillary buccal segments show a similar direction of change. Contemporaneously, the mandible very probably moves downward and forward, unrestricted in its growth. But the scientist asks, "How much of the maxillary change is due to the remodeling of the alveolar bone and how much to restriction at the various sites of maxillary growth, per se?" Similarly, in a strong Class III malocclusion with a pronounced mandibular prognathism, intraoral and extraoral force may be applied against the mandibular teeth and the mandible itself. In the correction of the malocclusion, how much is due to withholding of condylar growth, to restriction of modeling deposition of bone at the symphysis, to tooth movement and modeling changes in the mandibular dentition or to actual repositioning of the condyle in the glenoid fossa? We do not know. The response differs from individual to individual as growth gradients and directions vary, appliances vary, and patient cooperation ranges from good to poor.

Clinically, the author has had considerable success in the use of vertical extraoral forces to reduce steep mandibular plane and open bite problems, as have Straub[50] and others. Studies on the effects of the Milwaukee orthopedic brace and experiments on the macaque monkey show conclusive evidence of significant change induced by extraoral stimulus.[51] The exact nature of the change—whether condylar, basal bone or alveolar bone—must be studied further. Thus, the problem of analyzing what the orthodontist does with his appliances while the child is growing is exacerbated by too many variables and not enough constants.

13. WHAT IS THE AGE FACTOR IN TOOTH MOVEMENT?

As one of the many variables of orthodontic treatment, the age factor must be linked to the individual growth pattern, the timing of the pubertal growth spurt, the type of malocclusion, the mode of orthodontic correction, and so forth. There are certain general principles, however. It was pointed out in Chapter 2 that the treatment of a basal malocclusion, such as a Class II or Class III problem, must be undertaken during the growth period. Tooth movement and correction of Class II and Class III malocclusions depend on growth "assists" during actual treatment. In addition, the dentist may need growth during the period of mixed dentition if the problem is severe, or he may be able to correct the entire problem with the assistance of growth during the pubertal period. If growth increments are insignificant, he may have to resort to the removal of teeth.

Age, as such, is not a decisive factor in the actual movement of teeth. With proper pressures, teeth will move at almost any age. Deciduous teeth have been moved during the first couple of months of life. Octogenarians have had individual teeth shifted to allow placement of prosthetic appliances. In general, teeth move better during the vital growing period; tissues are more responsive, results more stable. It is only reasonable to assume that the reduced vitality of the tissues of the mature adult makes tooth movement a bit more circumscribed and retention of the results frequently only semipermanent. Care must be exercised at all ages with the application of orthodontic pressures. The application of force too early, while the apices of the incisors are wide open and before the roots have formed sufficiently, may very well round these roots off and prevent the full accomplishment of pattern. This is the danger when orthodontic treatment is started too early. Teeth in mature individuals respond more slowly to orthodontic pressures[20] (Fig. 10–22). Older individuals seem to be more prone to resorption. Apparently this is due to the penetration of the cementoid layer and the inability of the cells in this area, with their reduced vitality (as compared with the young growing child), to deposit new cementoid and protect the resorbing roots.

Since more and more orthodontic therapy is being performed on adults, it is wise to know the difference in tissue reaction. Because open marrow spaces are often absent, there is greater likelihood of indirect or undermining resorption. It is very important that light forces be used first to stimulate cell development. In tipping, the centroid is closer to the apex in adults than it is in children because of the completeness of the tooth and the fibrous anchorage.[12] Since the cementum tends to protect the tooth and is usually thicker in adults, bodily movement is quite possible and is a favorable form of movement in adults. Reitan recommends the use of a bite plate to relieve jiggling occlusal forces which may cause damage more easily in patients of this age group. Tipping movement apparently produces more damage at the alveolar crest in adults than in children—a factor recommending bodily movement whenever

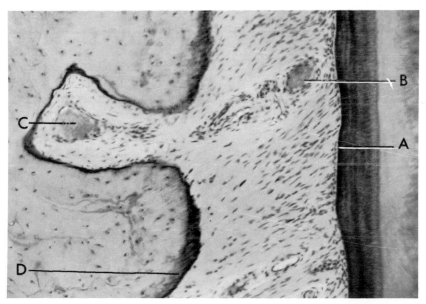

Figure 10–22   Area from alveolar bone crest of 37-year-old patient. A, Chain of cementoblasts along a thick layer of cementum. B, Interstitial space. C, Widened capillary in a cleft where bone resorption may start during initial stages of tooth movement. D, darkly stained alveolar bone surface, containing mucopolysaccharides. Note absence of osteoblasts along bone surface. Less activity means a longer interval between initial adjustment and tooth movement in adults. (Courtesy K. Reitan.)

possible.[37] Use of continuous light force is recommended for the adult group rather than interrupted force, as applied by the removable appliance, for example. There is need of continuous force to stimulate constant development of osteoblasts and osteoclasts in the adult. Finally, remember that in adults it is easier to damage the pulp and to devitalize teeth because the opening into the tooth is smaller and it is easier to disturb the entering vessels and nerves.

Another age-linked factor is the question of timing treatment with certain endocrine changes. Some observers feel that, as the endocrine system undergoes great changes during adolescence, changes in the calcium metabolism or tissue response may occur which might cause unfavorable response to orthodontic therapy.

14. WHAT ARE THE CHANGES DURING THE RETENTION PERIOD?

Relatively little research has been done on this phase of orthodontic treatment. Clinically, teeth that have been tipped or moved into positions of imbalance with muscular pressures and functional forces tend to return to their original position. If traumatic occlusion is not the driving force for this return, the tissue picture is essentially that seen in physiologic mesial drift. Retaining appliances interfere with the relapse of unstable tooth positions.

During the retention period it is often possible to see a thickened periodontal membrane as a result of the jiggling of the teeth by the retainer, which attempts to hold the teeth in one position, a position frequently not in balance with the environmental forces which are asserting pressures in a different direction. The jiggling causes alternate bone resorption and deposition and, as a result, the teeth never "tighten up." The removal of the retaining appliance permits the dominant environmental forces to move the teeth into a position of balance with all the involved pressures. Most post-retention changes are primarily of a tipping nature, with the apex showing relatively little change.[52-54, 64] The effect of the supra-alveolar fibers frequently is seen as the premolars particularly tend to rotate back toward their original malposition. Many orthodontists claim that there is less tendency toward relapse in their extraction cases — that is, where teeth have been removed during the course of orthodontic treatment. This is probably because the orthodontist has obtained better balance of the teeth with the environmental forces. The break in the transseptal supra-alveolar network at the extraction site may be contributory.

GENERAL PRINCIPLES OF TOOTH MOVEMENT

We have seen from the foregoing pages that teeth move when subjected to pressure. Depending on the kind of pressure, the manner in which it is delivered, the type of attachment on the tooth, the distance through which the force is active — to enumerate only a few of the factors — the tooth will move in a certain direction at a certain speed and assume a certain position with respect to contiguous structures. But it does not take very long for the dentist experimenting with tooth movement to find that Sir Isaac Newton anticipated the orthodontists' problems when he said, "Action and reaction are equal and opposite" — or, for every force applied, there is an equal and opposite force. A tooth does not move by itself any more than a man can pull himself up by his own bootstraps.

Depending on how the force is applied, different teeth have different resistance values to tooth movement. Recognizing this, the dentist can use certain teeth for "anchorage," in order to move other teeth into a more desirable position.

TYPES OF ANCHORAGE   uPORISTA

Thus, the term "anchorage" in orthodontics refers to the nature and degree of resistance to displacement offered by an anatomic unit when used for the purpose of effecting tooth movement. While the teeth are the most frequent anatomic units used for anchorage, other structures are available; for example, the palate, the lingual alveolar supporting bone in the mandible, the occiput and the back of the neck. Of course, there are different types of anchorage.

SIMPLE ANCHORAGE. Dental anchorage in which the manner and application of force tends to displace or change the axial inclination of the tooth or teeth that form the anchorage unit in the plane of space in which the force is being applied. In other words, the resistance of the anchorage unit to tipping is utilized to move another tooth or teeth.

An important factor here (and for all forms of anchorage) in assessing resistance values is the part of the tooth anchored in the alveolar bone. The number of roots and the shape, size and length of each root are vitally important. Another way to express this is the approximate surface area of the root portions. A tooth with a large surface area is more resistant to displacement than one with a smaller surface area. A multirooted tooth is more resistant to displacement than a single-rooted tooth; a longer-rooted tooth is more difficult to move than a shorter-rooted tooth; a triangular-shaped root offers greater resistance to movement than a conical or ovoid-shaped root. Other factors are involved such as the relation of contiguous teeth, the forces of occlusion, the age of the patient and individual tissue response variables. Since most dentists are familiar with the morphology of the roots of the different teeth, it is a good rule of thumb to pick anchorage or resistance units that have more root surface area than the tooth to be moved—that is, unless the dentist is interested in moving the anchorage unit also. Since all teeth are more susceptible to tipping movements than they are to bodily movements, it is obvious that simple anchorage, or resistance to a tipping force, has a lower anchorage or resistance value. It is important to check the inclined plane relationships and muscular forces in assessing the value of an anchorage unit (Fig. 10–23). Another factor here would be the *amount* of force. In the light wire, differential forces techniques, buccal segment anchorage units are established by keeping the applied force below the threshold needed to move the posterior teeth, while serving as a base for the delivery of light, continuous, low-friction force against the anterior teeth.

STATIONARY ANCHORAGE. Dental anchorage in which the manner and application of force tend to displace the anchorage unit bodily in the plane of space in which the force is being applied is termed stationary anchorage. If a tooth can be grasped with an appliance in such a manner that any movement requires the tooth to move without any change in its axial inclination, this resistance is considerably greater than to a tipping force. A good example of this type of anchorage is the retraction of maxillary incisors, using the first molars as the anchorage unit. By placing horizontal buccal tubes on the buccal surfaces of the molars and by having a continuous arch wire with spring force applied against the incisors, Newton's law is satisfied. There is an equal and opposite force to begin with.

TYPES OF ANCHORAGE

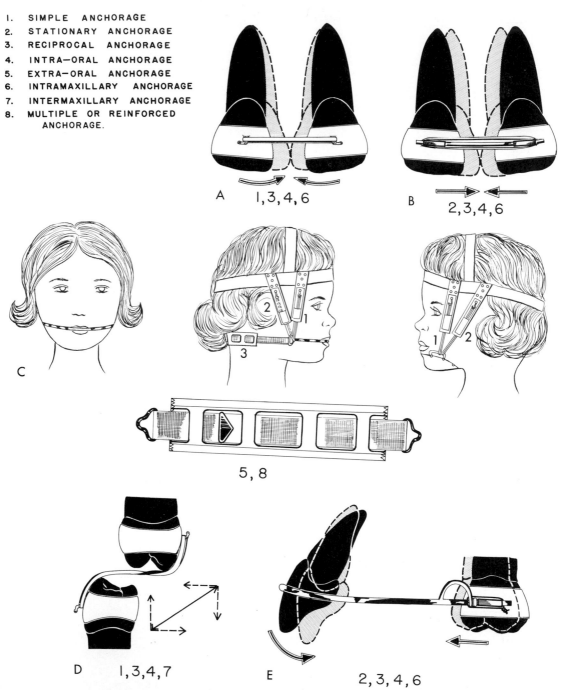

1. SIMPLE ANCHORAGE
2. STATIONARY ANCHORAGE
3. RECIPROCAL ANCHORAGE
4. INTRA—ORAL ANCHORAGE
5. EXTRA—ORAL ANCHORAGE
6. INTRAMAXILLARY ANCHORAGE
7. INTERMAXILLARY ANCHORAGE
8. MULTIPLE OR REINFORCED ANCHORAGE.

A   1,3,4,6

B   2,3,4,6

C

5, 8

D   1,3,4,7

E   2,3,4,6

Figure 10–23   Types of anchorage. Diagrams show that orthodontic anchorage is usually a combination of several types, as indicated beneath each picture. A, Diastema closure by elastic action, tipping crowns together. B, Bodily movement of incisors to close diastema. C, Extraoral force. D, Criss-cross elastics to correct cross-bite. E, Retraction of maxillary incisors by tipping them lingually. Molar resistance is of a bodily nature. Under C, you will note three directions of extraoral force pull: 1 is vertical for open bites; 2 is oblique for mandibular prognathism; 3 is horizontal, or cervical traction. Direction is important with force magnitude within tooth moving range, less important with orthopedic force.

But the root configuration and area of the molars provide considerable resistance to displacement. If the displacement of the molars is so guided that it must be *en masse* as the buccal tube guides it horizontally along the arch wire and prevents the tooth from tipping, then the anchorage value of these two teeth is increased considerably. If the pressure against the incisors is transmitted as a simple tipping force, their relative resistance to movement is decidedly less; they will respond quickly and can probably achieve the desired position before the molar anchorage units show any appreciable change (Fig. 10–23). Even here it is not as simple as it seems. Since the teeth normally move downward and forward in a growing face, somehow their resistance value is less in this direction than when they are being forced backward, or upward and backward, against the normal path of positional change. Thus, growth would reduce the anchorage value of the molar units somewhat.

Another factor is the occlusion. If the maxillary incisors are being retracted against the interfering force of the mandibular incisors, this raises their resistance to retraction appreciably and, together with the reduced value of teeth resisting downward and forward pressures, the molar teeth may come forward more than desired by the dentist.

Resistance to bodily tooth movement by a depressing force is the greatest of all. Because of the heavy demands of function, the periodontal membrane can withstand relatively powerful forces. Actual depression requires the rupturing of principal fibers. Relative depression by withholding the anchorage unit while the remaining teeth are erupting normally can be accomplished. But if the opposing tooth has not elongated or if the contiguous teeth have not encroached on the space of the depressed tooth, it will quickly erupt and regain normal occlusal level. Many anchorage units that are set up for bodily or stationary resistance also incorporate a depressing factor which increases their resistance value.

RECIPROCAL ANCHORAGE Anchorage in which the resistance of one or more dental units is utilized to move one or more opposing dental units is reciprocal anchorage. Usually this term is employed where both resistance units are malposed and the dissipation of the equal and opposite forces tends to move each unit toward a more normal occlusion (Fig. 10–23 A, B, D). The previous illustration of retracting maxillary incisors or using the molars as an anchorage unit is also a form of reciprocal anchorage. Only in that case, the resistance values are not equal because of the bodily resistance of the molars as opposed to the tipping action of the incisors. Reciprocal anchorage is also employed in the correction of Class II malocclusion where intermaxillary elastics are used from the maxillary to the mandibular arch, but an attempt is made here to establish unequal resistance values. (See Intermaxillary Anchorage.) Another simple form of reciprocal anchorage is the correction of posterior cross-bite by the use of through the bite elastics (Fig. 10–23 D). In a strict sense, all force must follow Newton's first law of being equal and opposite and is therefore reciprocal. If the dentist is aware of this broader interpretation, he may choose to limit the interpretation of reciprocal anchorage in orthodontics to pitting one malposed tooth against another to move both to a more normal occlusion. It should be obvious by now that anchorage can be a combination of several forms (i.e., reciprocal stationary, reciprocal simple, and so forth).

INTRAORAL ANCHORAGE Intraoral anchorage is anchorage in which the resistance units are all situated within the oral cavity. It has already been pointed out in our original definition of anchorage that while the teeth are the usual anatomic units employed, this is not always true. (See Extraoral Anchorage.) Even within the oral cavity, the palate, the muscular forces and the inclined planes of the teeth may be a form of intraoral anchorage. Usually, however, "intraoral anchorage" refers to a type of orthodontic therapy in which both the resistance or anchorage units and the teeth being moved are contained within the oral cavity.

EXTRAORAL ANCHORAGE. Extraoral anchorage is anchorage in which one of the anchorage units is situated outside the oral cavity. The use of cranial, occipital and cervical areas to bolster the intraoral resistance units is one of the oldest forms of orthodontic therapy. The dentist need not be concerned about the movement of the anchorage unit (Fig. 10–23 C). Extraoral anchorage is usually employed in the correction of basal or maxillomandibular jaw mal-relationships; this would mean in Class II and Class III therapy (see Chaps. 14 and 18). Despite the efficiency of modern intraoral orthodontic appliances, there has been a widespread use of extraoral force, as more and more orthodontists realize that they are dealing with problems that cannot be solved by tooth-bearing appliances alone.

INTRAMAXILLARY ANCHORAGE. Intramaxillary anchorage is anchorage in which the resistance units are all situated within the same jaw. If appliances are placed only in the maxillary or mandibular dental arches, they are considered intramaxillary resistance units. The illustration used to describe stationary anchorage is also an example of intramaxillary anchorage. Intramaxillary anchorage is obviously intraoral; it may be reciprocal, stationary, or of a simple type of resistance.

INTERMAXILLARY ANCHORAGE. Intermaxillary anchorage is anchorage in which the units situated in one jaw are used to effect tooth movement in the other jaw. In actuality, intermaxillary anchorage, being also reciprocal, serves to effect tooth movement in both jaws. The orthodontist used to think that if he could set up one jaw so that its resistance would be stationary with any movement in a bodily manner, he could move teeth in the other jaw without displacing the anchorage unit. He now knows that this is not possible for any protracted period. Most intermaxillary anchorage is in the form of elastic traction (Fig. 10–23 D). Since intermaxillary anchorage is reciprocal, embodies both simple and stationary factors and is intraoral, it is obvious that it is a form of multiple anchorage.

MULTIPLE ANCHORAGE. Multiple or reinforced anchorage is anchorage in which more than one type of resistance unit is utilized. An analysis of anchorage values in the correction of almost any orthodontic problem would demonstrate that the dentist is dealing with multiple anchorage factors. It may be multiple dental anchorage alone, where only teeth are involved, or there may be use of the palate through a bite plane or guide plane, or there may be extraoral appliances. Tissue- and tooth-borne anchorage such as a palatal removable appliance with clasps over molar bands — so that resistance is both tooth and soft-tissue types — is an example of multiple anchorage. Removable tissue- and tooth-borne and extraoral appliances to augment dental units provide good examples of reinforced anchorage. As the dentist has come to realize that the term anchorage is only a relative thing — that "anchor" teeth move as well as the teeth against which moving forces are primarily directed — he will recognize the need for anchorage reinforcement wherever possible.

BIOPHYSICAL CONSIDERATIONS

The neophyte can learn the hard way that anchorage is a problem, since anchorage units are dragged into abnormal positions. Knowledge of potential biologic response is only part of the answer. Certain physical and mechanical laws are involved. For a full discussion, Chapter 3, by Burstone, in *Current Orthodontic Concepts and Techniques,* is recommended.[55] Storey and Jarabak also go into considerable detail on physical properties and responses of the various types of wires and configurations of wires that are used.[56, 57]

As Burstone writes, an orthodontic appliance has both active and reactive members. For these elements, the objectives are (1) to control the center of rotation of the tooth, (2) to maintain desirable stress levels in the periodontal membrane and (3) to maintain a relatively constant stress level. To accomplish these objectives, Burstone lists three important characteristics which involve the active (tooth-moving part) and the reactive (anchorage part), namely (1) the moment-to-force ratio (2) the load-deflection rate and (3) the maximal force or moment of any component of an appliance.[55]

*The moment-to-force ratio determines the control that an orthodontic appliance will have, in both active and reactive units. It controls the center of rotation of a tooth or group of teeth. Simple orthodontic mechanisms, such as crisscross elastics for the correction of a crossbite or removable appliances such as a Hawley retainer, produce only forces; hence, only tipping movements of teeth will occur. More complex mechanisms using precise attachments between the tooth and the wire have the potentiality of producing varying ratios of moments and forces, and thereby an infinite number of types of tooth movement can be produced.[58]

The load-deflection or torque-twist rate is an indication of the force required per unit deflection. It also measures the rate of decay of the force or torque (moment) as teeth move under the influence of an appliance. Active members of an orthodontic device ideally should have low load-deflection rates. A low load-deflection rate insures a minimum rate of decay in a continuously active force system; the lower the rate, the more closely the system approaches constancy in force. On the other hand, where anchorage is the major consideration, the reactive appliance elements should be relatively rigid, possessing high load-deflection rates.

The maximum elastic moment or load is the greatest force or moment that can be applied to a member without producing permanent deformation. If the maximum elastic load or moment is too low, the orthodontic appliance will permanently deform at forces that are lower than the optimum force needed. A safety factor should exist, so that the optimum force is considerably higher than the maximum elastic load. This will prevent permanent deformation of appliances during their activation or accidental overloading during mastication.

These three characteristics are found within the elastic range of an orthodontic wire and are called *spring characteristics.* There are a number of variables in spring characteristics. These are: mechanical properties of metals, manner of loading, wire cross-section, length of wire, amount of wire, stress raisers, sections of maximal stress, direction of loading and the attachments on the tooth proper. Knowing the interrelationships of these structural and functional factors pertaining to the orthodontic appliance, the orthodontist should be able to decide on a basic configuration of arch wire and attachments that will develop a force system for the specific malocclusion correction (Table 10–1). Some of these appliance possibilities are illustrated in Chapter 11. They may differ in design but, as Burstone indicates, the appliance should have optimal elastic load and load-deflection rate. It also must be capable of delivering the desired moment-to-force ratio. A stress or potential stress analysis is required to prevent appliance failure or breakage. The best possible compromise with a functioning

*This portion of Chapter 10 was written by Dr. Charles Burstone, Professor of Orthodontics, University of Connecticut.

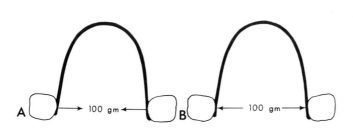

Figure 10–24 A lingual arch is shown which is used to expand the upper right and left first molar. A, The activation force system. A 100 gm force is exerted against the lingual arch in a lingual direction. Since right and left forces are equal, the lingual arch is in equilibrium. B, The deactivation force system. Forces are equal and opposite to the activation forces and are in the direction that the teeth will move.

oral environment as far as hygiene and comfort are concerned, the best possible material and the proper dimensions of arch wires, loops, springs, etc., are part of the biological engineering that is modern orthodontics.[55]

When an appliance is inserted in the mouth, a set of forces is produced—the activation force system (Fig. 10–24A). The activation force system describes the forces exerted by the clinician, in placing the appliance or after it is inserted, on the forces exerted by the brackets or teeth on the various wires. An equal and opposite set of forces is simultaneously produced—the deactivation force system. The deactivation forces are those exerted against the brackets and teeth from orthodontic wires and are the forces responsible for tooth movement (Fig. 10–24B). The activation force system is very important, since it enables the

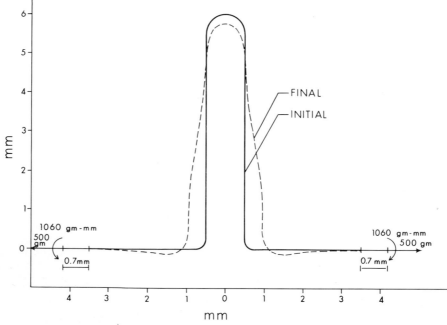

Figure 10–25 Equilibrium diagram of a .016″ stainless steel vertical loop retraction spring (from Burstone and Koenig). The vertical loop is activated 1.4 mm horizontally. To place the horizontal arms into an edgewise bracket, moments of 1060 gm-mm and a force of 500 gm are produced at each bracket. Solid line—initial configuration; dotted line—activated configuration. Teeth will move in directions opposite to the activation forces shown.

clinician to construct an equilibrium diagram for the appliance. Once an orthodontic wire is inserted, it reaches a state of equilibrium. It is possible to solve for unknown forces and moments using the laws governing equilibrium ($\Sigma T_x = 0$, $\Sigma F_y = 0$, $\Sigma_m = 0$). In this way, many undesirable side effects during treatment can be avoided by a careful biomechanical analysis of the appliance that will be used for a specific problem (Fig. 10–25). It is important in constructing an equilibrium diagram to have all forces and moments acting on a wire included and to make sure that only activation and not deactivation forces are used.

elastic deformation　　An amount of structural change in an object caused by a force. The amount of deformation is such that the object will return to its original, unstressed shape, once the deforming force is removed.

modulus of elasticity　　A constant of proportionality to measure stiffness of a material, derived by dividing a stress equal to or less than the proportional limit by its resulting strain value: (stress) ÷ (strain).

moment　　Measure of the tendency to produce movement around a particular axis. A *moment* may be measured as follows: (initiating rotational force) × (distance from point of force application to the axis point of rotation).

plastic deformation　　An amount of structural change in an object caused by a force. The amount of deformation is such that the object will not return to its original, unstressed shape, once the deforming force is removed.

proportional or elastic limit　　The maximum amount an object may be stressed without induction of permanent deformation.

strain　　The structural alteration of an object produced by a force per unit area (stress).

stress　　Application of force over a given area of an object. The force may be expressed either internally or externally. Placement of *stress* on an object produces deformation termed *strain*.

REFERENCES

1. Rudolph, C. E.: An evaluation of root resorption occurring during orthodontic treatment. J. Dent. Res., 19:367–371, 1940.
2. DeShields, R. W.: A study of root resorption in treated Class II, Division I malocclusions. Angle Orthodont., 39:231–245, 1969.
3. Zwarych, P. D., and Quigley, M. B.: The intermediate plexus of the periodontal ligament; history and further observations. J. Dent. Res., 44:383–391, 1965.
4. DeAngelis, V.: Observations on the response of alveolar bone to orthodontic force. Am. J. Orthodont., 58:284–294, 1970.
5. Frost, H. M.: Tetracycline bone labeling in anatomy. Am. J. Phys. Anthrop., 29:183–195, 1968.
6. Frost, H. M.: Laws of Bone Structure. Springfield, Ill., Charles C Thomas, 1964.
7. Epker, B. N., and Frost, H. M.: Correlation of bone resorption and formation with the physical behavior of loaded bone. J. Dent. Res., 44:33–41, 1965.
8. Dijkman, J. F. P.: Krachten verdelingen bij orthodontische behandelingen. University of Nijmegen, 1969.
9. Schour, I.: The growth pattern, growth rhythm and ring analysis of the tooth. Anat. Rec. (Suppl.), 67.45–46, 1937.
10. Baer, M. J., and Ackerman, J. L.: A longitudinal vital staining method for the study of apposition in bone. Studies on Anatomy and Function of Bone & Joints. Berlin, Springer-Verlag, 1966.
11. Sandstedt, C.: Nagra bidrag til tandregleringens teori. Stockholm, P. A. Norstedt & Söner, 1901.
12. Graber, T. M.: Tissue changes induced by orthodontic tooth movement. Washington University Dent. J., 5:55–60, 1938.
13. Oppenheim, A.: Die Veränderungen der Gewebe insbesondere des Knochens bei der Verschiebung der Zähne. Österreich. Ung. Vjschrift, f. Zahnheilk., 27:302–358, 1911.
14. Stuteville, O. H.: Injuries to the teeth and supporting structures caused by various orthodontic appliances and methods of preventing these injuries. J.A.D.A., 24:1494–1507, 1937.
15. Sicher, H.: Tooth eruption: the axial movement of continuously growing teeth. J. Dent. Res., 21:201–210; 395–402, 1942.
16. Graber, T. M.: Unpublished research.

17. Oppenheim, A.: Human tissue response to orthodontic intervention of short and long duration. Am. J. Orth. & Oral Surg., 28:263–301, 1942.
18. Furstman, L., Bernick, S., and Aldrich, D.: Differential response incident to tooth movement. Am. J. Orthodont., 59:600–608, 1971.
19. Reitan, K.: Effects of force magnitude and direction of tooth movement on different alveolar bone types. Angle Orthodont., 34:244–255, 1964.
20. Reitan, K., and Kvam, E.: Comparative behavior of human and animal tissue during experimental tooth movement. Angle Orthodont., 41:1–14, 1971.
21. Schwarz, A. M.: Über die Bewegung belasteter Zahne. Zeitschrift f. Stomatol., 26:40–83, 1928.
22. Sicher, H.: Bau und Funktion des Fixationsapparates der Meerschweinchenmolaren. Zeitschrift f. Stomatol., 21:580–594, 1923.
23. Sicher, H.: The principal fibers of the periodontal membrane. Bur, 55:2–8, 1954.
24. Sicher, H.: Changing concepts of the supporting dental structures. Oral Surg., 12:31–35, 1959.
25. Reitan, K.: Some factors determining the evaluation of force in orthodontics, Am. J. Orthodont., 43:32–45, 1957.
26. Sicher, H.: Personal communication, March 12, 1972.
27. Weinstein, S.: Personal communication, Dec. 29, 1967.
28. Oppenheim, A.: Verbürgt die Verwendung kontinuerlich wirkender Kraft den optimalsten biologischen und klinischen Erfolg? Zeitschrift f. Stomatol., 31:723–735, 1933.
29. Reitan, K.: Continuous bodily tooth movement and its histological significance. Acta Odont. Scandinav., 6:115, 1947.
30. Reitan, K.: Tissue rearrangement during retention of orthodontically rotated teeth. Angle Orthodont., 29:105–113, 1959.
31. Erikson, B. E., Kaplan, H., and Aisenberg, M. S.: Orthodontics and transseptal fibers. Am. J. Orthodont. & Oral Surg., 31:1–20, 1945.
32. Hixon, E. H., Aasen, T. O., Arango, J., Clark, R. A., Klosterman, R., Miller, S. S., and Odom, W. M.: On force and tooth movement. Am. J. Orthodont., 57:476–489, 1970.
33. Häupl, K., and Psansky, R.: Histologische Untersuchungen über die Wirkungsweise der in der Funktions-Kieferorthopädie verwendeten Apparate. Deutsche Zahn. Mund. Kieferheilk., 5:214–224, 1938.
34. Fränkel, R.: Personal communication, Aug. 6, 1971.
35. Jarabak, J.: Development of a treatment plan in the light of one's concept of treatment objectives. Am. J. Orthodont., 46:481–514, 1960.
36. Hixon, E. H., Atikian, H., Callow, G. E., McDonald, H. W., and Tacy, R. J.: Optimal force, differential force, and anchorage. Am. J. Orthodont., 55:437–457, 1969.
37. Reitan, K.: Clinical and histologic observations on tooth movement during and after orthodontic treatment. Am. J. Orthodont., 53:721–745, 1967.
38. Baumrind, S.: Reconsideration of propriety of "pressure-tension" hypothesis. Am. J. Orthodont., 55:12–22, 1969.
39. Baumrind, S., and Buck, D. L.: Rate changes in cell replication and protein synthesis in the periodontal ligament incident to tooth movement. Am. J. Orthodont., 57:109–131, 1970.
40. Schwarz, A. M.: Tissue changes incident to orthodontic tooth movement. Internat. J. Orthodont. & Oral Surg., 18:331–352, 1932.
41. Reitan, K.: Movement of teeth in Lundström, A. (ed.): Introduction to Orthodontics, New York, McGraw-Hill, 1960.
42. Glickman, I.: Inflammation and trauma from occlusion, co-destructive factors in chronic periodontal disease. J. Periodont., 34:5–10, 1963.
43. Reitan, K.: Om enkelte mekaniske og histologiske problemer ved rotasjon av tenner. Norsk. Tannl. Tid., 49:381–393, 1939.
44. Breitner, C.: Bone changes resulting from experimental orthodontic treatment. Am. J. Orthodont. & Oral Surg., 26:521–547, 1940.
45. Baume, L.: Cephalo-facial growth patterns and the functional adaptation of the temporomandibular joint structures. Trans. Eur. Orth. Soc., 1–19, 1969.
46. Charlier, J. P., Petrovic, A., and Linck, G.: La fronde mentonniere et son action sur la croissance mandibulaire. L'Orthodont. Franc., 40:100–113, 1969.
47. Lemoine, C., Charlier, J. P., and Petrovic, A.: Reaction condylienne à la deviation mandibulaire provoquée chez le rat. L'Orthodont. Franc., 39:147–151, 1968.
48. Miotti, B., Graziati, G., and Michieli, S.: Étude expérimental sur les effets des forces mécaniques appliquées en ortopedie dento-faciale: L'Orthodont. Franc., 39:625–629, 1968.
49. Graber, T. M.: Current Orthodontic Concepts and Techniques. Chapter 10, Philadelphia, W. B. Saunders Co., 1969.
50. Straub, Walter, J.: The successful treatment of skeletal open bite cases with steep mandibular plane angles, complicated by tongue thrust syndrome. Audiovisual clinic, St. Louis, American Association of Orthodontists, 1965.
51. Moyers, R. E., and Elgoyhen, J. C.: Crécimiento, craneo-facial (Factores no geneticos). Ortodoncia, 35:18–29, 1971.
52. Rateitschak, V. K. H., and Herzog-Specht, F. A.: Reaktion und regeneration des parodonts auf orthodontische Behandlung mit festsitzenden Apparaten. Sweiz. Monatschrft. Zahnheilk., 75:741–755, 1965.

53. Graber, T. M.: Postmortems in post-treatment adjustment. Am. J. Orthodont., 52:331–352, 1966.
54. Bouyssou, M., Lepp, F. H., and Zerosi, C.: Resorptions dentaires et biologie osseuse. Éditions Sciences et Lettres. Liège, Belgium, 1965.
55. Burstone, C. S.: Biomechanics of the orthodontic appliance in Graber, T. M. (ed.): Current Orthodontic Concepts and Techniques, Philadelphia, W. B. Saunders Co., 1969.
56. Storey, E., and Smith, R.: Force in orthodontics and its relation to tooth movement. Aust. Dent. Jour., 56:11–18, 1952.
57. Jarabak, J. R.: Technique and Treatment With the Light Wire Technique. St. Louis, C. V. Mosby, 1963.
58. Burstone, C. J., Baldwin, J. J., and Lawless, D. T.: Application of continuous forces to orthodontics. Angle Orthodont., 31:1–14, 1961.
59. Winzar, C. F.: Rotated anterior teeth. Aust. Dent. J., 12:417–420, 1967.
60. Nielsen, I. L.: Transsection of supra-alveolar fibers on orthodontically rotated teeth in monkeys. Tandlaegebladet, 75:1330–1340, 1971.
61. Anstendig, H. S., and Kronman, J. H.: A histologic study of pulpal reaction to orthodontic tooth movement in dogs. Angle Orthodont., 42:50–55, 1972.
62. Moore, G. J., McNeill, R. W., and D'Anna, J.: The effects of digit sucking on facial growth. J.A.D.A., 84:592–599, 1972.
63. Joho, J. P.: The effect of extraoral force on the maxilla of the Macaque. Master's thesis, University of Washington, Seattle, 1971.
64. Riedel, R. A.: Retention, in Graber, T. M. (ed): Current Orthodontic Concepts and Techniques. Philadelphia, W. B. Saunders Co., 1969.
65. Parker, G. R.: Transseptal fibers and relapse following bodily retraction of teeth—a histologic study. Am. J. Orthodont., 61:331–344, 1972.

chapter 11

ORTHODONTIC APPLIANCES AND TREATMENT PHILOSOPHY

A long time ago, Edward H. Angle, one of the outstanding pioneers of modern orthodontics, said, "All you can do is to push or pull or turn a tooth. I have given you an appliance. Now for God's sake, use it!"[1] Indeed, Angle gave us a number of appliances, and so did many pioneers in orthodontics. At the outset, we should emphasize what Weinstein has said so succinctly, "There is only one disease—malocclusion. The medicine is force, and there are a number of ways to apply that force!"[2]

DEVELOPMENT OF APPLIANCES

As has been learned from previous chapters, pressure on a tooth causes certain changes in the supporting structures. If the pressure is of the proper intensity and duration and if there are no restraining environmental or functional forces, the tooth, or teeth, will move.

Most of the early appliances were of the removable type (Fig. 11–1). Actually, they were modified dentures. The early fixed appliances were usually crude metal bands that were ligated to the teeth with brass or silver wire. They were outstanding for their inefficiency and their ability to trap food (Fig. 11–2). Kingsley,[3] Angle,[4] Case[5] and others soon realized that for any effective tooth movement some means must be devised to control the individual teeth. This led to the development of attachments that were soldered on modified crowns or bands.

The earliest attachments were nothing more than spurs that would hold a wire. The average appliance consisted of two molar "anchor" bands, or modified crowns, with long tubes or sheaths on the buccal surface, parallel with the occlusal plane, and a heavy labial arch wire that followed the contour of the

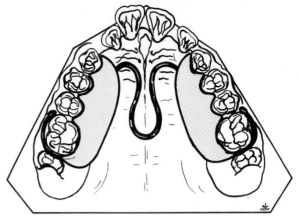

Figure 11-1 Coffin type vulcanite plate with central spring, used to expand the upper arch. Earlier modifications covered teeth completely with vulcanite, and there were no clasps. This type of appliance is still used in cleft palate therapy for segmental expansion.

upper or lower dental arch (Fig. 11–3). Individual teeth that were irregular were banded with copper, brass or silver strip material, and spurs were soldered to permit the rotation and tipping of these teeth.[6] Rotation was accomplished by tying or ligating the individual teeth to the arch wire. All movement was accomplished by tipping the teeth out toward the arch wire. The fact that a malocclusion was or was not in a state of balance with the available space in the jaw and muscle forces did not concern the early orthodontists. It was Angle's strong conviction that if the teeth were placed in their proper occlusal relationship, normal function would develop the supporting bone to hold them in this position. Thus, the major concept of orthodontics in those early years was one of expansion outward to a greater arc to eliminate individual tooth irregularities.

Spurs were soon modified to form hooks, and hooks became the forerunners of the modern "brackets." Pioneer orthodontists who worked with ligature wires and crude bands with spurs soon learned that simple tipping of the teeth

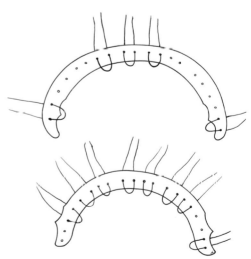

Figure 11-2 "Bandelette" plates used to "straighten" teeth by tying them to crude metal plates with brass or silver wire. This type of appliance can be traced to Pierre Fauchard.

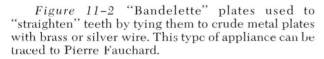

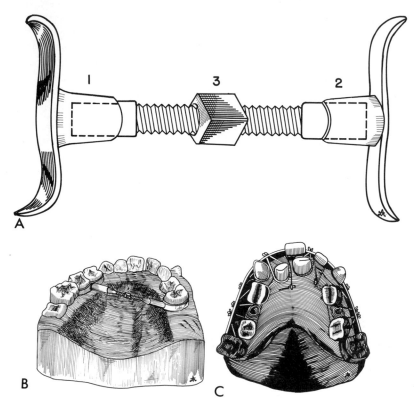

Figure 11–3 A, Jackscrew used by Guilford, Farrar, Kingsley and others to expand upper arch, by making ends (1 and 2) move apart. This is done by turning threaded nut at (3). B, Metal bands have been placed on the teeth to be moved, but the jackscrew reciprocal force principle is still being used. C, A vulcanite palate is combined with crowns on the molars, a soldered labial bar and silk thread ties to effect changes in tooth position.

did not provide the desired tooth movement, and they saw many of their cases collapse after supposedly successful treatment. It became apparent that to achieve the proper tooth position and axial inclination of the teeth, one must have better control of each individual tooth—control that would permit the movement of the root of the tooth as well as the crown.

PIN AND TUBE APPLIANCE. One of the most effective early appliances was developed by Edward H. Angle and was called the pin and tube appliance[7] (Fig. 11–4). Each band on the tooth had a vertical tube that paralleled the long axis of the tooth. The arch wire had pins soldered in such a position as to influence the total position of each tooth. The appliance was extremely difficult to use, requiring a high degree of precision and skill. However, in the hands of a few men it was an outstanding advance in orthodontic therapy.

RIBBON ARCH APPLIANCE. Succeeding the pin and tube appliance was the "ribbon arch appliance," as developed by Edward H. Angle.[8] In this instance, the hook was modified to receive a rectangular arch wire (Fig. 11–4 B). This ribbon arch fitted very closely into the machined bracket. Heretofore, round arch wires had been used, but the inability to control the apices of the teeth during tooth movement was rather apparent. With the use of the rectangular or ribbon arch, adjustments could be made that exerted strong pressures on the apices of the teeth and stimulated movements not possible with round wire therapy. The philosophy of treatment changed little with the more efficient attachments. Expansion was still the therapeutic goal in the majority of cases treated. Yet, the efficiency of the attachment was such that the ribbon arch was revamped and now serves as the mainstay of the Begg technique — locking pins and all (pp. 539, 540).

BAKER ANCHORAGE. Many men noticed that a large percentage of patients seeking orthodontic treatment had relatively straight teeth, but the upper and lower teeth were not related properly. In most of these cases, the upper teeth protruded excessively and the lower teeth and jaw seemed to be underdeveloped. Obviously, the mere expansion of the upper and lower arches would not achieve the desired correction. Some means had to be found to correct the protrusion of the upper teeth and the underdevelopment of the lower teeth and jaws. This was achieved by so-called "Baker anchorage,"[9] a method of using intermaxillary rubber bands (Fig. 11–5). By pitting the upper arch against the lower arch, it was possible to effect an adjustment of the teeth. The lower teeth and jaw would move forward and the protruding upper incisors would move back. In a small percentage of cases where the lower jaw was in front of the upper jaw, the same approach could be used. In this instance, the upper teeth could be brought forward and the lower teeth backward, to achieve a normal occlusal relationship.

LABIAL AND LINGUAL ARCHES. Intermaxillary therapy was also accomplished, using a simple maxillary labial arch tied into two molar anchor bands and a mandibular lingual arch that was either soldered to the molar bands or

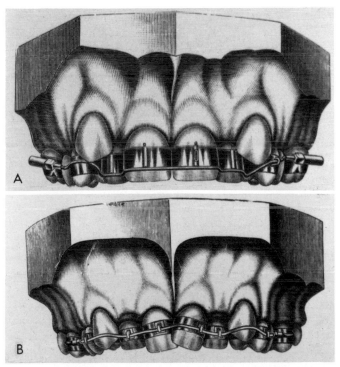

Figure 11–4 A, Pin and tube appliance introduced by Edward H. Angle in 1911. Soldered vertical pins on arch engaged vertical tubes on bands. B, Ribbon arch appliance introduced by Angle in 1916. Vertical slot in bracket accepts either round or rectangular wire, which in turn is held in place by lock pin.

INTERMAXILLARY ANCHORAGE

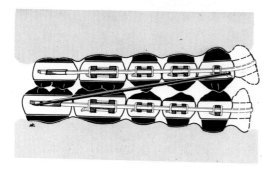

A   **CLASS II**

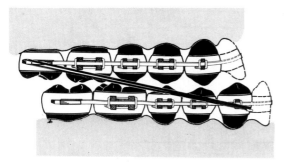

B   **CLASS III**

Figure 11–5   Baker intermaxillary anchorage to adjust jaw relationship and teeth through the use of rubber elastics from maxilla to mandible. A, For Class II malocclusion; B, for Class III malocclusion.

attached by a special appurtenance which permitted the removal of the arch for cleaning and adjusting. As with the philosophy of expansion, there was little concern over the fact that the lower teeth might be moved into abnormal positions and out of balance with the associated musculature by this type of therapy. The primary consideration was to establish a normal occlusion, irrespective of environmental and functional forces.

The lingual arch was developed to a relatively high degree of efficiency by John Mershon.[10] With the use of finger springs or auxiliary springs, he was able to achieve movement of individual teeth in the lower arch. At the same time, this arch could serve as a base for elastic traction (Fig. 11–6 D, H). Subsequent experience has shown that the lingual arch serves best as a space maintainer or for use as part-time elastic traction. As a base for tooth-moving appurtenances it offers only improved esthetics — it is less obvious—and little efficiency. Unfortunately, a number of so-called orthodontic laboratories currently recommend the labiolingual appliance setup for a great percentage of cases which actually are not amenable to correction with the appliance. The resultant is an iatrogenic malocclusion, created by the dentist.

Combinations of the labial and lingual arches were refined by Oliver.[11] He introduced a fixed guide plane to be used in conjunction with intermaxillary elastics, to eliminate functional retrusions, to take advantage of whatever growth was occurring and to relieve any possible environmental restrictions on the developmental pattern. The guide plane had the added advantages of decreasing the excessive overbite so often associated with Class II, Division 1 malocclusions and of inhibiting the abnormal tongue thrust habit that frequently increases these malocclusions. The original hopes of stimulating condylar

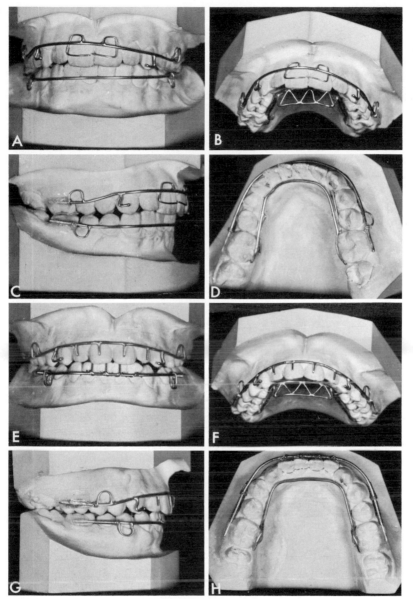

guide plain.

Figure 11–6   Labiolingual appliances. A, Upper and lower labial arches with elastic hooks at canines and finger springs off upper arch to tip incisors lingually. B, Oliver guide plane in conjunction with labial arch. C, Lateral view, labial arches, with Oliver vertical spring loop at molar, elastic hook at canine and finger springs at maxillary central incisors. D, Lower labial and lingual arches, with finger springs on lingual arch to move premolar teeth. E, Upper labial arch with vertical spurs to upright incisors and lower labial arch, with incisors ligated to arch wire. F, Guide plane used in conjunction with labial appliance for Class II malocclusions. G, Lateral view of labial arches, showing use of coil spring between lower vertical loop and molar. H, Lower labial and lingual arches, with mandibular incisors ligated to labial arch. (Courtesy O. Oliver.)

growth through the use of a guide plane were not to be rewarded with clinical results, however. Many patients developed "dual bites" (or "Sunday bites") after removal of the guide plane, and gradually dropped back from their learned anterior positioning of the mandible to true centric occlusion, with the condyle in proper relation to the articular eminence, instead of forward. Proper timing of growth and sufficient increments in the proper direction are essential here, even as they are with the Andresen activator, a removable appliance which utilizes the same jaw positioning principles.

EXTRACTION IN CONJUNCTION WITH ORTHODONTIC THERAPY.   Some orthodontists were quite disturbed about their failure to produce a normal occlusion by means of expansion and the use of intermaxillary rubber bands. In many instances, placing the teeth in the correct occlusal relationship to one another did not seem to develop normal bony support, and the teeth returned to their original positions of malocclusion after the retaining appliances were removed. Where there was crowding, the removal of one or two teeth frequently seemed to make the problem of correction much easier, and the results appeared to be more stable. In other cases, where there was a marked protrusion of the upper incisors, it was found that the lower teeth could not be moved far enough forward to engage the upper teeth correctly, or, if they were moved forward, they were tipped so badly that they no longer had proper bony support, and they would collapse as soon as appliances were removed. In some of these instances, the removal of upper first bicuspids seemed to permit the establishment of a normal occlusion with greater ease and post-treatment stability.[3, 5, 12, 13] Thus, the philosophy of extraction in conjunction with orthodontic therapy was introduced. It met great antagonism from the followers of Angle, steeped as they were in the philosophy that it was vital to maintain all teeth and to establish these teeth in ideal occlusion if the results were to be considered successful.

In defense of Angle, it must be said that extractions have produced iatrogenic malocclusions, too — deep overbites, collapsed lower anterior segments, pockets, spaces and tissue damage — when not done judiciously. It would be nice to think of this as a past event in dental history. Unfortunately, the current application of this observation is only too valid, particularly in the hands of men not trained in orthodontic case analysis diagnosis and the exact role of growth and development. Gnathologic concepts, based primarily on occlusion and a full complement of teeth, largely emulate the time-honored Angle philosophy — some 70 years later!

EDGEWISE ATTACHMENT.   To gain better control over the individual teeth, the edgewise attachment was introduced in the middle 1920's by Edward H. Angle[14] (Figs. 11–7 to 11–9). This attachment had greater versatility than its predecessor, the ribbon arch attachment, and many men soon switched to "edgewise." The term "edgewise" refers to the fact that the bracket was machined so that the rectangular arch wire had to be inserted with its long dimension horizontal, instead of vertical as in the ribbon arch bracket. The arch wire was tied in place with ligatures, rather than being held by lock pins which often broke and defied removal. This attachment has been modified and forms the major fixed appliance bracket in use today. The edgewise attachment was not able to achieve routinely stable results satisfactory to those men who followed the Angle philosophy of no extractions, of expansion to achieve normal occlusion and of pitting the upper arch against the lower arch irrespective of the environmental and functional factors.

UNIVERSAL APPLIANCE.   Spencer Atkinson and his followers felt that the answer lay in even greater control of individual teeth, and they developed the

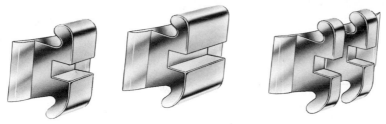

Figure 11-7 The edgewise bracket attachment comes in a variety of modifications. The original single bracket (left) has been widened for molar teeth and for greater rotational control (center). The twin edgewise modification (right) is available in different widths and is used most frequently because of its greater versatility, reduced frictional component and adaptability to various light-wire techniques. (Courtesy Rocky Mountain Dental Products Co.)

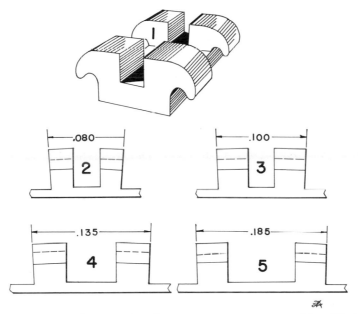

Figure 11-8 Twin edgewise brackets come in varying widths. Choice of width depends on width of tooth on which bracket is being used, on convexity of labial or buccal surface and on rotational demands. (After Unitek drawing.)

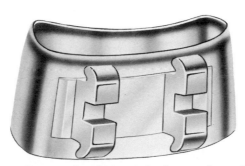

Figure 11-9 Twin edgewise bracket attached to preformed seamless orthodontic band. Seamless bands come in different sizes and shapes to fit any tooth in the mouth. They may be procured plain or with any of the common bracket attachments. (Courtesy Rocky Mountain Dental Products Co.)

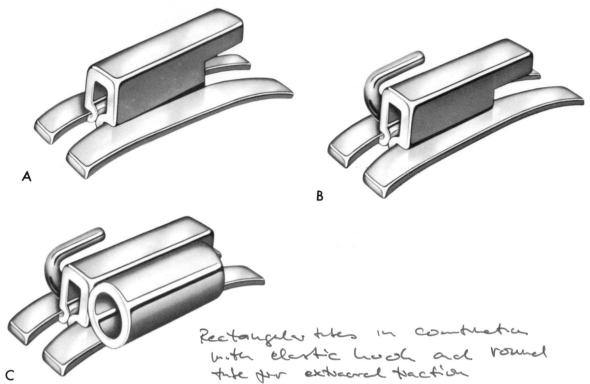

Rectangular tubes in combination with elastic hook and round tube for extraoral traction

Figure 11–10   Rectangular molar tubes for edgewise technique. A, With distal projection; B, with distal projection and elastic hook; C, combined edgewise and round tube for extraoral traction arch. Elastic hook also welded to assembly. All tubes have curved flanges to permit better adaptation to band. (Courtesy Unitek Corp.)

universal appliance which is, in reality, a combination of the edgewise and the ribbon arch attachment (Figs. 11–11, 11–12). But the use of rectangular and round arch wires, while giving exceedingly fine control of the individual teeth, did not seem to solve many of the problems of post-treatment stability.[15, 68] This is, of course, no criticism of the appliance itself, but rather a recognition of the limitations imposed by the very nature of tissue response and the problems of retention, rotational control, relapsing overbite and predominance of the morphogenetic pattern, which transcend any appliance philosophy, regardless of its versatility and degree of complexity—and the universal technique *is* both versatile and complex.[67] Current use of the attachment, with modern diagnostic methods, provides comparable results in any technique.

TWIN-WIRE ATTACHMENT.   The twin-wire attachment was introduced by Joseph Johnson in the 1930's.[16] The philosophy behind its use was that by virtue of *two* light wires placed in the same bracket, more physiologic tooth movement could be obtained than with *one* heavy wire. Indeed, the twin-wire attachment and bracket permit rapid reduction of rotations with relatively little discomfort to the patient (Fig. 11–13).[31] The fact that there were other problems of anchorage and lack of control of canine and premolar teeth after correction of rotations should also be considered in the light of the largely expansionist original Johnson philosophy, which pitted two molars and four incisors banded in the upper arch against a lower lingual arch.

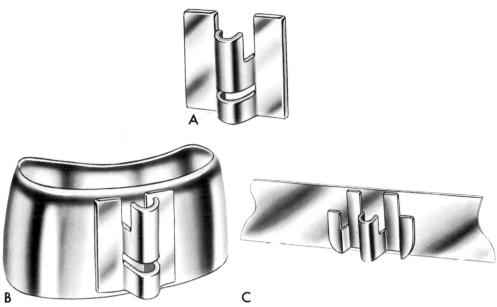

Figure 11–11 Universal bracket. A, Ready to weld on band. B, Universal bracket welded to preformed incisor band. C, Double wing universal bracket for greater tooth control. (Courtesy Rocky Mountain Dental Products Co.)

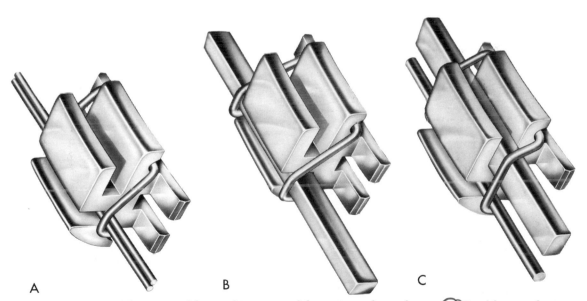

Figure 11–12 Three possible combinations of the universal attachment. A, Double round wire, tied to place in lower slot. B, Single rectangular wire in place in lower slot. C, Round wire, lower slot; rectangular wire, upper slot, tied in with steel ligature. Note the additional band side slot which increases bracket versatility. (Courtesy Unitek Corp.)

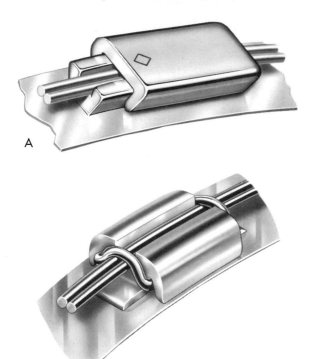

Figure 11–13 Twin-wire brackets. A, Regular twin-wire bracket, showing a portion of the band, the channel, two fine gauge arch wires and the covering and locking cap being slid into place. B, The twin-tie bracket which uses wire ligature to hold arch wires in place instead of a channel cap. Greater versatility is claimed for this type, since teeth completely out of the dental arch may be ligated directly. (Courtesy Unitek Corp.)

Today the twin-wired appliance finds less use in orthodontic specialty circles, largely because of its nonextraction orientation and greater difficulty in controlling teeth and achieving torque when teeth have been removed.

DIFFERENTIAL LIGHT FORCES. A number of attachments and mechanical variations have been introduced for orthodontic treatment by Kesling,[37] Brandt,[17] Swain,[19] Begg,[18] Jarabak,[38] Bowles and others.[20] This allows the orthodontist quite a selection, indeed. Currently, the Begg bracket and technique are being used in many areas. A modification of the old ribbon arch bracket of Angle, it has been turned upside down and refined for use in a new light-wire differential forces philosophy. Its use has been stimulated by the limitations of the twin-wire appliance, the frictional component of classic edgewise treatment, the production of iatrogenic malocclusions and the writings of P. R. Begg[36] (Figs. 11–14, 11–15, 11–16). This will be discussed later in this chapter.

Because of our highly mobile society, because of the many more children receiving the benefits of orthodontic treatment and because of the time-consuming nature of the treatment itself, there is a much larger number of transfer cases. There are currently some 117 possible bracket attachments, which poses a problem for continuation of treatment to the transfer orthodontist who might be unfamiliar with the attachment in use. Some standardization is imperative. There will always be a variety of orthodontic philosophies or methods of treatment, but a concerted effort must be made to provide a sufficiently versatile attachment so that transfer patients will not undergo major appliance changes, heavier financial obligations and the problems of trying to find a "Tweed man," a "Begg man" or a "Jarabak man" every time there is a move. The Bowles multiphase attachment is a significant step in the right direction. Designed in

1953 and used by an increasing number of orthodontists since then, the multi-phase bracket permits the use of any technique, eliminating the need for appliance change from location to location (Fig. 11–17). Bowles writes, "The multi-phase, designed to effect standardization of most philosophies, yet maintain the unique characteristics of labio-lingual, twin-wire, universal, differential light forces and edgewise technics, may be described as the common denominator."[20] In the multiphase technique, a single anterior bracket is usually used, with a choice of a molar width bracket, or different widths of twin multiphase brackets available, as with the edgewise. A double buccal tube or sheath is used routinely to permit use of extraoral force (Fig. 11–10). The ingenious bracket design accommodates all currently used gauges of wire, singly or in combination, as desired. Routine use of it with universal, twin-wire, edgewise or differential light forces, together with freedom of modification of mechano-therapy as the treatment progresses and the individual preferences of the operator demand, lends a high degree of versatility to the appliance. The Broussard bracket is also a combination bracket and permits varying treatment philosophies.

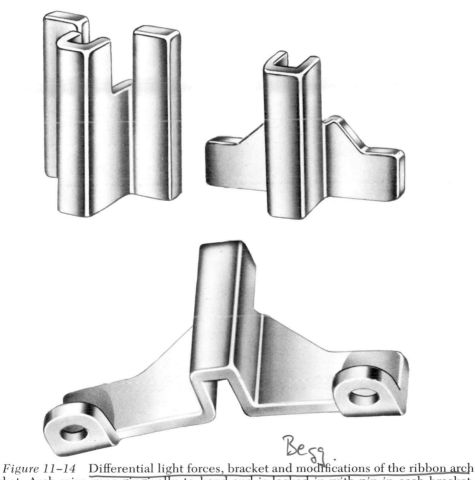

Figure 11–14   Differential light forces, bracket and modifications of the ribbon arch bracket. Arch wire runs gingivally to band and is locked in with pin in each bracket. Addition of eyelets (right) gives additional rotational control and versatility. (Courtesy Rocky Mountain Dental Products Co.)

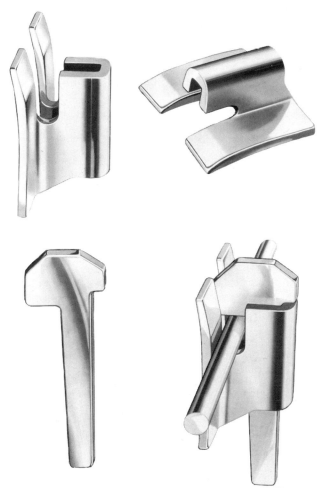

6,4 - 0,5 cm

Figure 11–15 Most popular bracket currently for Begg light wire technique is stamped from stainless steel and is easily spot welded. The original milled bracket required soldering to the band. The bracket is available with arch wire slots to accept either 0.016 or 0.020 inch round wire. When a safety lock pin, as in lower left, is employed, free mesiodistal tipping and sliding are automatically provided. The shoulder on the pin developed by P. C. Kesling is on the labial to prevent pin from traveling too far through slot. By preventing the head from contacting the arch wire, free mesiodistal movement is not hampered by a friction bind (lower right). (Courtesy T. P. Laboratories Inc.)

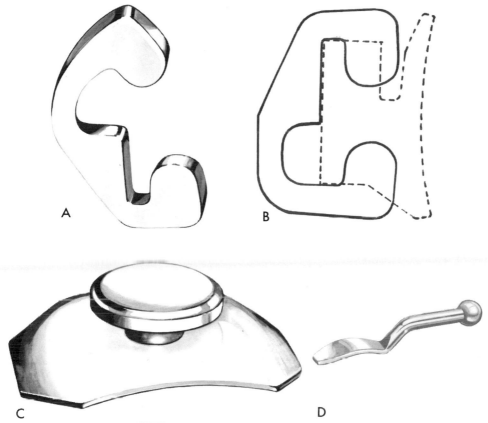

Figure 11–16 A, By-pass clamp used on premolars and canines in the Begg technique. It ensures free sliding of the arch wire and permits rotation of the tooth with elastic thread when desired. Note ends are wide apart, to permit slipping over the bracket. B, By-pass clamp in place on bracket. Clamp may be inverted to adjust for level of tooth as it erupts. C, Lingual button, normally welded to the lingual surfaces of premolars and canines that require rotating. It is also used on lingual of molars for light elastics. Thin flange and low profile enhance easy adaptation and comfort. D, Ball-end molar hook, usually welded to lingual surface of molar band for use with elastics or ligature ties. Ball end hook increases retentive ability and patient comfort. (Courtesy, T. P. Laboratories, Inc.)

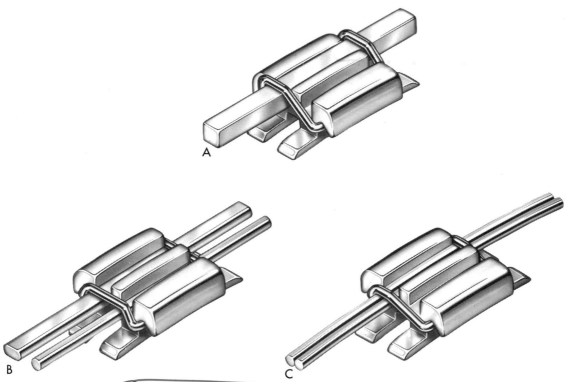

Figure 11–17 Bowles multiphase bracket, developed to be used with edgewise, universal and twin-wire techniques interchangeably. A, Edgewise; B, universal; C, twin-wire. (Courtesy Unitek Corp.)

TREATMENT PHILOSOPHY

PAST CONCEPTS OF THERAPY

Despite the large number of possible band attachments brought on the market, the philosophy for many orthodontists was pretty much one of expansion to a greater arc to correct the rotations and of pitting one arch against the other (upper against the lower) to achieve the correct occlusal relationship. It was claimed that the use of these appliances stimulated lower jaw growth, that it caused changes in the condyle of the mandible and that the mandible was brought forward by the use of intermaxillary elastics and remained in this position due to upward and backward growth of the condyle. These claims of appliance success were based largely on clinical impressions. Most judgments of relative success or failure were made immediately after tooth-moving appliances had been removed and before the teeth had an opportunity to establish an equilibrium with all forces acting on them. Growth was an unpredictable factor, and it clouded the issue by making it almost impossible to determine how much of the apparent success of orthodontic treatment was due to growth and how much was due to appliance manipulation. Many orthodontists had their patients wear retaining appliances indefinitely after the removal of tooth-moving appliances, and attributed any change back toward the original malocclusion to "the wisdom teeth" or to the lack of patient cooperation in wearing the removable retainer as instructed.

CONTEMPORARY THERAPEUTIC CONCEPTS

It has become increasingly apparent to many discerning orthodontists that the problem in therapy is not so much a matter of what attachment or mechanical approach is used. Of greater importance is the basic philosophy relating to orthodontic goals. Really, in a biologic medium, there is no place for a cult or "system" philosophy that treats malocclusions by the numbers. Most malocclusions result from the patient's morphogenetic pattern—a strong hereditary predisposition. Of prime importance in analyzing the various symptoms associated with malocclusions is recognition of the fact that tooth relationships often reflect jaw relationships. The mere moving of the teeth to a normal interdigitation does not ensure the establishment of normal jaw relationship. Many factors must be considered, not the least being hereditary pattern, ethnic origin, growth and development, function and tissue reaction to mechanotherapy. Where there is marked crowding of the teeth it has become obvious that the position of the teeth reflects nature's attempt to establish a balance between the available space in the jaws, the size of the teeth and the constantly molding and balancing effect of the musculature. To disturb this balance, where growth cannot be counted on as an ally, is to invite failure. In many instances, orthodontic therapy of this type can produce dire consequences that will later require the services of the periodontist or even the prosthodontist.[67]

The incidence of iatrogenic malocclusions has increased. The delayed reaction inherent in therapy makes the whole affair a long drawn out process and is conducive to the production of inadequate results. It must be emphasized again here, as it has been in so many sections in this book, that the limitations of orthodontic treatment are stringent and that damage is the handmaiden, unless proper training and experience are the basis for the rendering of orthodontic services. For the specialist, therapeutic modifiability is an orthodontic way of life. He must be prepared for all treatment demands and contingencies. The possibility of tooth sacrifice must be an integral part of any orthodontic philosophy, regardless of whether it is a Class I, Class II or Class III malocclusion. Tooth sacrifice means multibanded techniques and precise tooth control, with appliances that demand the utmost in diagnostic acumen, training and experience. There is no place for second class or second rate health service.

REMOVABLE APPLIANCES

Coincident with the development of fixed appliances have been the use and evolution of various types of removable appliances. Most of these have been modifications of the time-honored Coffin plate (Fig. 11–1) and, generally speaking, the philosophy behind their use has been similar to that of fixed appliances in use at that particular time.[91] Thus, expansion was a major goal of most removable appliances wherever individual teeth were crowded. Extraction as an adjunct found little use because of inability to control individual tooth position and inclination.

A survey of the literature shows that removable appliances are still being used to a much greater extent in countries outside the United States. One reason for this appears to be socio-economic. Appliances are less expensive, can be constructed by a technician from plaster casts, require less frequent adjustments and permit the dentist to see more patients in his practice. Whether these advantages outweigh the superior tooth-moving abilities of fixed appliances is questionable. If the philosophy is to give some treatment to the greatest number of patients, the use of removable appliances surely is justified. If the goal is to render the best possible service to each patient, then fixed appliances should be used. In many instances, the ideal is a combination of both fixed and removable appliances.[50] The big mistake that has been made is to fit the patient and the form of treatment to the appliance, not vice versa. Thus, a frank arch length deficiency case becomes a case for expansion treatment, since the removable appliance cannot cope with tooth movement adequately. Socioeconomic criteria are important, but should not be used to rationalize inadequate and ineffectual therapy and one's own choice of appliance. This admonition is necessary now because of the strong renaissance of the use of removable appliances in the hands of inadequately trained general practitioners.

The removable appliances can be divided into two broad groups: (1) appliances that effect actual tooth movement through adjustments of springs or attachments within that appliance (active plates) and (2) appliances that

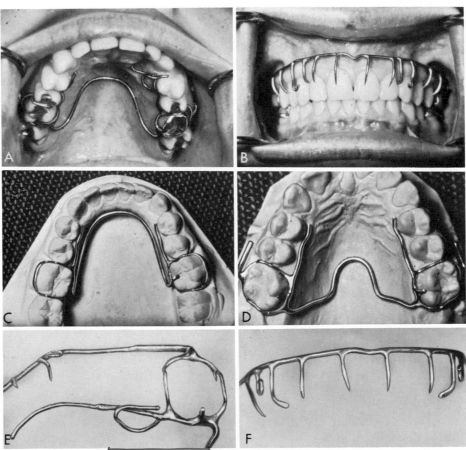

Figure 11-18   A, Crozat appliance, palatal view; note lingual extensions and heavy palatal base bar. B, Labial view of Crozat appliance, with vertical spurs from heavy labial base wire to effect rotational and inclination changes. C, Lower Crozat crib. D, Modified maxillary Crozat appliance. E, Crozat skeleton detail. Continuous molar clasp has rest. Lingual extension has an auxiliary spring to change individual tooth position. F, High labial base wire with vertical spurs. (Courtesy R. B. Smythe.)

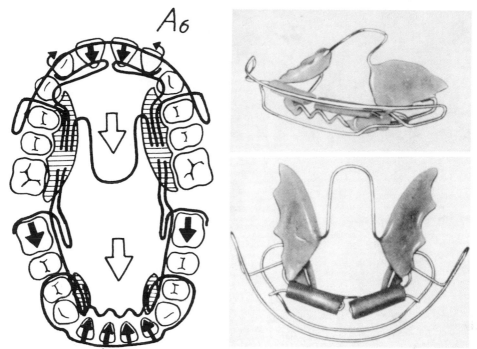

A₆

Figure 11–19 Bimler appliance, with continuous labial arch in lower appliance and U-shaped connecting Coffin spring. The anchorage afforded in the buccal segments permits tooth movement for the anterior teeth. Additional springs may be added on the labial wire for anterior tooth movement, as desired. (Courtesy H. P. Bimler.)

stimulate reflex muscle activity which in turn produces the desired tooth movement.[22] *(miofuncionele)*

USE OF APPLIANCE FORCE. There are a variety of removable appliances that utilize the inherent force placed in the appliance by adjustments. With the exception of the Crozat and Bimler appliances which are partly cast and partly wrought wire and almost completely tooth borne (Figs. 11–18 and 11–19), most of the removable appliances are largely tissue borne. A palatal appliance makes use of adhesion to the palate to provide part of the anchorage needed for the desired tooth movement. The simplest type of appliance is the so-called bite plate (Fig. 11–20).[23] (This will be discussed in greater detail in Chap. 16.) Its major purpose is to stimulate eruption of the posterior teeth and to decrease the amount of anterior overbite. To this basic acrylic palatal structure, wire appur- *dodcen'* tenances may be attached.[24] If the anterior teeth are spaced excessively, a simple labial wire may be used to retract them. Clasps, of which there are many types, may be added around the molar teeth (Fig. 11–21). Space may be opened up for a tooth to erupt; molars may be tipped back. Frequently the use of rubber elastics facilitates the desired tooth movement with the removable appliance (Fig. 11–21). As these appliances become more complex, the plastic itself is divided, and part of it actually moves to accomplish the desired tooth movement. The illustrations demonstrate various types of appliances. That these appliances can produce desired results is shown by the casts taken before and after treatment (Fig. 11–22). One of the most common forms of removable appliance is that developed by Martin Schwarz and used extensively throughout Europe (Fig. 11–23). Like the Heath X-plate, the Schwarz appliance utilizes tissue

(Text continued on page 549)

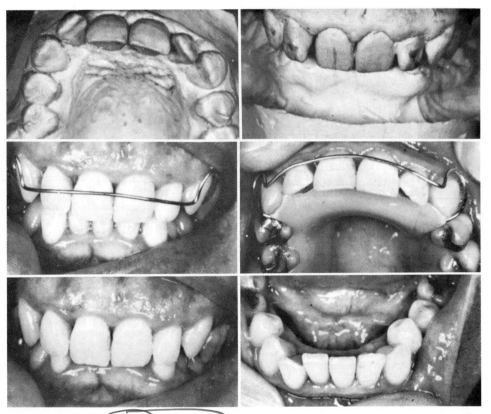

Figure 11-20 (Hawley bite plate) with acrylic palatal portion, circumferential, arrow or ball type clasps for retention in molar area and labial loops and wire to permit anterior tooth movement and retention. In this instance the maxillary right lateral incisor is being rotated and the damaging effects of the overbite are reduced by indefinite nocturnal appliance wear.

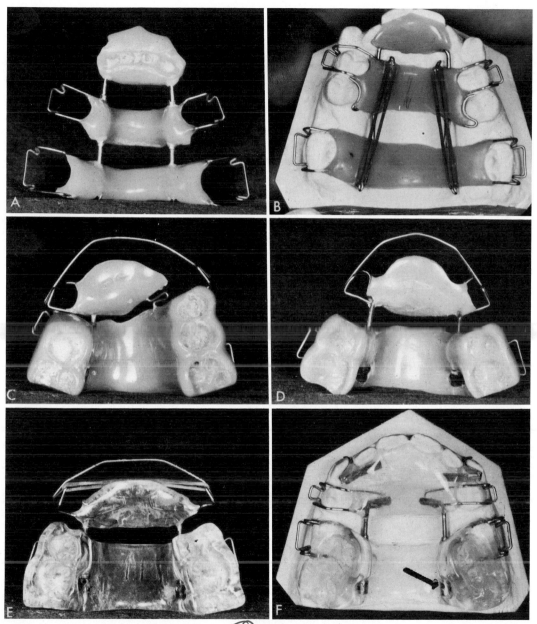

Figure 11–21 Removable appliances. A, Sliding midsection to retract premolar teeth with elastics, as in B. C and D, Posterior acrylic base portion, held in place by arrow clasps and patient's occlusion. Anterior sections may be advanced or retracted by springs or jackscrew adjustment. E, Elastic attaches to labial bow to close incisor spaces. Entire labial portion may be moved by jackscrew adjustment. F, The first premolar teeth are retracted into the second premolar extraction space, and at the same time auxiliary attachments engage the mesial portions of the canines. These teeth are moved distally by means of threaded screw end adjustments (see arrow). Retention of the appliance is aided by occlusion with opposing teeth. (Courtesy J. Heath, Sr.)

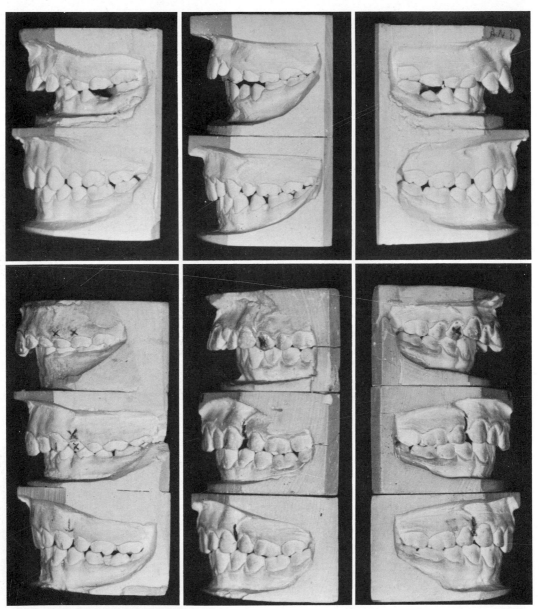

Figure 11–22 Results obtained using "X-plate" (Fig. 11–21) and planned program of serial extraction. (Courtesy J. Heath, Sr.)

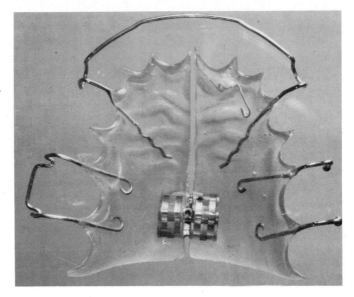

Figure 11–23 Modified Schwarz plate, with arrow type clasps on left and ball type clasps on right for retention. Split palate has adjustable jackscrew for expansion. Labial wire serves partly for retention and partly to move teeth. If incisors are to be retracted, acrylic resin must be cut away from the lingual aspect. Finger springs may be added directly to the acrylic or to the labial wire.

borne anchorage and appurtenances of wire for tooth movement. Effective use can be made in conjunction with fixed appliances.

USE OF MUSCULAR FORCE

The second group of removable appliances stems from the original efforts of Pierre Robin of France and modifications of the monobloc by Andresen[25] of Norway. Andresen believed that the musculature played a major role in the positioning of the teeth, and reasoned that it was possible to make use of this force to move teeth by creating new reflexes in the perioral neuromusculature. He constructed his "activator" in such a manner that the weight of the appliances together with the guiding effect on the teeth during deglutition influenced the position of the teeth and their contiguous alveolar bone. By guiding the mandible into a forward position with the appliance, he hoped that the new reflexes created would help maintain this position. At the same time, the forces created by the muscles attempting to return to the original mandibular position would be acting on the maxillary denture, retruding these teeth. The activator, or "monobloc," as it is called, has been modified by many practitioners (Fig. 11–24). Häupl[26] has further developed this system of "functional jaw orthopedics," as he termed it. Schwarz[27] of Vienna also modified the activator, incorporating various attachments to move the teeth while the musculature is effecting its tooth positioning.[22] Extensive research on monkeys, using the activator, has shown the broad potential of this type of appliance, if used properly.[28, 69]

The propulsor, introduced by Mühlemann and developed clinically with significant success by Hotz,[29] utilizes the same principles as the monobloc. However, there is a tissue borne portion of the appliance, so that the retrusive forces on the maxillary anterior segment are transmitted directly to the alveolar bone. In the mandible, the appliance is also partly tissue borne on the lingual side of the lower incisors. The attempt is to engage basal bone, to eliminate functional retrusions and to take advantage of any favorable growth that may occur in the mandible as the maxillary arch is being held by the retrusive force

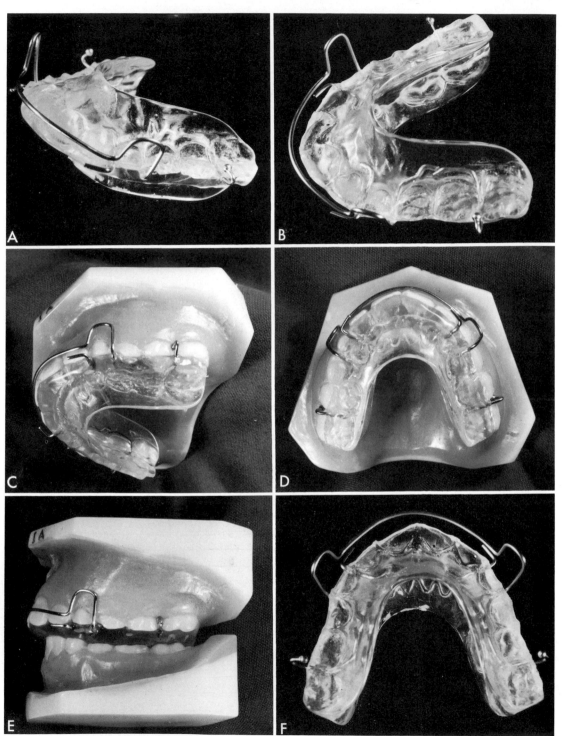

Figure 11-24 A to F, Different views of activator or monobloc appliance. Unit construction influences dental arches through the effect of function. (Courtesy A. Björk.)

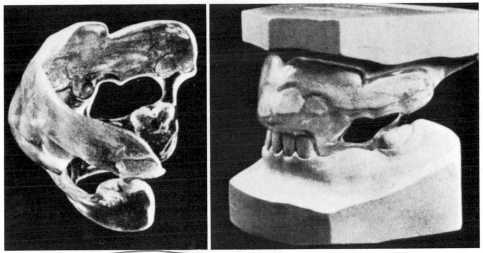

Figure 11–25   (Left) Propulsor; (right) in place on cast. The connection between the buccal flange in the maxillary portion and the lingual flange in the lower portion serves to prevent the appliance from being displaced at the beginning of treatment. It does this by opening the bite. After retraction of maxillary anterior segment, the contact areas that interfere with occlusal development are ground away, allowing the posterior teeth to erupt and eliminate the overbite and excessive interocclusal clearance. (Courtesy R. Hotz.)

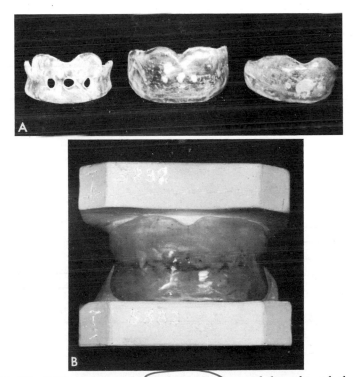

Figure 11–26   Different types of oral screens: A, with breathing holes; B, in place on model to show relationships. (Courtesy F. Kraus.)

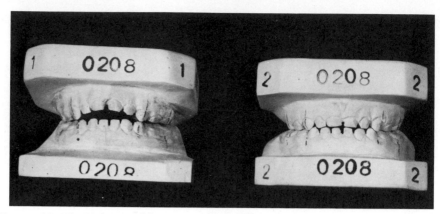

Figure 11–27   Habit problem responds uniformly well with oral screen therapy if patient is diligent. (Courtesy F. Kraus.)

of the orofacial muscles. As Hotz shows so well in his textbook, the maxillary incisors may also be retruded and there is a retardation of the horizontal maxillary alveolar movement anteriorly during appliance wear. In addition, the construction of the appliance permits eruption of teeth in the buccal segments while it is worn, which is an advantage over the activator (Fig. 11–25).

The oral screen (Figs. 11–26, 11–27) makes limited use of the basic concept of functional jaw orthopedics and is used with some degree of success to retract spaced maxillary incisors.[30]

ADVANTAGES OF REMOVABLE APPLIANCES

The advantages of removable appliances are obvious. It is possible for the dentist to treat many more patients with this type of appliance than with the much more time-consuming fixed appliances. The appliance utilizes the expanse of the palate or the alveolar bone inferior to the lower teeth for anchorage. The patient's own muscular activity is employed to produce a more physiologic type of tooth movement; the appliance is usually worn only at night and at home, and thus does not interfere with speech or create an esthetic problem. Since it is usually easier to keep such an appliance clean than it is to keep a fixed appliance clean, dental caries or decalcification is less of a problem during orthodontic treatment. Advantage can be taken of growth during treatment. Adjustment appointments are less frequent.

DISADVANTAGES OF REMOVABLE APPLIANCES

The greatest disadvantage of removable appliances is the strong, almost total dependence on patient cooperation. These appliances, with the exception of the Crozat and Bimler appliances, are bulky, relatively difficult to get used to and provide a mental, if not physical, barrier for those children who breathe through their mouths. While it makes use of growth occurring during treatment, lack of growth at that time strongly limits the value of the appliance. Removable appliances may be quite satisfactory for gross movements; but to correct the rotations of individual teeth, to move teeth bodily and to produce optimal interdigitation, it is frequently necessary to resort to fixed appliances to "finish" a case.

The length of time of removable appliance wear is usually considerably longer than with fixed appliances. In some cases, in which reliance on growth and development is necessary, this might be an advantage, but in most instances it is not. The level of patient cooperation is gradually reduced, and chances of damage or loss of appliances significantly greater. Tissue and growth changes reduce the chances for proper fit of the appliance. Achievement of the desired objective is far from being easier with removable than with fixed appliances. If anything, it requires more background, more biologic sense, more training, more experience, equal skill and a willingness to turn to fixed appliances, to tooth sacrifice or to both, if the treatment progress indicates this. In the majority of cases, therapy cannot be completed as well as with fixed appliances. In too many instances the situation is analogous to that of traveling from New York to Chicago and running out of gas in Cleveland. How to get to Chicago now? Maybe we'd better stay in Cleveland!

Finally, Reitan has shown conclusively that the jiggling effect of part-time force on teeth, with the appliance shoving the teeth one way and the functional forces pushing in the opposite direction may produce permanent damage. At the very least, excessive mobility is a consequence. Intermittent force of this type may actually stop tooth movement, with deposition of bone on the pressure side. Such reactions can hardly be called physiologic tooth movement. (See Chap. 10.)

FIXED APPLIANCES

There are many different types of fixed appliances in use today, just as there are many removable appliances. Different problems demand different amounts and types of mechanical aids.

THE ORTHODONTIC BAND. The basic element of all fixed appliances is the orthodontic band. This is made of either precious metal or chrome-cobalt stainless alloys, especially fabricated to produce the greatest strength and durability with a minimum of bulk. The band material must be soft enough to permit close adaptation to the contours of the teeth and yet strong enough to withstand the stresses of mastication and deglutition. As high a polish as possible is placed on the surfaces to reduce the adhesion of food debris. Band material is tasteless and will not tarnish.

Orthodontic bands come in strips, rolls, precut blanks, with the attachment already in place, in the center of the band, or in preformed, contoured and seamless forms of varying sizes and shapes. Bands for the anterior teeth are usually 0.003 or 0.004 inch thick and 0.125 inch wide. Canine and premolar bands are usually 0.004 inch thick and 0.150 inch wide. If not preformed, most canine and premolar bands are blanks and are precontoured because of the greater difficulty of making a well-fitting band. Molar bands also come in precontoured blanks of 0.005 to 0.006 inch thickness and 0.180 to 0.200 inch wide.

Since band fitting is the heart of orthodontics and since poorly fitting bands can cause permanent damage to the teeth and investing tissues, every effort must be made to fabricate and place bands as perfectly as possible. No compromise can be justified at any time. Modern technology has answered the demand for better fitting bands by the development of anatomically correct seamless bands for all teeth in a wide variety of sizes. The seamless band fitting materially reduces the chair time required, permits more effective use of auxiliary personnel and cuts down on the likelihood of future re-cementation. Seamless bands usually fit better and hold up better under the pounding of function than bands pinched, welded or soldered from band material. This is particularly true for the part-time orthodontist who hasn't had intensive training in technique (Fig. 11–28).

Each band has some sort of attachment or "bracket" to receive the arch wire and to transmit the adjustment force to the tooth in the proper, precise and effective manner. As was pointed out in the first part of this chapter, a number of attachments have been developed and discarded over the years. Some former "systems" or techniques, such as the labiolingual and ribbon arch have been modified extensively. Even the edgewise bracket technique, introduced over 40 years ago, has undergone changes in size, shape and number. No longer can (or should) a man say he is "a labiolingual man," "an edgewise man" or "a universal man," implying that he practices an appliance technique built specifically around the particular attachment. Elements of all so-called orthodontic philosophies are incorporated with the use of most brackets or attachments. Pure edgewise, pure twin-wire and pure Begg are about as pure as "pure Aryan." Such a sobriquet today would only ensure that the individual so labeled was purely unthinking—a disciple blindly following an orthodontic cult, as enamored with the orthodontic "leader" as the children were with the Pied Piper of Hamlin.

The most widely used attachments for orthodontic bands are the edgewise, modified ribbon arch (Begg), universal, twin-wire, and multiphase. The edgewise bracket has been modified by "twinning," by inserting vertical slots, by coupling it with ribbon arch bracket features and by changing the size of the center slot, which was formerly only 0.022 inch square, and now may be obtained in 0.018 or 0.016 inch square.[39] A partial count reveals that there are at

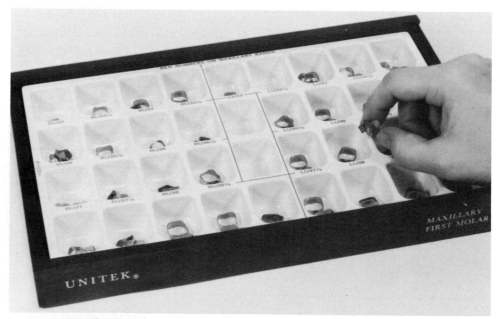

Figure 11–28   Seamless preformed bands are available from a number of commercial sources. Since they are available in different sizes, faithful attention to tooth anatomy makes this a good choice for a strong, well-fitted band, with a minimum of time expended on work in the dental chair. (Courtesy Unitek Corp.)

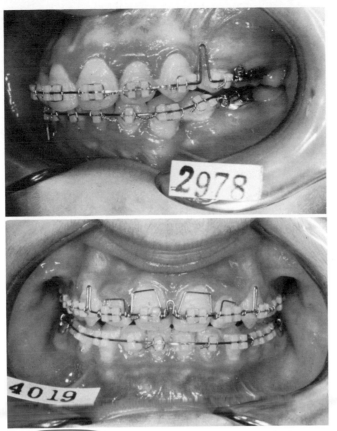

Figure 11–29. Plastic brackets, attached directly to the tooth surface by an epoxy resin. Ease of handling, rapidity of appliance placement, cosmetic improvement are strong recommendations for this type of "bandless" fixed appliance. Regular arch configurations, ligatures, etc., are used here, as with any regular twin-edgewise bracket set-up. (Courtesy F. Miura.)

least 117 possible bracket types and modifications, many of which are identified by the name of the modifying orthodontist. This "battle of the brackets" has created some confusion. Yet, all do essentially the same thing and can be employed for torque, tipping, bodily movement or rotations by modifying the arch wire or adding appurtenances (Figs. 11–31, 11–32). In addition to the so-called brackets which serve to hold and transmit arch wire force, spurs, buttons or rotating "eyelets" may be employed. With the development of new adhesives, the various attachments that are now welded or soldered to the band may be attached directly on the tooth. Epoxy resins and plastic brackets now are being used on maxillary incisors and canines, as well as maxillary premolars. Problems still exist for mandibular incisor teeth, and teeth in the lower arch generally because of the shearing effect of function on the contained arch. Cosmetically, the resin-bonded attachments are an improvement[32] (Fig. 11–29). They eliminate the tedious band fitting procedure and greatly reduce the decalcification and gingival damage that all too frequently are "the scars of the operation" in orthodontics.[32, 65, 67]

Whether brackets are on bands or attached directly to the enamel, precise positioning is the order of the day. Generally, brackets belong in the center of the facial surface of each tooth crown. They should be so placed that a straight

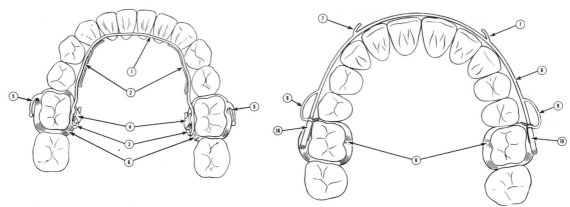

Figure 11–30   Elements of the labiolingual appliance. (Left) (1) 0.036 or 0.040 inch arch wire; (2) 0.020 or 0.022 inch auxiliary spring; (3) 0.028 inch lingual locking wire; (4) half-round or Mershon and vertical posts, 0.090 inch in length; (5) intermaxillary elastic hooks, 0.030 inch; (6) 0.006 by 0.180 inch band material or preformed molar bands. (Right) (7) Intermaxillary elastic hook, 0.030 inch wire; (8) labial arch, 0.036 or 0.040 inch; (9) vertical spring loop, 0.025 or 0.028 inch; (10) horizontal buccal tubes to fit arch wire. (Courtesy Williams Gold Refining Co.)

leveling arch wire will establish correct incisal and occlusal height automatically.

THE ARCH WIRE. The major force producing part of fixed appliances is usually the arch wire, or tooth-moving springs or spurs attached to that wire. The arch wire may be heavy and relatively unyielding to serve as a base for appurtenances or ligation, as in the labiolingual appliances (Figs. 11–6, 11–30), or it may be light and very flexible, with varying geometry, to iron out individual irregularities as the arch wire itself is inserted directly into the attachment of choice (Fig. 11–31). The wire may be rectangular or square in cross section and

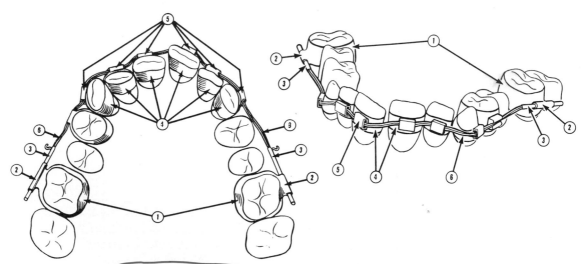

Figure 11–31   Twin-wire appliance. (1) Molar band, 0.006 by 0.180 inch material or preformed, contoured or loop bands. (2) 0.036 inch horizontal buccal tubes. (3) End tube-buccal tube, 0.036 inch outside diameter. (4) Attachment bands. (5) Twin-arch channel and cap (or twintie channel bracket). (6) Twin-wire 0.011 or 0.012 inch. Coil spring sections are usually used on the maxillary arch for driving molars distally; the lower appliance of the classic twin-wire technique is usually a lingual arch of the Mershon type.[31] Since this is often inadequate, many modifications of the mandibular appliance have been made. (Courtesy Williams Gold Refining Co.)

machined to fit snugly into the bracket slot, so that various bodily, root moving or torque forces may be employed (Fig. 11–32). The wire may be unadorned and straight, or it may be "looped"; it may have various soldered or welded appurtenances or "piggy-back" auxiliary springs to produce specific tooth movements (Fig. 11–42). To activate and sometimes to control arch wire force, elastics may be used within the same arch (intramaxillary) or between the arches (intermaxillary) (Fig. 11–40). The wire may actually be laminated together to form an arch "bundle," the result being a stranded or twisted force-producing unit, composed of very light, highly elastic individual wires. Together these stranded arches are capable of producing a light, continuous, long-acting force, and they are quite resistant to permanent deformation (Fig. 11–33). As the science of metallurgy has progressed, the combinations of metals within the wires have changed. Formerly, most wires were of gold or gold and platinum alloys. Now, almost all arch wires are combinations of stainless steel with chrome, cobalt, nickel, etc. In some stainless wires, there is actually no steel at all.[72]

With the light wire or differential light forces techniques, high intensity spring wire of a small gauge (0.012, 0.014, 0.016 or 0.018) is used. Numerous loops are then bent into the arch wires to produce a lighter, more gentle and continuous force, and yet effect torque and rotational changes. Vertical loops were introduced by Robinson[34] in 1915 and recommended by Griffin[35] in 1930 (Fig. 11–34) but did not achieve widespread use until metallurgy caught up

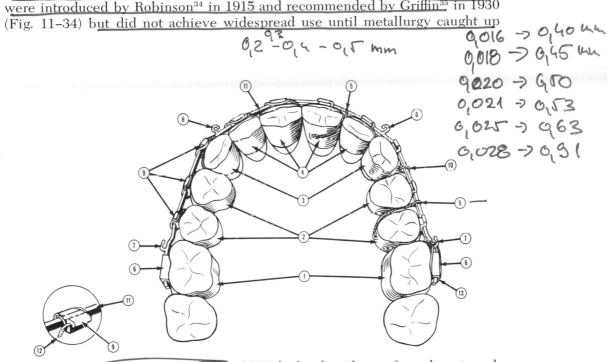

Figure 11–32 Edgewise appliance. (1) Molar bands, either preformed, contoured, loop bands or from 0.006 by 0.180 inch band material. (2) Contoured premolar bands or preformed bands. (3) Contoured or preformed canine bands. Single or twin edgewise brackets may be attached already, or welded after forming band. (4) Anterior attachment bands with single or twin edgewise brackets. (5) Steel ligature tie to eyelet on lingual for rotation. (6) 0.022 by 0.028 inch rectangular buccal tube. (7) Tieback hook or spur. (8) Intermaxillary hook, 0.025 or 0.028 inch wire. (9) Edgewise brackets of choice, depending on convexity of buccal surfaces and control needed. (10) Steel ligature tie to eyelet on distal of canine, for rotation. (11) Round or edgewise arch wire, depending on phase of treatment. If edgewise, it may be 0.018 or 0.021 by 0.025 or 0.022 by 0.028 inch dimensions. (12) Edgewise arch tied into bracket with twisted pigtail tucked under arch. (13) Ligature tie over tieback spur to maintain arch position.[33] (Courtesy Williams Gold Refining Co.)

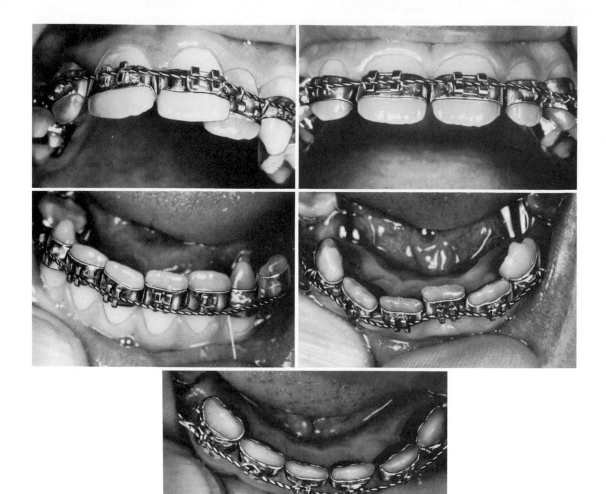

Figure 11–33 Stranded or "twist-flex" wire, made up of three light wire segments of a high spring type light wire, 0.0175, 0.0195 and 0.0215 inch dimensions are available to fit various brackets and demands for magnitude of adjustment. A minimum of adjustment is placed in the arch wire. When deformed, it tends to return to original straight configuration. Wire was not tied completely in bracket in original maxillary arch adjustment (above), but bottom series of three views shows arch standing away from lingually malposed teeth first, then being ligated completely into brackets and the alignment of the incisor teeth three weeks later as adjustment has worked out.

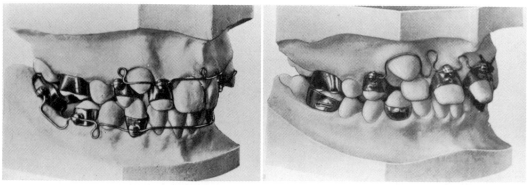

Figure 11–34 Vertical spring loops as used by Griffin to provide light, gentle forces.

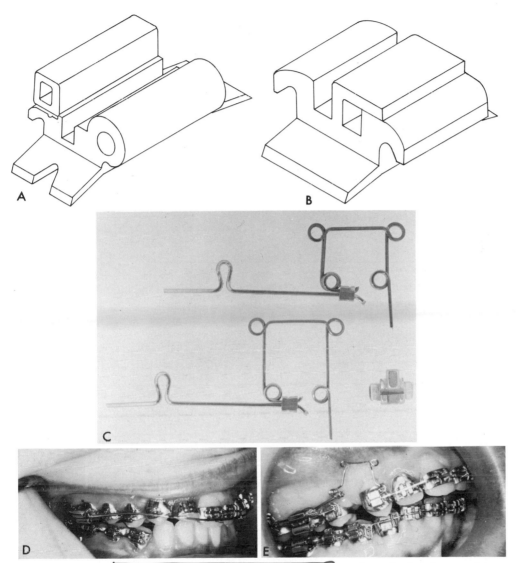

Figure 11–35 Burstone segmental arch technique. A, molar tube-bracket combination. B, premolar bracket-tube combination for greatest versatility. C, Anterior retraction assemblies, showing rectangular posterior segmental arch, and multi-looped retraction springs. Canines alone, or entire anterior segment may be controlled with this arrangement. The canine bracket-tube combination is shown in lower right corner. D, rectangular base arch for incisor intrusion. E, anterior retraction assembly in place, using horizontal bracket-tube on canine. En masse movement of anterior segment is achieved since six anterior teeth are tied together by a segmental arch. (Courtesy Charles J. Burstone.)

with the light continuous force concept by providing the right type of wire. The present differential light forces techniques, as developed and popularized by Begg,[36] Kesling,[37] Williams,[59] Jarabak,[38] Rosenstein,[39] Stoner,[40] Burstone,[41] Lindquist[40] and others make use of vertical and horizontal loops which incorporate a helical coil, or modifications of the push and pull loops of Bercu Fischer[43, 73] (Fig. 11–35).

ASSISTING ELEMENTS. To help the arch wire and bands in the function of moving teeth, certain "assists" have been developed. Highly resilient open and closed coil springs are very effective.[44] To provide "stops" or places on the arch wire to ligate, special locks can be placed without removing the wire from the mouth. Various size rubber bands as well as well as elastic thread are effective tooth-moving devices, when used properly; steel ligature is essential for a number of appliances to tie the arch into the brackets and to rotate turned teeth. Sometimes a removable appliance is used in conjunction with the fixed appliances either to retract individual teeth or to serve as a bite plate. Perhaps one of the best ways to understand how these appliances are being used is to analyze the approaches to treatment in Class I, Class II and Class III therapy. For a more detailed analysis of appliance fabrication and details of therapy, the reader is referred to a series of texts on specific orthodontic "philosophies." The two-volume text on the major orthodontic techniques, edited by the author, might be a good starting point.[19, 23, 40, 41]

TREATMENT OF CLASS I MALOCCLUSIONS

ARCH LENGTH DEFICIENCY

In Class I malocclusions the major problem is arch length deficiency (except in open bite malocclusions). There just is not enough room to accommodate all the teeth in their correct positions. As a result, some teeth may be rotated, others prevented from erupting, and still others may be forced into abnormal positions inside or outside the normal dental arch. In these cases the jaw relationship is good, facial balance is usually quite satisfactory, and perioral muscle function is usually normal. Where these problems were formerly corrected by expanding the dental arches to a greater arc to accommodate all the teeth on the same perimeter of basal bone, it is now realized that to move the teeth into the resisting musculature is to invite failure after the tooth-moving appliances are removed. Those muscle forces that operate in functional jaw orthopedics and provide the activator or monobloc with the ability to move teeth also may act on any teeth that are moved into a position where they are no longer in balance with all environmental and functional forces.[50] Unless the dentist is fairly sure that he can depend on growth and development to provide the additional space required, or unless he can change muscle patterns of activity, he had better use the philosophy of expansion in orthodontic tooth movement most sparingly in Class I malocclusions. In certain specially chosen cases, where diagnostic criteria indicate to the orthodontic specialist that he may need basal expansion of the maxillary segments themselves — not just expansion of the teeth — Korkhaus,[45] Derichsweiler,[46] Wertz,[47] Isaacson[48] and others have corrected maxillary arch width deficiencies with rapid expansion of the midpalatal suture, using a fixed splint (Figs. 11–36, 11–37).

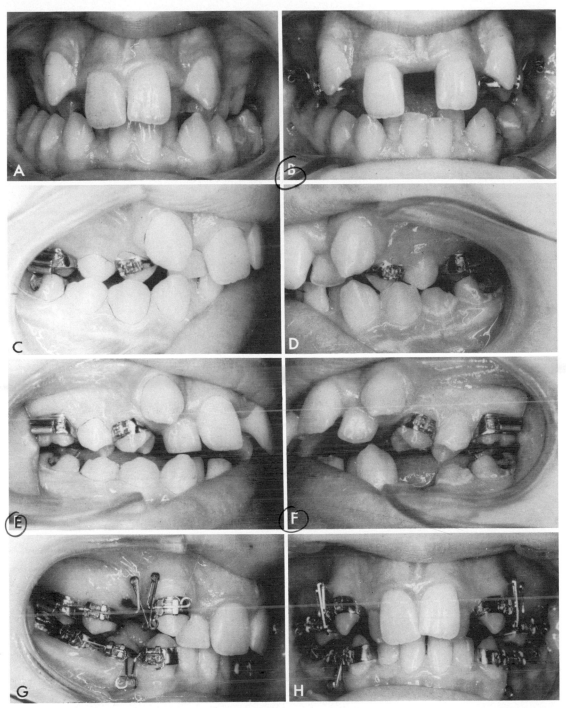

Figure 11–36 Correction of a severe maxillary narrowness (A, C and D) by means of opening the midpalatal suture demonstrates overcorrection (B, E and F), spontaneous closure of created maxillary midline diastema (H) and continuing therapy (G and H). The abutment bands cemented to the first premolars were removed, these teeth were extracted, and retraction of the canines was begun with the appliance utilized as a stabilizing device. The buccal segments were further supported by direct-pull face-bow traction to the maxillary molars. (From Wertz, R. A.: Skeletal and dental changes accompanying rapid midpalatal suture opening. Am. J. Orthodont., 58:41–46, 1970.)

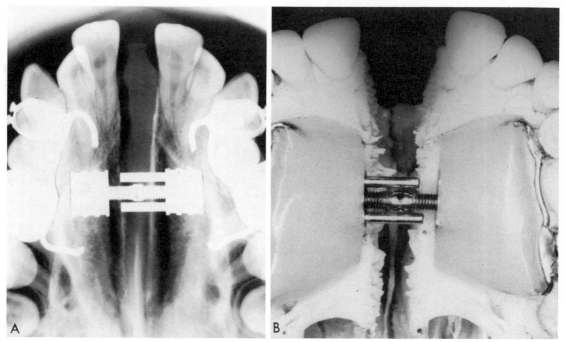

Figure 11–37   Occlusal view of opened suture in an actual case (A) as compared with mixed dentition dry skull material (B). Nonparallel opening of midpalatal suture is routine response to midpalatal separation. The opening appears to be at about a 2 to 1 ratio, with the anterior opening being widest. The image of the vomer is clearly seen in the posterior aspect. (From Wertz, R. A.: Skeletal and dental changes accompanying rapid midpalatal suture opening. Am. J. Orthodont., 58:41–46, 1970.)

This procedure is well documented in a 60-case study reported by Wertz in 1970.[47] He found that rapid maxillary expansion was definitely accomplished in all cases but, with advancing maturity, rigidity of the skeletal components limited the degree of orthopedic correction in older patients. Studied in profile, downward displacement of the maxilla was rather routine, but forward displacement to any degree was limited to isolated cases. Recovery of displacement during the period of stabilization varied so that only about 50 per cent of the cases demonstrated this post-treatment reaction. Mandibular displacement and subsequent recovery were usually noted. Studied in the frontal plane, the maxillary halves arced laterally with the fulcrum located close to nasion, and skeletal widening progressed inferiorly. Apparently, alveolar bending accounted for proportionately increased lateral denture displacement relative to that of the skeleton. Stability in this plane of space was judged as excellent. The maxillary central incisors always moved mesially and generally uprighted following stabilization. Such decrease in the SN-*1* angle aids in accounting for the rapid closure of the large midline diastema produced with this orthopedic movement. Concomitant shortening of gained arch length was evident, and increased muscular tension produced by the maxillary expansion together with interseptal fiber reaction is offered as reasoning for this behavior. Occlusally, the midpalatal suture opened in a nonparallel manner, with the widest opening being at ANS and diminishing posteriorly such that the opening was 3 to 2 and sometimes 2 to 1 when comparing ANS to PNS opening (Fig. 11–37).

SERIAL EXTRACTION

The best clue that an orthodontist has in Class I malocclusions is the shape of the arch that the patient presents with the original problem. To disturb arch shape and size is to court failure. This means that it is necessary to remove teeth in most severe Class I malocclusions. If teeth are removed, much of the irregularity may actually be reduced automatically by the spontaneous drift of the remaining teeth into the empty space. Serial extraction offers a great opportunity for the orthodontist who recognizes Class I malocclusions early and can thus provide the space needed for self-adjustment. Since the dentist in general practice will be called upon to extract deciduous teeth early in these cases, he should be quite familiar with the concept. The responsibility for serial extraction procedures, however, should remain with the orthodontic specialist. He is obviously best qualified to make the decision, based on his knowledge of growth and development, on his studies of headplates, cephalometric analyses, panoramic radiographs and on his clinical experience. Serial extraction can produce iatrogenic malocclusions that may be worse than the original problem, if not handled properly. Almost all serial extraction management problems require full appliances even though treatment time is reduced (Fig. 11–38). This is the most impelling reason for orthodontic control of guided extraction procedure. (This will be discussed in greater detail in Chapter 15.)

In most instances the orthodontist is confronted with irregular teeth, the need for tooth sacrifice and the demand for appliance therapy. Seldom will the removal of teeth alone completely effect the desired orthodontic result. Orthodontic therapy in Class I malocclusions means tooth control. Teeth that drift often merely tip into spaces, and the resulting abnormal axial inclinations, poor apical positions and improper contacts invite future periodontal troubles. *En masse* tooth movement is essential. This almost invariably means a multibanded technique and rules out the use of removable appliances, except as adjuncts.

Even though most dentists will not want to handle multibanded extraction cases, they will want to know what the orthodontist is trying to do and how the appliances work (Fig. 11–41). Most of the teeth are banded at one time or another during treatment. Rotations are corrected, proper axial inclination established and maintained, roots paralleled on either side of the extraction space as spaces are being closed, and arch form is maintained as nearly as possible to duplicate the configuration of the original arch form at the time the patient presented with the malocclusion.

RELATIONSHIP OF TOOTH TO BASAL BONE

A most important requirement for the success and stability of Class I orthodontic correction is the maintenance of a proper tooth-to-basal bone relationship. Effective control of individual teeth is essential. The orthodontist must be able to control his anchorage, to change the tooth inclinations at will and to be sure that he has not created new problems that did not exist with the original malocclusion. The removal of first premolar teeth, second premolar teeth or, possibly, second molar teeth may be essential in the establishment of a normal and healthy occlusion.[51-53] Not all Class I malocclusions are frank tooth sacrifice cases at the beginning of treatment. Needless extraction is as

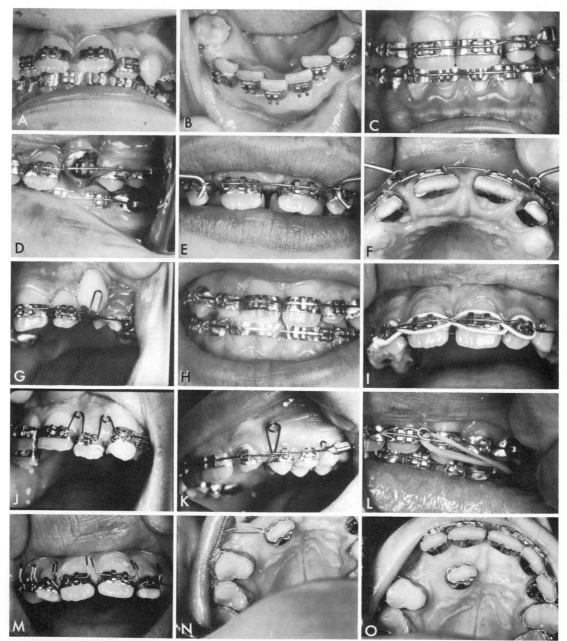

Figure 11–38 Appliances and appurtenances seen at various stages of Class I orthodontic treatment. A and B, Teeth banded for insertion of arch wire. C, Upper and lower round steel arches with twin edgewise brackets on bands. D, Use of gold overlay that has been used to bring high canine down to arch. E and F, Extraoral force arms inserted into horizontal loops bent in arch wire. G, Vertical loop exerting pressure on high canine. H, Edgewise upper and lower arches in place. I, Elastic thread being used to close spaces. J, Open helical coil loops being used to move lateral incisor labially. K, Closed helical coil loop often used in closing extraction spaces. L, Use of intermaxillary elastics to help close spaces in each arch. M, Simple vertical loops to provide gentler force for unraveling incisors. N and O, Canine in palate banded and being tied toward arch as push-coil spring opens sufficient space.

bad as not removing teeth when indicated. In the past, many orthodontists have extracted teeth because of preconceived ideas of incisor inclination alone and found to their chagrin, that spaces were hard to close, that overbite was difficult to correct and that demands of torque of maxillary incisors were so great that root resorption became a major concern. Many potential tooth sacrifice cases are started without removing any teeth, and treatment response is appraised first. The hope is that the third molars may be removed later, providing needed arch length for post-treatment stability and adjustment. Thus, therapeutic modifiability is an essential requisite of most treatment plans. Diagnosis is tentative and subject to treatment response. Periodic cephalograms and laminagraphic panoramic views are required in this continuing dynamic assessment. (See Chap. 8.) Present differential light forces techniques move teeth effectively, with minimal tissue damage. Figures 11–39 through 11–41 show Jarabak[38] light forces technique drawings for extraction Class I malocclusions. Figures 11–42 and 11–43 show extraction cases treated with the Begg principles and appliances.[19]

(Text continued on page 572)

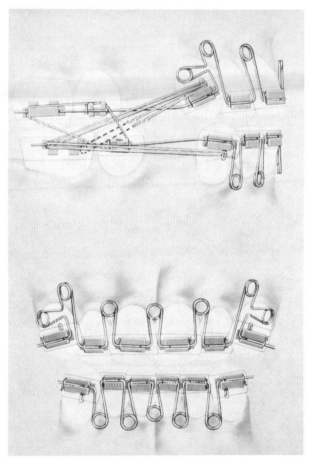

Figure 11–39   Class I extraction case, with high deflection helical spring loops being used to increase intercanine arch length by distally driving the four canines simultaneously. The elastics being used in this phase of treatment comprise the extrinsic force system. (From Jarabak, J. R., and Fizzell, J. B.: Technique and Treatment With the Light-Wire Appliances. C. V. Mosby Co., 1963.)

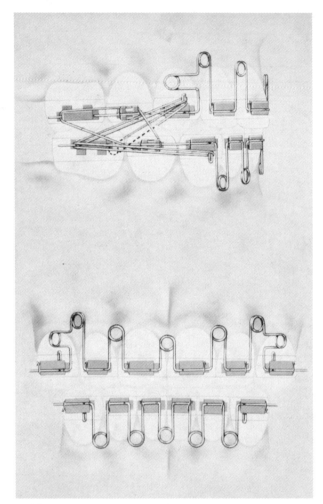

Figure 11–40 Class I extraction case shown in previous illustration. Spaces have been closed up and appliance is deactivated. There are four elastics on each side: (1) triangular upper first molar-upper second premolar to lower second premolar (2) Class II type from lingual aspect of lower molar to intermaxillary hook at maxillary canine, (3) Class II type from distal end of lower molar to intermaxillary hook at maxillary canine and (4) intermaxillary type from distal end of lower molar tube to hook at mandibular canine. These are vital in assisting arch wire, eliminating overbite, stimulating vertical development of posterior teeth, closing extraction spaces, stabilizing anchorage and achieving correct interdigitation. (From Jarabak, J. R., and Fizzell, J. B.: Technique and Treatment With the Light-Wire Appliances. C. V. Mosby Co., 1963.)

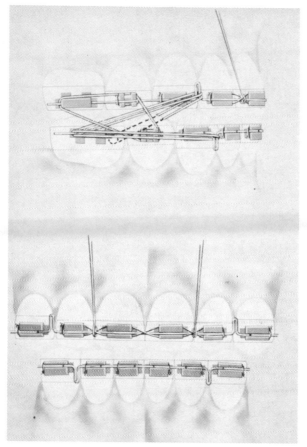

Figure 11–41   Class I extraction case (Figs. 11 39 and 11–40) showing final steps of seating inclined planes and establishing a functional overbite and overjet by using 0.016 × 0.016 inch square arches, in conjunction with an extrinsic high-pull extraoral force system. (From Jarabak, J. R., and Fizzell, J. B.: Technique and Treatment With the Light-Wire Appliances. C. V. Mosby Co., 1963.)

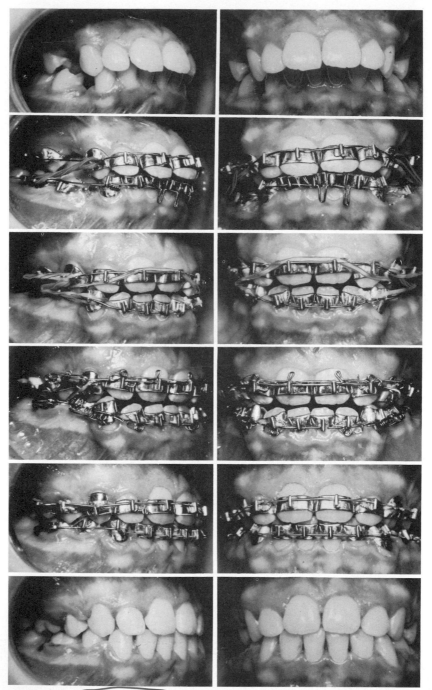

Figure 11–42 Begg technique in Class I bimaxillary protrusion extraction case. (Top row) Before appliance placement; (second row) beginning appliances, Stage I; (third row) six months later, end of Stage I and beginning of Stage II; (fourth row) two months later, end of Stage II, beginning of Stage III with piggy-back torquing mechanism in place; (fifth row) ten months later, end of Stage III. Appliances are ready to be removed. (Bottom row) Immediately after appliance removal. No positioner has been placed. Space closure with elastics and minimal friction characterizes Stage I. Overbite is eliminated. Note overtreatment and lingual tipping of incisors at the end of Stage II. Axial inclinations and uprighting through auxiliary springs completes Stage III. (Courtesy R. Williams.)

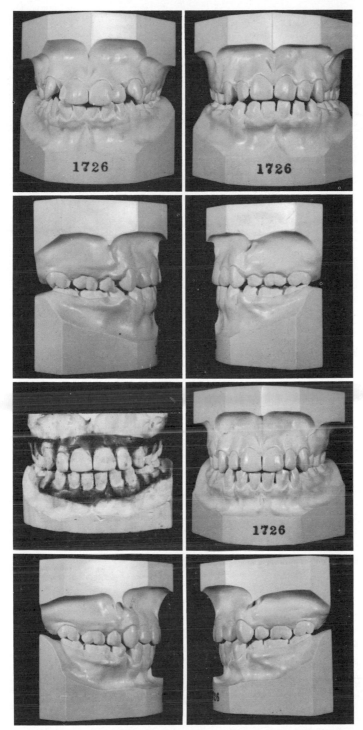

Figure 11–43A   Class I, four first premolar extraction case, treated with Begg differential light forces technique. (Top row) Before and after appliance removal, demonstrating bite-opening and overtreatment. (Second row) After appliance removal. Teeth are then reset in wax, in desired position for a plastic tooth positioner (third row, left). In third row, right, and fourth rows, casts show the "settling in" nine months later. This demonstrates advantage of overtreatment and use of positioner, counteracting the relapse tendency. See Figures 11–43B and 11–43C for more views of same case. (Courtesy B. F. Swain.)

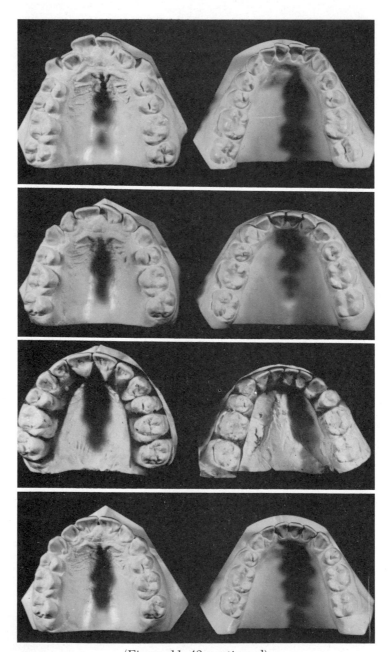

(Figure 11–43 continued)

Figure 11–43B   Same case as in Figure 11–43A, illustrating overtreatment and use of positioner, or elastoplastic appliance. (Top row) Before treatment. (Second row) Immediately after appliance removal, showing overtreatment. (Third row) Wax setup for positioner. (Bottom row) Nine months later, showing adjustment. (Courtesy B. F. Swain.)

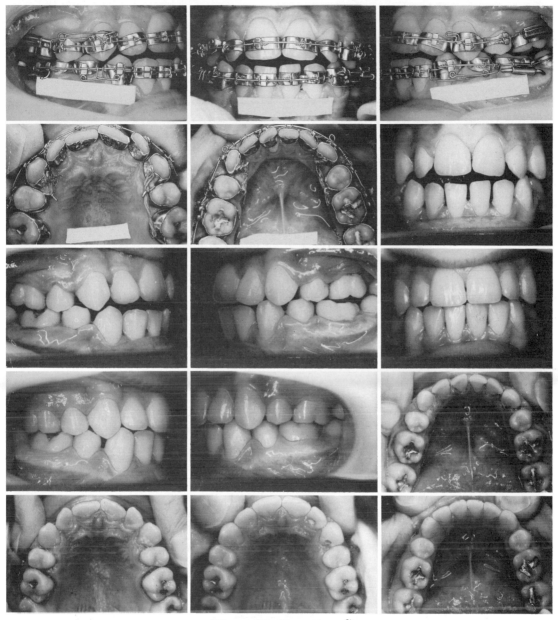

(Figure 11–43 continued)

Figure 11–43C Differential light forces technique, using Begg-Chun Hoon bracket. This allows control in three planes of space with employment of Begg light-wire principles through vertical slot and edgewise control technique with horizontal groove. (Top row) Appliances in place just before removal. Note uprighting and paralleling springs in canine-premolar region, overtreatment, etc. (Second row) Patient at same time, and frontal view immediately after appliance removal. Lingual elastic is in place to demonstrate space closure and rotational control of first molar (left). First two pictures of third row, occlusal views of lower arch in fourth row (right) and occlusal view of upper arch (fifth row, left) were also taken at this time when appliances were removed and they demonstrate overtreatment. The five views taken nine months later, after the wearing of a positioner, are: the third row frontal view (right), fourth row views (left and center) and fifth row views (center and right). The pictures are arranged to permit a comparison of comparable views before and after the 9-month interval. The frontal views (second and third rows, right) show the closing down of the bite. The right and left lateral views (third and fourth rows, left and center) also demonstrate settling in and space closure. The maxillary occlusal views (fifth row, left and center) demonstrate dramatically the effect of overcorrection and positioner wear during the 9-month interval. The mandibular occlusal views (fourth and fifth rows, right) show less change.[19] (Courtesy B. F. Swain.)

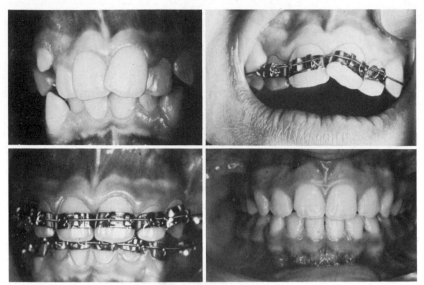

Figure 11–44   Class I malocclusion before, during and after orthodontic treatment. Four first premolars were removed.

TREATMENT OF CLASS II, DIVISION 1 MALOCCLUSIONS

In addition to rotations, root paralleling, overbite and space problems encountered in Class I cases, we see perversions of muscle function, problems of overjet, incisor inclinations and actual maxillomandibular basal malrelationship in Class II, Division 1 cases. In other words, more than irregular teeth and lack of space are involved. In most instances there is an actual anteroposterior discrepancy in the jaw relationship. Unquestionably, the challenge is greater here for the orthodontist.

CONCEPT OF THE APICAL BASE

To better understand the nature of the challenge and the problems encountered in Class II, Division 1 malocclusion therapy, an outline of the development of the concept of apical base is essential. Apical base to the clinician means the arbitrary juncture of the alveolar bone at the apices of the teeth with the basal bone of the maxilla and mandible. It is the adequacy of this bony support and the relation of the bony support in the maxilla to that of the mandible that conditions the ultimate therapeutic objectives in orthodontics.

In 1923 Axel Lundström of Sweden made some remarkably cogent observations concerning apical base relations and orthodontic treatment.[49]

1. Function does not determine the size of the apical base.
2. Mastication has little to do with the apical base size.
3. Orthodontics does not develop normal apical bases.
4. Spontaneous development of apical bases may occur.
5. Problems of malocclusion are problems of apical base.

Recognizing the limitation of Class II therapy, a University of Illinois group made the following observations in 1938:

1. Occlusal plane inclinations tend to return after treatment. This tendency diminishes as age advances.

2. A change in mandibular plane position contributes to the orthodontic result in a number of cases. This change usually comes from downward and backward mandibular rotation, but occasionally there is an anteroposterior shift.

3. Changes in axial inclination of the teeth tend to revert after orthodontic therapy.

4. Bone changes are restricted to the alveolar process.

5. Post-treatment changes primarily are the shifting of the occlusal plane back toward the original inclination and the tendency for re-assertion of the original incisor axial inclination.

6. Success depends on a correlation between growth and treatment.[54]

TREATMENT PROBLEMS AND PROCEDURES

When one recognizes that abnormal jaw relationship and abnormal functional forces are involved, it is not difficult to understand the reason for the strong relapse tendency in many Class II malocclusions. Unless there is an improvement in the anteroposterior jaw relationship and an elimination of muscle perversions, the changes wrought in individual tooth position will be inadequate to eliminate the malocclusion. The role of heredity is indeed strong.

MAXILLARY AND MANDIBULAR GROWTH

To adjust the anteroposterior jaw relationship it is necessary to institute orthodontic therapy during the time when there are significant increments of growth in the upper and lower jaws. This is the reason why orthodontists emphasize the importance of growth and development. Success of therapy depends on correlation with this vital process. Correlation with the pubertal growth spurt is perhaps even more rewarding for the orthodontist, and so timing of growth is critical. In Chapter 2 it was pointed out that the maxilla and the mandible grow downward and forward. Anything that can be done to enhance or take advantage of this growth-linked phenomenon should be carried out by the orthodontist, if he is to adjust the anteroposterior malrelationship. Growth directions vary, even as do growth increments, of course. Diagnostic decisions and therapeutic manipulations should take into account original inheritance-linked cephalometric projections.

In Class II malocclusions the mandible is retruded and the maxillary teeth and the maxillary alveolar process appear to be anteriorly displaced. Most studies have shown that actually only the maxillary anterior teeth are displaced labially. The maxilla and its alveolar process are in relatively normal relationship to the other parts of the face and cranium, at least in the posterior segments. It is the mandible that is retruded in its relationship to the remaining craniofacial structures. If examined by itself, the mandible may appear perfectly normal. Seldom are there any characteristics that would lead an observer to think that this is a "Class I mandible," a "Class II" or "Class III mandible." It is primarily the positional relationship of that bone with its opposing member that is abnormal.

STIMULATION AND RETARDATION OF GROWTH

Ideally, what we would like to do is stimulate growth in the mandible so that it could "catch up" with the maxilla. For many years orthodontists thought they were doing just that with their mechanical appliances. There are still men in many parts of the world who feel they are accomplishing this objective. Most trained observers, however, believe that orthodontic appliances cannot stimulate any more growth than is going to occur according to pattern. Appliances can remove restrictions or retardations in the accomplishment of growth patterns; they can allow the fullest accomplishment of a particular pattern; they can eliminate functional retrusions, but to produce growth increments beyond the predetermined, genetic potential does not seem to be possible with present orthodontic procedures.

The orthodontist handles his problems much like the orthopedic surgeon attacks the congenital club foot deformity. In the past the orthopedic surgeon would try to lengthen the shorter leg so that it would equal the normal leg in length.[55] This failed in most instances. The surgeon learned that by stapling the epiphyses and the diaphyses he could retard the growth of the good leg so that the net result would be two legs of the same length. What is done in a Class II type malocclusion, then, is to restrict the downward and forward movement of the alveolodental structure in the maxilla, while the same structures in the mandible along with the mandibular basal bone move forward through growth and development.

Dentofacial orthopedic techniques, emulating the orthopedic surgeon in his use of the Milwaukee brace, can now guide maxillary and mandibular growth, by changing direction, if not by retarding growth, per se. Since two thirds of all malocclusions commonly treated by orthodontists are basal malocclusions, with the teeth reflecting the jaw malrelationship, correction of anteroposterior relations is paramount. The orthodontist is literally the orthopedic surgeon of the craniofacial complex.[55]

ROLE OF EXTRACTION. With good timing and significant growth increments during orthodontic treatment, fairly satisfactory results can be obtained (Figs. 11–45, 11–46). Sometimes, where there is inadequate growth or where arch length problems are present, a further adjustment is necessary—that of tooth removal. This may mean the removal of two maxillary first premolars, two maxillary second molars or, if there is an acute arch length problem in the mandible or excessive labial inclination of the mandibular incisors, four first premolars are removed (Figs. 11–47, 11–48, 11–49). The space created by the removal of teeth allows the elimination of individual tooth irregularities and the adjustment of the maxillary and mandibular anterior segments toward a normal overbite and overjet relationship.

ROLE OF EXTRAORAL FORCE. Force applied against the maxillary teeth by means of an extraoral appliance is an excellent way to restrain the downward and forward progression of the maxillary alveolodental complex in severe Class II, Division 1 malocclusions. The use of extraoral force for such problems is not new. Such appliances were used in both Class II and Class III therapy before 1900 (Figs. 11–50, 11–51). With the advent of the use of intermaxillary elastics, "skullcap therapy" was discarded for a seemingly better and easier approach. The test of time proved this decision premature and extraoral force was resurrected, refurbished with new materials, and it now occupies an important place in Class I therapy to reinforce anchorage, and in Class II and Class III therapy to effect jaw relationship changes.[51–53, 55]

Timing orthodontic treatment with the most favorable growth direction and increments, the proper direction of force application and the magnitude of force for orthopedic control of basal malrelationship have made it possible for extraoral appliances to become an important part of all Class II and Class III therapy (except in the Begg technique, where it is not recommended).

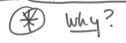

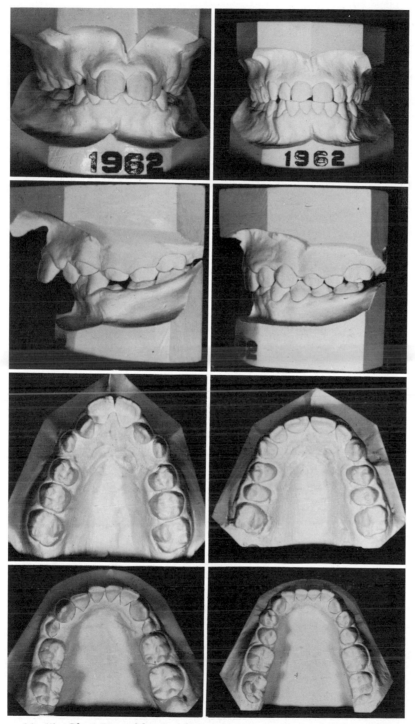

Figure 11–45   Class II problem with usual compensatory muscle activity. Extraoral appliances against maxillary arch, proper treatment timing with favorable growth direction and amounts, and good patient cooperation combined to produce the result in the views on the right. No mandibular appliances were worn.

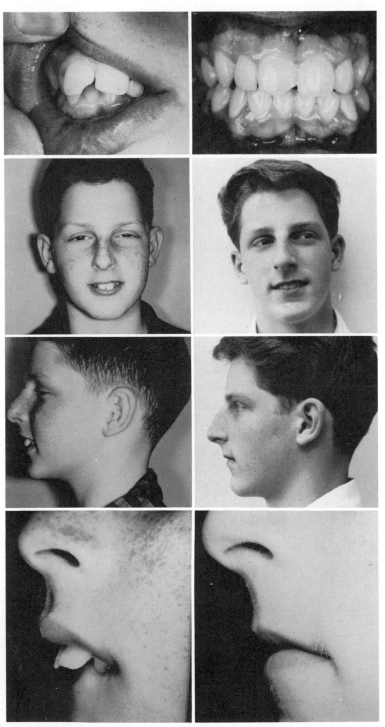

Figure 11–46 Same patient as in Figure 11–45. (Left) Before treatment; (right) after extraoral force therapy. Change in muscle balance indicates greater likelihood for a reasonably stable result.

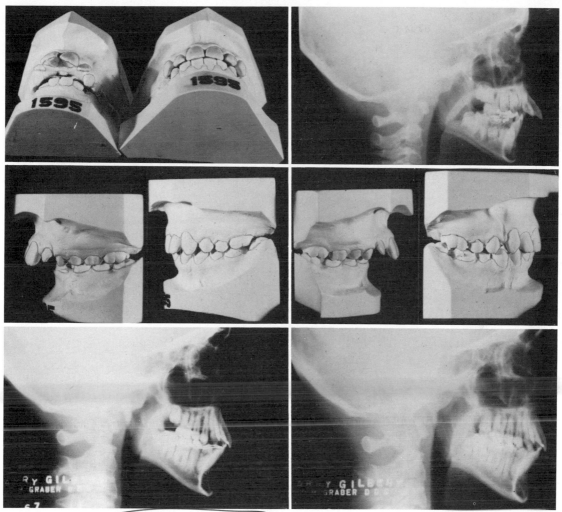

Figure 11–47. Severe Class II, Division 1 malocclusion in mixed dentition. As cephalometric tracings show, the prospects for appreciable *amounts* of growth are good, but the steep mandibular plane, and large apical base dysplasia do not offer much hope on a favorable *direction* of growth (Fig. 11–49). After considerable extraoral orthopedic guidance, with vertical growth, the maxillary second molar teeth were removed to allow retropositioning of the maxillary arch, in conjunction with orthopedic withholding of the maxillary complex itself. The changes produced are illustrated by casts before and after treatment, and headplates before and after treatment, and after retention. The lower fixed lingual retaining arch, with occlusal extension to prevent over-eruption of mandibular second molars, was removed after the eruption of maxillary third molars.

Extraoral force by itself is inadequate. Intraoral appliances are necessary to receive and direct this force. *In the great majority of cases the control of the extraoral mechanotherapy should be in the hands of the orthodontic specialist.* Total orthodontic diagnosis is a requisite for *any* therapy, and this means not only a careful clinical examination, but study casts, headplates, a cephalometric appraisal, a panoramic radiographic survey and correlation of all data to make a differential diagnosis. Periodic repetition of these records is essential during active treatment, permitting the therapeutic modifiability so often necessary. It is obvious that the demands of Class II, Division 1 therapy would overtax the average dentist. It is important, however, that he be acquainted with the principles of this type of treatment so he may better guide the patient's total oral

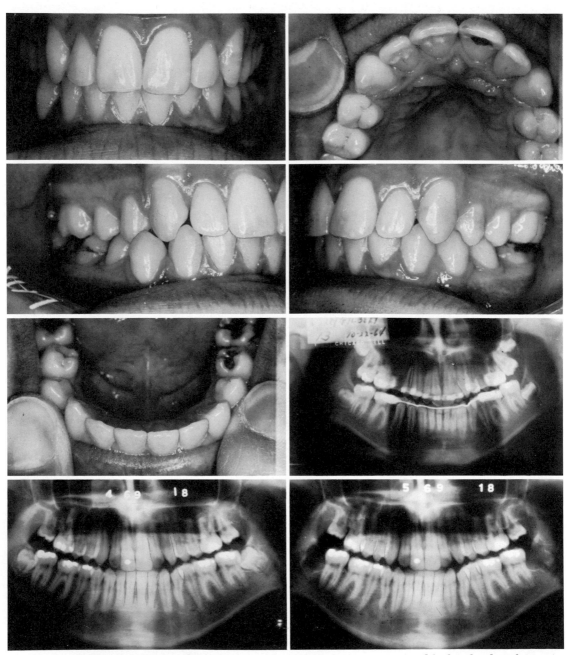

Figure 11–48   Intraoral and panoramic views of Figure 11–47. Mandibular third molars were removed to balance earlier removal of maxillary second molars.

Case:L.G. age:	9	10	11	12	14	16	17	18	19	20
SNaA	78.0	79.0	78.0	76.0	75.0	74.0	74.0	73.5	75.0	73.5
AB Diff	10.0	8.5	8.0	7.0	5.5	5.0	5.0	4.5	5.5	5.0
NaS–GoGn	41.0	40.0	41.0	42.0	43.0	42.0	41.0	42.0	42.5	42.0
U1–NaS	107.0	83.0	80.5	79.5	90.5	94.5	93.5	96.0	94.5	92.5
L1–GoGn	86.0	90.0	90.0	97.0	97.0	101.5	100.0	98.5	97.5	96.5
U1–NaPog(mm)	19.0	7.0	8.0	7.5	9.0	9.0	9.0	9.0	10.0	9.0

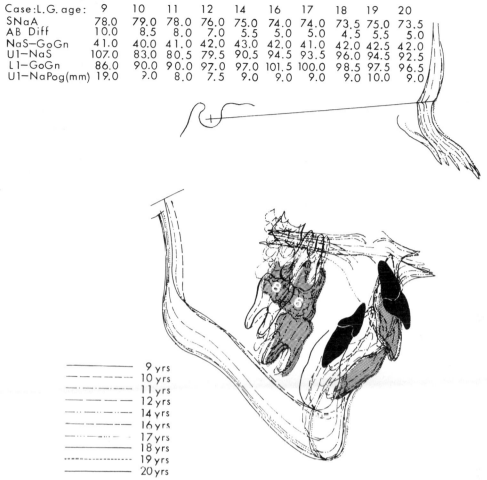

————— 9 yrs
– – – – 10 yrs
–·–·–·– 11 yrs
– – – – 12 yrs
–··–··– 14 yrs
– – – – 16 yrs
–·–··– 17 yrs
————— 18 yrs
············ 19 yrs
————— 20 yrs

Figure 11–49   Cephalometric tracings of patient in Figure 11–48. Despite extraoral force therapy continued over a protracted period, the greatest benefit was to prevent forward maxillary growth after maxillary incisors had been tipped lingually. The vertical direction of mandibular growth remained until the pubertal growth spurt between 13 and 14 years. The removal of maxillary second molars one year before removal of appliances expedited the establishment of normal buccal segment relationship, requiring less of a contribution from hoped-for horizontal mandibular growth increments.

health, i.e., with respect to orthodontic specialty service, that he understands what has to be done, when to do it, the limitations imposed, etc.

If the Class II, Division 1 malocclusion is severe enough and if it appears likely to become more pronounced through abnormal functional forces of the perioral musculature, with the lower lip cushioning to the lingual side of the maxillary incisors during function and at rest, a first assault on the problem may be made during the mixed dentition period. Growth increments are not as great or predictable at that time, and seldom does therapy eliminate the malocclusion permanently, but it can reduce the anteroposterior apical base discrepancy and eliminate the attendant muscle perversions — or at least reduce their pernicious deforming influence and functional retrusion of the mandible. Cervical extraoral force treatment apparently enlists and modifies the functional matrix. As Figure 11–52 shows, the mandible is thrust forward as the chin drops

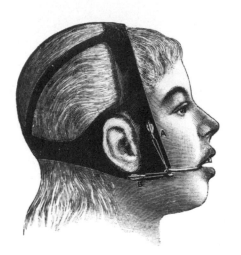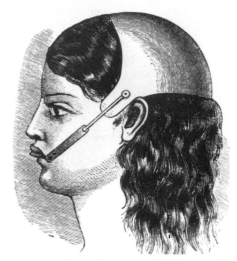

Figure 11–50   The type of "skullcap" designed and used by Kingsley for maxillary protrusions in the 1890's.

against the chest and as its reflexive activity keeps the airway open. If there is any validity to the functional matrix concept of growth dominance, then such activity can be beneficial to mandibular growth during orthodontic guidance. In most of these serious malocclusions that have been treated during the mixed dentition period, final correction when the premolars erupt is usually more likely to be successful, stable and of shorter duration than if nothing had been done at all until this time.

Despite the great reliance on mixed dentition treatment by some, great care must be exercised that the maxillary canines are not by-passed or deflected into an abnormal eruption path. Indeed, the decision to treat or not to treat may frequently be made on the position and status of the maxillary canines. A discretionary decision on therapy requires considerable diagnostic acumen and an appreciation of the possibilities and limitations of treatment and since a

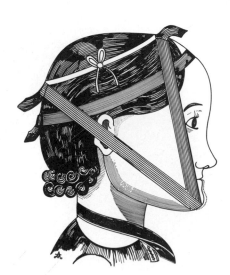

Figure 11–51   Extraoral bandage used to retard mandibular growth in Class III malocclusions in the 19th century.

second period of mechanotherapy is usually necessary, it is obvious that ortho-dontic guidance is a long-range program, covering a period of 6 to 8 years in the average patient.

Mixed dentition treatment should be kept as simple as possible. If extra-oral force alone is used, the patient may wear only two maxillary molar bands and a fixed or removable labial arch that receives and transmits the extraoral retrusive force to the dentition (Figs. 11–53, 11–54). There are a number of types of extraoral appliances (Fig. 11–55). Various types of arches may be used: some in which the extraoral arms attach directly into the integral arch wire and some which have separate inner and outer bows and double tubes (Fig. 11–56). In some cases the orthodontist deems part-time extraoral force inadequate (these appliances are usually worn only at night), and he augments the retrusive force against the maxillary arch with part-time intermaxillary elastic traction from the

(Text continued on page 585)

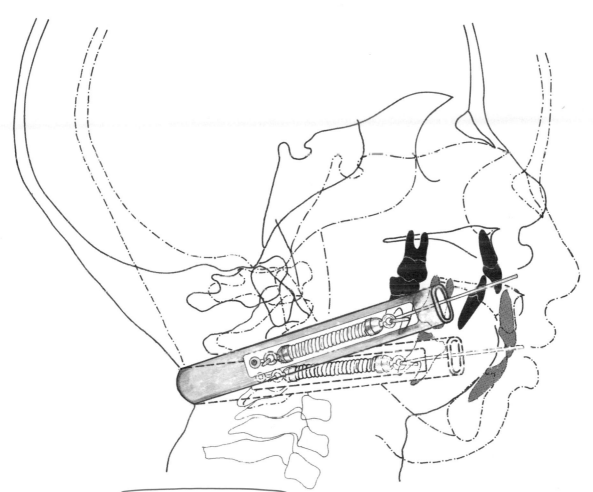

Figure 11–52 Reflexive mandibular thrust associated with cervical extraoral force therapy. Mandible moves forward to keep airway open, as a result of tissue displacement pressures. Such "activator-like" movement is probably beneficial to the total maxillomandibular basal adjustment. Retruding effect of posterior temporalis and deep masseter muscle fibers is eliminated by this neuromuscular phenomenon.

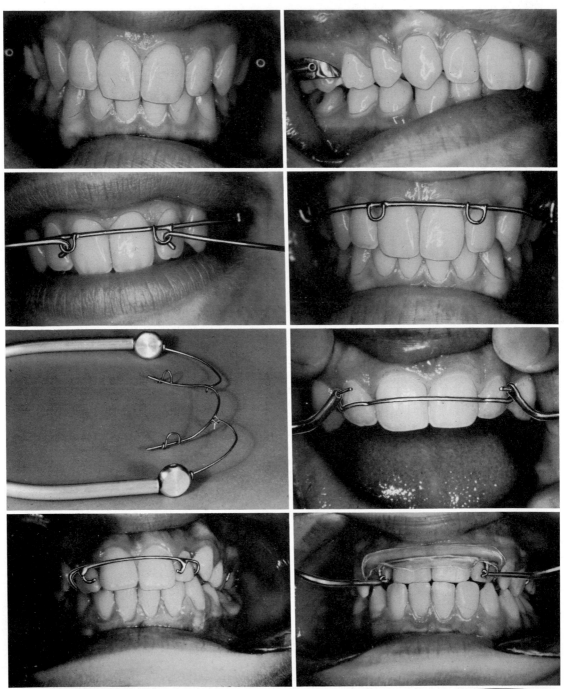

Figure 11–53   Delivery of orthopedic force to maxillary dentition through heavy labial arch. A precalibrated spring-loaded cervical tube, or a conventional cervical strap or headgear may be used to provide force. Vertical spring loops at molars serve as stops, or to retract arch (Fig. 11–54). A removable palatal appliance may be used for lesser amounts of extraoral force when retention is the main objective (third row, right, and bottom row). Acrylic added to the labial bow reinforces and stabilizes the removable appliance for reception of extraoral force arms.

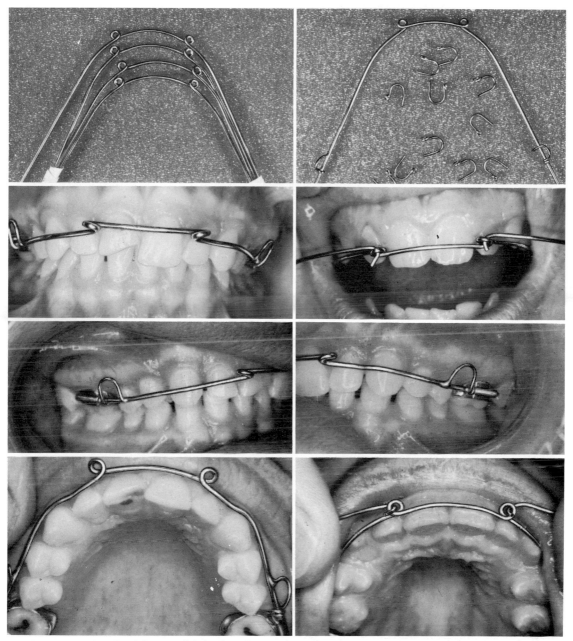

Figure 11–54 Prefabricated labial arch wires, with loops for reception of extraoral force arms, and ready-made vertical spring loops make for rapid appliance fabrication. (Courtesy Unitek Corp.)

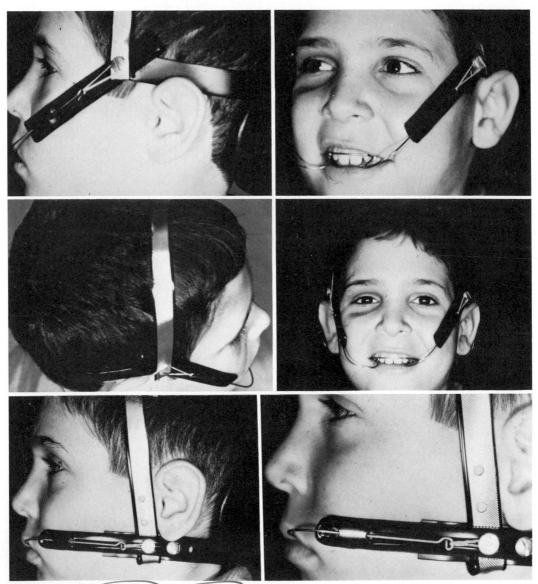

Figure 11–55. High-pull and low-pull headgear (bottom row) permits change in direction of pull. Generally, the high-pull type is used in conjunction with full appliances, and thus exerts an intrusive force on maxillary incisors for overbite control. This direction of pull is also more favorable when augmenting torque force that has been applied intrinsically.

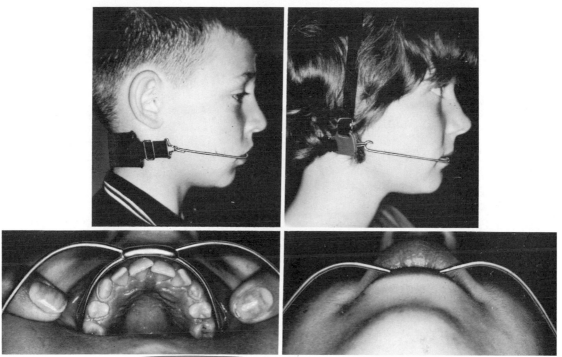

Figure 11–56. Conventional cervical strap and headcap, to serve as extraoral base for utilization of labial bow arch wire. Inner arch is stopped at molars, slightly advanced, away from maxillary incisors segment. (Courtesy W. R. Mayne.)

mandibular arch. Usually only a fixed lower lingual arch provides the mandibular anchorage.

ADJUNCTS TO EXTRAORAL FORCE. Formerly, elastic traction was the sole means of correcting Class II malocclusions. But, as noted earlier in this chapter, constant forward pull on the mandibular dental arch resulted in excessive labial tipping of the lower incisors, with permanently deleterious results. Part-time intermaxillary rubber band therapy, with good mandibular arch form and a properly made lower fixed lingual arch that is closely adapted to the cinguli of the anterior teeth, is considerably less likely to disturb the mandibular denture balance. Its value in augmenting extraoral force is immeasurable in many cases. And, of course, there are mild Class II, Division 1 problems, requiring a minimum of anteroposterior adjustment, where intermaxillary elastic traction alone may be all that is necessary.

In some first-period, mixed dentition treatment problems where maxillary incisors are relatively upright and spaces are minimal, it is wise to band these incisors and torque the apices lingually, in conjunction with extraoral therapy (Fig. 11–57). Here again, great care and considered judgment must be exercised with regard to the position of the unerupted maxillary canines. Many "high cuspids" have been ignored and by-passed by overzealous clinicians, bent on reducing the protrusion of the upper front teeth, only to find the canines blocked completely out of the arch and erupting high in the vestibular fornix. This means either moving the maxillary incisors anteriorly again to pick up the canines, or removing the maxillary first premolars. If these cases are properly selected and carefully treated, neither alternative is necessary.

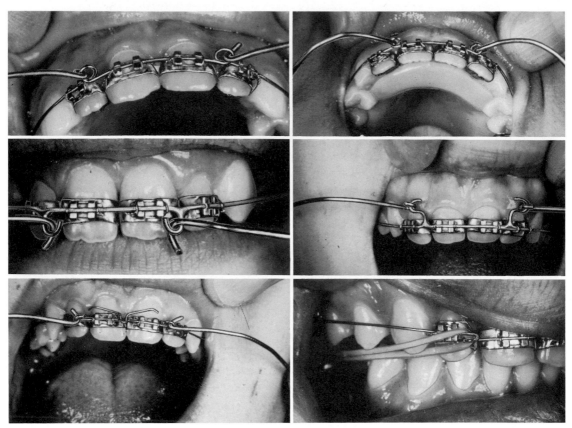

Figure 11–57   Insertion of extraoral force arms into arch wire, when anterior teeth are banded, as is the case in most Class II, Division 1 malocclusions. Loops between central and lateral incisors are horizontal in the round arches, but are usually soldered below the wire (second row, left) when a rectangular arch is used. If a torque adjustment is made, soldering the loops above the arch permits the extraoral force to enhance the torque adjustment (middle row, right). Torquing auxiliaries may be soldered on the arch wire (bottom row left). If part-time elastic traction is indicated, the horizontal loops may also be used as an elastic hook. The arch wire is stopped at the molar tube, to prevent it from moving through the tube, after spaces are closed. Bite plate may be used in conjunction with orthopedic force, preventing overclosure, stabilizing the maxillary dentition and helping to transmit the force to the maxillary base proper, thereby preventing the excessive lingual tipping of the maxillary incisors (top row, right).

THERAPY IN CONJUNCTION WITH PUBERTAL GROWTH

Class II, Division 1 therapy in the permanent dentition often requires the removal of premolar teeth whether there was a first period of treatment or not. Growth changes during the pubertal period are most beneficial, and if therapy can be timed precisely with the pubertal growth spurt, the possibility of tooth sacrifice may be reduced. The principal problem lies in predicting just when this spurt will occur for a particular individual. For girls, it is easier to predict, since puberty usually occurs between 10½ and 12 years. For boys, puberty comes later and the age spread is much greater. A range of from 12 to 17 years is probable in any appreciable sample. Even when treatment can be successfully timed with maximum growth activity, it is still not possible to project accurately the *direction* of mandibular growth. If it is primarily forward, this is fortunate, but many patterns show a primarily vertical tendency; or they will grow vertically and then change to a forward direction with no apparent reason. (See The Dynamics of Facial Growth, Chap. 2.)

TYPES OF APPLIANCES USED

With sacrifice of dental units, appliances used are much more complicated. Almost all maxillary and mandibular teeth much be banded. The arch wire delivers the desired force when ligated or pinned into the bracket. (See Chapter 10, Biophysical Principles.) Anchorage is set up, tooth irregularities eliminated, arch relationship corrected, and abnormal perioral muscular habits eliminated through the media of the appliances, in conjunction with the use of extraoral appliances which attach to the conventional intraoral orthodontic appurtenances (Fig. 11–58). Following the removal of tooth-moving appliances, retaining appliances may be placed to enhance the stability of the orthodontic result, holding the teeth passively while the tissue around them reorganizes and assumes a normal character (Fig. 11–68).

OUTLINE OF THERAPY

Using two cases as examples, the student can see how most routine Class II, Division 1 therapy is done.

EXAMPLE 1. A girl eight and a half years of age is referred by a dentist to an orthodontist. She has a severe Class II, Division 1 malocclusion, excessive overbite and overjet, spacing of the upper incisors and the strong tendency for the lower lip to cushion to the lingual aspect of the maxillary incisors. The upper arch is narrow and the lower incisors tend to be flattened and forced lingually by the abnormal muscle function. The orthodontist takes complete diagnostic records (Chap. 8), and if he finds that the roots of the maxillary incisors are sufficiently formed, he may then decide to institute a first period of treatment, using primarily an extraoral force approach (Figs. 11–53 to 11–55). The maxillary first molars are banded, and horizontal tubes are placed on the buccal side of these bands. An arch wire can either be tied in and the extraoral appliance attached to this wire during the night, or a single unit consisting of both the arch wire and an external "bow" can be used and the whole attachment inserted and hooked up to an extraoral appliance at night or when the patient is at home (Fig. 11–53).

Twelve to eighteen months of this type of treatment often reduces the severe anteroposterior discrepancy, closes the spaces and retracts the maxillary incisors out of the danger zone, and eliminates the deforming abnormal muscle habits. Sometimes, a lower fixed lingual appliance with lower maxillary first molar bands and hooks on the buccal side is used to augment the extraoral force, providing a base for the attachment of intermaxillary elastics (Fig. 11–60). Much depends on the particular problem. If the result can be accomplished without the use of intermaxillary elastics, this is usually the method of choice. Where intermaxillary traction is used, great care must be exercised that it is not overused, with a resultant sliding forward of the mandibular teeth off the base and into positions of imbalance with environmental forces.[52] More than half-time elastic traction to a mandibular lingual arch invites trouble. Even the "rounding out" of the flattened mandibular anterior segment may not be possible without tipping the lower incisors through the labial plate into positions of unstable procumbency.

In mixed dentition treatment, many orthodontists prefer to eliminate the muscle perversions first and let the molding effect of normal function reshape the dental arch area before aligning the teeth themselves in the permanent dentition phase of therapy.

EXAMPLE II. For the second example of Class II, Division 1 therapy, a girl of eleven years with a Class II, Division 1 malocclusion is selected. If the problem is not severe

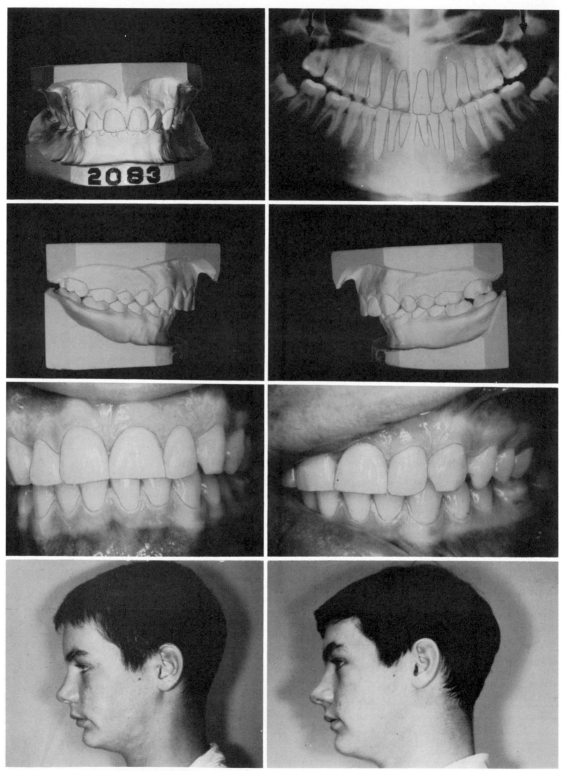

Figure 11–58   A good example of the effectiveness of orthopedic force when there are favorable growth increments and the direction is horizontal. Despite the deep bite and the upright maxillary incisors before treatment, no lingual tipping is seen, because of orthopedic levels of force, beyond tooth-moving range. Cephalometric tracing (Fig. 11–59) shows the strong maxillary base withholding effect.

Case: R. H.	Age: 13	16	17.5	19	20
SNaA	84.0	83.5	83.0	83.0	84.0
AB diff.	7.0	3.5	3.5	3.0	3.0
NaS-GoGn	26.0	23.5	23.5	24.0	21.0
U1-NaS	92.5	98.0	98.0	100.0	102.5
L1-GoGn	101.5	102.0	102.0	103.0	104.5
U1-NaPog (mm)	7.5	4.5	4.5	5.0	4.5

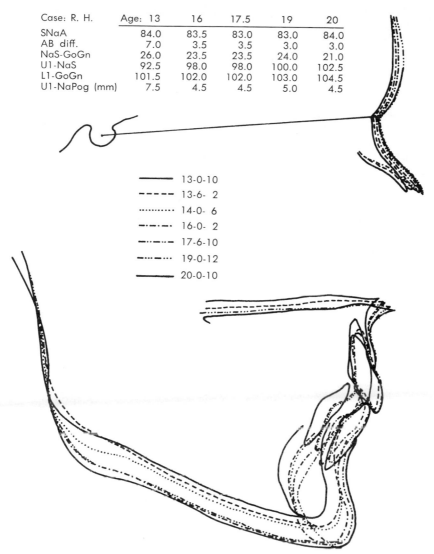

———	13-0-10
- - - - -	13-6- 2
··········	14-0- 6
-·-·-·-	16-0- 2
-··-··-	17-6-10
-···-···-	19-0-12
———	20-0-10

Figure 11–59 Serial cephalometric analysis of the effect of orthopedic force in a severe Class II, Division 1 malocclusion, when growth increments and direction are favorable and patient cooperation is excellent. Interrupted force was applied to prevent excessive lingual movement of incisors, which were already too upright at the beginning of treatment. A palatal bite plate augmented the stabilization of the maxillary dentition.

or if this has been a severe problem that has been reduced partially through a mixed dentition period of therapy, a period of mechanotherapy is instituted at the beginning of the pubertal growth spurt, if possible. With girls, this frequently coincides with eruption of the premolar and second molar teeth.

Assuming that this is the first assault on the orthodontic problem and that the treatment was timed properly to coincide with the adolescent growth contribution, the patient can expect to wear tooth-moving appliances for a year and a half to two and a half years to produce the desired result. Even if it is the second assault on an originally severe problem, it is not likely that treatment time will be appreciably shorter. Much depends on the amount and direction of growth, on whether teeth had to be removed during treatment and on the patient's cooperation. As in the mixed dentition period of treatment, the primary objective is the establishment of normal anteroposterior jaw relation-

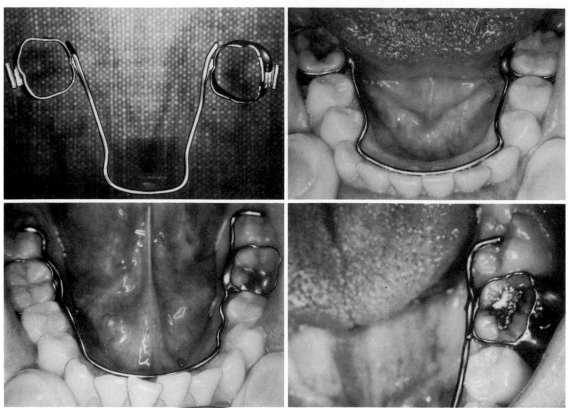

Figure 11–60   Lower fixed-removable lingual arch that is passive and adapted to the cinguli of the mandibular incisors. Buccal hooks or tubes serve to hold elastics for part-time intermaxillary traction to augment extraoral force. If maxillary second molars have been removed, then extensions to the central fossa of the mandibular second molars must be made (lower photos) to prevent over-eruption of these teeth.

ship, reflected by proper interdigitation of the teeth and normal overbite and overjet, and the elimination of abnormal perioral muscle function. Even the most competent orthodontist is not always able to accomplish this multipurpose objective. And when he does, the predominance of the morphogenetic pattern, together with post-treatment adjustment, frequently causes certain retrogressive changes.[67]

If there is an arch length deficiency or a need to retroposition the maxillary dentition appreciably more in order to establish a correct maxillomandibular relationship than can be expected from growth alone, teeth are removed, e.g., two premolars in the upper arch, two upper and two lower premolars or two upper second molars. This decision obviously requires a differential diagnosis based on definitive criteria (Figs. 11–47 to 11–49).

TREATMENT OF CLASS II, DIVISION 2 MALOCCLUSIONS

With Class II, Division 2 malocclusions muscle perversions generally are not a factor (see Chap. 5). Maxillomandibular basal discrepancy is usually less. But these favorable attributes are counterbalanced by the characteristic lingual inclination or "rabbitting in" of the maxillary central incisors, the excessive overbite and the predilection toward functional mandibular retrusion in the occlusal position (Fig. 11–61). Predominance of the morphogenetic pattern is equally strong or perhaps stronger than that in Class II, Division 1 malocclusions.

If the Class II relationship is not due to a functional retrusion and if the mandibular incisors are crowded and arch length is also a problem in the maxillary arch, the therapeutic demands are of the first magnitude. Even with the most efficient tooth-moving appliances (incorporating torque control) in the hands of the most competent orthodontist, a full resolution of the orthodontic problem is frequently not possible. With the removal of the retaining appliances, many patients exhibit a tendency toward a relapsing overbite, a return of mandibular incisor crowding and a reassertion of the original Division 2 characteristics of the maxillary incisors.[67]

TREATMENT PROCEDURES

Actual treatment procedures are usually a combination of conventional Class I and Class II mechanics.[44] Most orthodontists strive first to align the maxillary incisors, establishing the correct axial inclination of the central incisors through root torque. If a functional retrusion is present, there is usually a partial reduction of the Class II molar relationship. The balance of treatment is then carried out essentially as if this were a Class II, Division 1 malocclusion. A large percentage of the cases with arch length deficiency, however, require tooth sacrifice (Fig. 11–61). Precise control of individual teeth is essential if normal arch relationship, proper axial inclination and a correct overbite are to be established. To the clinician, growth somehow seems to be less of a factor in the success or failure of Class II, Division 2 cases than it is in Class II, Division 1 cases. Perhaps this is because anteroposterior apical base relationship is more balanced with less compensatory muscle abnormality and because the arch form of both upper and lower dental arches is more nearly normal in the original

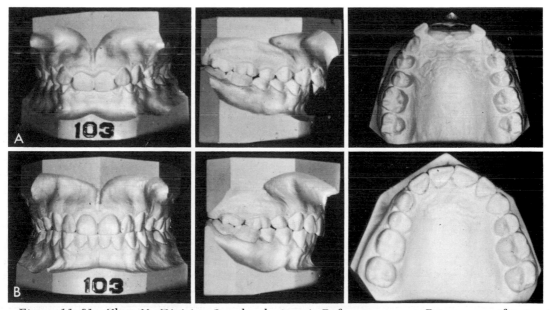

Figure 11–61 Class II, Division 2 malocclusion. A, Before treatment; B two years after treatment. Two maxillary first premolars were removed as one phase of orthodontic guidance.

malocclusion. It seems that more than in any other type of case, post-treatment retaining appliances are essential in Class II, Division 2 problems. (This will be discussed in greater detail later in this chapter.) Some overbite return is almost always to be expected.

TREATMENT OF CLASS III AND OPEN BITE MALOCCLUSIONS

Most orthodontists are very thankful that the percentage of Class III and gnathic open bite malocclusions is relatively small. As with Class II, Division 2 cases the hereditary pattern is apparent in the majority of cases, and in the remainder it is not unlikely that an endocrine malfunction is contributory.

TREATMENT PROBLEMS

The strong mandibular prognathism and a seeming maxillary retrusion often demand corrective measures beyond the scope of tooth-moving appliances. Although the orthodontist is apparently successful in the correction of Class II malocclusion by guiding the maxillary teeth and supporting structures into a more favorable relationship with the opposing mandibular teeth, he does not seem to have the same control over the mandibular teeth and supporting structures in Class III malocclusions. The teeth merely reflect an obvious basal maxillomandibular malrelationship (see Chap. 5). Attempts to inhibit mandibular growth often meet with less success with conventional *intraoral* appliances. Such success may be temporary as terminal growth and maturation increments re-establish the mandibular prognathism. This is truly an orthopedic problem. The challenge is to emulate the orthopedic surgeon, using orthopedic forces of sufficient magnitude to effect a basal change. At the very least, if the horizontal growth dominance can be converted to a more vertical vector, the maxillary growth may be able to keep pace so that correction is a possibility and the chances of success are appreciable. The author has used orthopedic force and extraoral appliances in large numbers of Class III patients in the deciduous and mixed dentition stages with beneficial results, often completely correcting an anterior cross-bite with no appliances at all inside the mouth.[55] Claims made by some clinicians who have never used headcaps that temporomandibular joint problems are created with chincap therapy are without foundation. In not a single case in the author's experience has there been temporomandibular joint dysfunction (Fig. 14–31). Similar success has been observed in anterior open bite cases, where chincap treatment has closed down the open bite. That this can happen has been amply demonstrated by the Milwaukee brace, and also has been observed in patients required to wear braces for whip lash and other injuries.[56] (See Figs. 2–84 and 6–36.)

"PSEUDO" CLASS III MALOCCLUSIONS. Occasionally an orthodontist may be lulled into a false sense of satisfaction as he corrects a "pseudo" Class III malocclusion. In such cases there is a functional protrusion as the incisors meet in an end-to-end relationship at point of initial contact and the mandible is then guided forward into an anterior cross-bite relationship by tooth guidance. The dramatic change in two to three months from Class III to normal occlusion is accomplished merely by tipping the maxillary incisors labially a little and

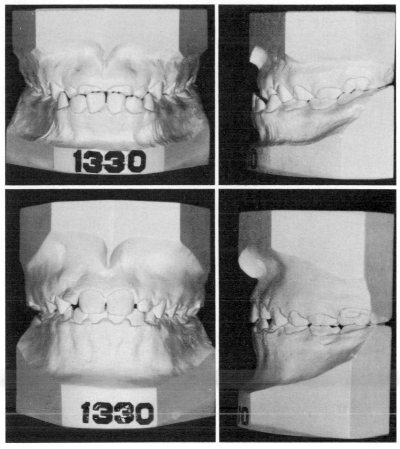

Figure 11-62   Pseudo Class III malocclusion, corrected in three months by tipping maxillary incisors labially and mandibular incisors lingually, with intermaxillary elastics as the primary motivating force.

retracting the mandibular incisors, eliminating the premature tooth contact and guidance (Fig. 11-62). True Class III malocclusions with normal paths of closure cannot be expected to respond in this manner. Even in so-called "pseudo" Class III cases, continued wearing of a chincap and extraoral force is advisable to maintain the correction on the anterior cross-bite.

In Chapter 10 of *Current Orthodontic Concepts and Techniques* by the author there is a complete discussion of orthopedic force in open bite Class II and Class III malocclusions. The philosophy is that if a normal jaw relationship can be established, then tooth movement will be less extensive, less damaging and more stable.[55] The alternative of surgical reduction is always there, after completion of growth makes orthopedic guidance no longer possible (Fig. 11-63).

TYPES OF APPLIANCES USED

As a rule, conventional appliances for Class III correction incorporate intermaxillary elastics with assistance from extraoral force against the mandible. Tooth sacrifice is often required in the mandibular arch. Full orthodontic

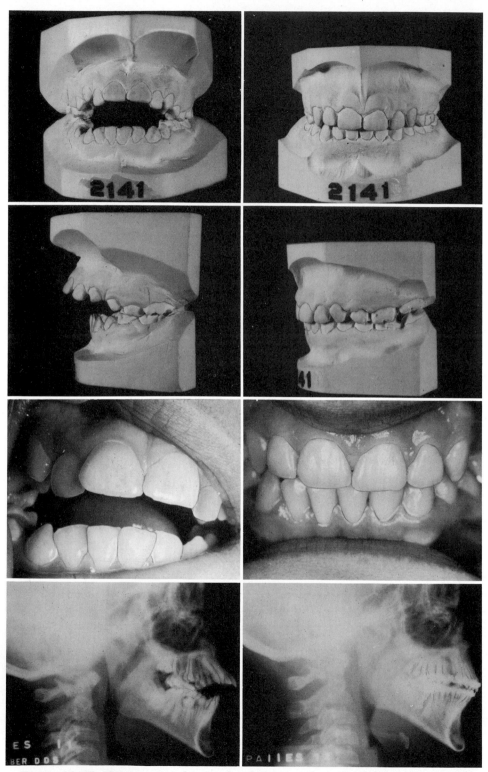

Figure 11–63   Severe open bite malocclusion. Orthopedic force with a strong vertical component was used, in conjunction with conventional fixed appliances and the removal of maxillary first premolars. Result has been stable for a number of years after retention.

appliances are usually required to gain maximum control of individual teeth. The length of treatment for Class III malocclusions is usually greater than for any other type. In the mixed dentition, an attempt is generally made to correct the anterior cross-bite if it is not too severe. This is often done in conjunction with the wearing of a chincap and the use of extraoral force (Figs. 11–64, 11–65). A second period of treatment in the permanent dentition follows, with removal of mandibular first bicuspids, or possibly a mandibular incisor in severe cases. Continued intermaxillary and extraoral force are usually necessary in an assault on the basal mandibular prognathism. Orthopedic extraoral appliances are left on well into the adolescent period to restrain latent mandibular growth.

Because of the demands of long-range guidance and orthopedic control of mandibular prognathism, referral of Class III malocclusions should be made during the early deciduous dentition or when first recognized. Some of the most successful cases are those in which orthopedic therapy has eliminated the basal malrelationships in three to six months. Subsequent tooth system adjustment and muscle function adaptation have made any further mechanotherapy unnecessary. Now that we realize our problems lie beyond the teeth and investing tissues, growth guidance in the deciduous and mixed dentitions offers one of the most exciting prospects for the future.

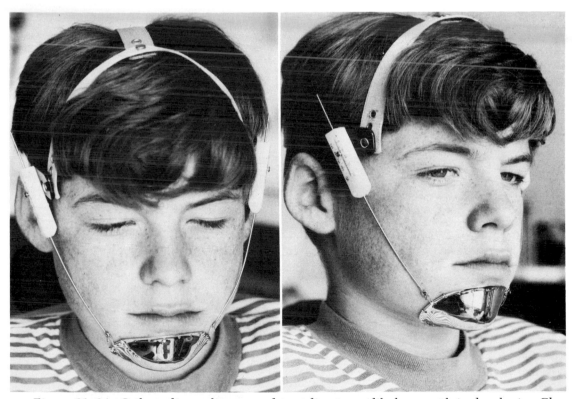

Figure 11–64 Orthopedic appliance used to redirect mandibular growth in developing Class III malocclusion. Force is delivered by spring-loaded module or by elastic straps or bands of the magnitude of 2 to 3 pounds. Orthopedic appliance must be worn for open bite and Class III malocclusions for 12 to 16 hours per day for best results, emulating the orthopedic control of long bone growth. Chin irritation is a constant concern, and chincaps should be lined with soft tissue. Plastic caps are available commercially, in various sizes, and they may be easier to use than the swaged and polished metal chincaps. (See Figures 14–30 and 14–31.)

800 - 1200 grama. 1 - 1,5 kg 12-16 h/dan

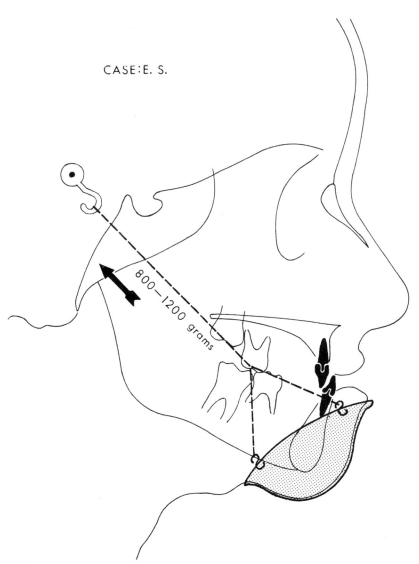

CASE:E. S.

800 – 1200 grams

Figure 11–65 Orthopedic control of Class III malocclusions. Force magnitude of 2 to 3 pounds for 12 to 16 hours per day is required to effect the desired changes. Dento-facial orthopedics is successful only in the growing child. Longrange guidance by the specialist is desirable in these problems, starting in the deciduous dentition. Usually 2 to 3 short periods of orthopedic guidance are necessary before the end of puberty.

RETENTION AFTER ORTHODONTIC THERAPY

"After malposed teeth have been moved into the desired position they must be mechanically supported until all the tissues involved in their support and maintenance in their new positions shall have become thoroughly modified, both in structure and in function, to meet the new requirements" (Angle).[4]

THE RETENTION PROBLEM

As discussed in Chapter 10, a great change takes place in the periodontal membrane and contiguous bony structures during tooth movement. The orthodontist sees this clinically in the excessive mobility of teeth under appliance pressures. It is just good sense to "splint" or stabilize the teeth, as the orthopedic surgeon does with the fracture of a long bone, until the tissue reorganizes and is able to "take over." Yet we seem to know less about this phase of orthodontic management than any other. Much of the knowledge that we have is empiric and the retention procedures are largely arbitrary, being based on a general rule and not the demands of the particular case. There is no question that the stability of the end-result is a major requisite. No matter how long teeth are splinted in abnormal positions with a retaining appliance, the tissue will not reorganize to hold them if they are not in balance with environmental forces. To obtain a balance is not always possible; this is a dynamic situation and changes with growth and development, function, restoration of carious teeth, loss of teeth and other phenomena.[58]

UNFAVORABLE RESULTS OF RETENTION

The retaining of teeth in abnormal positions with fixed or removable appliances can cause permanent damage to both teeth and investing tissues as the retainer attempts to hold them in one position, achieved by tooth-moving appliances, and functional forces drive them toward another. The "jiggling" increases the thickness of the periodontal membrane; there is alternate bone deposition and resorption and continued mobility of the teeth in question. The supporting structures sooner or later succumb to the insuperable demands of the artificially established occlusion, and there is a deterioration of the teeth of these investing tissues.[67] In all fairness, if it is not possible for the orthodontic specialist to achieve structural balance, full functional efficiency and desired esthetic harmony, how can the part-time orthodontist do it with a wrought wire removable orthodontic appliance that the patient has to wear indefinitely to prevent collapse of the expanded dentition? Again, we meet the iatrogenic malocclusion which produces pathologic conditions and endangers the longevity of the stomatognathic system as surely as the patient's original, untreated malocclusion might have done if left alone (Fig. 11–66).

POSTRETENTION ADJUSTMENT

It is normal in most cases to expect a postretention adjustment of some degree. The orthodontist can reduce this with selective grinding and careful equilibration of the occlusion, but the tendency still exists in many cases. It has been stated by some authorities that a 70 per cent correction of the original problem should be considered a success. For some problems this is undoubtedly

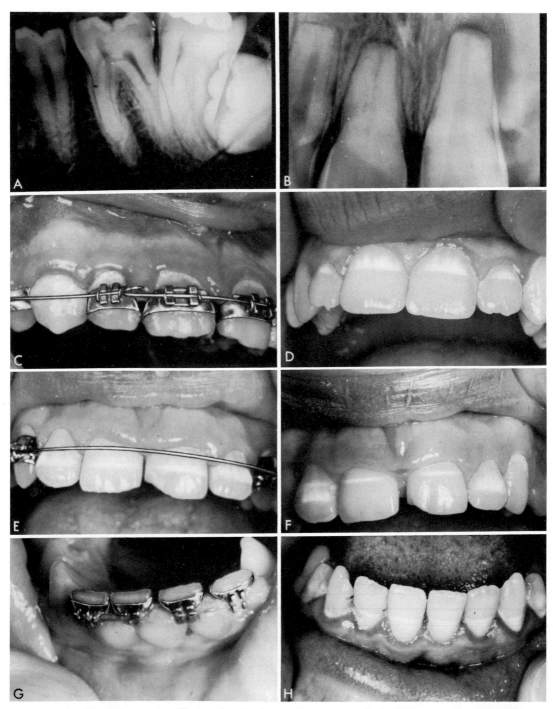

Figure 11–66 Iatrogenic effects of orthodontic therapy. A, "Ideal" therapy has tipped second molar distally, impacting third molar. B, Root resorption, a frequent consequence of torque adjustments. C, D, E, F and H, Decalcification due to poor prophylaxis and loose bands. G, Gingival hypertrophy.

true. The question still unanswered is, "Which problems?" Criteria are not yet adequate to make this determination in a significant percentage of cases that have undergone orthodontic treatment.

In the author's extensive clinical experience, even the best therapeutic results show tendencies to return to the original malocclusion to some degree. Crowding of the mandibular incisors, even with removal of four premolars during treatment, is not infrequent five to six years after all restraining appliances have been removed (Fig. 11–67). Relapsing overbite is all too frequent. The orthodontists are loath to admit this to themselves, and even more reluctant to show this to fellow dentists. Thus, the patients are really not aware of this "settling-in," "individualization," "predominance of the morphogenetic pattern" or relapse. It is imperative that all concerned—the specialist, the referring dentist and the patient—recognize the limitations imposed by the biologic medium in which we work. Obviously, such recognition should come prior to orthodontic therapy, not afterward.[67]

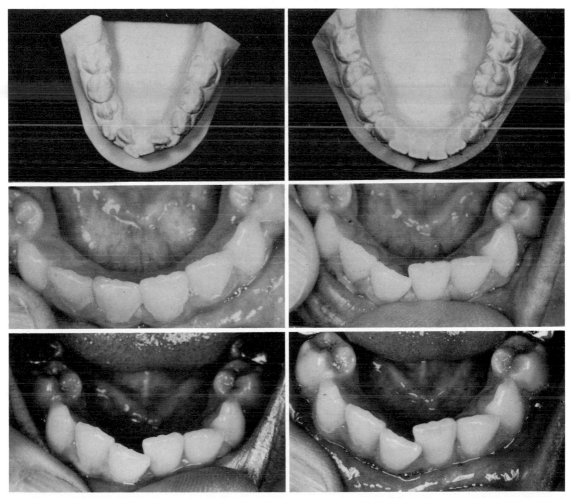

Figure 11–67 Post-treatment "adjustment," despite removal of four first premolars and excellent treatment response. Second premolars are rotating lingually, contacts with canines have been broken, and incisors show an obvious relapse. In many instances, overbite tends to return, hastening the relapse.

RESULTS REQUIRING RETENTION

With the removal of appliances and the reasonably successful establishment of a structural balance, the organization of the periodontal and alveolar structures is fairly rapid. Within 28 days the periodontal fibers realign themselves and adjust to the new tooth position. Selective osteoblastic and osteoclastic activity re-establishes the lamina dura as well as the supporting cancellous bony structure, with trabeculae aligned to the new structural and functional demands. But Reitan pointed out that the supra-alveolar and transseptal fibers change very slowly and that rotated teeth must be held for a very long time to prevent the relapse to the original malposition.[57] The method of retention depends on the type of tooth movement that has been accomplished. Some forms of tooth movement require no retention at all. For example, the correction of an incisor cross-bite is self-retaining because of the forces of occlusion. If the orthodontic result is stable, and the dentition is in balance with the muscular functional forces, there need be less dependence on retainers.

If a balance has not been established and if future growth and developmental changes, inclined plane contact and muscular force offer no hope toward achieving stability, retention must be permanent. However, as has been pointed out, permanent retention generally is an unhealthy condition. The teeth are constantly being jiggled, the periodontal membrane is thickened and a premature deterioration of the supporting structure is quite likely. The efficient tooth-moving appliances of today can achieve almost any tooth position, but retention is another matter. Particularly in Class I malocclusions with arch length problems where the environment forces have been ignored and the dental arches have been expanded to achieve normal tooth position, no form of retention is adequate to stabilize these teeth; nor can the inevitable relapse toward the original malposition be prevented after the retention appliances are finally removed. We know too little about this phase of orthodontic management. Empiricism seems to be the guiding rule; stability or instability the ruling forces. To paraphrase Hamlet, "to retain or not to retain, that is the question. Whether it is nobler in the mouth to suffer the rotations and relapsing overbite now, or to hold off indefinitely—that *is* the question!"[70]

REQUIREMENTS OF RETAINING APPLIANCES

The requirements of a good retaining appliance are:

1. It should restrain each tooth that has been moved into the desired position in directions where there are tendencies toward recurring movements.

2. It should permit the forces associated with functional activity to act freely on the retained teeth, permitting them to respond in as nearly a physiologic manner as possible.

3. It should be as self-cleansing as possible and should be reasonably easy to maintain in optimal hygienic condition.

4. It should be constructed in such a manner as to be as inconspicuous as possible, yet should be strong enough to achieve its objective over the required period of use.

To achieve these objectives most orthodontists use a removable upper retainer and a fixed or removable lower retainer. The removable type consists of an acrylic base in which are embedded molar clasps and a steel or nichrome labial bow (Fig. 11–68). The labial bow coverage is determined by what was done during active treatment (whether teeth were extracted or not, etc.). If a fixed retainer is used, it usually consists of part of the original appliance that

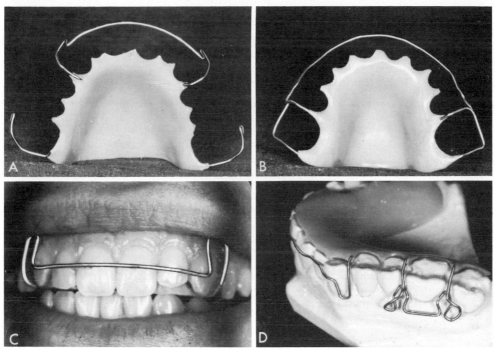

Figure 11–68   Hawley removable upper retainer. A, Type used for nonextraction case. B, For extraction case. Vertical loops are behind extraction site to help maintain second premolar-canine contact. C, Proper position for labial bow on incisors. D, Arrow type clasp that may be used instead of circumferential type for better retention. (See Chap. 16 for illustrations of different types of clasps and methods of obtaining minor tooth movement with the retaining appliance.)

has been rendered passive or a cemented upper or lower lingual arch (Fig. 11–60). Frequently the fixed retainer is only a lower canine-to-canine appliance (Fig. 11–69); where only one tooth is of concern, a band and spur type is used (Fig. 11–70).

Often a case is treated to the point where only minor corrections and settling will produce the desired final result. To achieve this goal, Kesling designed an elastoplastic positioner which is particularly valuable in extraction cases. An impression is made at the time fixed appliances are removed, teeth are cut off the model and re-set in the ultimate positions desired (using wax), and the positioner is then fabricated to this relationship (Fig. 11–71). While these appliances are usually made out of rubber or plastic (Fig. 11–72), they may also be constructed on hard or soft acrylic or vitallium.

Other elastoplastic materials are available. The elastoplastic technique is described in Chapter 16. Not only may minor tooth movements be accomplished by the elastoplastic device, but the appliance also serves as a retainer; or it may be used as a mouth guard during contact sports. With the proper equipment, this appliance is very simple to fabricate (see Figs. 16–46 to 16–47).

The chart on pages 602–603 outlines the retention objectives and the appliances that may be used.

The multiplicity of mechanisms, the profusion of philosophies and the welter of conflicting claims emanating from disciples of different orthodontic

RETENTION: OBJECTIVES AND APPLIANCES USED

OBJECTIVES	FIXED AND REMOVABLE APPLIANCES USED	COMMENT
Arch length and arch width changes	*Fixed* First molar to first molar, premolar to premolar or canine to canine cemented bands, with lingual adapted and soldered wire. *Removable* Acrylic palate or lingual horseshoe mandibular retainer, with or without clasps, rests or labial wire, as required. Elastoplastic intermaxillary positioner.	Lingual wire is better because of lessened caries susceptibility, less restraint of growth processes and better esthetics. Full palate better for maxilla because of greater stability and resistance to displacement. Rests are advisable for mandibular retainer. Lower fixed lingual appliance is superior to removable type. Properly used, can effect minor corrections and help "settling in." Bad taste and patient cooperation demands are disadvantages.
Rotation corrections	*Fixed* Cemented bands with soldered spurs to mesial or distal, labial or lingual. United bands (labial frenum cases). *Removable* Acrylic palate with labial wire. Elastoplastic intermaxillary positioner.	Often, overcorrection assists retaining appliance. Oral hygiene important to prevent decalcification around spur extensions. Excellent for maxillary anterior teeth. Most effective on incisor rotations. (See disadvantages listed above.)
Changed axial inclination	*Anterior segments* Acrylic palate and labial wire. Fixed labial or lingual retainer. *Posterior segments* Removable acrylic palate with labial wire, bands and spurs and united bands.	Properly fabricated, quite effective retainer. Seldom used for axial inclination alone. Fixed retainer for axial inclination used most in canine-first premolar region.
Mesiodistal relationship changes	*Fixed* Soldered inclined plane on maxillary lingual arch, soldered to cemented molar bands. Soldered inclined planes on molar bands.	Effective while in use, but may cause labial inclination of mandibular incisors and dual bite when removed. May be cast or wrought wire. Not used often and less effective than lingual "guide plane."

RETENTION: OBJECTIVES AND APPLIANCES USED *(Continued)*

OBJECTIVES	FIXED AND REMOVABLE APPLIANCES USED	COMMENT
	Removable Acrylic palatal retainer with clasps and inclined plane lingual to maxillary incisors.	Used most frequently, in conjunction with overbite correction and retention.
	Elastoplastic intermaxillary positioner.	Quite effective as long as it is used but, like fixed guide plane, may cause procumbency of lower incisors and dual bite.
	Part-time extraoral orthopedic force.	Of significant importance in basal malrelationships, when growth still remains.
Vertical dimension changes; overbite correction	*Fixed* Acrylic or metal splints cemented to posterior segments (diagnostic splints). Cast overlays, full mouth reconstruction.	Used primarily in temporomandibular joint disturbances prior to permanent reconstruction.
	Bite plane from fixed lingual arch, soldered to cemented first molar bands (guide plane).	Used when orthodontic procedures cannot effect a permanent change, whereas bite plane soldered to lingual arch is designed to stimulate and hold eruption of the posterior teeth — permanent correction.
	Removable Acrylic palatal appliance with clasps and horizontal or inclined plane lingual to maxillary incisors, separating occlusal surfaces of upper and lower buccal segments.	Used most frequently, both as treatment adjunct and for retention; also as diagnostic appliance in TMJ disturbances. Bite plate may be modified for other uses. Loses efficiency if not used during mastication.
Holding spaces created by therapy	*Fixed* Cemented bands with soldered bar in between. Functional and nonfunctional. Cemented band and cantilever type spur. Original tooth-moving appliance with ligated arch segment.	Most frequently used space maintainer. Contoured stainless metal crowns may also be used. Less effective over any long period of time. Satisfactory for short period of time.
	Removable Acrylic palatal or mandibular horseshoe appliance, with clasps and necessary spurs, or pontics in edentulous areas.	Particularly effective for maxillary anterior spaces. May be used as modified bite plate, or Hawley type retainer, with labial wire. Fixed retainers more desirable in mandibular arch.

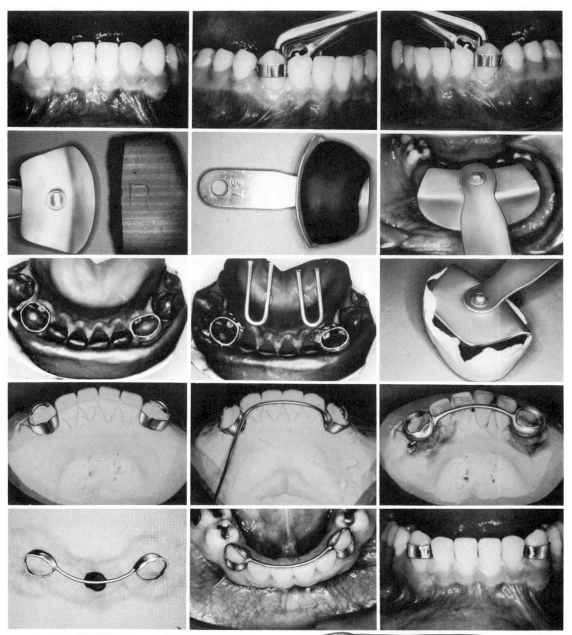

Figure 11–69 Steps in fabrication of mandibular canine-to-canine fixed retainer. (Top views) Orthodontic bands are formed on canines; then an impression is taken with the properly fitted and adapted canine bands in place on the teeth. Preformed bands may be used, if desired. The third row shows the canine bands seated in the impression, with paper clip reinforcement hooks ready to place to prevent breakage of teeth during the adapting of the lingual wire and soldering. (Fourth row) The poured up cast has been separated and the canine bands are in place, ready for adaptation of lingual wire. Wire is fitted, cut and soldered. (Bottom row) The finished canine-to-canine retainer is polished and cemented in place. (See Chap. 13 for description of molar-to-molar fixed or removable lingual arch retainers, Figs. 13–21, 13–22.) (Courtesy W. R. Mayne.)

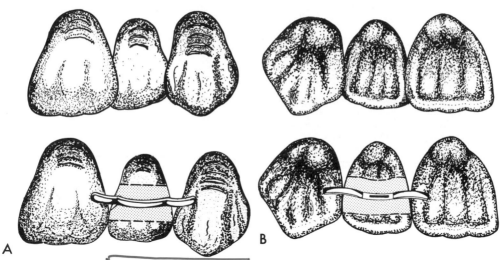

Figure 11–70 Band and spur retainer to hold incisor that was formerly malposed lingually (A) or labially (B), preventing it from returning to original position. The same type retainer is used for single rotations but with one spur placed on the lingual, the other on the labial side, to restrain any relapse tendency.

"leaders" makes a paraphrase of a well-known biblical sequence quite contemporary.

And they said to one another: Go to, let us build an institution, a tower, and let us establish ourselves and make us a name, lest we be scattered upon the face of the earth. And it came to pass that the people prospered and the structure grew, and the workers became as numerous as the grass of the field.

But behold, there rose up specialists; some there were who were *orthodontists*, some *prosthodontists*, some *exodontists*; others there were who were *endodontists*, *periodontists*, *radiodontists*, *full-mouth reconstructionists* and *pedodontists*. Then did each group cleave unto itself and forsake the others, and the work on the tower did begin to suffer.

And lo, confusion grew and multiplied throughout the land. Then arose a cry from

Figure 11–71 Teeth cut off plaster model and waxed in desired position for fabrication of rubber or plastic positioner, used as a finishing and retaining appliance (see Fig. 11–72). (Courtesy Professional Positioners, Inc.)

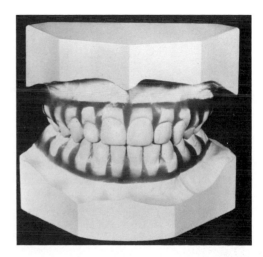

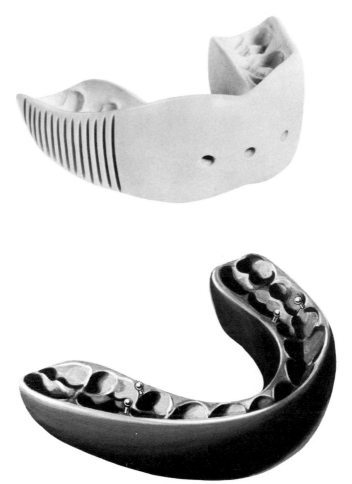

Figure 11–72 Elastoplastic positioners, fabricated from waxed setups, illustrated in previous figure. Minor tooth movements, space closure, overbite correction are all possible, if the patient wears the appliance as prescribed by the orthodontist. The bottom view shows a Position-ette® which is made of rubber. This modification is less bulky than the conventional tooth positioner. Activation and retention of the appliance are achieved by unique ball-end seating springs, which are usually located mesial to the maxillary first permanent molars. (Top view, courtesy Professional Positioners, Inc.; bottom view, T. P. Laboratories, Inc.)

the workers; let ivory be brought for the completion of the tower. And it came to pass that the specialists did multiply and did form themselves into lesser groups of specialized specialists as a multitude of leaders sprang from the ranks. For the orthodontists, each master claimed, "I am the salvation, follow me!" Splinter groups were formed, rallying around each bracket as a coat-of-arms and crying for all the world to hear, "This is the only way. Follow the master. Do not think; do not deviate; do not modify. Do not fraternize with nonbelievers. To change is to fail." Then all progress ceased for there was a strange confounding of language and they understood not one another's speech.

Then were the dentists without unity; then did their common heritage slip from them, and they became scattered like the leaves over the face of the earth.

And the tower fell into ruin and decay. Therefore is the name of it called Babel, because the speech of the people had become as diverse strange tongues and as the clashing of cymbals.[67]

REFERENCES

1. Noyes, F. B.: Personal communication.
2. Weinstein, S.: Personal communication. July 5, 1971.
3. Kingsley, N. W.: Oral Deformities: A Treatise on Oral Deformities as a Branch of Mechanical Surgery. New York, Appleton-Century Co., 1880.
4. Angle, E. H.: Treatment of Malocclusion of the Teeth. 7th ed. Philadelphia, S. S. White Mfg. Co., 1907.
5. Case, C. S.: Dental Orthopedia. Chicago, C. S. Case and Company, 1921.
6. Weinberger, B. W.: Orthodontics—An Historical Review of Its Origin and Evolution. St. Louis, C. V. Mosby Co., 1926.
7. Angle, E. H.: Evolution of orthodontia—recent developments. D. Cosmos, 54:853–867, 1912.
8. Angle, E. H.: Some new forms of orthodontic mechanism, and the reasons for their introduction. D. Cosmos, 58:969–994, 1916.
9. Angle, E. H.: Further steps in the progress of orthodontia. D. Cosmos, 55:1–13, 1913.
10. Mershon, J. V.: A practical talk on why the lingual arch is applicable to the orthodontic problem. Dent. Rec., 46:297–301, 1926.
11. Oliver, O. A., and Wood, C. R.: Lingual, labial appliances and guide plane. Internat. J. Orthodont., 18:1182–1190, 1932.
12. Grieve, G. W.: Manifest evidence of the cause of relapse in many treated cases of malocclusion. Internat. J. Orthodont., & Oral Surg., 23:23–34, 1937.
13. Tweed, C. H.: Clinical Orthodontics. 2 vols., St. Louis, C. V. Mosby Co., 1966.
14. Angle, E. H.: The latest and best in orthodontic mechanism. D. Cosmos, 70:1143–1158, 1928.
15. Fastlicht, J.: The Universal Appliance. Philadelphia, W. B. Saunders Co., 1972.
16. Johnson, J. E.: A new orthodontic mechanism: the twin wire alignment appliance. Internat. J. Orthodont., 20:946–963, 1934.
17. Brandt, Sidney: Experiences with the Begg technique. Angle Orthodont., 32:150–166, 1962.
18. Sims, M. R.: The Begg philosophy and fundamental principles. Am. J. Orthodont., 50:15–24, 1964.
19. Swain, B. F.: Begg differential light forces technique in Graber, T. M. (ed.): Current Orthodontic Concepts and Techniques. Philadelphia, W. B. Saunders Co., 1969.
20. Bowles, V. D.: Personal communication, Sept., 1971.
21. Adams, C. Philip: The Design and Construction of Removable Orthodontic Appliances. 4th ed., Bristol, England, John Wright & Sons, 1969.
22. Schwarz, A. M., and Gratzinger, M.: Removable Orthodontic Appliances. Philadelphia, W. B. Saunders Co., 1966.
23. Neumann, B.: Removable appliances in Graber, T. M. (ed.): Current Orthodontic Concepts and Techniques, Philadelphia, W. B. Saunders Co., 1969.
24. Hawley, C. A.: A removable retainer. Internat. J. Orthodont. & Oral Surg., 2:291–298, 1919.
25. Andresen, V.: Nogle Variationer af Actovatorene til Funktions-Kaebeortopedisk Behandling. Svensk Tandlak. T., 36:411–422, 1943.
26. Häupl, K.: Gewebsumbau und Zahnveränderung in der Funktions-Kieferorthopädic. Leipzig, Herman Meusser, 1938.
27. Schwarz, A. M.: Lehrgang der Gebissregelung, Vienna, Urban, 1953.
28. Harvold, E. P., and Vargervik, K.: Morphogenetic response to activator treatment. Am. J. Orthodont., 60:478–490, 1971.
29. Hotz, R.: Orthodontie in der Taglichen Praxis. Berne, Hans Huber, 1970.
30. Kraus, F.: Prevence a Naprava Vyvojovych vad Orofacialni Soustavy. Prague, Statni Zdravotnicke Nakladatelstvi, 1956.
31. Shepard, E. S.: Technique and Treatment With the Twin-wire Appliance, St. Louis, C. V. Mosby Co., 1961.
32. Miura, F., and Masuhara, E.: New direct bonding system for plastic brackets. Am. J. Orthodont., 59:350–361, 1971.
33. Thurow, R. C.: Technique and Treatment With the Edgewise Appliance. 3rd ed. St. Louis, C. V. Mosby Co., 1972.
34. Robinson, R.: A system of positive and painless tooth movement. Internat. J. Orthodont. & Oral Surg., 1:497–509, 1915.
35. Griffin, E. M.: Technique of Resilient Arch Assemblage. Newark, Alpine Press, Inc., 1930.
36. Begg, P. R.: Begg Orthodontic Theory and Technique. Philadelphia, W. B. Saunders Co., 1965.
37. Begg, P. R., and Kesling, P. C.: Begg Orthodontic Theory and Technique. Philadelphia, W. B. Saunders Co., 1971.
38. Jarabak, J. R., and Fizzell, J. B.: Technique and Treatment With the Light-Wire Appliances. St. Louis, C. V. Mosby Co., 1963.
39. Rosenstein, S. W., and Jacobson, B. N.: Class I extraction procedures and the edgewise mechanism. Am. J. Orthodont., 57:465–475, 1970.
40. Lindquist, J., and Stoner, M. M.: The edgewise appliance today in Graber, T. M. (ed.): Current Orthodontic Concepts and Techniques. Philadelphia, W. B. Saunders Co., 1969.
41. Burstone, C.: Biomechanics of the orthodontic appliance in Graber, T. M. (ed.): Current Orthodontic Concepts and Techniques. Philadelphia, W. B. Saunders Co., 1969.

42. Heydt, K. von der: Can the challenge of modern orthodontic standards be met with the Begg technique? Am. J. Orthodont., 51:321–341, 1965.
43. Fischer, Bercu: Clinical Orthodontics. Philadelphia, W. B. Saunders Co., 1957.
44. Graber, T. M.: The edgewise appliance in routine practice. Am. J. Orthodont., 46:1–23, 1960.
45. Korkhaus, G.: German methodologies in maxillary orthopedics in Kraus, B. S., and Reidel, R. A. (eds.): Vistas in Orthodontics. Philadelphia, Lea & Febiger, 1962.
46. Derichsweiler, H.: Die gaumenrahtsprengung. Forstchr. Kieferorthop., 14:234–255, 1953.
47. Wertz, R. A.: Skeletal and dental changes accompanying rapid midpalatal suture opening. Am. J. Orthodont., 58:41–46, 1970.
48. Isaacson, R. J., Wood, J. L., and Ingram, A. H.: Forces produced by rapid maxillary expansion. Angle Orthodont., 34:256–270, 1964.
49. Lundström, A.: Malocclusion of the teeth regarded as a problem in connection with the apical base. Stockholm, A. B. Fahlcrantz, 1923.
50. Hasund, A.: The use of activators in a system employing fixed appliances. Trans. Eur. Soc. Orth., 329–342, 1969.
51. Graber, T. M.: The role of upper second molar extraction in orthodontic treatment. Am. J. Orthodont., 41:354–361, 1955.
52. Graber, T. M.: Extra-oral force—facts and fallacies. Am. J. Orthodont., 41:490–505, 1955.
53. Graber, T. M.: Maxillary second molar extraction in Class II malocclusion. Am. J. Orthodont., 56:331–353, 1969.
54. Brodie, A. G., Downs, W. B., Goldstein, A., and Myer, E.: Cephalometric appraisal of orthodontic results. Angle Orthodont., 8:261–265, 1938.
55. Graber, T. M.: Dentofacial orthopedics in Graber, T. M. (ed.): Current Orthodontic Concepts and Techniques, Philadelphia, W. B. Saunders Co., 1969.
56. Logan, W. R.: Recovery of the dentofacial complex after orthopedic treatment for scoliosis. Trans. Eur. Soc. Orth. 197–208, 1968.
57. Reitan, K.: Tissue rearrangement during retention of orthodontically rotated teeth. Angle Orthodont., 29:105–113, 1959.
58. Rosenstein, S., and Jacobson, B.: Retention: an equal partner. Am. J. Orthodont., 59:323–332, 1971.
59. Williams, R. T.: The Begg Theory. Audio-visual sequence. St. Louis, American Association of Orthodontists, 1964.
60. Jacobson, B., and Rosenstein, S.: Kephalometrie: ein wichtages kieferorthopadisches werkzeug. Information Orthodont. Kieferorthop., 3:36–52, 1970.
61. Jarabak, J. R.: Principles of Light-Wire Appliances. Audio-visual sequence. St. Louis, American Association of Orthodontists, 1963.
62. Burstone, C. R.: Root Movement. Audio-visual sequence. St. Louis, American Association of Orthodontists, 1963.
63. Jarabak, J. R.: Management of Class II, Division 2 Type of Malocclusion. Audio-visual sequence. St. Louis, American Association of Orthodontists, 1965.
64. Sandusky, W. C.: The Tweed Technique. Audio-visual sequence. American Association of Orthodontics, 1965.
65. Retief, D. H., Dreyer, C. J., and Gavron, G.: The direct bonding of orthodontic attachments to teeth by means of an epoxy resin adhesive. Am. J. Orthodont., 58:21–40, 1970.
66. Newman, G. V.: Epoxy adhesives for orthodontic attachments: progress report. Am. J. Orthodont., 51:901–913, 1965.
67. Graber, T. M.: Postmortems in post-treatment adjustment. Am. J. Orthodont., 52:331–352, 1966.
68. Stoller, A. E.: The Universal Appliance. St. Louis, C. V. Mosby Co., 1971.
69. Elgoyhen, J. C., Riolo, M. L., Graber, L. W., Moyers, R. E., and McNamara, J. A.: Craniofacial growth in juvenile Macaca Mulatta. Am. J. Phys. Anthropol., May, 1972.
70. Riedel, R. A.: Retention, in Graber, T. M. (ed.): Current Orthodontic Concepts and Techniques. Philadelphia, W. B. Saunders Co., 1969.
71. Fogel, M. S., and Magill, J. M.: The Combination Technique in Orthodontic Practice. Philadelphia, J. B. Lippincott, 1972.
72. Andreasen, G. F.: Selection of the square and rectangular wires in clinical practice. Angle Orthodont., 42:81–84, 1972.
73. Sims, M. R.: Loop systems—a contemporary reassessment. Am. J. Orthodont., 61:268–270, 1972.
74. Andreasen, G. F.: Treatment approaches for adult orthodontics. Am. J. Orthodont., 62:166–175, 1972.
75. Silverman, E., Cohen, M., Gianelly, A. A., and Dietz, U. S.: A universal direct bonding system for both metal and plastic brackets. Am. J. Orthodont., 62:236–244, 1972.
76. Thompson, W. J.: Current application of Begg mechanics. Am. J. Orthodont., 62:245–271, 1972.

chapter 12

DENTAL CARE
DURING ORTHODONTIC
THERAPY

Too often a patient under orthodontic therapy assumes that routine dental care will not be necessary. Nothing could be farther from the truth. The dentist should see patients under orthdontic treatment at 4-month intervals to look for developing caries, areas of decalcification at the gingival margin that are the result of collection of food debris and poor oral hygiene, loose or deformed bands, impairment of soft tissue health or anything the orthodontist might have missed.

One of the best ways to begin a 2-year teamwork effort of patient-dentist-orthodontist is for the orthodontist to write a full report to the patient's parents and to the dentist, explaining the problems and the recommendations. Then everyone knows the problem and the potential service. If there are any questions, this is a good time to ask them.

CARIES AND DECALCIFICATION DURING THERAPY

Properly made orthodontic bands cover many caries-susceptible interproximal areas, but caries may still occur in unprotected areas. The orthodontist may overlook these lesions as he makes appliance adjustments. If food debris remains around appliances for any length of time, the telltale white lines at the periphery of each band or bracket, if attached directly to the enamel, remain as mute testimony when the appliances are removed (Fig. 12–1). These decalcification lines will persist throughout the lifetime of the individual. Particularly in the lower first molar region, where the pounding of the occlusion often breaks the cement seal and allows the cement to be washed out, areas of decalcification are fairly common on the buccal surface of the teeth. There is no need for these "scars of the operation" if the dentist-orthodontist team continues to work together during active mechanotherapy. Protection of enamel surfaces by application of topical fluoride is one example of teamwork, which results in reduction of caries and less decalcification during active orthodontic treatment.[1]

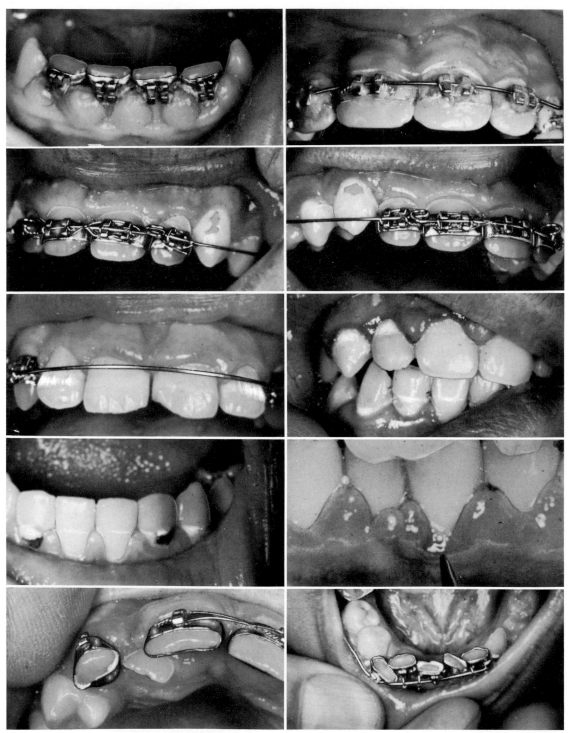

Figure 12–1   Iatrogenic damage to teeth and investing tissues. Tissue proliferation, decaying food debris, decalcification and pockets are constant companions. Poorly fitting bands and an attempt to accomplish an impossible treatment objective can only cause harm, not improvement.

LOOSE OR DEFORMED BANDS

The orthodontist should be urged to re-cement lower first molar bands at 6-month intervals. Almost the same situation exists with the upper incisor bands (Fig. 12–1). These are constantly being pounded on the lingual side by incision, so that the cement is frequently loosened and washed out. The lingual surfaces of the central incisor bands may be reinforced by an additional layer of metal or by flowing solder over the surface. Seamless or preformed bands are less likely to need this reinforcement, however. As with first molar bands, upper incisor bands should also be re-cemented periodically.[2] If appliances are made properly, and if the orthodontist checks them carefully, bands in other areas of the mouth usually do not have to be re-cemented during the average period of orthodontic management. Care must be exercised to see that the periphery of a band is not peeled away from the tooth, which can happen when the patient is chewing on a hard object. The damage to the band will result in a break in the cement seal. If the dentist sees an obvious cement bulk between the tooth and the band, an inquiry to the orthodontist is in order. A poorly fitting band, where the tooth is literally "an island in a sea of cement," invites trouble. The dentist has the continuing responsibility for the patient long after orthodontic therapy is completed. Thus, first and foremost, he must safeguard the patient. A diplomatic request for re-cementing a poorly fitting band can hardly be refused by a conscientious orthodontic specialist[3-5] (Fig. 12–1).

CARE OF SOFT TISSUE

One of the most important services that the dentist can render while his patient is under orthodontic treatment is to take proper care of the soft tissue. Most orthodontic patients are under treatment at a time when their tissue is prone to show deviations from the normal.[6] At puberty, hormonal disturbances frequently are reflected in the gingival tissue. Orthodontic appliances are foreign bodies, and while the tissue does an admirable job in most instances — adjusting to the irritant by forming a keratinized layer wherever an appliance impinges on the tissue — in many instances the irritation of the appliances produces inflammation, redness, swelling and pain. If these irritations are allowed to go unchecked, a permanent fibrous gingival reaction can be a sequela of orthodontic therapy (Figs. 12–1, 12–8).[10, 12]

NECESSITY FOR PROPER ORAL HYGIENE. Proper oral hygiene during orthodontic treatment cannot be overemphasized. Children naturally shirk their brushing duties, even without appliances, and it thus requires the combined efforts of orthodontist, dentist, hygienist and parent to establish a proper routine. If this is not done, decalcification, caries, more frequent loose bands and soft tissue damage are likely to occur. This is only one reason why the dentist should see his patients under orthodontic treatment at 4-month intervals, or more frequently. Periodic periapical radiographic examination should be made, even with the bands in place. Tooth contours can still be seen beneath areas covered by bands, and any suspicious areas on the radiographs justify asking the orthodontist to remove the band for a further check. Root resorption may also be intercepted before it becomes excessive (Fig. 12–2). A panoramic survey also will help both the dentist and the orthodontist to see the tissue response — favorable and unfavorable. Too often the dentist says, "I can't see anything with the bands on — no use taking x-rays." This is not true; there is much that can and should be seen.

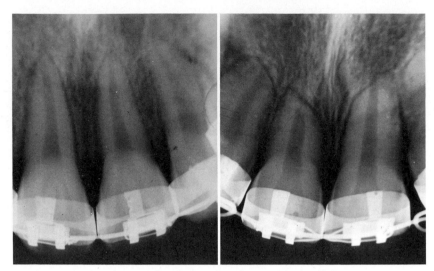

Figure 12–2   Two periapical radiographs of same patient, taken six months apart. In the picture on the left (at the beginning of treatment and before lingual root torquing action) the integrity of the roots is complete. In the picture on the right, six months later, considerable resorption has occurred. Routine periapical radiographs during orthodontic treatment are a "must" to prevent iatrogenic damage.

Where tissue has been irritated by the orthodontic appliances and where a planned program of oral hygiene has not been able to cope with the problem, the dentist must employ all possible measures to control the inflammation. Careful scaling, removal of debris from pockets, and sometimes actual removal of fibrous proliferation by surgery or electrocautery are necessary. Cases of suspected vitamin deficiency, though rare, should be noted and supplemental dietary aids should be recommended to the patient. Dilantin medication greatly enhances gingival hyperplasia. It may be necessary to ask the physician for substitute medication in severe cases where the tissue actually covers the bands.[7] Gingival care may be indicated at monthly intervals, supplemented by the patient's efforts at home.[11, 13]

METHODS OF HOME CARE.   It is difficult to keep the gingival tissue pink and healthy around orthodontic appliances. A well-planned "home-care" program is most important throughout the period of orthodontic treatment. Even the simplest orthodontic appliances become excellent foci for the build-up of food and debris. Areas around appliances are difficult to clean and hence provide ideal spawning grounds for dental plaque. It is no wonder that too often the gingival tissue proximal to orthodontic appurtenances is swollen, soft, hyperemic, and so forth.

The problems are evident, and their solutions, theoretically simple. The name of the game is dental plaque removal. Any way that the patient can remove debris and plaque from his teeth, without injury to the delicate appliances and soft tissues, is allowed. The following method, however, has proved to be most effective.[8] The patient is given a soft, multitufted tooth brush (Fig. 12–3). He is then instructed to start with his upper teeth, placing the bristles at about a 45 degree angle to the tooth, i.e., pointing toward the gums. The brush should be held so that it covers the wires and "the gum where it meets the tooth." With small circular motions the brush is rotated and vibrated so that debris is removed from the appliances and the tissues. It must be emphasized to the patient that he cover the "gum line" with his brushing, for it is there that most patients leave debris, with decalcification as the result. The patient is then instructed to brush the buccal and labial surfaces of the lower teeth in a similar manner. The lingual aspects of the teeth are brushed likewise. In the lingual anterior regions the handle is held in a vertical position relative to the arch. This position allows the patient better access to the lingual surfaces of all his anterior teeth and minimizes "missed" areas. The occlusal surfaces are brushed last. The patient is told to brush systematically, i.e., start at one side of his mouth and continue around the arch. The same "system" should be followed at each brushing session so that all areas in the mouth are covered (Fig. 12–4).

The patient should use a mirror to check the results of his efforts at each brushing. A disclosing solution or tablet is to be recommended for patients who cannot seem to clean the critical areas. Commercial kits are available which include the soft, multitufted brush, a dentifrice and disclosing tablets.[9] Either the orthodontist or the attending dentist should see that the patient has a kit – and uses it. A new development, a Plaque-lite, may also be used.

In some cases, where the patient appears to be unable to attain an adequate level of oral hygiene, special home care techniques may be in order. For various reasons, some children do not possess the motor skills necessary to use a manual toothbrush properly. In this case, an electric toothbrush unit, with soft, multi-tufted heads may be recommended. The patient should be instructed in its use so that he will cleanse all areas, especially the important free gingival margin region. Another, but less effective prophylactic device directs a jet stream of water (or a mixture of water and mouthwash) at the teeth and investing tissues (Fig. 12–5). This unit has the advantage of dislodging debris from beneath and around the appliances with little chance for appliance damage. A note of caution is in order, since high water pressure may force debris into tissue pockets, contributing to rather than alleviating the hygiene problem.

Massage has been recommended by some authorities as a means of increasing circulation in the soft tissues, thereby maintaining a better state of gingival health. Some orthodontists have found that vigorous digital gum massage by the patient for a period of five minutes in the morning and evening controls soft tissue proliferation (Fig. 12–6). A soft rubber interdental stimulator may

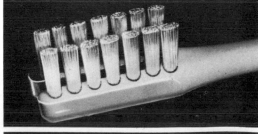
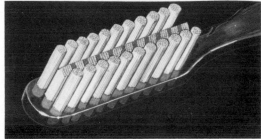

Figure 12–3 Specially designed toothbrush for patients wearing orthodontic appliances. Conventional three-row brushes may be modified in this manner by shortening the middle row of fibers. (Courtesy Unitek Corporation.)

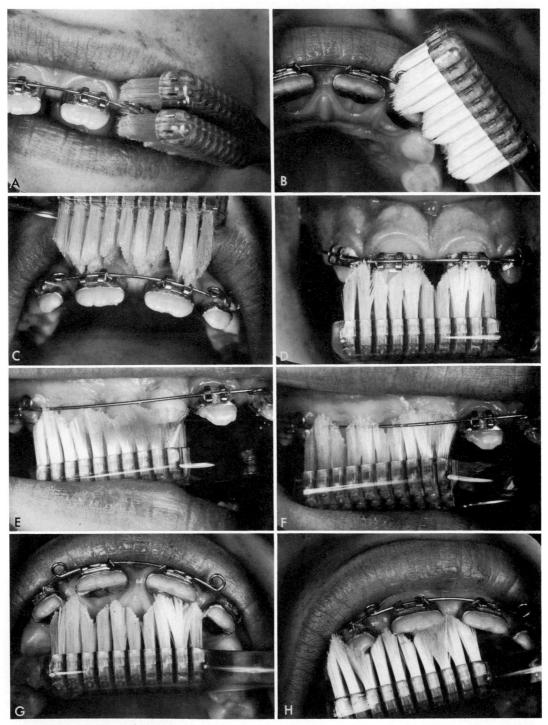

Figure 12–4 One of various possible positions for brush placement for oral prophylaxis following each meal. Middle row may be cut or special brush obtained to allow brush to straddle arch wire as the patient moves the brush along the arch wire (A and B). One row of bristles may be inserted under the arch wire from above (C) and below (D) and the brush rotated and vibrated. In the buccal segments, one row engages the occlusal surfaces while the other row slides between the arch and the teeth and bands (E and F). For the lingual surfaces, the long axis of the brush should parallel the occlusal plane as the brush is moved in a circular fashion, working the bristles into the proximal areas (G and H). Better access for anterior lingual surfaces may be obtained by holding the brush perpendicular to the arch plane.

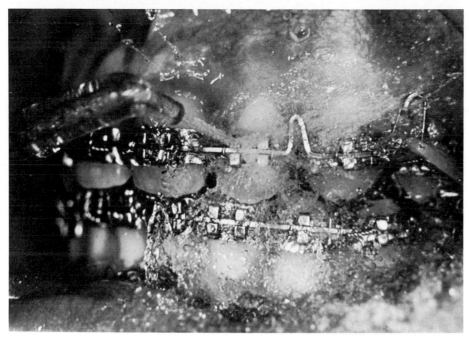

Figure 12-5   Water-Pik for oral prophylaxis. Jet stream of water or water mixed with mouthwash dislodges debris around appliances, without disturbing delicate appurtenances or interfering with the adjustments placed in the arch wire. Tissue tone may also be improved by the massaging effect of the jet stream. (Courtesy Aqua-tec Corp.)

Figure 12-6   Rubbing the index finger back and forth along the gingival margin as a massage may be often beneficial for orthodontic patients. Dipping the finger first in an astringent mouthwash may help to add a "fresh" feeling to the tissue.

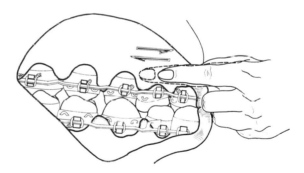

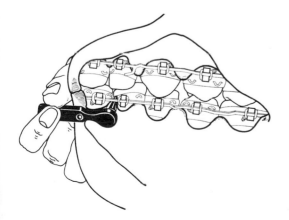

Figure 12-7 With proliferation of the interdental papillae during orthodontic treatment, routine use of a stimulator helps to increase circulation and prevent formation of pendulous fibrous areas.

also be helpful for massaging and cleaning the interproximal areas (Fig. 12–7). Care must be taken not to disturb the orthodontic appliance with it.

It must be stressed again that an adequate program of oral hygiene, to be followed by the patient while at home, is a team effort of the orthodontist, dentist, hygienist and parent. A home care program, with a strong tooth-brushing regimen is of prime importance.[11]

When an orthodontist places tooth-moving appliances he should instruct his patient what to do and what not to do, how to brush the teeth and gingival tissue and what foods to avoid. Much of this information can be placed on the back of his appointment card as a reminder to the patient at each visit. A number of patient education pamphlets are now available, both from the American Dental Association and from commercial sources, which tell the patient the "do's" and "don'ts" during orthodontic treatment. These should be given to the patient by the orthodontist when he starts active treatment. In addition,

---

Please Read—   THE PATIENT'S RESPONSIBILITY

Co-operation on YOUR part is as important as the professional services.

For the best results you must carefully follow instructions and keep your appointments. See your dentist every 4 months.

The teeth should be brushed after every meal. Avoid eating sweets between meals unless the teeth can be cleaned immediately thereafter.

AVOID chewing ice, hard or sticky candy, gum, popcorn, playing with or dislodging appliances.

AVOID scuffling or rough play where you are likely to receive a blow in the face or to catch the appliances upon the clothing thereby dislodging or breaking them.

Please notify the office IMMEDIATELY if the appliances are loose, lost or broken. School-time appointments are usually necessary.

A charge will be made to cover the cost of replacing lost or broken appliances. SO BE CAREFUL.

---

*Dear*_____

I am sending this memorandum to you because I have not been successful in impressing _____ *with the importance of keeping the teeth and orthodontic appliances properly brushed and clean. This is of vital importance. The alternative is dental decay or, at the very least, white decalcified areas around the bands that will remain for the entire life of the teeth. It apparently is necessary that you supervise the brushing and home care. Otherwise, orthodontic treatment must be discontinued.*

Sincerely,

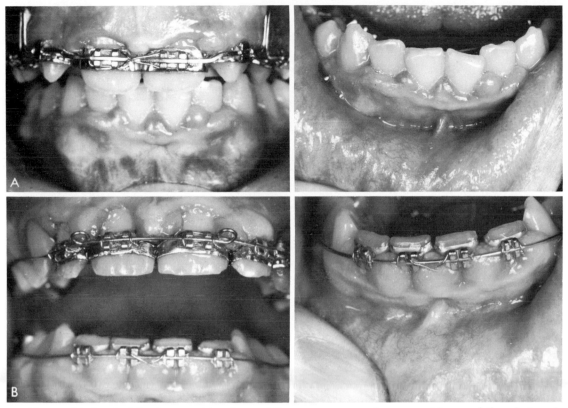

Figure 12-8 A, Gingival proliferation of the type commonly seen with a multibanded technique and inadequate home care; note the proliferation in the lower arch, although no appliances have been worn on these teeth. B, Advanced proliferation is tending to become fibrous. Gingivectomy will be likely after removal of appliances, but a good oral hygiene program can control the proliferation somewhat during orthodontic care.

slide-tape and film-strip record sequences are now used in many offices to provide patient education and to reduce the unfavorable sequelae.

If he is not successful in teaching the proper oral hygiene routine to the young patient, he may have to send reminders to parents such as the cards at the bottom of page 616, used in one form or another by some orthodontists.

DANGERS TO APPLIANCE INTEGRITY

The dentist should do all he can to assist in keeping the appliances intact and working properly, and should counsel the patient on diet and proper oral hygiene techniques. Orthodontic appliances are made out of strong materials, highly polished to reduce surface tension, and if they are properly placed they should withstand the normal functional forces with a minimum of breakage. However, with some types of malocclusions abnormal functional forces exist that make it almost impossible to maintain the appliance intact.

For example, teeth that are locked in cross-bite are difficult to band. When these bands are constantly pounded by the occlusion, either the cement seal is broken and the band loosened or the bracket or attachment is bent or broken.

In problems of deep overbite, such as Class II, Division 2 malocclusions, there is often a shearing stress on the band attachments; either the bands are broken or the attachments are injured. Frequently the attachment and labial portion of the band are pulled away from the tooth, providing an ideal trap for debris, even though the band may still seem tight. The use of a bite plate or removable bite block reduces this breakage, but the danger always exists. While orthodontic appliances can withstand the impact of a normal bolus of food, they are no match for a bout with taffy apples or a mouthful of caramels. Despite strong admonitions to the contrary, these items are often found on the menu of a youngster wearing orthodontic appliances. Another constant danger to the integrity of the appliance is the tendency for the child to constantly finger it. The net result is metal fatigue and a broken appliance or, at the very least, a bent arch wire. Such accidents change the intensity and direction of force that is placed to do a particular job. This is particularly true of light-wire, multilooped appliances that distort easily and then release their stored force in another direction— usually the wrong one. Obviously, considerable damage can be done if this situation is left unattended.[2] It is highly desirable that, in the event of accident, the orthodontic patient call his orthodontist as soon as possible for an emergency appointment. Since it is not always possible to reach the orthodontist, the general dentist should not hesitate to step in. It is recommended that he familiarize himself with some of the problems that may arise and the simple steps to be taken to help his patient.

EMERGENCY ORTHODONTIC APPOINTMENTS

LOOSE BANDS

REMOVAL.   All loose bands should be carefully removed. If allowed to remain, the collection of food debris beneath the band may well cause permanent damage to the tooth, leaving the telltale decalcified white surface to disfigure it (Fig. 12–1). Bands are held on the arch wire either by lock pins holding the arch in a slot (ribbon arch bracket for light-wire techniques) where the pin may be clipped and removed to pull off the loose band; by metal caps, which can be slid off the band attachment allowing the band to be removed; or by steel ligature wire that is wrapped over the arch wire and under the band attachment. This can be either unwound or clipped with a ligature cutter if the dentist has one (Fig. 12–9). A crown and collar shears will often serve as a substitute.

MODIFICATIONS OF BANDS.   After the loose band has been removed, the tooth should be pumiced and all debris removed. Since a band that has worked loose often needs modification and perhaps the insertion of a thickness of band material on the lingual side at the seam to restore a snug fit before re-cementation, it is usually better to have the orthodontist perform this step. There is the additional demand of placing the band exactly where it should be on the tooth so that the bracket or tube is in optimal position for proper tooth control. This is of prime importance to the orthodontist and should be his responsibility. Few patients or parents realize that the average dentist has not had training or experience in orthodontics, and they will frequently demand services beyond the scope of routine practice. There should be no hesitancy on the dentist's part to explain his reluctance to make an adjustment in existing appliances or

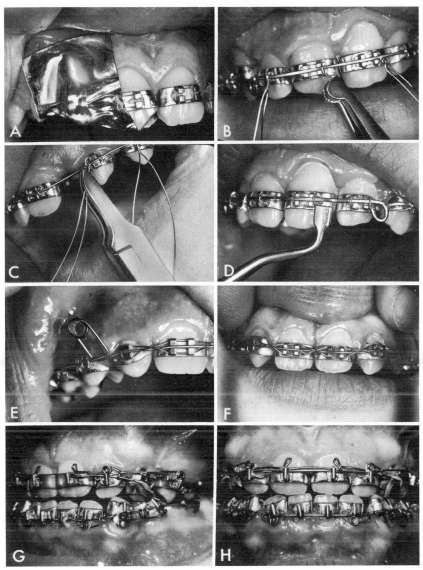

Figure 12-9 A, Aluminum foil adapted over orthodontic band that has just been cemented. A harder, uncontaminated cement set is the result, with no soggy cotton rolls. B, The twisting of a steel ligature, tying in the arch to the bracket. How or office pliers may be used. C, Ligature "pigtails" are clipped with a ligature cutter to a length of about one quarter inch. A crown and collar shears can be used if a ligature cutter is not available. D, Pigtails should be tucked under the arch wire with a flat amalgam plugger. E, Vertical loops frequently are displaced and either bury themselves in the mucosa of the cheek or the gingivae. They may be bent away with office pliers and wax put on them until an appointment is made with the orthodontist. F, Figure-of-eight ligatures are frequently used to close spaces and consolidate segments. Brushing and mastication loosen them, as in illustration. They may be pulled tight by twisting the pigtail on the end a couple of turns, preventing them from being dislodged completely from the brackets. G and H, The beginning of the third stage of the Begg technique, in which a modified and inverted ribbon arch bracket is used. Arch is "pinned" in and these pins may need tucking under. Uprighting springs and "piggy-back" torquing mechanisms can become dislodged or distorted. Cover with wax and refer immediately to the orthodontist.

to modify or repair them "to save a visit." Better patient-dentist-orthodontist relations will result.

REPLACEMENT OF BANDS.   There are times when a band that fits well and requires no modification comes loose and must be re-cemented. In this case, the band may be washed with soap and water, sterilized in alcohol and dried. The tooth is then isolated with cotton rolls and the band cemented after it has been filled with crown and bridge cement. The cementation is quite similar to that of a multisurface inlay. After the band has been forced to place, with the ball of the index finger serving as a plunger to force excess cement past the gingival margin of the band and driven to fit in its proper position on the tooth, using a round amalgam plugger, a piece of tin or aluminum foil should be adapted over the tooth to allow the cement to set (Fig. 12–9). This step prevents contamination with saliva and ensures a harder set, with the heat contained longer instead of dissipated. Excess cement may be removed with a universal type scaler, moving the point *parallel* with the gingival and incisal margins of the band. (See Chap. 17 for a more complete discussion of band fitting and cementation.)

Sometimes a patient will come in complaining of a soreness in a particular area, not knowing that the band is loose because it is tied to the arch. The band moves up and down during function, lacerating the periodontal attachment, causing considerable soft tissue irritation. Lower premolar bands are particularly susceptible. Medication may be applied after the band is removed — preferably a combination of a topical anesthetic and an oxidizing agent. Since the "bobbing band" may have cut the gingival attachment and created an area susceptible to infection, it is better not to re-cement the band immediately when obvious irritation is present. Saline rinses for a couple of days will permit recovery and restoration of the integrity of the investing gingival mucosa.

DISPLACED OR BROKEN ARCH WIRES AND ATTACHMENTS

Sometimes a choice morsel of a "forbidden food" has dislodged the arch wire from the buccal tube on the molar, and the patient comes in with the end of the wire sticking in the cheek. Any wire that has been dislodged can usually be replaced in the buccal tube by temporarily deforming the wire and then straightening it with office pliers after the end has been inserted back in the tube on the molar. The arch wire may have worked around to the opposite side and be sticking out the distal end of the molar tube. All too frequently the patient, parent or dentist merely clips off the offending end, which results in considerable time lost in the construction of a new arch wire. Since the arch wires are literally power storehouses, clipping an arch wire may allow unaccounted forces to cause quite considerable improper tooth movement and tissue damage if the patient is not seen immediately to remove the active fragment and have it replaced with a full and properly adjusted arch wire.

Occasionally there is irritation of the cheek at the distal end of the arch wire. Since the buccinator mechanism or muscular band tends to turn medially just distal to the last tooth, the mucous membrane of the cheek is particularly susceptible to any sharp object at this point. Care must be exercised to see that the end of the arch wire is turned in sharply toward the gingival tissue, or at least rounded off so that it poses no threat. On an emergency appointment, usually all that needs to be done is to make sure that the arch wire is indeed turned in sufficiently (distal to the buccal tube on the molar) and to prescribe hot saline rinses.

The cheek may also be irritated by a loop or spur on the arch wire (Fig. 12–9). The cheek tends to proliferate at the point of irritation and invaginate into loops. If there is an infection, actual swelling of the cheek may be seen, and the cervical lymph nodes can become enlarged and tender. The parotid papilla (which marks the opening of the duct of the parotid gland) is particularly sensitive to appliance irritation, and every attempt should be made to round all surfaces in contact with it. Most commonly it is the end of the maxillary arch wire that causes irritation here.

A large percentage of orthodontic appliances now being used employ brackets that are tied to the arch wire by steel ligature. These steel ligature ties are made in such a manner that a twisted "pigtail" is left to be tucked under the arch wire next to the band (Fig. 12–9). This pigtail may be dislodged by mastication, may not have been tucked in sufficiently or may be moved by digital manipulation. Most emergency appointments involve nothing more than tucking the pigtails back under the arch wire to stop irritation of the gingivae or mucous membrane of the lips and cheek. The complaint may be caused by the end of a coil spring (Fig. 12–10). Where there appears to be a sharp edge on an orthodontic appliance and it cannot be smoothed down with a pumice impregnated rubber disk, sugarless chewing gum can be used in an emergency. The patient is advised to chew this until it is soft and then to adapt the gum over

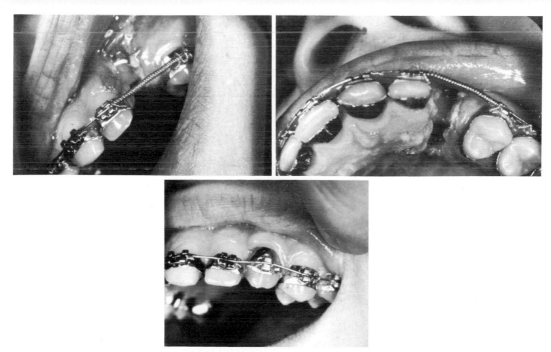

Figure 12–10 Orthodontic appliance being used to create space for an impacted canine that has just been uncovered. Note the ligature wire "pigtails" at each bracket. These may be dislodged by mastication and should be tucked back under the arch wire and against the band. The coil spring may also rotate and irritate the cheek. The end is rotated back lingually. If the lingual surface of a band irritates the tongue, it is smoothed down with a small mounted stone and rotated from the band toward the tooth. Coil spring is removed as soon as space is created and canine brought down into position (lower view).

the offending part of the appliance. Soft utility wax or baseplate wax can also be used for this purpose.

When a patient comes into the office with part of his arch wire already broken, it is wise to remove the remaining portion, if possible. This means undoing the attachment between the arch wire and the individual brackets or eyelets on each band by slipping off the caps, in a twin-arch appliance, removing the lock pin, in a Begg appliance, or clipping the ligature tie, in appliances like the edgewise, twin-channel tie, universal, multiphase, differential forces and similar types. (See Chap. 11.) If it is not possible to detach the arch wire, then the remaining sharp edge should be bent toward the tooth to prevent further irritation of the mucous membrane. Wax or sugarless gum may be used to help in this instance, too. It should be made quite clear to the patient that he must still see his orthodontist *at the earliest opportunity.*

With light-wire techniques, "piggy-back" or accessory appurtenances are often used in addition to the regular arch wire. These may be torquing auxiliaries, root uprighting or paralleling springs, or special space-closing adjuncts. If these come loose, they may usually be removed by freeing the ends or covering them with wax until the patient can see the orthodontist. Don't cut them off. (See Chap. 11.)

REMOVABLE APPLIANCES

ABRASION. Occasionally an abrasion may develop under a removable appliance that is being used either in conjunction with fixed appliances or by itself to effect changes or retain a result accomplished previously by fixed orthodontic appliances. Most commonly this occurs on the palatal-incisal periphery of the upper appliance and on the lingual periphery of the lower removable appliance. Such complaints may be handled much like those from a new denture patient. Often nothing more than spot polishing is necessary. A vulcanite type bur may be used to reduce the appliance at the point of soreness. Then the periphery should be polished with pumice and a felt cone or rag wheel (Fig. 12–11). It is often wise to apply tincture of benzoin, or a mixture of a topical anesthetic and medication to the irritated area and to advise saline rinses until the irritations clear up.

RETAINER REPAIR

BENT OR BROKEN ATTACHED WIRES. On removable retaining appliances, the attached wires are frequently bent out of shape by "pocket wear," and loops or clasps will impinge on the gingival tissue. Wire appurtenances should

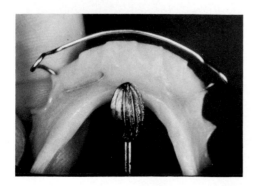

Figure 12–11 The lingual periphery of a lower removable appliance most frequently irritates the mucosa due to overextension. This may be reduced with a vulcanite bur and then polished.

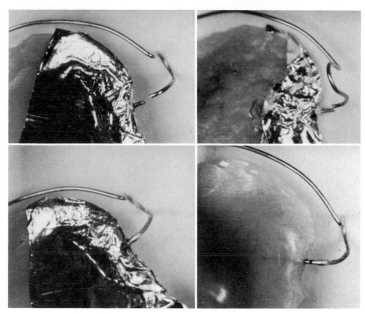

Figure 12–12 Broken labial wire being repaired for upper removable retainer. Acrylic has been cut back and covered with aluminum foil, with only the broken end protruding (top). Immediately after soldering, foil is still in place, protecting acrylic (lower left). After removing foil (lower right), acrylic should be polished to prevent irritation. This is an excellent place to use electric soldering

be checked carefully to make sure nothing is broken and then adjusted so that they lie in proximity to the tissue but not actually in contact with the mucous membrane. These adjustments can usually be done with contouring pliers, clasp-forming pliers or No. 139 wire-bending pliers.

BROKEN LABIAL BOWS. Frequently the labial bow of the removable appliance is broken. Most often this is at the junction of the acrylic and wire. Temporary repair may be done fairly easily without burning the acrylic, in the following manner (Fig. 12–12):

1. Cut away about one-eighth inch of acrylic, exposing the end of the labial bow wire embedded in the plastic.

2. Adapt two thicknesses of aluminum foil over the plastic, leaving only the free end of the broken wire projecting.

3. Apply flux to the free end of the wire projecting from the acrylic and heat carefully with a fine needle-point flame on the blowpipe until silver solder will flow on the tip. The foil reflects the heat away from the plastic and protects it from burning.

4. Flux the unattached end of the labial bow, hold it in the flame and "tip" it with silver solder. Reflux both the free and attached ends of the bow.

5. Hold the solder-tipped ends in close approximation directly over the needle-point flame until the solder liquefies and joins to form one mass. Withdraw carefully but immediately. Polish rough edges if any remain on the acrylic after removing the aluminum foil.

6. If an electric soldering machine or attachment is available for the welder, tack-weld a piece of band material to each broken labial wire end, holding wire ends in apposition. Apply flux-solder paste and place electric soldering electrodes on band material "splint" on either side of break in wire. After solder flows, cut off band material and polish.

EXTRACTION DURING ORTHODONTIC THERAPY

The importance of extraction of teeth as a frequent requirement in Class I orthodontic treatment is discussed in Chapter 11. Attention has also been called in the same chapter to the role of extraction in Class II and Class III orthodontic management. For the sake of a better understanding between patient, dentist and orthodontist, a short discussion is indicated in this section.

Since there is still considerable controversy in the orthodontic specialty itself concerning extraction as a treatment adjunct, it is understandable why both patients and dentists are confused by requests for removal of teeth by the orthodontist. Yet, if all concerned employ the same perspective and think ahead about the role of the third molars, about the high percentage of relapses that occur in treatment of Class I malocclusions where no teeth have been removed and about the investment in time and money by both the patient and orthodontist, the "four teeth now instead of four teeth later" argument should make sense in most instances.

PREMOLAR REMOVAL

In a great number of cases, removal of first premolars during the course of orthodontic treatment allows the normal eruption of third molars at a later date and prevents the collapse of the orthodontic result. But the orthodontist should not be given *carte blanche* on first premolar removal. Third molars may still not erupt and eight teeth (4 premolars and 4 third molars) are a great deal to remove. Before the decision is made, the dental health status of all teeth should be determined. It is not always possible for an orthodontist to look at a set of dental radiographs or to make a clinical examination and be completely sure of the prognosis of an apparently restored tooth. There are literally thousands of first permanent molar teeth and teeth in other areas of the mouth that remain in service because of pulp capping procedures or pulpotomies. Prognosis of longevity of these teeth is indeterminate in many cases; in some it is an outright gamble.

It is the responsibility of the dentist to let the patient and orthodontist know about any such teeth. It can prove most distressing to both the dentist and orthodontist to remove the first premolars and then have a first permanent molar "blow up" during orthodontic treatment. In many cases, although orthodontic mechanical demands may be greater and treatment time prolonged, the questionable first permanent molar—or second premolar, as the case may be—should be removed instead of the healthy premolar. Modern appliances can effect a satisfactory result in most cases, whether it is the first premolar, second premolar, first molar or second molar that is removed. The problem is to create space in the alveolar trough. It is easier to control space in some areas than in others, but as long as the space is there, an orthodontist can utilize it.

No extractions should be performed by the dentist without a written request from the orthodontist. There should be no hesitancy about calling and discussing the matter before performing the requested surgery. This should be done tactfully so as not to undermine the patient's confidence. If dental radiographs or panoramic surveys are not sent along with the extraction request, they should either be procured from the orthodontist or a new series made of the proposed extraction sites. No teeth should ever be removed without accompanying radiographs. It is better for the dentist to call the orthodontist than to be sorry later for having removed the wrong tooth.

IMPORTANCE OF RADIOGRAPHS

Great care must be taken in interpreting radiographs supplied by others. Some dentists mount their dental radiographs as if they were standing on the tongue; others prefer mounting them as if standing in front of the patient. This means that what is the left side of the mount for one dentist is the right side for another. A clinical check of teeth present and of restorations will usually resolve the question if it is not possible to tell from the dental radiographs. If there is any doubt, there should be further consultation between the dentist and orthodontist. It may be difficult to fix the responsibility if a mistake is made; the patient will suffer in any event. Panoramic radiographs reduce this chance for error, since they are marked with "L" (left) or "R" (right) automatically during film exposure.

The same care must be exercised in following instructions given by orthodontists for planned programs of serial extraction (see Chap. 15). Before deciduous teeth are removed, the status of the permanent successors must be determined. If radiographs reveal any unusual situation, the findings should be discussed with the orthodontist unless the dentist is certain that this information is common knowledge. A "hotline" must be maintained at all times between the orthodontist and the general practitioner or oral surgeon whenever tooth removal is required. It is better to postpone removal until another time than to wish you had postponed it later.

A request will be made occasionally to enucleate unerupted first or second premolars. The request may be valid, and there are probably cases that might benefit from such a radical procedure, but the possibility of damage to contiguous teeth and tissues is great and the technical demands usually beyond the scope of general dental practice. Such a decision must be weighed carefully and discussed with the orthodontist before implementing the request. It is wise to refer enucleation procedures to the oral surgeon. Don't be offended if the referral for enucleation of unerupted or impacted teeth is made directly to the oral surgeon. Fewer and fewer dentists in general practice want the responsibility for possible unfavorable sequelae, and more and more patients want surgery performed under a general anesthetic. The specially trained oral surgeon is better equipped for such services.

CARIES REPAIR DURING ORTHODONTIC THERAPY

Finally, there is the problem of restorative dental care during orthodontic therapy. Too many patients assume that the orthodontist will check for caries or any unusual dental condition while he is adjusting the appliances. Unfortunately, few men do, and then their examination is only superficial. They tell their patients to have periodic dental checkups during orthodontic treatment, but seldom follow this up to see if these checkups are actually being made.[2] Dental care thus grinds to a halt during orthodontic treatment — or during the period of greatest caries susceptibility for the average child. Properly made orthodontic appliances may protect part of the teeth from carious assault, and the increased and more efficacious hygienic procedures and reduced carbohydrate substrate should cut down on the caries index: but deep developmental pits have a way of becoming deep cavities in a hurry. Many a parent has been horrified to find that his child has a half dozen cavities after a couple of years of orthodontic treatment, and he blames the appliances. In reality, this may be less than would have occurred during this period if no appliances had ever been worn.

It is the duty of the dentist to *insist* on seeing his patients at frequent intervals during orthodontic treatment and to make the parents understand the divided responsibility problem. If patients miss their recall appointments, a blunt letter pointing out the possibilities of dental neglect and placing the responsibility on the parent should be sent. Such measures can only improve total dental health care, develop better understanding of dental health problems by the public and enhance relations between the general dentist and the orthodontist.

REFERENCES

1. Rogers, G. A., and Wagner, M. J.: Protection of stripped enamel surfaces with topical fluoride applications. Am. J. Orthodont., 56:551–559, 1969.
2. Wagers, L. E.: Clean and check procedure. J. Pract. Orthod., 3:370–374, 1969.
3. Graber, T. M.: Postmortems in post-treatment adjustment. Am. J. Orthodont., 52:331–352, 1966.
4. Muhler, J. C.: Dental caries—orthodontic applicances-SnF$_2$. J. Dent. Child., 37:18–21, 1970.
5. Balenseifen, J. W., and Madonia, J. V.: Study of dental plaque in orthodontic patients. J. Dent. Res., 49:320–324, 1970.
6. Rateitschak, K. H.: Orthodontics and periodontology. Int. Dent. J., 18:108–120, 1968.
7. Cunat, J. J., and Sebastion, G. G.: Diphenylhydantoin sodium: gingival hyperplasia and orthodontic treatment. Angle Orthodont., 39:182–185, 1969.
8. Proper oral hygiene during orthodontic therapy. American Association of Orthodontists, Patient Education Card, 1970.
9. Accepted dental therapeutics, American Dental Association, 1971.
10. Zachrisson, S., and Zachrisson, B. U.: Gingival condition associated with orthodontic treatment. Angle Orthodont., 42:26–34, 1972.
11. Cheraskin, E., and Ringsdorf, W. M.: Biology of the orthodontic patient: Relation of chronologic and dental age in terms of vitamin C state. Angle Orthodont., 42:56–59, 1972.
12. Furstman, L., and Bernick, S.: Clinical considerations of the periodontium. Am. J. Orthodont., 61:138–155, 1972.
13. Nizel, A. E.: Nutrition in Preventive Dentistry: Science and Practice. Philadelphia, W. B. Saunders Co., 1972.

chapter 13

PREVENTIVE ORTHODONTICS

MAINTENANCE OF A NORMAL OCCLUSION

How many times has a dentist said to a new patient, "If only I had seen you earlier, we could have prevented your problem. Now it will require strong measures. Even then we may not be successful." And, all too often, the reply comes back, "But doctor, I have always gone to the dentist at least twice a year and he never mentioned any trouble except cavities." It is not depreciating the value of restorative dentistry to say that it is only one facet of the total dental service. Equally important is *preventive dentistry* of which preventive orthodontics is just a part. Unlike certain phases of restorative dentistry, which are "one shot" services, preventive orthodontics, by its very nature, requires a continuing, long-range approach. Without this, the complex timetable of growth, development, tissue differentiation, resorption, eruption—all under the influence of continuous functional forces—cannot be assured. It is a tribute to the magnificence of human engineering that so many children do achieve a normal occlusion. But many hundreds of thousands do not because of the onslaught of caries and the lack of recognition of any one of a multiplicity of deterring phenomena. Preventive orthodontics means a *dynamic*, ever-constant vigilance —a routine, a discipline, for both the dentist and the patient.[1,2]

NEED FOR PATIENT-DENTIST RAPPORT. It is essential that a proper rapport be established between the dentist and the child and his parents at the first visit. Through the use of illustrations and models it should be made clear to the parents that a normal occlusion does not just "happen." They should understand how many things can go wrong and should appreciate the complexity of dental development. How much easier it is to prevent or intercept incipient problems rather than correct them at a later date. The American Dental Association makes literature available for all dentists for this important job of patient education. Use it by all means.

NECESSITY FOR DIAGNOSTIC RECORDS. The child should be seen by his dentist as early as two and a half years of age. This does not mean that services need be rendered. A clinical examination may suffice but, emphasizing the ever changing picture, diagnostic records (especially dental x-rays or a panoramic x-ray examination) should be obtained whenever possible, even at this early age. By the time the child has reached five years of age, the dentist should place him on a definite schedule for obtaining longitudinal diagnostic records. Bite-wing radiographic examinations should be made twice a year. Periapical radiographic examinations should be made once a year if there is any *hint* of a developing malocclusion. Otherwise, a full radiographic examination every two years is sufficient. If at all possible a panoramic radiographic examination should be made, since this record, more than any other diagnostic criterion, gives an appreciation of the *whole* dentitional development beneath the surface. Too often dental radiographs show only part of the picture—and a distorted part at that (Fig. 13–1). Study models are essential. Besides being a time-linked record of a particular morphologic relationship, they help the dentist interpret his radiographs.[2]

SIGNIFICANCE OF STUDY CASTS.   During the critical years from 6 to 12, it is not too much to obtain a set of study casts at yearly intervals. These need not be beautiful works of art in the sense that the bases are polished and geometrically trimmed. Indeed, only the occlusal and dental portions need be poured up in plaster. But they make an invaluable record for each patient (see Chap. 8). Much can be learned about similar problems in other patients by correlating all

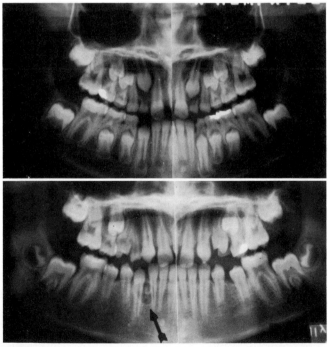

Figure 13–1 Serial panoramic radiographs taken 18 months apart demonstrate value of periodic examination. Clinical examination at first visit of 9-year-old girl showed only maxillary incisor diastema and retained deciduous lateral incisors. Panoramic view shows congenital absence of maxillary lateral incisors, with canines erupting mesially into space of missing teeth. As a preventive procedure, should deciduous lateral incisors be removed? Will deciduous canines resorb or be retained? In lower view, canines have erupted into maxillary lateral incisor position, with one deciduous canine lost and one still intact. Despite developing third molars, arch length is no problem in the mandibular arch, but a developing cyst is! This was not seen in first view taken 18 months earlier. Constant vigilance is essential.

diagnostic criteria and comparing sets of records. Occasional photographs help to personalize radiographs and study casts, and they help the patient to realize that these records are really a part of him. But they do more than that. They show in a general way the relationship of the various parts of the face. If there is a mandibular retrusion, this may be quite apparent on the photograph. The all-encompassing role of heredity and genetics is brought to the fore. The resulting compensatory and adaptive muscle activity which may serve to extenuate the developing malocclusion should be a matter of record. This becomes more important when it is not possible to obtain panoramic radiographs or oriented lateral and frontal headplates (cephalometric radiographs). (See Chap. 8, Diagnostic Procedures, Aids and Their Interpretation.)

ORTHODONTIC ALTERNATIVES IN OCCLUSION MAINTENANCE

The primary charge to the dentist who would render preventive orthodontic service is that he strive to maintain a normal occlusion for that particular age. This means that he is like the dispatcher at a busy airport who tries to see that each plane lands and takes off on time. Like the dispatcher, the dentist must prevent any accidents from occurring to each patient. Teeth must leave and arrive on time and there must be no obstacles in their path, just as each plane must stay on schedule. Maintenance of the best health of each tooth requires periodic checkups as does the maintenance of an airplane. Even as the control tower at the airport knows that a schedule must be kept on all runways — coordinating the blips on the radar screen to fit the constantly changing traffic pattern — so must the dentist realize that it is important to coordinate all arch segments consistent with the overall developmental traffic pattern. He may choose one of three alternatives: prevent anything abnormal from occurring, intercept an abnormal situation that is developing or correct an abnormality that has already developed. It is obvious that the first alternative is infinitely preferable. It is here that the dentist who does not have specialized orthodontic training can do his greatest service.[3]

Most people associate orthodontics with "braces," but if the orthodontist is to earn his "applied biologist" status, this is only part of the picture. Only 45 per cent of his practice should consist of full corrective, mechanotherapy cases. As Figure 13–2 shows, an ideal orthodontic service should devote 10 per cent to observation and prevention, 20 per cent to interceptive procedures, 25 per cent to partial corrective mechanotherapy and the balance to full treatment.

The observation group includes pretreatment and post-treatment patients, as well as patients with transient, developmental malocclusions and those with conditions that may benefit from preventive efforts.

The preventive group includes all patients in a patient education program. Such things as space control, space maintenance and space regaining, maintenance of a quadrant tooth-shedding timetable, functional analysis and oral habit check-up, muscle exercises, caries control, prevention of Milwaukee brace damage, and so forth, also are part of the preventive group.

Interceptive procedures are required for developing basal dysplasias (orthopedic guidance), cleft palate problems, anterior diastemas, habit problems, arch length deficiency problems, and so forth. Here, such things as habit control

IDEAL ORTHODONTIC SERVICE

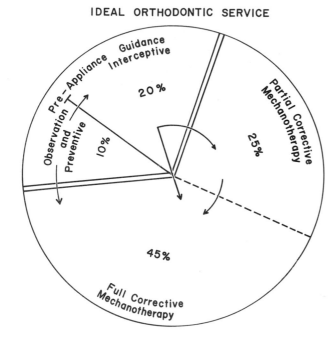

Figure 13–2   Ideal orthodontic service.

appliances, space regainers, occlusal equilibration, slicing, stripping and serial extraction procedures are important.

The partial mechanotherapy group includes two-stage Class II, Class III and open bite problems, vertical dimension problems, (bite plate, etc.), orthopedic intervention for basal malocclusions, space control, cross-bite correction, temporomandibular joint disturbances, retention and post-treatment manipulation, prerestorative uprighting of teeth, and so forth. Severe rotations may be corrected in the two-stage group.

Full mechanotherapy (45 per cent of the practice) is employed in conventional Class I, II and III corrections—extraction and nonextractions. Second phase treatment cases are also included as well as guided extraction cases, now ready after completion of autonomous adjustment.

The remaining chapters of this book are devoted to the 55 per cent of cases, exclusive of full multibanded orthodontic problems. The latter group is the basis for the two-volume text. *Current Orthodontic Concepts and Techniques,* edited by the author.

INDICATIONS OF FUTURE ORTHODONTIC PROBLEMS

A visual examination of the patient will quickly reveal a gross malocclusion, in which there is an anterior open bite, excessive overbite and overjet, cross-bite, basal malrelationship and other problems. Interceptive or even preventive procedures may sometimes be instituted in treatment of patients with these problems, but the decision as to timing and mode of treatment should usually be made by an orthodontic specialist, since he will ultimately have the responsibility for therapy. Thus, one form of preventive orthodontics is obvious—refer the patient for an orthodontic consultation whenever there is any question of a developing malocclusion. However, not all malocclusions are "surface evident." A large percentage of Class I malocclusions exist because of what happens during the critical developmental years, with most of the activity *below the surface.* Thus, the dentist should not be content with a cursory glance at the number of teeth present, a quick check of the caries problem and a couple of bite-wing radiographs. A complete and accurate radiographic examination should be made soon after the first visit. This may be either a panoramic radiograph together with bite-wing views, or a complete long-cone technique, periapical series together with bite-wing views. Periodic examinations should be scheduled at least once a year after the eruption of the permanent central incisors.

The most likely radiographic indicators of future orthodontic problems are:
1. Resorption pattern of the deciduous dentition.
2. Eruption cycle of the permanent dentition.

Much of our knowledge about resorption is empiric. As with tooth eruption, many theories have been advanced about the nature of this process. Just why the osteoclasts should attack the cementum and dentin of the roots of deciduous teeth at a specific time is not known. Since pressure stimulates osteoclastic activity in mesial drift and actual tooth movement, the most likely factor initiating resorption is the pressure from the erupting permanent tooth germ. Yet there is usually bone of relatively normal character between the permanent tooth germ and the deciduous root. As we delve into the mystery of physiologic chemistry, it is probable that the answer will be found in cellular, enzymatic or proteolytic activity. How can we explain the frequent spontaneous resorption of the root of the deciduous tooth where there is congenital absence of the permanent successor? Even though we do not know the exact mechanism of resorption we can follow its course rather precisely by routine radiographic examination.

The same is true of the eruption of the permanent teeth. Here, too, numerous theories have been proposed to describe the eruption phenomenon, with the actual growth of the root being the most likely inciting cause. As the root elongates against the resorption-resistant hammock ligament during the prefunctional eruption phase, the crown of the permanent tooth approximates the deciduous root. Little does the patient realize that beneath the quiet and nearly unchanging exterior, the vital processes are seething with activity, with growth of bone, cementum, dentin, pulpal mesenchyme and periodontal membrane tissues, all moving in orderly fashion as if some electronic brain were directing each step along the way. So many things can hardly be going on at once with so many intimately related and dovetailed changes without having something go wrong at one time or another. That this happens so seldom, that nature works itself out of so many seemingly blind alleys, never ceases to baffle observers. Following the progress of this extravaganza of nature on all fronts is a job in itself. But the dentist must do this to maintain the timetable of development in case something goes wrong.

ABNORMAL RESORPTION

Why is it that the mesial root of a deciduous molar may resorb and the distal root remain unaffected? Why is it that a permanent tooth will assume an abnormal eruptive path and yet not be in contact with any other tooth? Why is it that some deciduous teeth stop erupting and drop below the level of their

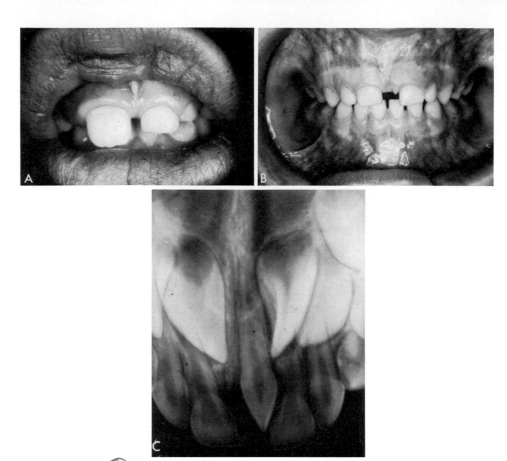

Figure 13–3 A, The left deciduous central incisor is still firm. Why? A preventive orthodontic orientation demands immediate investigation. The dentist may suspect a supernumerary tooth, congenital absence, abnormal path of eruption, delayed resorption or a bony barrier. In B, there is a diastema. Is this normal? It appears mostly left of the midline and has grown rapidly in a short time. The dentist must investigate and make his diagnosis now and not wait and see what happens. *C,* A radiograph shows a supernumerary tooth causing the diastema, abnormal resorption of the deciduous central incisor and rotation of the developing permanent central incisors. The supernumerary must be removed immediately. (B and C, courtesy W. R. Mayne.)

Figure 13–4 The top four pictures represent four quadrants of the same patient's mouth. B, Only the upper left second premolar is erupting normally. A, The upper right second premolar is being deflected by an abnormal resorption pattern; C, the lower right second premolar is congenitally missing, and the lower left second premolar is following an abnormal path of eruption. D, Preventive orthodontics requires immediate care. This may mean removal of maxillary second deciduous molars, or possibly the lower left second deciduous molar, and uncovering the crown of the left second premolar, depending on the total diagnostic picture. If crowding exists, tooth sacrifice in the permanent dentition is possible. Pictures E and F are also of the same mouth. The abnormal resorption pattern on F demands immediate removal of both second deciduous molars. In G and H, another preventive orthodontic problem is seen. The lower left second deciduous molar is dropping below the level of occlusion and is probably ankylosed. This is not true of the lower right second deciduous molar (G). But the lower right second premolar is definitely more malposed than the same tooth on the opposite side. Removal of second deciduous molars is preventive orthodontics.

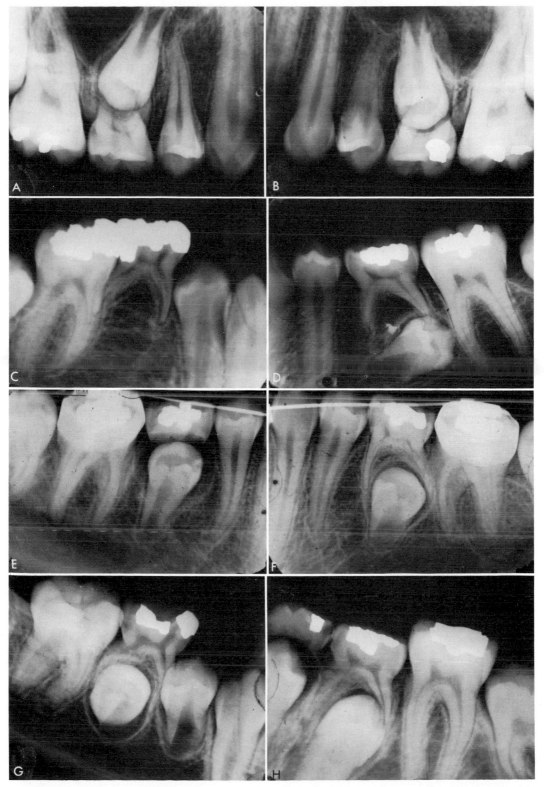

(*Figure 13-4*   See opposite page for legend.)

contiguous teeth (ankylosis)? Why is it that an erupting permanent tooth can apparently stimulate the resorption and shedding of a deciduous tooth but apparently be stopped by a thin bony barrier or the mucosa itself? We do not know the answers to these and many other questions, but these problems arise and must be solved over and over again for countless patients during the mixed dentition if the dentist is interested in more than just filling cavities, in reparative procedures, or in treating the patient after "the horse is out of the barn" (Figs. 13–1, 13–3, 13–4). This is the essence of preventive dentistry. (Chapter 7 provides an atlas of such conditions that the student will find of continuing value as a reference.[4])

ABERRANT RESORPTION PATTERNS

Abnormalities of resorption are associated most frequently with space deficiency problems, but they occur also in patients where there is plenty of space and seemingly every reason for uneventful shedding of the deciduous teeth. The deciduous canines and the second deciduous molars are particularly prone to aberrant resorption patterns. If the dentist sees such patterns in the dental radiographs and if he sees one segment exchanging deciduous teeth for permanent successors while the teeth are still quite tight in another, he had better ask himself why (Fig. 13–5). In an ideal sequence, right and left deciduous central incisors should be lost at about the same time, deciduous lateral incisors should be loose and lost at about the same time, all deciduous canines should be loose and lost within a short period, etc. If one deciduous canine is lost spontaneously and prematurely, the dentist should get radiographs and check immediately to see if this is not an abnormal manifestation or nature's

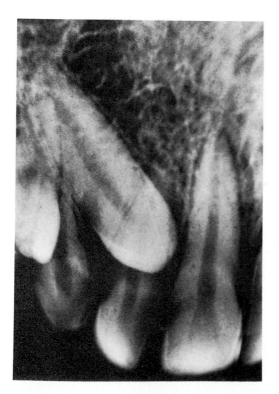

Figure 13–5 A retained deciduous canine in a 16-year-old patient. Periodic radiographic examination and removal of the deciduous canine at the proper time might have prevented the palatal impaction of the permanent successor or, at the very least, reduced the severity of the problem.

attempt to gain space for a future arch length problem. (See Chap. 15, Serial Extraction.)

CONTINGENCY OF EXTRACTION

As a rule of thumb, the shedding of the deciduous dentition should be kept on schedule by extracting the tooth or teeth on one side of the maxilla and mandible when they have been lost through natural processes on the other side. To wait longer than three months for nature to do the job, particularly when there is radiographic evidence of abnormal resorption, is to court future malocclusion. This does not mean that the dentist must fit each patient into the Procrustean bed of group normality—into the charts that have been derived from studies of thousands of children in which age levels have been set up for the loss of deciduous teeth and the eruption of permanent teeth. Each patient has his own "norm" and it is up to the dentist through careful study to determine what this is and to see that it is maintained in all four buccal and both maxillary and mandibular anterior segments. Longitudinal diagnostic records permit him to do just that. (See Chap. 8.)

ROLE OF SECOND DECIDUOUS MOLAR REGION

The second deciduous molar region is a particularly critical area.[5] Because the second deciduous molar is usually larger than its successor, abnormal resorption and prolonged retention may have a far reaching effect (Fig. 13–3). Erupting canines may be forced buccally or lingually or may actually be prevented from erupting at all because of the additional arch length taken up by the retained deciduous molar. Prolonged retention of mandibular second deciduous molars may make the space problem critical enough to cause a break in the continuity of the lower arch that leads to irregularity of the lower incisors. As shown in the discussion in Chapter 2, there is a transient crowding of the mandibular incisors in the normal course of events as they erupt. Autonomous adjustment reduces this crowding, as shown by longitudinal studies. (See Chap. 2.) However, if there is the additional strain on the arch length problem, preventing self-adjustment at the proper time, it may never take place; or the crowding may become more severe as the overbite tends to increase incisor irregularity. Abnormal resorption of any deciduous tooth may be a factor in the deflecting of the permanent successor into an abnormal path of eruption. Frequent radiographic examination allows the dentist to check the progress and intercede if necessary. (See Chap. 7.)

CASE I. The following case is an example of a situation that happens quite frequently.

Betsy B. is 11½ years old. She has lost all her deciduous teeth except an upper left deciduous canine and a lower left second deciduous molar. All the mandibular teeth in the lower right buccal segment have erupted, except the third molar. There is a retained deciduous molar on the lower left side, but since it is the only one left, it probably should be lost shortly (so the dentist says). The maxillary canines are not erupting yet, and only one 12-year molar has erupted; but after all, Betsy has a few months to go before she is 12. The occlusion seems normal and the dentist sees nothing to worry about. Betsy has never had more than bite-wing radiographs. Why take additional x-ray pictures when everything seems normal? The "baby" cuspid still left on the upper left side is loose, and should be lost soon.

Is the dentist justified in not being concerned? Let us take one single picture that the dentist did not take, a step requiring about 90 seconds of the patient's time — a panoramic radiograph. If Betsy is a statistic, the probability is that the panoramic view will justify the dentist's lack of concern. But Betsy happens to be an individual, and chagrin and embarrassment now replace the dentist's lack of concern (Fig. 13–6). The lower left second deciduous molar obviously is not about to be lost; there is abnormal resorption of the distal root and an abnormal eruptive path of the second premolar beneath it. Also, the second premolar is rotated and will take up additional arch length, if it ever erupts. Those maxillary canines that were about to erupt when viewed from "above the surface" are not likely to come in normally now, as the radiograph shows clearly. The eruptive paths of both maxillary canines are abnormal, and the upper right canine is probably erupting palatally and is impacted. "Just wait, Betsy, and come back in six months." Wait for what? And now, if the dentist wants to look for those erupting 12-year molars that are due to join their counterparts in the lower right buccal segment, he may also have to look twice. The lower left second molar is congenitally missing, as is the upper left second molar, and it appears that although the tooth in the upper right second molar position seems larger than a third molar, it probably is a third molar, and either the second or third molar is missing in this quadrant.

Prompt action by the dentist now can prevent or at least ameliorate the chances of preventing a malocclusion. Uncovering the imminently impacted maxillary canines may be sufficient to allow them to erupt reasonably normally, while they still have sufficient eruptive force to "go it alone." Removal of the retained mandibular deciduous second molar is clearly indicated. Even if the second premolar does erupt in a rotated position, it may be improved, shaped or left as is. All third molars erupting in the second molar spaces should be checked periodically. Overeruption of the mandibular right third molar will have to be prevented, since there is no opposing tooth. Such situations cause functional disturbances. A record made now may prevent trouble later.

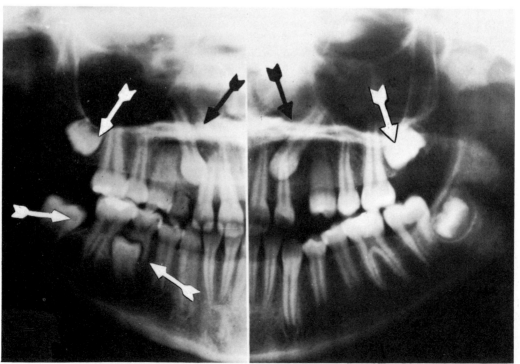

Figure 13–6   This 11½-year-old girl faces malocclusion if she is not treated promptly by the dentist.

Obviously, Betsy is not a statistic and should not be treated as one. Each case should be judged on its own merits and all possibilities explored when there is a variation in bilateral symmetry of the developmental pattern. The dentist will find practice more exciting and challenging, even as the patient finds it more rewarding.

CASE II. Another case in point is that of a 16-year-old boy with all his permanent teeth except in the maxillary right canine region where the deciduous canine is still in place (Fig. 13–5). Contacts are tight and the occlusion reasonably normal except for mesial drift in the upper right buccal segment. The patient has been under continuous dental care, and the restorative work is in excellent condition. But what is the situation in the right canine region? A radiograph shows that the permanent canine has been deflected to the lingual side and that there is abnormal resorption of the root of the deciduous canine. Because of the mesial drift of the right maxillary buccal segment, there is inadequate space at present to accommodate the permanent canine, even if the deciduous counterpart is removed. Could this have been prevented? In all probability, if the deciduous canine had been removed when the other three were lost (before the mesial drift of the right maxillary buccal segment) the permanent canine would have erupted normally. Preventive orthodontics would have saved this patient from the need of corrective appliances. The parent, on learning the facts, is angry with the dentist and has every right to be. This patient and innumerable others like him often have problems which are masked by statistics.

CRITICAL PERIOD OF TOOTH EXCHANGE

From the foregoing cases it should be evident that constant vigilance is essential during the critical period of tooth exchange. Leighton, in an excellent study including birth notes of a large group of children, found that there are a number of observations that may be made early, concerning tooth position and alignment and from which predictions may be made. By fostering study along these lines, truly preventive dentistry may be achieved, eliminating unnecessary and inappropriate treatment. Even when therapy is indicated, the treatment timing may be optimal.[6] Dentists must be on the lookout for anything that might stand in the way of the development of a normal occlusion. Abnormal resorption patterns, retained deciduous root fragments, supernumerary teeth, ankylosis of the deciduous tooth, a nonresorbing bony crypt, a soft tissue barrier and possibly an overhanging restoration in a deciduous tooth all may upset the timetable at one time or another. To make sure that they render the best possible service when they start out in practice, some dentists make themselves a check list of all possible detrimental factors. Like the pilot of the commercial air liner, they "check out" each factor each time they examine a new patient. This is a good idea, at least until these criteria become second nature for the dentist. Chapters 6 and 7 have been produced in great detail and with a multiplicity of illustrations. Intimate knowledge of all facets of the causes of malocclusion is essential if preventive orthodontics is to mean more than lip service.[7]

SPACE CONTROL IN DECIDUOUS DENTITION

An important part of preventive orthodontics is the correct handling of spaces created by the untimely loss of deciduous teeth. As more and more people become aware of the importance of the repair of the deciduous teeth, this problem is bound to arise less often, but at present it is a major one. Unfortunately, some dentists have been guilty of advising patients to disregard the repair of deciduous teeth, because they will be lost. Perhaps it is because children are sometimes more difficult to manage; perhaps it is because on a time-and-fee basis the results are less productive to the dentist; perhaps it is just because the dentist does not know that premature loss can, and often does, destroy the integrity of a normal occlusion.

This does not mean that as soon as a dentist spots a break in the continuity of the upper or lower arches he must rush in and place a space maintainer. Not by any means. Some teeth are lost prematurely at nature's behest. This is particularly true of the deciduous canines. In most of these spontaneous premature losses, the reason is the lack of space to accommodate all the teeth in the dental arches. This is nature's way of easing the critical space problem, at least temporarily. (The subject will be discussed in greater detail in Chapter 15 under Serial Extraction Therapy.) In this chapter, space maintainers and space control are discussed for cases involving the premature loss of deciduous teeth because of caries or accident.

INDICATIONS FOR SPACE MAINTAINERS

Whenever a deciduous tooth is lost before the time it would normally be shed, predisposing the patient to a malocclusion, a space maintainer should be placed. Occasionally loss of an anterior tooth may require a space maintainer for esthetic and psychological reasons. There are no hard and fast rules to go by in determining whether a malocclusion will result from the premature loss of a deciduous tooth. But there are some guiding principles that must be weighed very carefully before making a decision. It was pointed out in Chapter 2 on Growth and Development and in Chapter 10 on the Biomechanical Principles of Orthodontic Tooth Movement that teeth are constantly shifting in a growing and changing medium. These teeth are subject to manifold pressures and depend on one another for support in many instances. This is particularly true of proximal contact relationship and occlusal contact during function. It was pointed out that the position of the teeth represents a state of balance of morphogenetic and functional forces *at that particular time.* The role of the musculature in establishing and maintaining this equilibrium is paramount.

DETERMINING FACTORS GOVERNED BY COMPENSATORY OR ADAPTIVE RESPONSE. Finally, another factor to be taken into consideration is the inherent adaptive response of the human organism to changing conditions. When a deciduous tooth is lost ahead of time, the dentist must ask himself: (1) Has the balance been disturbed? (2) Will nature adapt to this change favorably or unfavorably? (3) Is the loss of a tooth, or teeth, likely to stimulate abnormal muscle function or habits? (4) Will the occlusion, through the inclined plane action of the opposing teeth, be sufficient to prevent migration into the edentulous area? (5) If a malocclusion is already present, will this have any effect on the space created by the loss of a deciduous tooth? (6) How does the loss of the deciduous tooth affect the eruption time of the permanent tooth? (7) If a space maintainer has to be placed, what kind should be used?[7]

Has the balance been disturbed? This question cannot always be answered easily since, as pointed out in Chapter 2, the loss of a tooth in a growing, expanding medium may be different from loss after the pattern has been completed. For example, the loss of a maxillary or mandibular incisor from the mouth of a youngster four or five years of age where generalized, so-called developmental spaces exist becomes primarily an esthetic consideration. If the occlusion is normal it is not likely that the space will close. It may be necessary later to check and see that the permanent tooth erupts on time and is not held back by a bony crypt or mucosal barrier, which sometimes results from premature loss, but the actual placement of a space maintainer in all probability would be unnecessary. Since the lower arch is the contained arch (it has been likened to the Gothic arch construction used so frequently in churches during the Middle Ages), the loss of a structural unit is more likely to require maintenance.[9] This is particularly true of the posterior segments where the balance has been disturbed due to the loss of proximal contact relationship, and where the opposing tooth is now free to overerupt into a malposition. Even if a disturbance in the equilibrium of the stomatognathic system is caused by the loss of a deciduous tooth, other factors must be considered before rushing in and placing a space maintainer.

Will the structures adapt to the changing conditions favorably or unfavorably? One of the remarkable attributes of the human organism is its ability to accommodate itself to environmental stimuli. Orthodontics itself has been considered by some men as an adaptive response to active pressures. Certainly the premature loss of a deciduous tooth in the maxillary or mandibular anterior segments usually poses no problem. The contiguous teeth take over the load of incision, and the mucosa covers over the hole left by the extraction until the permanent tooth erupts. Occasionally the bone that fills in this area may be unduly resistant to the eruption of the permanent tooth, and this should be watched. Or, the mucosa in adapting to the functional demands and pressures exerted by the bolus of food may become fibrous and more unyielding to the eruptive force, requiring the dentist to incise the resistant tissue to permit the tooth to erupt. Thus, both favorable and unfavorable sequelae may occur. If a posterior deciduous tooth is lost early, a patient may occasionally develop a tongue thrust habit in this area which serves to keep the space open — sort of a dynamic space maintainer. Not all muscle "tics" are favorable when associated with loss of deciduous teeth, which leads us to the next question.

Is the loss of a tooth or teeth likely to stimulate abnormal muscle function or habits? While the premature loss of deciduous teeth results in adaptive muscle activity that serves to hold the needed space in some cases, there are other cases in which this muscle activity enhances the malocclusion. The formation of abnormal muscle habits such as tongue or cheek biting (or possibly finger sucking if the missing tooth is an anterior one) may lead to an open bite and malocclusion. Space maintainers can prevent this from happening.

Will the occlusion, through the inclined plane action of the opposing teeth, be sufficient to prevent migration into the edentulous area? This question, of course, refers to the loss of deciduous canines and first and second deciduous molars. Since the cuspal morphology is usually much more poorly defined than in the permanent dentition and since occlusal contact in the centric position is only momentary and ineffectual, it is wishful thinking to expect the inclined planes in the deciduous teeth to maintain the space. Occasionally, sharply defined cusps that interdigitate precisely with their opposing teeth will hold the space. These cases are exceptions. With the tendency toward an end-to-end "bite" or flush terminal plane in the posterior segments in the deciduous and mixed dentition, until the loss of the second deciduous molars, the looked-for locking is clinically a rarity. In fact, with an end-to-end cuspal contact, the drifting of the teeth contiguous to the space may allow the creation of a Class II interdigitation. To prevent this, space maintainers are most important.

What does the premature loss of a deciduous tooth do to the eruption time of the permanent tooth? In most instances the eruption of the permanent tooth is accelerated, and it appears in the oral cavity ahead of the time that it would normally have erupted if the deciduous tooth had been shed normally. First premolars have erupted in children as young as 7 years of age, which is quite early[10]. The use of a removable, tissue-borne retainer sometimes stimulates earlier eruption.[11] Accelerated eruption of the permanent tooth is a good thing. Occasionally, however, the socket of the extracted deciduous tooth fills in with bone, supra-alveolar tissue forms a fibrous network covering this area, and either the bone does not resorb as rapidly as desired, or the mucosa does not break down ahead of the advancing permanent tooth, retarding the eruption indefinitely. This is just one of the many reasons why it is important to take periodic radiographs. Incision of the tissue or curettage of the resisting bone may be necessary. If the comparable teeth in the remaining three buccal segments have erupted and there is still no clinical evidence of the tooth for which the space is maintained, it is reasonable to assume that the tissue between the tooth and the oral cavity may be retarding its eruption. In any event, it does no harm to incise it.

If a malocclusion is already present, will this have any effect on the space created by the loss of the deciduous tooth? The answer depends on the type of malocclusion. In a patient with an arch length deficiency, the premature loss of a deciduous tooth may mean the rapid closing of the space to ease the crowding elsewhere. This may actually be desirable and will be discussed in Chapter 15 on Serial Extraction. If there is a tendency toward a Class II malocclusion, with abnormal perioral muscle function, the loss of a deciduous tooth in the lower arch may increase the overbite and overjet as muscle forces stimulate the drift of the teeth on either side of the space. With an incipient Class III malocclusion, the premature loss of the maxillary incisor may mean the difference between a normal overjet and an anterior cross-bite. Where the child has an end-to-end incisal contact on occlusion and active lip musculature, it is usually wise to place an anterior space maintainer. These are the cases where there are usually no spaces between the maxillary incisors so that the muscular forces tend to constrict the maxillary arch, and the mandible may then develop a convenience bite and slide into a prognathism on full occlusion, trapping the erupting incisors to the lingual side. If the malocclusion that is present is due to an enlarged tongue or abnormal tongue function, with generalized spacing throughout the arch, this would, of course, affect the decision on space maintenance. In all probability, maintenance would not be necessary.

If a space maintainer has to be placed, what kind should be used? Obviously, this depends on the tooth loss, the age of the patient, the state of health of the remaining teeth, the type of occlusion, patient cooperation and the manual dexterity and preferences of the operator.

PREREQUISITES FOR SPACE MAINTAINERS

There are certain prerequisites for all space maintainers, whether they are fixed or removable.

1. They should maintain the mesiodistal dimension of the lost tooth.
2. If possible, they should be functional, at least to the extent of preventing the overeruption of the opposing tooth or teeth.

3. They should be as simple and as strong as possible.

4. They must not endanger the remaining teeth by imposing excessive stresses on them.

5. They must be easily cleaned and not serve as traps for debris which might enhance dental caries and soft tissue pathology.

6. Their construction must be such that they do not restrict normal growth and developmental processes or interfere with such functions as mastication, speech or deglutition.

Depending on the tooth lost, the segment involved, the type of occlusion, possible speech involvements and cooperation, a particular type of space maintainer may be indicated.

SPACE MAINTENANCE IN MAXILLARY AND MANDIBULAR ANTERIOR SEGMENTS

In the maxillary anterior segments, space maintainers are not usually necessary, even with the drifting of the contiguous teeth, since normal growth and developmental processes usually increase intercanine width. In the very young child, however, a fixed space maintainer may be justified as an aid to proper speech. Lisping is very common with the absence of the maxillary incisors. The sibilant sounds are made more easily with the presence of all incisor teeth. The replacement of the maxillary incisors that have been lost early may also serve an esthetic as well as psychological purpose for the child who wants to look like his playmates (Figs. 13-7, 13-8). A removable palate type retainer with a tooth on it is quite satisfactory if the child is older and more mature, has learned proper speech habits, can adjust to the increased bulk and is reasonably cooperative (Fig. 13-9).

Tooth loss in the lower anterior segment is rather rare. Space maintenance

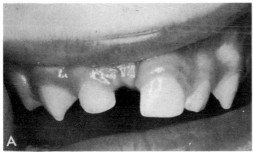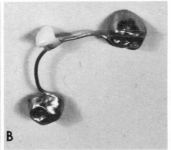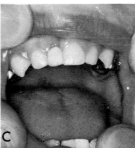

Figure 13-7 A, This two-year-old patient lost his maxillary right central incisor at 14 months of age. The clinical picture gives the impression that there has been an appreciable degree of loss in space due to the early loss of the tooth. Actually, what has occurred is that the two teeth adjacent to the area of premature loss have drifted into the vacant area. However, the distance from canine eminence to canine eminence has not diminished but will become larger to accommodate the larger permanent successors. B, An appliance was constructed for esthetic reasons, the parent being quite concerned by this unfortunate accident. An alginate impression was taken of the maxillary dentition with crowns in place on the abutment teeth. After the impression had been poured in hydrocal, an 18-gauge lingual wire was bent and soldered to the crowns. A small wire spur was soldered to the lingual arch wire to give the acrylic tooth additional stability. C, The appliance in place. (From Olsen, N. H.: Space maintenance. D. Clin. North America, July, 1959.)[12]

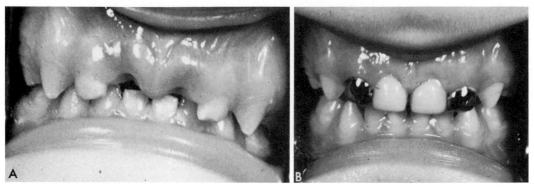

Figure 13–8   A, This 3½-year-old child who lost his two primary central incisors in an accident had difficulty with sibilant sounds. B, A fixed appliance employing a pin and sleeve on the lingual aspect was fabricated. Thin cast overlays using type C gold serve as the abutments. (From Olsen, N. H.: Space maintenance. D. Clin. North America, July, 1959.)

in this area is controversial. Part of the controversy is about the *type* of space maintainer, because it is relatively difficult to anchor a space maintainer on the tiny deciduous incisors. An added hazard is accelerating the loss of contiguous teeth, which serve to hold the maintainer. Since the lower arch is the "contained arch," however, and, like the stone Gothic arch, is more likely to collapse when a "keystone" is removed, and since the permanent teeth as they erupt usually need every available bit of space to achieve a normal position, the dentist would do well to maintain this space. Not to retain the space means that he must assume that the musculature and functional forces and the growth and developmental pattern will team together to overcome the loss. A fixed space maintainer is preferable despite difficulty of construction if confined to the contiguous teeth. The use of a metal crown with a cantilever pontic and rest on the approximating incisor is satisfactory. A canine-to-canine fixed lingual arch or deciduous molar-to-deciduous molar fixed lingual arch may work, depending on the age of the patient, possible growth in this area and similar factors. Sometimes the incorporation of a sleeve attachment is necessary so that growth will not be inhibited (Fig. 13–20). A removable space maintainer is not very desirable here because of its poor retention qualities, probable removal during mealtime and greater likelihood of being lost. In addition, lower anterior succedaneous teeth usually

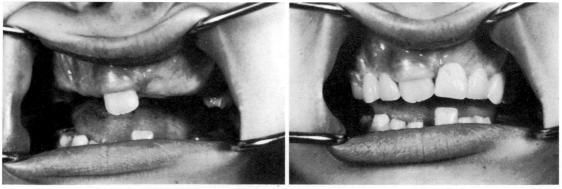

Figure 13–9   Removable upper space maintainer for patient with congenital absence problem combined with high caries susceptibility. Appliance will be worn until premolars erupt.

erupt lingually and move forward under the influence of the tongue. A removable horseshoe type of space maintainer will probably interfere with this movement. This is also true of a fixed lingual arch. Eruption of permanent lower incisors should be watched carefully, and the space maintainer must be removed at the first signs of eruption.

SPACE MAINTENANCE IN BUCCAL SEGMENT

It is in the buccal segments that space maintenance finds its greatest application and where the greatest discretion must be used in deciding when and how the space problem should be solved. As a student of oral anatomy and physiology knows, the deciduous canine and first and second deciduous molars are on the average 1 to 2 mm. greater in total mesiodistal width than the permanent canine, first and second premolars. In many children the width of the mandibular second deciduous molar makes this discrepancy even greater. It may be as much as 3.5 mm. Nance has referred to this as the "leeway" space. In other words, in a normal occlusion there is enough room for the permanent teeth to erupt in the buccal segments; and there is also a little space left over for the shifting of the mandibular first permanent molars mesially to establish a full and correct inclined plane interdigitation, and for the maxillary canine to drop a bit distally as it erupts into the mouth. Nature manages pretty well to use up this space during the exchange of teeth. The figures of 1.7 mm. on each side in the lower arch and 1.0 mm. in the upper arch are averages that have been derived from measuring a great number of individuals. It is incumbent on the dentist to measure the leeway space *in every case* where the question of space maintenance arises (Fig. 2–71).

Other factors that may influence the decision on space maintenance are the age of the patient, the sex of the patient, the status of the occlusion in general, the morphology of the cuspal inclined planes, the manner in which they lock during centric occlusion and during the working bite and the presence or absence of abnormal perioral muscle habits.

HYPOTHETICAL CASE OF BUCCAL SEGMENT SPACE MAINTENANCE

Using a hypothetical case for an example, the dentist finds that he must remove a mandibular first deciduous molar because of carious involvement of the pulp. For him, to maintain or not to maintain is the question. Before he makes his decision he must obtain all possible information.

INFORMATION REQUIRED. A complete intraoral radiographic examination is essential, preferably using the long cone technique to reduce magnification and distortion. The dentist should then measure the width of the deciduous teeth and all permanent successors in all buccal segments and record this figure. He may also do a mixed dentition analysis. At the same time, he should observe the relative amount of root resorption on the deciduous teeth, the state of development and eruption of the permanent successors, the position of the erupting permanent teeth and the character of the alveolar bone. A panoramic radiograph examination is also helpful, and gives an overall picture, including the status of the developing third molars, which are frequently missed on the intraoral examination. A careful analysis must be made of the occlusion of the patient to determine if it is normal or abnormal. Any peculiarities must be noted. The lack of sufficient arch length may mean that this is a serial extraction problem, depending on the degree of deficiency, on the size of the permanent teeth, on the age of the patient, the growth pattern and so on. If there is any doubt, the patient should be referred for an orthodontic consultation.

CRUCIAL FACTOR OF AGE.   The age of the patient is particularly important. Most girls, for example, are one and a half to two years ahead of the boys in their tooth exchange. Thus, the dentist can expect the eruption of the permanent teeth earlier in girls than in boys. Modifying this sex differential would be the individual's own developmental pattern, which could be slow, fast or just average. A good clue on this is the time it took to complete the deciduous dentition and the radiographic evidence of resorption and eruption in the tooth exchange areas. Assuming that the occlusion is normal, that adequate leeway space is present and that the inclined planes of the teeth are not completely flat and have some locking value, a rule of thumb can be established. If it appears that the permanent successor will erupt within a year or less after the loss of the deciduous tooth, space maintenance is probably not necessary, but frequent, periodic, watchful waiting is the order of the day. This means careful measurements of the edentulous area with a pair of dividers and a periapical radiograph of the erupting tooth at 2-month intervals.

QUESTIONS OF MOLAR RETENTION AND EXTRACTION.   If it is likely to be more than a year before the permanent successor appears, allowing for slightly earlier eruption because of the premature loss of the deciduous tooth, it is probably safer to retain the space created by the loss of the deciduous molar. Most clinicians feel that the loss of a first deciduous molar is less critical than that of the second deciduous molar. For one thing, the first premolars will erupt sooner; for another, the second deciduous molar seems to deter the unwanted mesial drift of the first permanent molar. Controversy still exists over whether it is more important to maintain an upper or lower first deciduous molar space. The author considers the lower space more critical because it is the contained arch, and there is a tendency for the overbite and functional forces to push the contiguous teeth into the space provided by the premature loss of the deciduous tooth. If the deciduous canine is small and the permanent canine large, it is advisable to hold the space for the missing tooth. Any loss of space might result in the permanent canine being deflected into a buccal or lingual position in the mouth.

PREMATURE LOSS OF DECIDUOUS CANINES AND MOLARS.   A great many unnecessary space maintainers have been placed for deciduous canines that have been lost early. If the occlusion is normal and the early loss is because of caries or accident, space maintenance may very well be necessary. But usually the premature loss of the canines is tied into a generalized arch length deficiency. This is nature's way of exfoliating teeth ahead of time so that there can be autonomous alignment of the incisors. The orthodontist in many cases helps with a planned program of serial extraction (see Chap. 15). It is poor dentistry to interfere with a naturally occurring program of serial extraction by placing a space maintainer. This only serves to prevent the alignment of the anterior teeth and clouds the issue as far as future orthodontics is concerned. Whenever a deciduous canine is lost early, the dentist must establish why it was lost and if there is a space deficiency. He must decide whether he should not take this as a clue from nature that serial extraction procedures are indicated for the whole mouth. Better still, he should refer the patient to an orthodontic specialist who will then decide, since he has the ultimate responsibility of tooth movement.

The loss of the first or second deciduous molar may mean the creation of a malocclusion unless the dentist makes a careful diagnostic study. A thorough radiographic investigation, a clinical examination of the occlusion in general and of the space available and a consideration of the age and sex of the patient are essential before arriving at a decision. As a general rule, first permanent molars tend to drift mesially into the space created by prematurely lost second deciduous molars. An error of commission (placing a space maintainer) is better than an error of omission (ignoring the loss), in most instances. In both the first and second deciduous molar areas, the danger of elongation of the opposing teeth is always present, and the dentist must take this into consideration in the design of a space maintainer.[8]

SPACE RETAINING APPLIANCES

In placing a space maintainer in any one of the four posterior segments, the dentist has the opportunity to use a functional or nonfunctional, a fixed or removable type of appliance. Since space maintenance should be considered in three dimensions, and not just the anteroposterior component that is uppermost in the minds of most practitioners, a functional type of space maintainer is usually preferable to prevent the elongation and possible shifting of the opposing teeth. This does not mean that this space maintainer must function in mastication like the tooth it replaces. It does mean that it must resist the forces of occlusion, function and muscular activity in a similar way.

FIXED MAINTAINERS

FUNCTIONAL TYPE. The surest way to hold a space is to bridge that space with an appliance that is cemented to the adjacent teeth. It must be durable enough to resist the functional forces and yet satisfy the previously listed requirements of a good space maintainer. There are several types of fixed functional space maintainers. If at all possible, some effort must be made to simulate normal physiology in the design of the appliance. The mere splinting of two teeth adjacent to an edentulous area in a vise-like grip of metal components may provide strength but will not satisfy the functional demands, though this is better than not placing a maintainer at all (Fig. 13–10).

In line with restricting the maintainer abutment teeth as little as possible, a "broken stress" type appliance is preferable. This need not mean a sacrifice of strength. It does mean that it may prevent intolerable loads from being thrust on the supporting teeth. The stress breaker should be designed to allow vertical movement of the supporting teeth consistent with normal functional demands and, to a lesser degree, adjustive labial or lingual movement. It is quite correct to maintain a constant mesiodistal relationship. For this reason, one of the most successful types of retainers is the band, bar and sleeve functional maintainer (Fig. 13–11). Additional tipping vectors are still imposed on the anterior or posterior tooth that carries the soldered bar. These need not be excessive if the operator carefully checks the occlusal contact of the opposing tooth during centric, working and balancing bite conditions for the bar in the space being maintained. It is particularly important to check the working and balancing bite relationships, because premature contact in the space maintainer area means jiggling of the abutment teeth and accelerated loss, if not appliance breakage.

FIXED FUNCTIONAL SPACE MAINTAINER

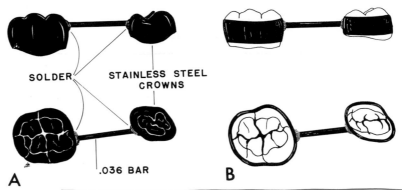

Figure 13–10 Crown-and-bar and band-and-bar fixed functional space maintainer. Bar is soldered on both ends to abutment attachments. This is the simplest functional type of maintainer, if not the most desirable. Full metal crowns for the abutments are generally to be preferred and are less likely to require recementation later.

Regardless of the variation in design of the bar attachment, excellent anatomically correct stainless-steel crowns are available in many sizes for the abutment teeth (Fig. 13–12). The bar can be stainless steel or one of the nickel chromium alloys. The use of a fluoride flux and silver solder makes a quite satisfactory joint (Fig. 13–11). To keep chair time to a minimum, an impression is made of the segment involved and it is poured up in plaster. The gingival portion is trimmed away from the teeth on either side of the space to a distance of 2 mm. An effort should be made to maintain the contour of the tooth as it would appear beneath the gingival tissue. The proper size stainless-steel crown form is chosen, contoured and fitted carefully by scribing the gingival margin (Fig. 13–13). The most frequent mistake is to cut the proximal portions of the band too severely. After the crowns have been carefully fitted, a vertical tube is soldered on one crown and the L-shaped bar fabricated to fit the edentulous area. If it has been possible to obtain an opposing model, the working and balancing bite positions can be determined so that the bar does not interfere. If not, these positions may be determined in the mouth and the bar bent slightly to adjust for any interferences. The horizontal end of the bar is soldered to one of the crowns.

Before cementing the appliance in place, a slit is made on the buccal side of both crowns and the material overlapped at this point to reduce the circumference of the gingival portion of the crown. When the patient bites the maintainer strongly to place, the gingival portion of the band opens up to the correct circumference as determined by the patient's own tooth. The buccal slit is then spot welded or soldered at this point (Fig. 13–14). This reduces unnecessary impingement and irritation of the gingival tissue.

The final trimming and polishing of the gingival periphery of the stainless-steel crowns can be done, and the occlusion should be checked in the centric, working bite and balancing bite positions. The abutment crowns of the space maintainer "open the bite," and the only occlusal contact is made in this area.

This need not concern the dentist because the remaining teeth will quickly erupt to this occlusal level, obviating the necessity of cutting down the abutment teeth. Check again that the space-spanning bar does not contact prematurely. The appliance is cemented to place as a unit, with the bar inserted in the vertical tube.

NONFUNCTIONAL TYPE. The most popular type of nonfunctional space maintainer consists of the same steel crown components as the functional type, but with an intermediate bar or crib arrangement that follows the contour of the tissue (Figs. 13–15, 13–16). If this is designed properly, the tooth for which the space has been maintained erupts between the maintainer arms. In many instances only one crown is made; for example, in the space maintenance for a first deciduous molar. In this case the second deciduous molar may be crowned with a cantilever crib approximating the mucosa and making contact with the deciduous canine tooth. This is less desirable than the 3-unit, non-functional space maintainer. In general, any type of nonfunctional space main-tainer is less desirable than the functional type previously described.

FUNCTIONAL SPACE MAINTAINER

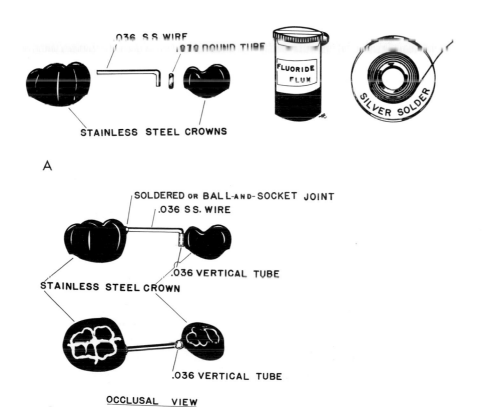

Figure 13–11 Broken stress functional space maintainer. There is freedom of move-ment of the vertical portion of the bar in the vertical tube. For even greater freedom, a ball-and-socket joint may be made where the horizontal end of the bar joins the abut-ment crown. This is usually not necessary, however. The bar should be at the proper occlusal height to prevent overeruption of the opposing tooth.

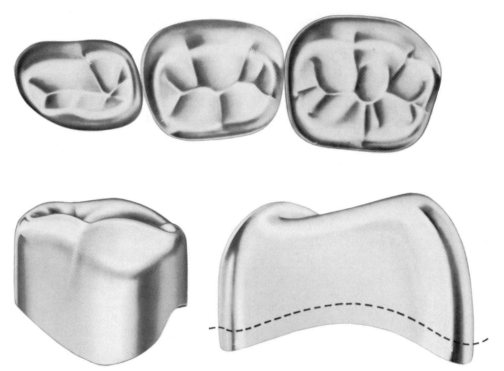

Figure 13–12   Stainless-steel metal crowns make excellent abutments for space maintainers and regainers, habit appliances, partly impacted teeth and broken down teeth that are difficult to band. They are generally superior to orthodontic bands for such purposes and thus are preferred. (Courtesy Unitek Corp.)

One type of nonfunctional space maintainer that permits minor adjustments for space control while the tooth in question is erupting has been designed by W. R. Mayne (Fig. 13–17). Using either an orthodontic band or a full metal crown for the first permanent molar, a 0.036 inch mesially extending cantilever arm initially engages the first deciduous molar. When it is lost, it can be bent to contact the erupting first premolar and to guide it mesially to create adequate space. Minor adjustments may be made on the erupting second premolar, moving it lingually or distally.

CANTILEVER TYPE.   Occasionally a second deciduous molar will be lost before the first permanent molar erupts. The first permanent molar then is likely to erupt mesially to its normal position and to trap the second premolar, with widespread repercussions. There is often a midline shift to the affected side of the arch, the interdigitation of the opposing cusps may be disturbed, and functional prematurities created. It is possible to place a cantilever type space maintainer that will prevent the mesial migration of the first permanent molar and to safeguard the space for the second premolar, thus preserving the integrity of the occlusion (Figs. 13–18, 13–19). A precise radiographic technique is essential in the construction and placement of this type of space maintainer. Periodic radiographic checkups are required to follow the progress of the erupting first molar and second premolar. Occasionally it is necessary to change the design of the space maintainer after the first permanent molar has appeared clinically.[12]

FIXED LINGUAL ARCH.   Where there is bilateral loss of deciduous molars, a fixed lingual arch is often most satisfactory (Fig. 13–20). An impression is

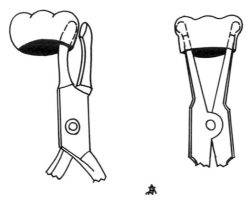

Figure 13–13   In markedly bell-shaped teeth, metal crowns should be contoured by flaring out part of crown at greatest convexity.

made of the involved arch and a model poured in plaster. The gingival portion around the first permanent molars is cut away to the depth of 2 to 3 mm. Metal crowns or orthodontic bands are then fitted carefully. In the mandibular arch the full metal crown is preferred, because the constant pounding of the occlusion on the buccal surface of an orthodontic band tends to break the cement bond, permitting decalcification or the loosening of the appliance itself. Orthodontic bands can be placed on the maxillary first permanent molars with less likelihood of this happening. If the metal crowns are used, the buccal surface should be slit and the crown overlapped when placing the appliance in the mouth. Spot welding is done at the proper circumferential dimension as determined by the tooth. This technique has been described for the fixed functional space maintainer.

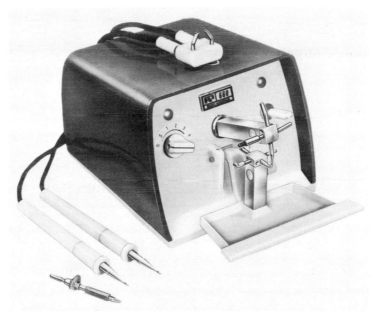

Figure 13–14   Simple type of spot welder, ideal for space maintainers or habit appliances, matrices, etc. (Courtesy Rocky Mountain Dental Products Co.)

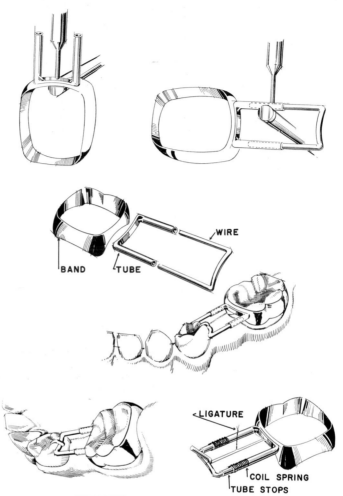

Figure 13–15. Gerber space maintainer. This type of appliance may be fabricated directly in the mouth during one relatively short appointment and requires no laboratory work. A seamless orthodontic band or crown is selected for the abutment tooth and fitted, and the mesial surface is marked for placement of "U" assembly, which may be welded or soldered in place with silver solder and fluoride flux. The wire "U" section is fitted in the tube, the appliance placed and wire section extended to contact the tooth mesial to the edentulous area. A marking file or pencil is used to establish proper position. Assembly is removed and welded or soldered at this point (upper right). Expanded center and lower left views show occlusal rest added to wire section to reduce cantilever effect. If appliance is to be used as a spring-loaded space regainer, tube and wire "U" assembly are not welded. An eyelet may be welded to the flattened part of the tube next to the band; weldable tube stops are soldered on wire portion (lower right); and open coil spring sections are cut to fit over wire between "stops" and ends of "U" tube. The length of the push coil springs is established by placing the band-tube-wire assembly in the mouth, extending the wire to the desired length, in contact with the mesial tooth, and measuring the distance between the tube stops on the wire and the end of the "U" tube. To this distance add the amount of space needed in the regainer, plus 1 to 2 mm. to ensure spring activation, and cut springs to this length. Load springs, tie floss or steel ligature through eyelet and over "U" wire to hold stored force in compressed spring. Be sure to compress springs enough to allow the assembly to fit the edentulous area. After cementation, cut the ligature and remove to activate regainer. (Courtesy Unitek Corp.)

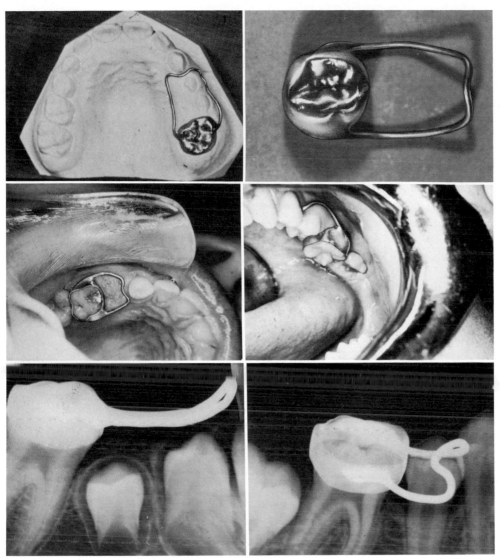

Figure 13–16 Crown-and-crib and band-and-crib cantilever type space maintainers. Crib should follow tissue contour and have enough width buccolingually to allow premolars to erupt unimpeded. In middle and lower right pictures, space maintainer was not removed at the right time. The mesial end is actually trapped beneath the contact in the middle right picture and must be cut apart before removing. (Middle pictures, courtesy W. R. Mayne.)

After the crowns or bands have been fabricated, a 0.036 or 0.040 inch nichrome or stainless steel lingual arch wire is adapted carefully to the cast so that the wire itself is well to the lingual side of where the unerupted teeth are expected to make their clinical entry. The U-shaped portion of the lingual arch wire should rest on the cingulum of each mandibular incisor, if possible, to prevent the mesial tipping of the mandibular first permanent molars and lingual retrusion of the incisors themselves. In both the fixed molar-to-molar and the removable molar-to-molar lingual arches, closer adaptation may be achieved by using the electrodes of an electric welder or electric soldering machine, as shown in Figure 13–21. The carbon electrodes are placed on the lingual wire,

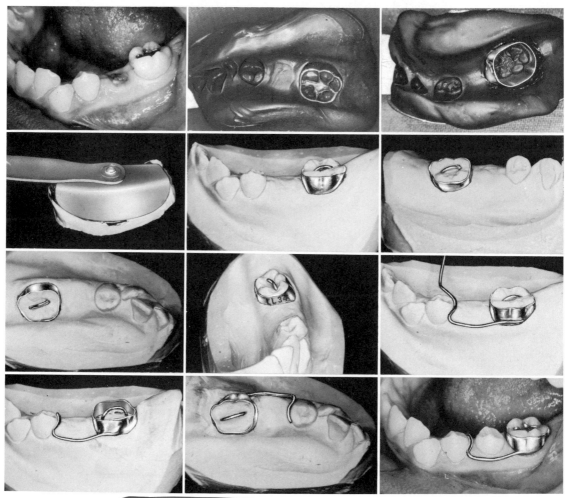

Figure 13–17 (Mayne space maintainer.) Impression is taken with band on first permanent molar. Band is seated in impression (upper left) and poured up in stone after a paper clip reinforcement is placed in compound in the center of the molar band. (See second row as clip protrudes from stone.) Stainless-steel 0.036 inch wire is soldered buccally, bent lingually at the distal surface of the first bicuspid (third row), clipped lingually distal to the first bicuspid, and polished. Wire may be bent to move bicuspid mesially to regain space for erupting second bicuspid. The same construction would work if the mesial tooth were a first deciduous molar. Design does not interfere with eruption of permanent successor. Disadvantage is that retainer is nonfunctional, but this is of no concern if occlusion prevents overeruption of opposing tooth. (Courtesy W. R. Mayne.)

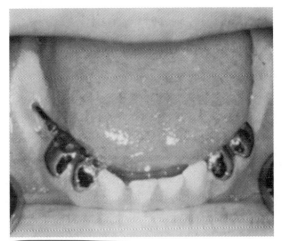

Figure 13–18 Cantilever type space maintainer where the tooth approximating the area of premature loss has not erupted. The two abutments are either cast together or soldered to form a "bulkhead attachment." The distal vertical flattened arm enters the tissue just mesial to the first permanent molar and engages the mesial surface of this tooth. The maintainer will be modified after molar eruption. (From Olsen, N. H.: Space maintenance. D. Clin. North America, July, 1959.)

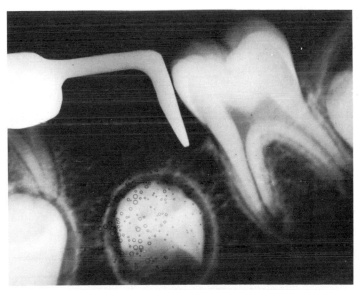

Figure 13–19 A periapical radiograph is required before cementation, to be sure that the distal vertical arm is in correct relationship to the mesial marginal ridge of the unerupted tooth. (From Olsen, N. H., Space maintenance. D. Clin. North America, July, 1959.)

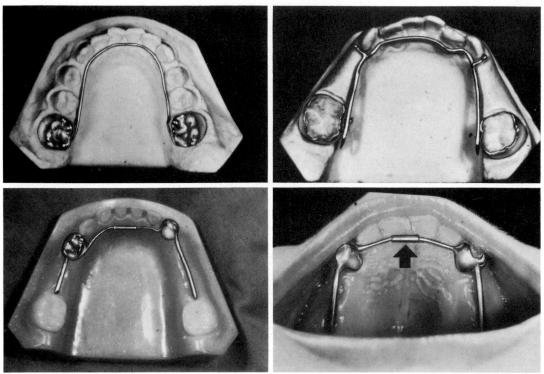

Figure 13–20 Mershon type lingual arch (upper left and right). Spurs distal to canines (right) will be cut when premolars erupt. Cantilever design (lower left) is less desirable. As soon as first molars erupt sufficiently, they should be banded and a union made between the bar and the bands. Note the sleeve arrangements in both lower pictures to allow lateral growth. In the picture on the lower right, the posterior bars are functional and soldered to crowns at the mesial of the first permanent molars.

and the wire between the electrodes is allowed to heat to a dull red to permit better adaptation and relief of stresses. The electrodes are carried around the arch in successive steps, repeating the heat treatment. In this manner, a passive lingual arch is ensured. There is considerable danger that the molar teeth will move, or at least be subjected to undue trauma unless this step is done. This is particularly true in the fixed-removable type of lingual arch where it is difficult to obtain a perfect alignment of tube and post in a completely passive state.

In the maxillary arch, the lingual wire can follow the palatal contour, lingual to where the mandibular incisors occlude during the centric and working bite positions (Fig. 13–20). After the lingual wire has been adapted carefully, the free ends are soldered to the lingual surfaces of the crowns or bands using a fluoride flux and silver solder. The appliance is then polished and cleaned for cementation. The patient should be checked periodically subsequent to the placement of the space maintainer to make sure that the lingual wire is not interfering with the normal eruption of the canine and premolar teeth. At times, mastication causes the maxillary lingual arch to impinge on palatal tissue and to incite proliferation which "buries" the anterior portion of the arch. The wire may then be bent away from the palatal tissue without removing the appliance, if care is exercised.

FIXED-REMOVABLE LINGUAL ARCH. Although a soldered molar-to-molar lingual arch is more stable, it is also less versatile. Various horizontal or vertical attachments are available, permitting the dentist to remove and adjust the lingual

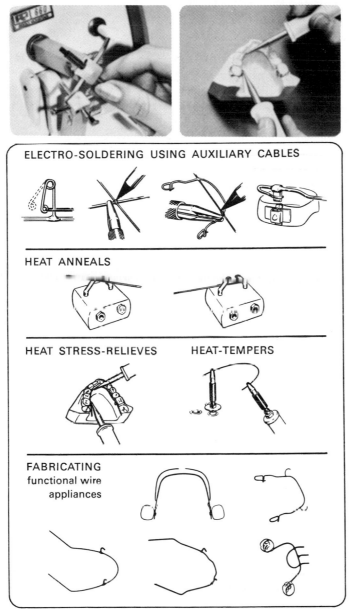

ELECTRO-SOLDERING USING AUXILIARY CABLES

HEAT ANNEALS

HEAT STRESS-RELIEVES   HEAT-TEMPERS

FABRICATING
functional wire
appliances

Figure 13–21   Some of the auxiliary uses of a spot welder, such as shown in Figure 13–14. (Courtesy Rocky Mountain Dental Products Co.)

(Mershon) arch. The most widely used attachment is the half-round tube and post arrangement which is designed to allow the vertical removal of the lingual appliance. The technique of fabrication is illustrated and described in Figures 13–22 and 13–23. The arch is held in place by a locking spring which fits under the gingival end of the vertical half-round tube. To remove the appliance, the spring is merely adjusted lingually on its free end with a heavy scaler, allowing the post to withdraw from the tube. After the lingual arch is replaced, the spring is pushed back underneath the tube with an amalgam plugger. As Figure 13–23 shows, auxiliary springs may be added for space control.

REMOVAL OF FIXED MAINTAINERS. The prolonged retention of a functional type fixed maintainer prevents the full eruption of the tooth beneath it and may deflect this tooth to the buccal or the lingual aspects. Special precautions must be taken with the use of the cantilever type space maintainer. As the tooth to which it is anchored becomes progressively looser due to resorption and the pounding of functional forces, the free end of the bar traumatizes the tissue where it is buried, and it can cause bone destruction at the mesial portion of the first permanent molar. If this happens well in advance of the expected eruption of the second premolar, then a new space maintainer of a different type, incorporating the first permanent molar, should be placed. In no event should this type of space maintainer be allowed to remain after the clinical appearance of the second premolar. In the case of the nonfunctional type of space maintainer, it can be a bit embarrassing to have the patient return with the tooth or teeth erupted and the free arm buried in the interproximal tissue (Figs. 13–16, 13–24).

Where orthodontic bands are used for abutment teeth, particularly in the mandibular arch, the cement can be "washed out" by the pounding of occlusal forces, allowing debris to collect and causing decalcification or caries beneath the band. Prolonged retention of a space maintainer enhances this possibility. Thus, the proper timing of the removal of a space maintainer is not much less important than the selection of a proper time for its placement. If the patient fails to keep a recall appointment, it is the responsibility of the dentist to see that the parent is informed of the importance of periodic checkups and of the possible damage that may occur if the appliance is left in too long.

Many space maintainers are made by laboratory technicians totally unaware of the demands of retention, function and the overall occlusal picture. It is no wonder that the situations illustrated in Figure 13–24 occur. Complete responsibility for the design of the space maintainer should remain with the dentist.

REMOVABLE SPACE MAINTAINERS

Removable types of space maintainers have certain definite advantages. Being tissue-borne, they impose less stress on the remaining teeth. They can be functional in the truest sense. By virtue of their tissue stimulation in the edentulous area, they often accelerate the eruption of the teeth beneath them. Usually they are considerably more esthetic than the fixed type space maintainer (Fig. 13–9). They are easier to fabricate, requiring less chair time. They are generally easier to keep clean. They cannot be left in too long, in contrast with the fixed type space maintainer. On the liability side are the greater dependence on the patient's cooperation, the bigger chance of loss or breakage, and a little more trouble for the patient to get used to them when they are placed initially. Oral hygiene can be a problem with removable appliances, too, if they are not removed and cleaned routinely. Occasionally a combination

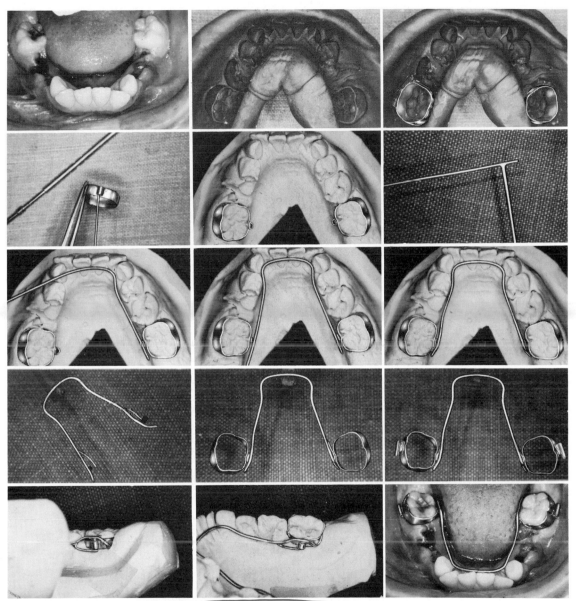

Figure 13–22   Fabrication of lower fixed-lingual retainer. Impression is taken with molar bands in place, seated in impression (top, right) and poured up in stone. Second row illustrates half round tubes and post material. After post is soldered to 0.040 nichrome or stainless-steel lingual arch wire, post is cut off at proper length, inserted in one half-round tube, and arch wire is formed to approximate the lingual surfaces. Note position of wire on cinguli of incisors (third row). Second half-round tube is soldered on opposite side and arch wire is inserted in tubes and checked for parallelism. Locking springs are soldered on arch (fourth row) and buccal tubes may also be welded or soldered, if needed later. Lingual lock and half-round tube detail are shown in bottom row. Appliance is then cemented to place. (Courtesy W. R. Mayne.)

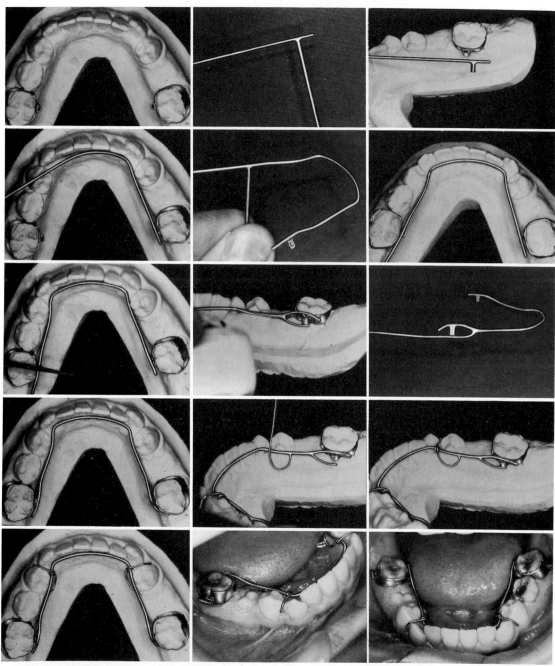

Figure 13–23   Fabrication of lower fixed lingual space maintainer to permit insertion and removal by virtue of half-round tube and post on lingual side of molar bands. Using post material makes it easier to solder than with precut posts (top row). Posts are then cut with separating disks at proper length. Locking mechanism (third and fourth rows) may come around mesial or distal aspect, to hold post in tube. Proper placement of posts is assured by marking arch with file before soldering second post (third row). Finger springs may be added on. Wrap-around loop type is preferred to give maximum spring and minimum distortion (fourth and fifth rows). Buccal tubes may be placed on molar bands, if orthodontic therapy is likely later. (Courtesy W. R. Mayne.)

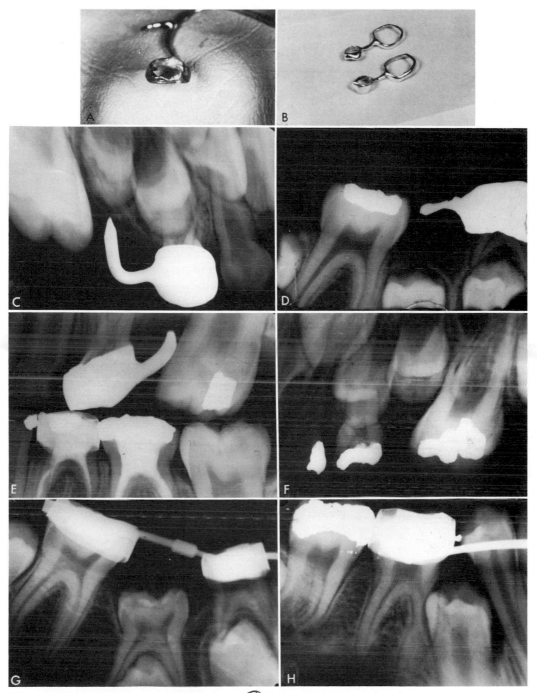

Figure 13-24   Inept space maintenance. A, Space maintainer placed with too narrow gingivo-occlusal dimension and totally inadequate retention. Appliance would not stay in. B, Poorly designed and executed space maintainers. Castings are so narrow gingivo-occlusally that cement cannot hold them under the stress of mastication. C, Cantilever "shoe" is too short and of no service. Radiograph suggests that serial extraction may be needed. D and E, Poorly made space maintainers that serve no purpose. F is same case as in E, with maintainer removed. This is obviously a serial extraction problem and no space maintainer should have been placed at all. G, Space maintainer over ankylosed second deciduous molar. Since no radiograph had been taken by dentist, he was unaware of this situation. H, Space maintainer was placed too late and tooth sacrifice is now indicated.

fixed and removable appliance is indicated. The use of partial or full crowns with lugs to assist in the retention of the removable appliance increases the functional efficiency of the removable space maintainer (Fig. 13–25). These appliances become in essence removable partial dentures, requiring the same high degree of attention to soft tissues, occlusion, and so forth, that the dentist gives his adult prosthetic patients.

TREATMENT FOR CARIES: A PREVENTIVE ORTHODONTIC PROCEDURE

Ordinarily, the dentist would not think of restoration of lost tooth material as an orthodontic consideration. But restorations can be and often are to the detriment of the teeth and investing tissues. The "snap ligature" concept of restorative dentistry can make a malocclusion out of a normal occlusion. It is imperative that the proper mesiodistal dimension of the restored teeth be maintained. It is common practice to place a gutta-percha or temporary stopping filling until the permanent restoration can be inserted. The pounding of the occlusion on this rubbery mass serves to increase the arch length at this point. If the permanent restoration perpetuates this arch length increase, there will be a break in the arch continuity at this point or somewhere else—usually in the anterior segment. An additional danger is the use of a mechanical separator to allow the placing of the restoration matrix. Frequently the teeth are not only driven apart in a mesiodistal direction, but they are elongated into positions of premature contact. The permanent restoration perpetuates the traumatic posi-

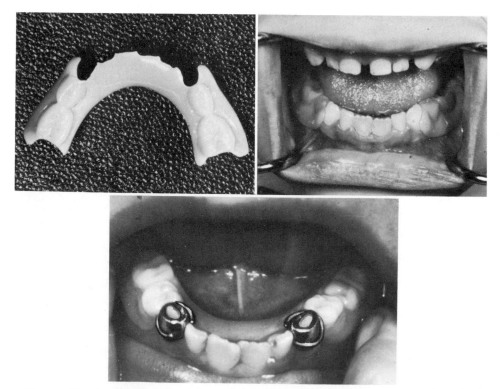

Figure 13–25   Removable space maintainers. Crowning abutment teeth and placing lugs on the buccal surface increases retention of clasps from removable appliance (lower view).

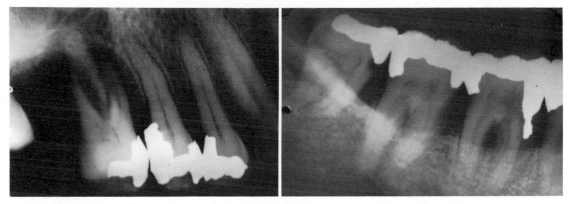

Figure 13–26 Advanced periodontal breakdown, at least partly attributable to overextension of proximal restorations and to amalgam overhang.

tion and the investing tissues suffer accordingly. The dentist must be careful not to overseparate teeth, either by the use of temporary filling materials that are "high" or by mechanical separation. Proper mesiodistal dimension is essential (Fig. 13–26). It is not too much to expect the dentist to record the original mesiodistal dimension after making the measurement with a pair of fine-line dividers. A millimeter overextension on a restoration can have far-reaching effects, particularly if there are three or four proximal restorations in one segment. The "ping" of the ligature snapping through the newly established contact may sound most pleasant to the operator. The "ring" of the advice of an orthodontist to the patient at a later date will be considerably less pleasant (Fig. 7–78).

The contact size and position are no less important than the correct mesiodistal dimension. Improperly placed contact points or points that have become surfaces aggravate a developing malocclusion. Underextension can be as bad as overextension, allowing drift of contiguous teeth, packing of food, etc. The dentist has very little latitude in making the proper size correction. There are thousands of people today with crowded mandibular incisors, functional prematurities and traumatic occlusion resulting from improper mechanical "filling of the holes." Also important is the re-establishment of the proper inclined plane relationship as restorations are placed. The anatomic carving of the restoration thus has more than an esthetic appeal. Normal function may demand it; stability of the occlusion requires it.[13]

RELATION OF ORAL HABITS TO PREVENTION OF MALOCCLUSION

Chapter 14 will deal in greater detail with the subjects of finger and thumb sucking and abnormal lip and tongue activity where, as interceptive procedures, appliances are necessary to prevent further damage and allow autonomous correction of the developing malocclusion. In the present chapter on preventive procedures we assume that the child has a normal occlusion. But, as pointed out in Chapter 6, prevention starts with proper nursing, proper choice of a physiologically designed nursing nipple and pacifier to enhance normal function and deglutitional maturation. Proper kinesthetic, neuromuscular gratificational activity at this time may well prevent abnormal finger, lip and tongue deforming action later.

It is just as important to see that the surrounding soft tissues maintain normal development and function as it is to watch for normal development in the teeth and bone. A loose tooth, a high restoration or a prematurely lost tooth can initiate an abnormal muscular "tic" or habit which can cause a malocclusion. Constant tongue thrust into an edentulous area may cause an open bite that remains in the permanent dentition. There are tongue exercises that may prevent a malocclusion, by ensuring the normal deglutitional maturation.[13, 14] (See Chap. 6.) An uncomfortable oral condition frequently stimulates a child to place his fingers in his mouth, and this can well lead to finger sucking or nail biting which endanger the normal development of the occlusion. It behooves the prudent dentist to question the parent and patient carefully about all abnormal eating, speaking and swallowing habits. Warning the patient about possible ill effects is frequently sufficient to stop the habit before it becomes permanently harmful. If, for example, the youngster has the tendency to bite on his lower lip as a means of releasing excess energy or nervous tension, the dentist can prescribe lip exercises of short duration on arising and before retiring which may serve as an effective tensional release (Fig. 13–27). Where there is a general flaccidity of perioral musculature, blowing exercises may stimulate normal activity. In conjunction with a speech therapist, the dentist may work with the child on tongue position[13, 14] Many a lisp is intimately tied to a tongue thrust habit that is also working against the normal eruption of the anterior teeth. Nail biting need not create malocclusions, but in conjunction with other predetermining factors it may be contributory. Thus, nail biting should be on the dentist's check list. If the dentist has the patient's confidence and respect, his influence can be considerable as he cooperates with the parents to eliminate these annoying roadblocks to their child's psychological and social maturity.

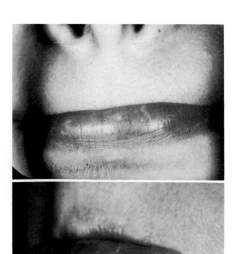

Figure 13–27 The "T" zone. Children's tensions that so often lead to muscle tics or undesirable perioral habits, such as finger sucking, lip biting, nail biting, cheek sucking, bruxism and clenching, find effective release in this lip exercise, where the upper lip is sucked down and contracted against the maxillary anterior segment, with the lower lip placed on top and pressed against the upper lip. Fifteen to 30 minutes a day serves as a preventive orthodontic procedure in children with short, hypotonic upper lips.

OCCLUSAL EQUILIBRATION IN THE PRIMARY AND MIXED DENTITIONS: A PREVENTIVE ORTHODONTIC PROCEDURE

In line with the organization of orthodontic service into three basic categories — preventive, interceptive and corrective — occlusal adjustment through judicious grinding is included here as a preventive orthodontic procedure. This does not mean that it is any less important as an interceptive adjunct (the actual technique of equilibration is discussed in detail in Chapter 14 under Equilibration of Occlusal Disharmonies). But the old axiom, "An ounce of prevention is worth a pound of cure," is apropos. Discovering occlusal disharmonies *before* they have had a chance to create malocclusions is entirely within the realm of day-to-day practice for the discerning, able dentist. Although there is a psychogenic component to bruxism, functional prematurities are significant causative agents. All functional disturbances should be eliminated. The wearing of a bite plate at night will do little good unless occlusal aberrations are removed during the day. Routine diagnostic records, like plaster casts, dental radiographs and recording of clinical signs as the patient closes from postural resting position to full occlusion, provide many clues. To augment these diagnostic armamentaria a thorough knowledge of just what is normal, a sensitive set of finger tips, some very thin articulating paper and some soft baseplate wax will be found of value (see Chap. 14).

Functional prematurities are frequent in the primary dentition.[15] Most of these are transitory and incident to the eruptive process. After the deciduous teeth have achieved full occlusal contact, however, they should be checked carefully. Beginning functional interferences, precursors to mandibular shifts or crossbites may be observed quite early. Following the technique outlined in the next chapter, articulating paper and a wax bite will quickly call attention to questionable cusps or inclined planes. An analysis of facets of wear of erupted teeth will provide additional information. One should not wait until a frank malocclusion exists. The occlusal dynamics should be "checked out" each time young child patients are recalled. A few moments of selective grinding may prevent countless hours of orthodontic mechanotherapy later on. Particularly important is a careful analysis of occlusal relationships following the placing of proximal restorations. Overextended restorations or overly tight or misplaced contacts may cause elongation and trauma to the affected tooth.

DISKING

Closely related to occlusal equilibration is the occasional need for disking of oversized first or second deciduous molars to allow eruption of contiguous permanent teeth. If it appears, for example, that a maxillary canine will not have quite enough space in the dental arch and it will thus erupt to the labial side and if the second deciduous molars are large and firm with the second premolars not ready to erupt, the needed arch length may be obtained by slicing the proximal end of the second molar. This "robbing Peter to pay Paul" procedure (Figs. 13–28, 13–29) is effective if the timing is good. If the roots of the second deciduous molar are fairly well resorbed, however, it is preferable to remove the tooth a little ahead of time.

In instances where second premolars are congenitally missing and second deciduous molars are retained, there is, of course, an increase in arch length because of the greater mesiodistal width of the molar tooth. To prevent a break in contact or rotation of the incisor teeth, the second deciduous molar can be

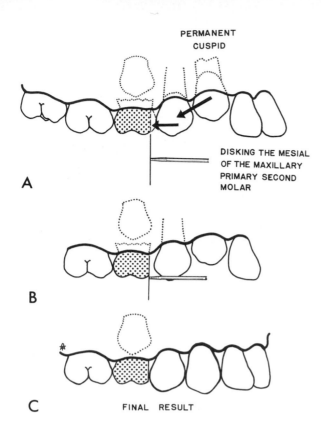

A

B

C FINAL RESULT

PERMANENT
CUSPID

DISKING THE MESIAL
OF THE MAXILLARY
PRIMARY SECOND
MOLAR

Figure 13–28 Disking of a large second deciduous molar to provide needed arch length for eruption of the permanent canine. Similar procedures are recommended where the second premolar is congenitally missing and the second deciduous molar occupies more space than its successor normally would. (After H. P. Hitchcock.)

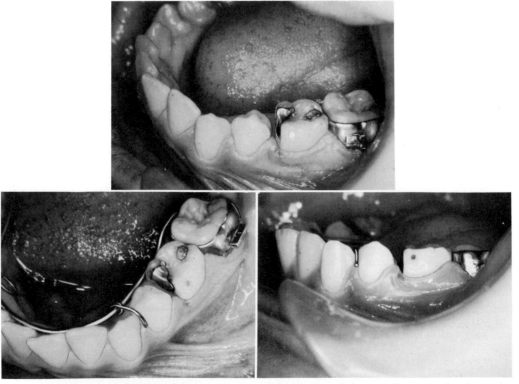

Figure 13–29 An example of space maintenance with a lower molar-to-molar lingual arch, together with disking of the second deciduous molar on the mesial aspect, to allow the first premolar to erupt. Note the spur distal to the canine (lower pictures) to maintain space. (Courtesy W. R. Mayne.)

664

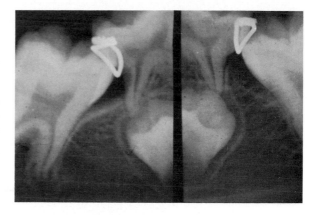

Figure 13–30 Large second deciduous molars, with marked distal convexity, blocking eruption of first permanent molars. Before disking the distal of the second deciduous molar (Fig. 13–28), brass separation wire tightly wrapped around the deciduous molar-first permanent molar contact may force the erupting tooth enough to the distal to by-pass the contact convexity. Disking should be tried only if this procedure does not work.

reduced in width by disking so that it approximates the size of its missing successor. The situation is analogous to overextended proximal restorations, which create the same break in arch continuity.

A large second deciduous molar may interfere with normal eruption of the permanent first molars. Sometimes the use of brass separating wire wrapped tightly around the contacts will force the erupting first molar enough distally to slip past the contact convexity of the second deciduous molar (Fig. 13–30). (The separating wire technique is illustrated in detail in Chap. 14, Figs. 14–6 to 14–9.)

THE LABIAL FRENUM

With the newborn, the labial frenum is literally attached to the crest of the alveolar ridge. In the normal course of events as the teeth erupt and as alveolar bone is laid down to increase the vertical dimension, the frenum attachment gradually migrates superiorly with respect to the ridge. A careful dissection would show that the fibers from this attachment could be traced through the mucosa between the maxillary central incisors and into the lingual papilla. Often the fibers approximate or actually insert into the intermaxillary suture. In the early years, the frenum fibers normally terminate in this manner so that a strong pull on the upper lip will elicit a blanching of the tissue lingual to the upper incisors. Ordinarily, the fibers are confined to a rather narrow band and are not heavy enough to materially influence the incisor position. In some individuals, however, this band of nonelastic, unyielding fibers is heavier and serves as a barrier to mesial migration of the central incisors during eruption, leaving a diastema of noticeable proportion.

Frenum diastemas are frequently hereditary. This does not mean that if a space exists between the incisors in the parent the child will always have a similar space; nor does the mere fact that the frenum is attached between the spaced incisors prove it causes the space. Some observers consider the spacing itself the hereditary characteristic and the presence of the frenum incidental. They feel that the fibers that anchor lingually to the incisors remain intact because there has not been any pressure from the central incisors moving toward the midline. In other words, is the diastema there because of the frenum or is the frenum there because of the diastema? (See Chap. 7.) It is not possible to solve this "chicken and egg dilemma" (Fig. 13–31). Very likely, both are part of an overall pattern and neither is completely dependent on the other.

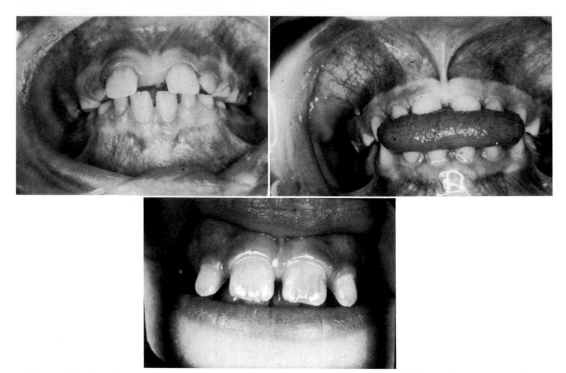

Figure 13–31   Diastemas (upper left) are not always associated with heavy frenum attachments (upper right). The tongue may also be a factor (right) or spacing may be a transient developmental phenomenon (lower). (Upper pictures, courtesy W. R. Mayne.)

Wanton clipping of the labial frenum is akin to the needless removal of tonsils which will regress spontaneously later, if left alone. Yet millions of tonsils have been parted from their owners. There are certainly more factors causing maxillary incisor diastemas than the labial frenum. Weber lists microdontia, macrognathia, supernumerary teeth (especially the mesiodens), peg laterals, missing lateral incisors, heavy occlusion of the lower incisors against the lingual surfaces of the upper incisors, midline cysts and such habits as thumb sucking, tongue thrust, lip sucking or biting. (See Chaps. 6 and 14.)[2]

From a hereditary standpoint, however, there is a strong tendency for the reopening of an anterior diastema, even after orthodontic closure and prolonged retention, even when the frenum fibers are dissected from the lingual attachment. As one of the facets of preventive orthodontic service, the dentist should prepare to judge the role of the frenum for each patient where there is an anterior diastema. As he observes his child patients routinely, he should carefully check the frenum attachment in each one and record any unusually heavy attachments (see Chap. 7). Where there is a hereditary diastema, as evidenced by spacing in the mouth of parents or siblings, it is good preventive orthodontics in selected cases after specialty consultation to carefully dissect the frenum fibers from the crest of the alveolar ridge. In many instances the incisors will migrate together autonomously as the canines erupt.[16] Even where the space does not close fully, simple orthodontic procedures may complete the closure with a reasonable chance of success, provided that the occlusion is normal otherwise. As with space maintenance, an error of commission is better than an error of omission. Before stepping in with surgery, however, one should be sure that the diastema is not a transient "ugly duckling" stage of development as the canines and lateral incisors maneuver for erupting space in the alveolar process (Fig. 13–31). If there is any doubt, one must wait until the permanent canines have fully erupted before incising the frenum.

PREVENTION OF DEFORMATION OF THE DENTITION BY MILWAUKEE BRACE TREATMENT

The effect of pressures on growing bone has been discussed in Chapter 2. The severe deformation of teeth and jaws by an orthopedic appliance used to correct idiopathic scoliosis of the spine is also illustrated. To prevent these iatrogenic malocclusions, the dentist should establish a "hot-line" with the orthopedic surgeon—and orthodontist. Specially designed intraoral splints, activators, positioners and dentofacial orthopedic appliances may prevent malocclusion, or at least reduce the deleterious effects. Modified Hawley bite-plates, described in greater detail in Chapter 16, are often effective. Most important is the proper use of the Milwaukee brace itself, with a two-finger space between the chin rest and the mandible and not the 5 to 6 pounds of constant pressure applied by an overly extended brace, as has too often been the case in the past.[17, 18]

REFERENCES

1. Leighton, B. C.: The early signs of malocclusion. Trans. Eur. Orth. Soc., 353–368, 1969.
2. Weber, F. N.: Orthodontic education for the nonorthodontist: why, where, and how. Am. J. Orthodont., 48:436–443, 1962.
3. Daughtry, C. W.: Mixed dentition guidance. S. Carolina Dent. J., 28:4–13, 1970.
4. Wilding, R. J. C.: Early loss of deciduous teeth. A review of the literature. Diastema, 2:57–58, 1969.
5. Au, E. T. K.: The effect of premature loss of primary and permanent teeth. J. Hawaii Dent. Ass., 2:9–12, 1969.
6. Leighton, B. C.: The value of prophecy in orthodontics. Dent. Pract., 21:359–372, 1971.
7. Gecker, L. M., and Weil, R. B.: The family dentist's opportunity to preserve normal occlusion. New York J. Dent., 40:57–60, 1970.
8. Engh, O.: Space maintainers. When and how. Norske Tannlaegeforen. Tids., 80:81–90, 1970.
9. Owen, D. G.: The incidence and nature of space closure following the premature extraction of deciduous teeth. Am. J. Orthodont., 59:37–49, 1971.
10. Chitre, D. A., and Shourie, K. L.: The effect of premature loss of deciduous molars and role of space maintainers. J. Indian Orthodont., 1:12–14, 1968.
11. Sake, H.: The use of removable space maintainers and their retainers in pedodontics. Shikwa Gaku., 69:169–176, 1969.
12. Olsen, N. H.: Pediatric dentistry in Grabb, W. C., Rosenstein, S. W., and Bzoch, K. R. (eds.): Cleft Lip and Palate. Boston, Little, Brown and Co., 1971.
13. Rinderer, L.: Care of the deciduous teeth, orthodontic diagnosis and treatment expectations. Rev. Belg. Med. Dent., 24:123–128, 1969.
14. Garliner, D.: Some ancillary results of the correction of abnormal swallowing habits. New York J. Dent., 39:158–164, 1969.
15. West, E. E.: Treatment objectives in the deciduous dentition. Am. J. Orthodont., 55:617–632, 1969.
16. Dausch-Neumann, D.: Diastema with missing deciduous incisors. Fortschr. Kieferorthop., 30:82–88, 1969.
17. Freunthaller, P.: Prevention of deformation of the dentition by Milwaukee brace treatment. Oest. Z. Stomat., 64:89–93, 1967.
18. Stöckli, P., and Gisler, G.: Ergebnisse kieferorthopädischer Begleitbehandlung bei Skoliosepatienten. Deutsch. Zahn. Mund. Kieferheilk., 52:1–8, 1969.

chapter 14

INTERCEPTIVE ORTHODONTICS

A number of procedures were described in Chapter 13 that could very well be called interceptive. The criterion for selecting the problems discussed in Chapter 13, however, was that the occlusion was within normal limits at that time, and those procedures were intended to keep it that way. In the present chapter, a number of procedures will be described to intercept a malocclusion that *has already developed* or is developing, and the goal is to restore a normal occlusion. In many instances the problems discussed in Chapter 13 are the beginning stages of a number of the problems discussed in this chapter. For this reason, a certain amount of repetition is necessary.

The difference between preventive and interceptive orthodontics lies in the timing of the services rendered. In interceptive orthodontics the dentist is dealing with malocclusion as a *fait accompli*, at least to a minor degree. If he renders the proper service with dispatch, autonomous adjustment will restore normal occlusion. If he waits too long, then there is no question that he must resort to the limited corrective orthodontic procedures described in Chapters 16 and 17. More likely, comprehensive orthodontic service will be necessary and requires the efforts of the specialist.

DEVELOPMENTAL SCHEDULE OR TIMETABLE MAINTENANCE

Timing and degree of interception are the main problems at this stage. An abnormal resorption or eruption pattern has already created a malocclusion. The dentist must eliminate the causes, and if self-adjustment cannot restore normal occlusion, he must resort to limited corrective procedures. The removal of supernumerary teeth, the elimination of bony or tissue barriers to erupting teeth, the removal of ankylosed teeth—these are interceptive procedures as well as preventive procedures (Chap. 13) within the realm of general dental service (Fig. 14-1).[18] Study models and full dental radiographs or a panoramic radiograph are essential. A conference with the parents and with the patient, stressing the need

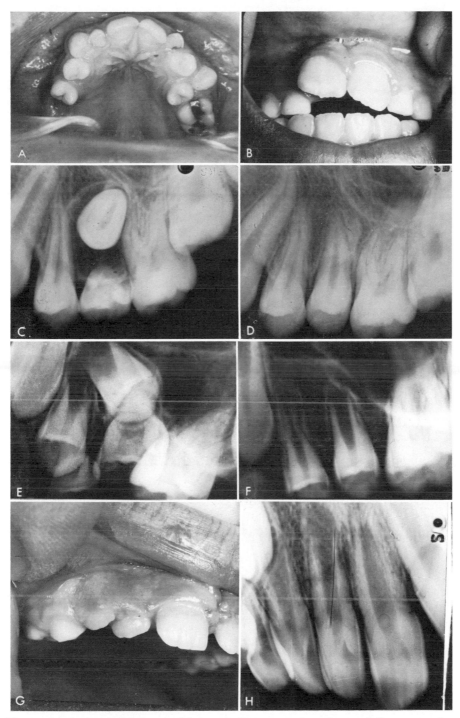

Figure 14–1 Interceptive problems. A, Transposed canine and first premolar and drifting of contiguous teeth make a crippling malocclusion that could have been prevented largely by interceptive orthodontics. B, A long active finger habit could have been intercepted before the anterior open bite was created. C, The removal of a coronal cyst and retained deciduous molar allowed the second premolar to turn around and erupt down into normal position (D), while a similar interceptive approach (E and F) removed an ankylosed molar, permitting normal eruption of the premolar beneath. G and H, The erupting supernumerary lateral incisor should be removed immediately to allow normal eruption of the canine. (Pictures C and D, courtesy H. Fischer.)

for continuing service and explaining the essential dental facts so that they understand the services rendered, is equally important.

EQUILIBRATION OF OCCLUSAL DISHARMONIES

Premature contacts that have not been eliminated in their incipiency (Chap. 13) can develop into tooth guidance problems, with both the mandible and the individual teeth reflecting the abnormal function. To check on occlusal harmony or lack of harmony, the patient should be observed carefully as he closes from wide-open mouth to postural resting position and, more particularly, from postural resting position to full occlusion. (See Chap. 3 on Physiology of the Stomatognathic System and Chap. 9 on Unfavorable Sequelae of Malocclusion.) Postural resting position is a balanced, unstrained relationship of mandibular condyle, articular disk, articular eminence, articular capsular structures and ligaments, and of the controlling musculature. This balanced relation should not be disturbed as the mandible moves into full occlusal contact. In other words, habitual occlusal position should be the same as centric occlusal position and one of a number of possible centric relations. This is not true in many types of malocclusions, and more than occlusal equilibration is necessary to correct them. But with a normal occlusion, selective grinding may make the difference between normal and pathologic supporting tissue response.

ANTERIOR MANDIBULAR DISPLACEMENT.   One form of tooth guidance in the deciduous and mixed dentition is the anterior mandibular displacement. The patient closes from physiologic resting to point of initial contact (premature contact in this case). At initial contact there is an edge-to-edge incisal relationship usually due to lingual malposition of the maxillary incisors or incipient mandibular prognathism. Since the maxillary incisors are literally " in the way," and the posterior teeth still out of contact, the condyle slides forward on the articular eminence and the posterior teeth make occlusal contact as the labial-incisal margin of the maxillary incisors glides down the lingual surfaces of the mandibular incisors (Fig. 11–62). By beveling the labial incisal of the mandibular incisors and the lingual incisal of the maxillary incisors a more nearly correct overjet is established (Fig. 14–2). The mandibular thrust no longer occurs from the point of initial contact to full occlusion. The dentist must be quite sure, however, that he is not dealing with a true Class III malocclusion and that this is indeed a convenience swing because of local tooth guidance. Otherwise, the grinding will do little more than impose excessive trauma on the maxillary and mandibular incisors. In many instances limited orthodontic procedures are required in conjunction with occlusal equilibration. There is some indication that these patients are more prone to bruxism, and the patient may already have "ground" his dentition into a neutral bite, eliminating the functional aberrations.

In the deciduous dentition the flatter inclined planes are less likely to cause tooth guidance than the steeper planes in the permanent dentition, but it can happen. The dentist must make sure that there are no anomalous enamel "pearls" or morphologic variations that can cause a malocclusion.

CROSS-BITE CONDITIONS.   Tooth guidance can also deflect the mandible laterally or posteriorly as well as anteriorly, in the initial contact—full occlusion range. Where there has been a prolonged finger sucking habit, with associated perioral muscle forces of abnormal functional character, the maxillary arch is frequently narrowed and a unilateral cross-bite is common on the left or right side.

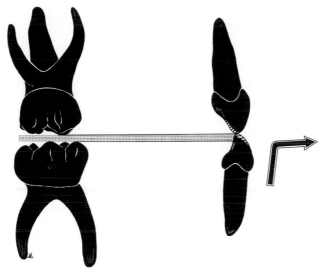

INITIAL CONTACT — PREMATURE CONTACT

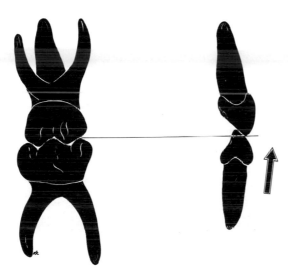

INITIAL CONTACT — CENTRIC OCCLUSION

Figure 14–2 Occlusal equilibration for pseudo Class III malocclusion in the deciduous dentition. Tooth guidance and an anterior mandibular thrust can be eliminated, restoring a normal path of closure.

Careful study shows that narrowing is usually bilateral and the cross-bite is a convenience swing to one side or the other. Prolonged cross-bite conditions also accentuate individual tooth malpositions so that asymmetry of the arch becomes a fact. In the initial stages, however, the upper arch can be quite symmetrical despite the cross-bite. The belief is widespread that unless these cross-bites are eliminated, not only will they lead to asymmetry of the dental arches, but an actual facial asymmetry may result in the adult. Obviously, cross-bites should be eliminated whenever possible. A number of these cross-bites require corrective procedures, which will be described in detail in Chapter 17. In some of them, however, judicious occlusal grinding is enough to eliminate the guiding force.

Since a "high" tooth can cause a deflection of the mandible during closure, calling for certain proprioceptive responses and a learned pattern of activity, the elimination of the inciting factor breaks the proprioceptive pattern and permits re-direction of the manifold associated forces toward a normal path of closure and centric relationship.

AIDS TO EQUILIBRATION

The following armamentaria are recommended for occlusal equilibration:

1. Ultra-thin articulating paper.
2. Sheet baseplate wax (soft).
3. Anatomic articulator to mount study casts.
4. Small, round, pear-shaped and knife-edged mounted stones for both straight handpiece and contra-angle handpiece.
5. Pumice-impregnated disks, or pumice and rubber cups on a mandrel.

To better use these aids, a sensitive set of finger tips is most valuable to check for excessive mobility as the patient taps in habitual centric, balancing and working bites. A good sense of hearing helps pick up "double-taps" and mushy contacts, when interferences or tooth guidances exist. A stethoscope placed on each temporomandibular joint will record crepitus or clicking, though this can be felt in most instances by placing the finger tips gently in front of the patient's ear. A wax bite taken in full habitual occlusion is a good place to start after it has been determined that equilibration is indicated. A sheet of baseplate wax is softened, bent over on itself and shaped roughly into a paraboloid form following the dental arch contour (see Chap. 8). The softened wax is placed over the maxillary occlusal surfaces, and the patient bites directly into it into full habitual occlusion. The wax is chilled and then examined by holding it up to the light. Where the wax has been completely perforated, one should check for a premature contact. Articulating paper will assist in establishing the exact contact area for opposing teeth, marking the cusps and planes involved. These same areas should then be marked on the study casts which have been mounted on an anatomic articulator, and the teeth and cusps should be noted on the patient's written record for future reference. It is wise to scrape away the apparent prematurities on the study casts to make sure that one is on the right track. Only then should the actual teeth be equilibrated.

The dentist, when working intraorally, should always proceed slowly and remove only a slight amount at a time, rechecking by using articulating paper and by having the patient tap his teeth together lightly. In a malocclusion with premature contacts, a mushy, dull thud or double tap is heard as the patient brings his teeth together, in contrast with a crisp and a sharp retort from all the teeth contacting at the same time in normal centric occlusion. The teeth are carefully palpated in each segment as the patient taps them together over and over. By doing this repeatedly, the dentist soon learns which teeth are under premature stress and which are excessively mobile, corroborating the auditory observation. Constant articulating paper checks are necessary to verify the auditory and digital study.

In the primary dentition the tooth guidance usually requires less spot grinding than later on to establish a normal relationship. Inclined planes are not as deep and, in conjunction with growth and development, the adjustment to a new position is comparatively easy. In the mixed dentition, greater care must be exercised to avoid removing too much tooth material from the permanent teeth.

If orthodontic therapy is contemplated, equilibration should be withheld until the desired tooth position is obtained. Most competent orthodontists carefully check the occlusion and equilibrate their finished result to enhance the stability of the therapeutic objective. In the permanent dentition even greater dependence must be placed on articulated study models, and a careful plan must be evolved before instituting the actual grinding procedures. Checking for interference must be extended to an analysis of the "working bite" and the "balancing bite." The most careful auditory, digital, wax and articulating paper records should be obtained before the grinding procedure.

While the detailed techniques of occlusal equilibration are beyond the scope of this text, the recognition of the problems is not. (For additional information on occlusal equilibration see the references listed in the Appendix.) As pointed out in Chapter 3 on the Physiology of the Stomatognathic System, there must be harmony between temporomandibular joint function and occlusal relationships during mastication, deglutition, respiration and speech. Further, the dentist must strive for creation of molar and incisal paths of closure from postural resting position that are uniform and harmonious with the inclination of the condylar path. At least it must be possible for the combined hinge and translatory functions of the temporomandibular joint, as limited by the fibrous capsule and joint ligaments and postarticular connective tissue, to compensate for the individual tooth positions as modified by selective grinding.

DEVELOPING ANTERIOR CROSS-BITE

It is quite normal for the maxillary lateral incisors to erupt slightly to the lingual side of the line of the central incisors and to come forward as the clinical crown is exposed and as tongue function makes itself evident. Occasionally, even with adequate arch length, the lateral incisors erupt too far lingually and the clinical crown is forced completely to the lingual side of the opposing lower incisor, as the upper and lower teeth are brought into habitual occlusion. This tendency may be more manifest in the so-called straight-faced individual, with less overbite than average, and is, of course, seen where there is a familial Class III tendency. Maxillary central incisors normally bulge on the labial side above their deciduous counterparts, and are less likely to be trapped on the lingual side by the occlusion. But such accidents of eruption do occur, and the observant dentist may frequently intercept these developing cross-bites before full fledged malocclusions occur (Fig. 14-3). As with the relatively simple corrective procedures, which are discussed in detail in Chapter 17, sufficient space is an essential prerequisite. Patient cooperation is critical. By perusing his routine diagnostic records the conscientious dentist may anticipate a developing cross-bite. Eruption path, resorption patterns, timetable of teeth exchange, history of an accident to the immediate area, facial pattern type, and hereditary pattern all may give a clue of "things to come." Instructing the patient on what to look for, on normal development and on what may go wrong may assist the dentist in intercepting developing cross-bite, as well as other facets of malocclusion.

THERAPEUTIC TECHNIQUES

Assuming that this is a simple local problem with adequate space for the tooth in cross-bite to be moved into its correct position, several approaches are

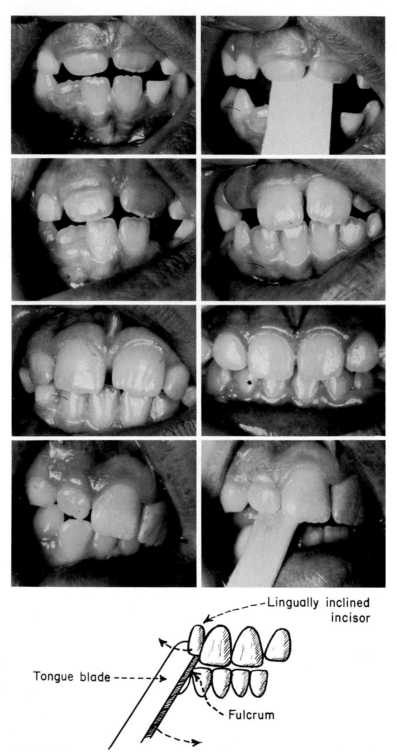

Figure 14–3 It is easier to intercept a developing anterior cross-bite than to correct it after it is established. Frequent observation by the dentist at this critical time and the use of a tongue blade for one or two hours a day over a three-week period produced the result seen in the three top rows. The mechanics of tongue blade action is illustrated in the bottom row of photographs and in the diagram.

possible. If the dentist is fortunate enough to anticipate and intercept the developing cross-bite as the permanent teeth erupt, the use of a tongue blade may be quite sufficient. Let us take as an example the most common type of cross-bite—the lingual malposition of a maxillary central incisor. The child is instructed to place a tongue blade in such a manner that it rests on the mandibular incisors opposing the tooth in cross-bite. With the mandibular incisal margin serving as a fulcrum, the oral portion of the tongue blade is rotated upward and forward to engage the lingual surface of the lingually malposed tooth. The patient is advised to bite with a constant pressure on the wood incline and at the same time to exert a slight but constant pressure with his hand on the blade so as to prevent blade displacement. The proper use of the tongue blade for an hour or two a day for 10 to 14 days is usually sufficient to deflect the lingually erupting maxillary incisor "across the fence" into a proper relationship. The tongue blade exercise may be prescribed for television time so that it does not become an onerous duty. It is advisable that the parent be present during the exercise to ensure constant application. Sometimes the tongue blade is too wide and engages more than one tooth. If it does, the blade may be whittled down to the correct width. Equally satisfactory are the wooden blades that are inserted as handles in ice cream bars. Actual finger pressure, pushing the lingually posed tooth outward, can be exerted during the day while the child is in school. Every little bit helps, even though the time periods of force application may not exceed 5 to 10 minutes at a time. To enhance the patient's cooperation—a critical factor in the success or failure of therapy—it has been found a good trick to "prescribe" an ice cream bar, complete with handle, for the proposed therapy.

Usually the dentist is not fortunate enough to see the child at the moment of developing cross-bite. Confronted with a *fait accompli*, corrective procedures must be more vigorous. While it is physically possible to correct the cross-bite with protracted periods of tongue blade therapy, the strong antagonistic force of the occlusion tends to negate these efforts. Several possible corrective procedures will be discussed in Chapters 16 and 17.

ANTERIOR DIASTEMAS

In Chapter 2 Broadbent's "ugly duckling" stage of incisor development was described in the section on tooth eruption. As the lateral incisors erupt, they often literally slide down the distal root surfaces of the central incisors to achieve their position. In the initial stages this bilateral action tends to force the apices of the central incisors toward the midline. The crowns flare distally, creating a developmental diastema. The flaring may remain after the lateral incisors erupt but will usually close as the canines repeat the flaring effect on the lateral incisors as they erupt into full clinical position. Thus, the spaces close by themselves without mechanical assistance. Indeed, mechanical assistance during the ugly duckling stage is fraught with great danger. The uprighting of the incisors can cause root resorption and likely deflection of the canines into positions of malocclusion (Fig. 14–4). A thorough study of diagnostic records guards the dentist from this serious error. A discretionary and questioning attitude toward some of the literature from so-called orthodontic laboratories which shows highly polished but archaic appliances performing an impossible correction will be of help, also.

The role of the labial frenum in the spacing between the maxillary incisors

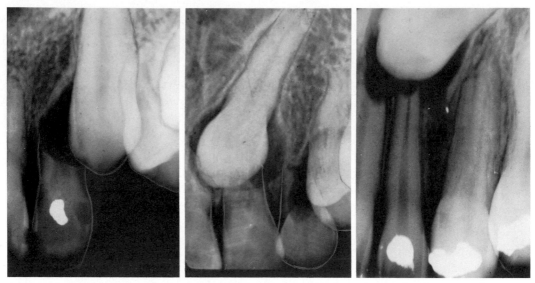

Figure 14–4   Severe root damage in three separate cases as a result of inept and premature orthodontic therapy which moved incisors into crown of erupting maxillary canines. All three patients were treated by general practitioners using appliances designed by so-called orthodontic laboratories to close anterior diastemas.

has been discussed (see Chaps. 7 and 13). In some cases an unyielding fibrous attachment may be present. Clipping this attachment may then allow the normal mesial migration of the incisors into proper proximal contact. This situation occurs in a distinct minority of cases; a number of other factors may be involved.

When viewing an anterior diastema, an important differential diagnosis must be made. Many diastemas are not transitory developmental phenomena. Frequently maxillary central incisors erupt with a 2 to 3 mm. space between them, encroaching on the necessary space for the maxillary lateral incisors. If left alone, a malocclusion is likely to develop. Because of lack of space the maxillary lateral incisors erupt to the lingual side, often in cross-bite. The erupting canines tend to migrate mesially and assume positions labial to the apices of the lateral incisors. It is then too late to close the diastema and move the lateral incisors into normal position, because in doing so the roots of these teeth may be damaged. The ideal situation is to move the maxillary central incisors into contact as they erupt and leave sufficient space for the laterals to assume a normal position in the dental arch. A word of caution—the apices of the erupting central incisors are wide open, and conventional orthodontic pressures have been known to cause a rounding off or foreshortening of these teeth as a result; therefore, the force that is used must be as close to physiologic levels as possible.

THERAPEUTIC TECHNIQUES

THE ORTHODONTIC PRESCRIPTION.   Space closure can be effected simply and expeditiously with removable appliances. These are discussed in Chapter 16. If patient cooperation is reasonably satisfactory, diastema closure is rapid and relatively painless. The removable appliance may be used as a retainer. If the frenum is indeed an adverse factor, as discussed in Chapter 13, it may be clipped in conjunction with removable appliance therapy during this mixed dentition stage.

Simple fixed appliances may also be used, but greater care must be exercised with the wide open apices, and there is a greater possibility of tissue damage. Tooth control is superior, and so is the therapeutic result. If, for example, the maxillary central incisors have erupted, leaving a diastema between them, and encroaching on space needed for maxillary lateral incisor eruption, the central incisors may be banded (Fig. 14–5), and horizontal tubes may be welded on the labial surface. Tubes of 0.032 to 0.036 inch size are desirable. A small section of round wire of the same size is placed in the tubes, and the ends are bent gingivally to prevent the wire from slipping out and irritating the soft tissue. The patient may then place a light rubber dam elastic over the ends of the arch segment. The reciprocal force will bodily slide the teeth together, apices as well as crowns (see Chap. 10). The segment may be shortened and ligated with stainless-steel wire to retain the incisors until the maxillary lateral incisors make their clinical appearance. With the new epoxy bonding agents and plastic attachments, it is not even necessary to band the incisors. Direct attachment of tubes or brackets eliminates gingival irritation of partly erupted teeth. A removable Hawley type appliance may be used as a retainer. Great care must be exercised in retracting maxillary incisors during this critical tooth exchange period. It is incredibly easy to deflect erupting canines, to close space for the canines, and thus bring about an iatrogenic malocclusion, requiring the services of a specialist.

CONTROL OF ABNORMAL HABITS

Abnormal deglutition, retained infantile mechanisms, tongue thrust, finger sucking and other abnormal perioral muscle activities have been discussed in some detail in Chapter 6. The damaging consequences of these habits are apparent. One of the most valuable interceptive orthodontic services that the dentist can render is to eliminate pernicious thumb, finger, tongue or lip sucking habits before they cause harm to the developing dentition. It is unfortunate that he does not see the infant early enough to assist in deglutitional and nursing problems. If he did, there would be fewer thumb, finger, lip and tongue habits to concern him, since the dentist could intercept the assault on the integrity and

Figure 14–5   Diastema closure with simple fixed appliance. Elastics slide teeth together along arch wire segment. Tubes prevent rotation and maintain axial inclination of incisors. Light elastics are to be preferred.

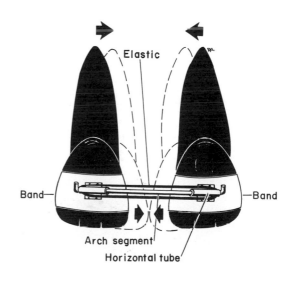

accomplishment of a normal dentition. Patient education is the answer here. Parents then know what to expect, and may thus prevent future orthodontic problems by intelligent handling of the physical and emotional demands of the growing child.

DEGLUTITIONAL PROBLEMS

Parents should be made aware of the damaging consequences of prolonged visceral (infantile) swallowing and nursing activity beyond the time that it would normally be superseded by a more mature (somatic) behavior. The great need for emotional, psychological and sensual gratification of the infant is more abstract, but no less important than the very concrete demands for nutritional fuel. Both appetites—that of the psyche and that of the intestinal tract—are important. To ignore the need for warmth, well-being and euphoria means that there is a greater likelihood of prolonged infantile deglutitional activity and of compensatory response in the nature of substitutive gratification. The "built-in" pacifiers are the tongue, the thumb and the lips. If natural nursing is really not possible— and there are actually very few cases in which this is really so, if the mother is willing to devote the time and attention to it—a reasonably physiologic substitute must be used. Sufficient time still must be spent in holding the developing infant, in fondling, caressing and loving him. Properly designed pacifiers are to be recommended and are a real deterrent to prolonged retention of infantile behavior facets (Fig. 14–29) (see Chap. 6, Figs. 6–61 to 6–63).

THUMB AND FINGER SUCKING AND ASSOCIATED HABITS (THE "BUILT-IN PACIFIERS")

Considerable space has been devoted to swallowing, tongue thrust, finger sucking and lip habits in Chapter 6. The retention of the infantile sucking and deglutitional posture as a malocclusion conditioner is described. The "vicious circle" activity associated with open bite and nature's compensatory and adaptive activity are profusely illustrated. When the child is seen with a malocclusion and a persisting finger sucking habit, it is easy to interpret this symbiotic relationship and arbitrarily assign cause and effect. It may be correct to say that finger sucking is one factor in deformation of the teeth and supporting structures, but it is just that—only one factor in a syndrome that consists of various admixtures of tongue thrust, abnormal deglutition, lip biting, hyperactive mentalis muscle, hypoactive upper lip muscles and probably hyperactive buccinator activity as well. To assign specific values to any one element in the production of the total malocclusion would be difficult, indeed. Nevertheless, it is often a good interceptive procedure to place an appliance which is designed to reduce and eliminate deforming activity.

Not all abnormal finger and oral muscle habit problems require appliance intervention. Not all habit problems create any damage; these cases should be left alone and observed periodically. Occasionally a frank discussion of the problem with the child may at least eliminate the finger sucking component, and the other elements may be superseded by more mature physiologic activity. As Worms, Meskin, Isaacson, Tulley, etc., have shown, the malocclusion may be a time-linked problem that is autonomously eliminated with developmental maturation.[1-10]

It has been found clinically beneficial by the author to have some patients use the lip and tongue exercise mentioned in Chapter 13 and described later in

Chapter 14, for example, running the tongue rhythmically back and forth over the lips for five to ten minutes before retiring. This often provides sufficient gratification and relaxation, making the demand for finger sucking at bedtime less forceful. Warm milk or soft music on retiring also tends to reduce the desire to suck.

If definite damage exists (a full-fledged malocclusion), a thorough case history should be obtained, preferably with the child out of the room (see sample, pp. 680 to 681). If the sucking habits are only one facet of a galaxy of symptoms of an abnormal behavior problem, a consultation with a psychiatrist is the first consideration. However, these cases are in the minority. In most instances the children are reasonably well adjusted and adequately healthy. If patient, parental and sibling cooperation can be assured, an appliance should be considered. Current learning theory indicates that the psychological aspect has been exaggerated by psychiatrists and pediatricians. (See Chap. 6.)

PLACEMENT OF HABIT-BREAKING APPLIANCES. The optimal time for appliance placement is between the ages of three and a half and four and a half years, preferably during the spring or summer when the child's health is at its peak and the sucking desires can be sublimated in outdoor play and social activity. The appliance serves several purposes. First, it renders the finger habit meaningless by breaking the suction. The child may, of course, place his finger in his mouth but he gets no real satisfaction from it. Thus, the finger sucking becomes analogous to coffee without caffeine or cigarettes without nicotine. Great care is exercised to inform both the child and the parents that the appliance is not a restrictive measure, that it is not used to prevent anything but merely to straighten the teeth, improve the appearance and provide a healthy "chewing machine." Second, by virtue of its construction, the appliance prevents finger pressure from displacing the maxillary incisors farther labially, from creating more open bite and from causing a greater likelihood of adaptive and deforming tongue and lip function. Third, the appliance forces the tongue backward, changing its shape during postural resting position from an elongated mass to a wider, more nearly normal tongue. As a result, the tongue tends to exert more pressure on the maxillary buccal segments and the narrowing of the maxillary arch by the abnormal swallowing habit is reversed; the peripheral portions again overlie the occlusal surfaces of the posterior teeth, preventing the overeruption of these teeth. If the patients are normal, healthy children, few unfavorable sequelae are observed except for a temporary sibilant speech defect which usually disappears while the appliance is being worn or immediately after it is removed.

FIXED HABIT EDUCATION

FINGER SUCKING PRESCRIPTION: APPLIANCE USED IN THERAPY. The orthodontic prescription for habit re-education takes several forms. One of the more effective means is a fixed crib. An alginate impression is taken on the first visit, and a plaster cast is poured from it. If the proximal contacts are quite tight in the maxillary second deciduous molar area, it is advisable to place brass separating wires at this visit (Figs. 14–6 to 14–9). The appliance is then fabricated on the cast for placement at a subsequent appointment. Generally speaking, the maxillary second deciduous molars make excellent abutment teeth. Full metal crowns, which are available in assorted sizes, are preferred to conventional orthodontic bands. The mesial portion of the first permanent molar, if present, and the distal portion of the first deciduous molar are then trimmed away on the cast from contact with the second deciduous molar (Fig. 14–10). A millimeter or

Address: _____   Name: _____
_____   Tel: _____

ORAL HABIT PROBLEMS

Referred by: Dentist ☐   Physician ☐   Other ☐   Specify: _____
Age: ☐☐ yrs. ☐☐ mos.   Birth weight: ☐☐ lbs.   Sex: Male ☐   Female ☐
Premature: ☐   Congenital anomalies: ☐   Specify: _____

Home
　　Siblings: No. brothers ☐☐   Ages brothers: _____
　　　　　　　No. sisters   ☐☐   Ages sisters: _____
　　Child living with: Mother ☐   Father ☐   Other ☐   Specify: _____
　　Others in household: _____
　　Parents'　　　　　Mother: Calm　　☐　　　　　Father: Calm　　☐
　　temperament:　　　　　　Forceful ☐　　　　　　　　Forceful ☐
　　　　　　　　　　　　　　Tense　　☐　　　　　　　　Tense　　☐

Social behavior
　　Personality: Introvert　　　☐　　Play: Abnormal ☐　　School: Behind　　☐
　　　　　　　　Well-adapted ☐　　　　　　Normal　　☐　　　　　　Same　　　☐
　　　　　　　　Extrovert　　　☐　　　　　　　　　　　　　　　　Advanced ☐
　　Comments: _____
　　　　　　　　_____

General health
　　Present　　Good ☐　　　Under treatment ☐　　　Serious illnesses ☐
　　health:　　Fair　☐　　　Comments: _____
　　　　　　　Poor ☐　　　　_____
　　Annual colds and　　　Frequent　　☐　　Time of year: Winter　　☐
　　　other minor ailments: Occasionally ☐　　　　　　　　　Spring　　☐
　　　　　　　　　　　　　Rarely　　　☐　　　　　　　　　Summer　　☐
　　　　　　　　　　　　　　　　　　　　　　　　　　　Autumn　　☐
　　Response under　　　Antagonistic ☐　　Comments:_____
　　　stress:　　　　　　Docile　　　☐　　　　　　　_____
　　　　　　　　　　　Defensive　　☐　　　　　　　_____

Feeding
　　Breast-fed ☐　　How long: ☐☐ mos.　　Age at weaning: ☐☐ mos.
　　Bottle-fed ☐　　How long: ☐☐ mos.　　Age at weaning: ☐☐ mos.
　　Present eating　Good　　　　☐　　　Comments:_____
　　　habits:　　　Fair　　　　☐　　　　　　　_____
　　　　　　　　Indifferent　☐　　　　　　　_____
　　　　　　　　Poor　　　　　☐　　　　　　　_____

Sleeping

    Daytime: Regularly □   Night: No. hours   □□

                Irregularly □   Soundly   □

                Rarely   □   Frequent

                                            interruption □

Toilet

    Habits: Abnormal □   Comments: _____

            Normal   □   _____

    Age trained; Bowel   Completely

               movement □□ yrs. □□ mos.   trained   □□ yrs. □□ mos.

Oral habit

    Sucking: Thumb: Frequently   □   Fingers: Frequently   □

                    Occasionally □   Occasionally □

                    Rarely   □   Rarely   □

    Age habit began: □□ yrs. □□ mos.   Age discontinued: □□ yrs. □□ mos.

    Still continuous: □   Day □   Night □   School □   Watching T.V. □

    Associated   Twirling hair □   Caressing blanket □   Specify: _____

      habits: Pulling ear   □   Licking lips   □   _____

               Picking nose □   Other   □   _____

    Methods used to None   □   Specify: _____

      stop habit: Dental □   _____

                Other   □   _____

    Awareness Child aware   □   Other □

      by child: Nagged by siblings □   Specify: _____

                Nagged by mother □   _____

                Nagged by father □

    Others with   No one □   Father □   Other □

      similar habit: Sibling □   Mother □   Specify: _____

Therapy

    Child's desire   Yes: With treatment   □   Unconcerned □

      to cease habit: Without treatment □   No desire   □

    Parental attitude: Mother: No treatment   □   Father: No treatment   □

                              Treatment: Treatment:

                              Appliance   □   Appliance   □

                              No appliance □   No appliance □

General comments:

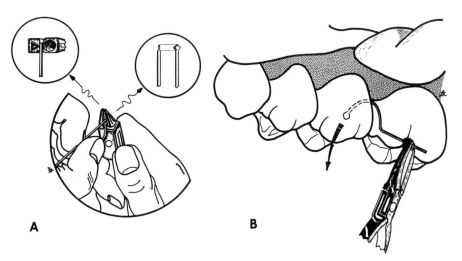

Figure 14–6.   Separating wire technique. A, Flattening the end of the brass separating wire before forming crescent of wire for interproximal insertion. B, Insertion of separating wire beneath contacts with How or office pliers.

two is quite sufficient. The gingival margin of the second deciduous molar is then cut back, following the contour of the tooth, to a depth of 2 or 3 mm. on the buccal, lingual and proximal surfaces. The correct size of stainless-steel crown is selected, contoured if necessary (Fig. 14–10), and the gingival portion trimmed with a crown and collar shears to fit the carved gingival contour on the cast. The most frequent mistake is to trim the proximal portions of the crown too severely,

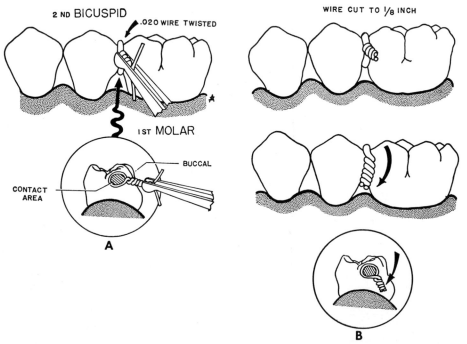

Figure 14–7   Separating wire technique. A, Twisting of brass separating wire to buccal, around contact area. B, Wire is then cut off, leaving a "pigtail" which is tucked gingivally into the interproximal area.

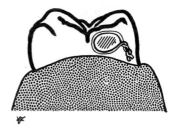

Figure 14–8 Contact relationship of separating wire mesial to maxillary first permanent molar.

reducing the gingivo-occlusal dimension too much. A slit is then made in the crown at the mesial buccal surface or distal buccal surface and the crown pushed sharply to place.

The palatal assemblage is made of 0.040 inch nichrome or stainless-steel wire. The U-shaped base wire is adapted by running it mesially at the level of the gingival margin from the second deciduous molar to the embrasure between the first deciduous molars and primary canines. At this point a sharp bend is made to carry the wire straight across to the opposite first deciduous molar–primary canine embrasure, maintaining the same gingival level. It is important not to follow the contour of the palate if the suction and kinesthetic-neuromuscular gratification are to be rendered meaningless. Remember how important a role the tongue plays in this picture. Unless tongue position is changed and thrusting diminished, chances for total success are very much diminished. More than one symptom must be treated, and the finger sucking is usually only one symptom—

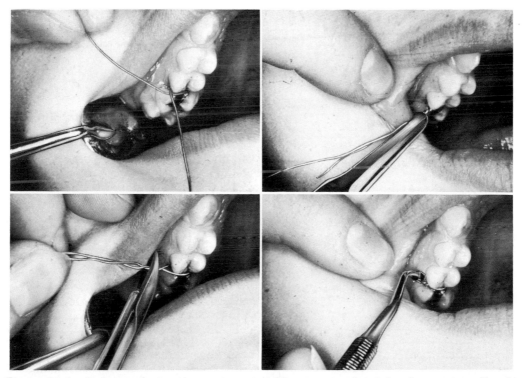

Figure 14–9 Steps in placing separating wire. Wire is twisted tightly after cutting off ends and then tucked in with an amalgam plugger.

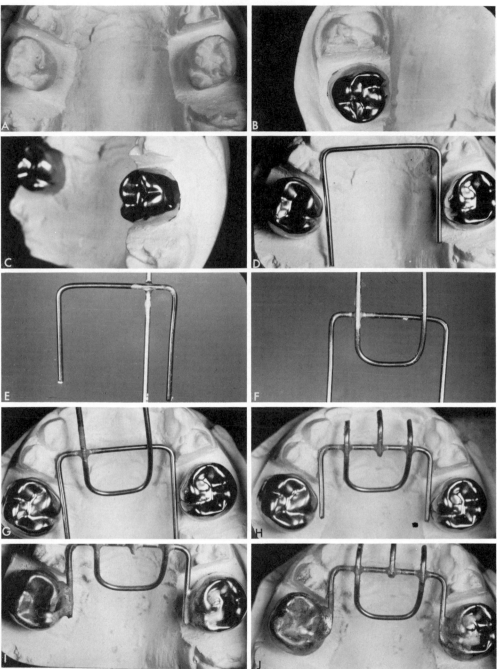

Figure 14–10   Fabrication of finger sucking re-education appliance. A, Second deciduous molars trimmed 3 mm. all around on gingival margin. B and C, Fitting stainless-steel metal crowns. D, Central base bar of 0.040 steel or nichrome crosses palate mesial to first deciduous molar at level of gingival margin. E and F, Loop and spurs formed by soldering straight 0.040 wire at 45 degree angle to legs of base wire, forming loop so that it extends back to anterior third of second deciduous molar, inclined toward palate at 45 degrees to occlusal plane (G). The other leg of the central loop is then soldered, a midpalatal spur is soldered to base bar, and all three spurs are bent toward palate (H). Steel crowns and base wire are heavily fluxed and soldered with silver solder (I) and the appliance is then removed from cast and this solder joint and spur ends are smoothed down (J). Appliance is now ready to polish. Make sure slit is made on buccal of each crown before trying in the mouth, so that there is minimal gingival impingement.

not the only factor. At the opposite canine–first deciduous molar embrasure the wire is bent back along the gingival margin to the crown on the second deciduous molar. The base wire should fit passively when placed on the cast.

The central assemblage consists of spurs and a loop of the same gauge wire. The loop extends posteriorly and superiorly at an angle of approximately 45 degrees to the occlusal plane (Figs. 14–10, 14–11). The loop should not project posteriorly beyond the line drawn connecting the distal surfaces of the second deciduous molars. The two legs of this central loop are continued past the same bar and bent toward the palate so that they just contact it lightly. With a fluoride flux and silver solder, the loop is now soldered to the main bar. A third anterior projection with the same curvature toward the palate is soldered between the two anterior projections of the central loop. The main bar and soldered assemblage is then soldered to the crowns on the second deciduous molars. An excess of solder is preferable for these joints. After the appliance is cleaned and polished, it is ready for insertion.

At the second visit the appliance is removed from the cast, and the gingival circumference is deliberately reduced by overlapping the crown at the buccal slit. Separating wires, if present, are removed and the appliance is placed on the second deciduous molars. The patient is instructed to bite firmly into occlusion. The crowns automatically open up to the desired circumference as dictated by the individual teeth and can be soldered or spot welded along the buccal slit that has been made. If the gingival tissue blanches unduly or if the patient complains of tenderness, the gingival portion should be trimmed further. The entire periphery should be beneath the gingival margin. The appliance is replaced after peripheral adjustment and the child instructed to bite as strongly as he can.

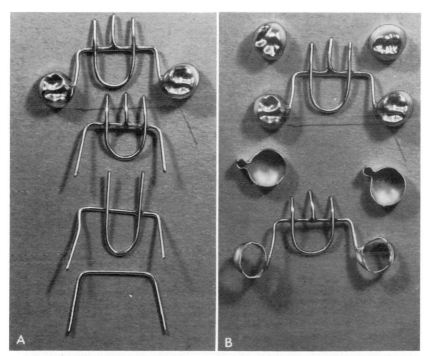

Figure 14–11 A, Steps in habit appliance construction from bottom to top: Base bar, base bar and loop, base bar, loop and spurs bent toward palate, central assemblage soldered on steel crowns. B, Two types of habit appliances: one with loop type molar bands and the other with steel crowns.

This helps adapt the occlusal contours and provides a further check for gingival impingement. One should be sure to check that the mandibular incisors are not occluding against the anterior projections of the central assemblage. If there is contact, these spurs should be shortened and bent back toward the palate. The abutment teeth are then isolated, cleaned and dried, and the appliance thoroughly dried and cemented to place by having the child bite the appliance itself into position. Most of the excess cement is wiped away immediately and the remainder removed with a universal type scaler five to ten minutes later. The crowns literally block open the occlusion and serve as the only maxillary contacts of the mandibular teeth. This need cause no concern as the remaining maxillary teeth erupt within a week into contact with their opposing mandibular counterparts.

The child is told only that the appliance is to straighten his teeth. At no time is it mentioned that an attempt is being made to break any habit. The parent is expected to provide the same information at home. Siblings are instructed in like manner. If a lingual cross-bite tendency exists in the deciduous molar area, the central bar can be expanded before cementing the appliance and sprung to place on the teeth when the appliance is cemented. The wire tends to regain its original expanded form, moving the first and second deciduous molars buccally. If retraction of the maxillary incisors is necessary and desirable at this time, horizontal buccal tubes may be soldered on the steel crowns and a 0.040 or 0.045 inch steel labial arch wire placed. Provision can be made for vertical closing loops and reception of arms from an extraoral appliance (Fig. 14–15). (See Chap. 18 for more complete discussion of extraoral force and incisor retraction.)

After the cementation, the child is told that it will take several days to become accustomed to the appliance, that he will have a little difficulty cleaning the food from beneath the appliance and that he must speak slowly and carefully because of the bar across the roof of his mouth. No mention is made of the finger. The parent is then told that there will be relatively little discomfort but that the residual speech impediment is to be expected for at least a week, affecting the sibilants particularly. Speech impairment may even be present during the entire course of therapy. The diet should be kept quite soft for the first couple of days. Some children may drool; some may complain that it is difficult to swallow.

After a 2- to 3-day adjustment period, most children are hardly aware of the appliance. Checkup appointments should be made at 3- to 4-week intervals. The habit appliance is worn for 4 to 6 months in most cases. A period of 3 months of total absence of the finger habit is good insurance against a relapse. In most instances the habit disappears after the first week of appliance wear. After the 3-month habit-free interval the spurs are cut off first (Fig. 14–12). Three weeks later, if there is no evidence of a recurrence, the posterior loop extension is removed; 3 weeks after that the remaining palatal bar and crowns may be taken off (Fig. 14–12). If there is a tendency toward a return to the habit, it is wise to leave at least a partial appliance in place for a greater period of time. If there is a combined tongue thrust and finger habit, the appliance is modified and left in for a longer time, also.

It cannot be emphasized too strongly that the habit appliance is not a punishment or purposely painful experience. There should be no sharp spurs. Structure is designed to prevent deformation of the premaxillary segment, to stimulate development of somatic swallowing and mature tongue posture and function, to allow autonomous correction of habit-induced malocclusion. Improperly designed appliances, which have spurs and follow the contour of the palate, may actually accentuate the malocclusion (Fig. 14–13).

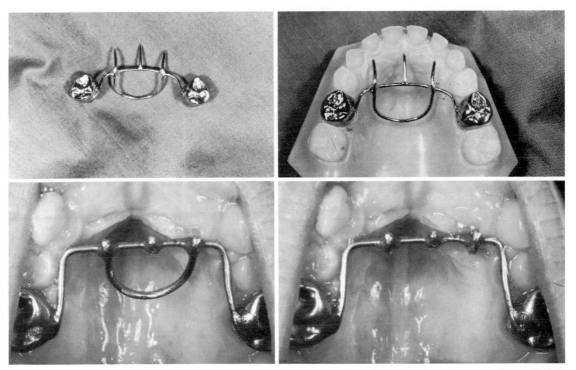

Figure 14-12 Finished habit appliance that has been placed on first deciduous molars (above). Appliance is removed gradually; first the spurs, then the loop and finally the entire appliance (below).

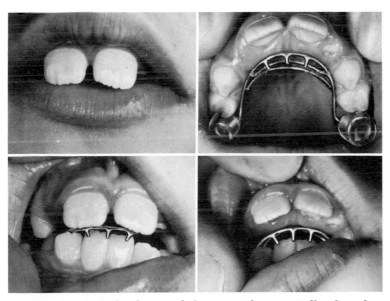

Figure 14-13 Improperly designed finger appliance. Bulk of appliance follows palatal contour, not breaking suction. Spurs engage labial surface of lower incisors, preventing them from moving labially, thus perpetuating the malocclusion, which the lower lip will accentuate as it cushions in the excessive overjet. Thus, this becomes an iatrogenic malocclusion. The appliance creates a more severe problem.

TONGUE THRUST

Not infrequently, the tongue is the only problem; there is no longer a finger habit, but 500 to 1000 times a day the tongue thrusts forward to accentuate the open bite or maxillary incisor protrusion.

TONGUE THRUST PRESCRIPTION: APPLIANCE USED IN THERAPY.   The tongue thrust appliance, a variation of the finger sucking appliance discussed above, tends to force the tongue downward and backward during swallowing. When the spurs are bent down so that they form a sort of picket fence behind the lower incisors during full occlusal contact of the posterior teeth, a more effective barrier to tongue thrust is assured. Since an analysis of the tongue thrust habit shows that the tongue is carried habitually low and does not seem to approximate the palatal contour as it would under normal conditions, a tongue thrust appliance should attempt to do two things: (1) eliminate the strong anterior thrust and plunger-like action during deglutition; (2) re-educate tongue posture so that the dorsum of the tongue approximates the palatal vault, and the tip of the tongue contacts the palatal rugae during deglutition, instead of sneaking through the incisal space. As the tongue is forced back within the confines of the dentition, it spreads laterally, with the peripheral portions overlying the occlusal surfaces of the posterior teeth. Interocclusal clearance is maintained, or created where it is deficient, in this manner and overeruption and narrowing of maxillary buccal segments is prevented. The mature swallowing act is stimulated by this type of appliance, as the tongue adapts to its new position and function.

To accomplish these purposes, when the finger habit is not a factor, it is better to eliminate the cross-palatal bar and posterior loop extension of the finger appliance and modify the design of the restraining crib (Fig. 14–14). The second deciduous molars serve as satisfactory abutments, usually. If first permanent molars are present and sufficiently erupted they are preferred.

Good alginate impressions are taken of both dental arches (in addition to those taken previously for study models) and poured up in plaster. It is best to mount the two working models on a hinge type, or anatomic, articulator. The plaster abutment teeth (either first permanent molars or second deciduous molars) are then trimmed down in the manner outlined for the interceptive finger sucking habit appliance. The proper size full metal crown is chosen and the gingival portion contoured to fit the carved tooth periphery on the cast. A buccal slit is made as outlined for the finger habit interceptive appliance. The 0.040 inch nickel chromium alloy or stainless-steel U-shaped lingual bar is then adapted by starting at one side of the cast and carrying the wire anteriorly to the canine area at the level of the gingival margin. The bar should make point contact with the most prominent lingual surfaces of the second deciduous and first deciduous molars.

Next, the casts are occluded and a pencil line is drawn across the maxillary cast to the canine on the opposite side. This line approximates the anteroposterior relationship of the mandibular incisal margins with respect to the maxillary dentition. The base wire is adapted to follow the contour of the palate just lingual to this line and carried to the opposite canine tooth. The bar is then bent and carried posteriorly along the gingival margin, contacting the lingual surfaces of the first and second deciduous molars and the metal crown on the first permanent molar.

Since the appliance is being placed to correct an open bite, occlusion is no concern at this point. Later, however, as the open bite is reduced, the dentist must be sure that the anterior portion of the base bar and its crib do not interfere with incision. This is the reason for constructing the base bar lingual to the man-

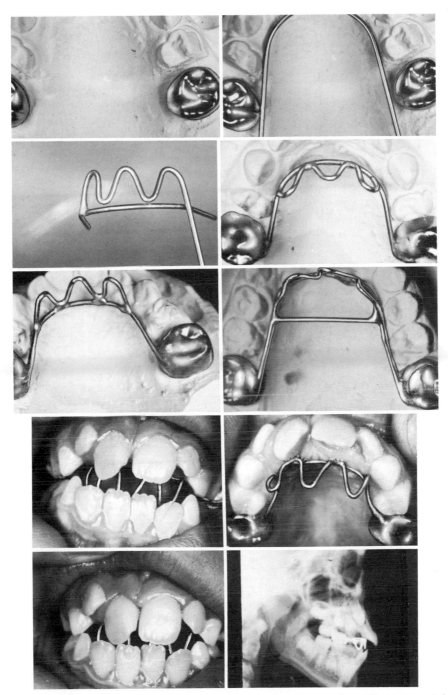

Figure 14–14. Tongue crib to eliminate infantile or visceral swallowing and thrusting and to stimulate mature or somatic tongue posture and function. As with finger habit appliance, full metal crowns are used. Crib portion is smooth and polished to prevent any irritation and to ease adaptation difficulties. A cross-palatal bar may be used occasionally but is not usually necessary. Bottom four views are of the same patient. Open bite closure in lower left view occurred over a 3-week period. (From Graber, T. M.: The "three M's": muscles, malformation, and malocclusion. Am. J. Orthodont., 49:418–450, 1963.)

dibular incisal margin. After the base bar has been carefully fabricated and assumes the desired position passively when placed on the maxillary cast, the crib can be formed. The same gauge wire is used as for the base bar. One end is soldered to the base bar in the area of the canine. Using No. 139 pliers or office pliers, three or four V-shaped projections are made so that they extend downward to a point just behind the cinguli of the mandibular incisors when the casts are occluded (Fig. 14–14). There should be no actual contact that might interfere with the eruption of these teeth. After each V projection has been carefully shaped so that the arms of the projections are approximately at the base wire, these are thoroughly fluxed with the fluoride paste flux and attached to the base wire with ample amounts of silver solder. The base wire itself is then carefully positioned on the cast and soldered to the metal crowns. After cleaning and polishing, one is ready to try the appliance in the patient's mouth and establish the correct peripheral circumference for the abutment crowns. If a bilateral

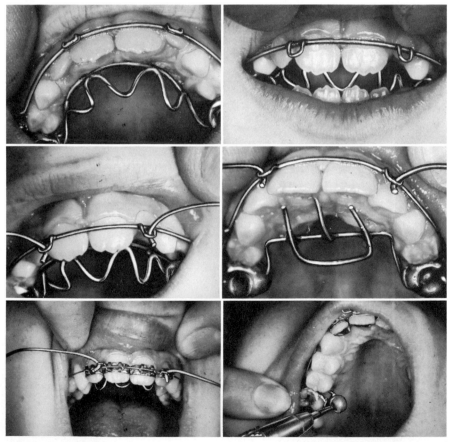

Figure 14–15 Orthodontic therapy in conjunction with tongue crib. Excessive overjet is also a sequential development of tongue thrust, and it may be accentuated by the tongue thrusting against the habit appliance itself. Extraoral force may be necessary to eliminate maxillary protrusion tendency with tongue (top) or finger habit appliances (middle right). Actual banding of maxillary incisors is often necessary (lower views). After open bite correction, habit appliance is removed, bands polished, and orthodontic therapy completed in a conventional manner. Orthodontic specialist consultation and guidance and actual therapy are to be recommended in most problems of this type. (From Graber, T. M.: The "three M's": muscles, malformation, and malocclusion. Am. J. Orthodont., 49:418–450, 1963.)

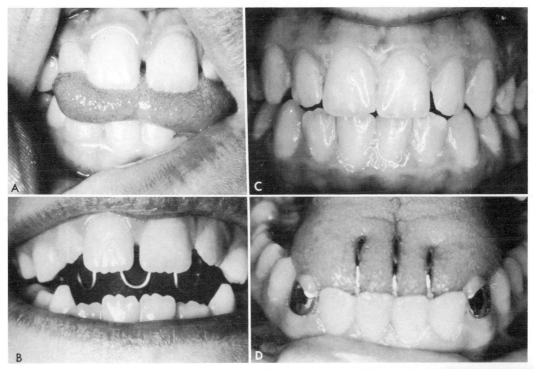

Figure 14–16   Tongue thrust habit (A), with appliance and correction of open bite (B and C). Palatal appliance, as in Figure 14–15, was used. D shows a lower anti-tongue thrust appliance, with spurs soldered to a lower canine-to-canine lingual arch. The spurs curve lingually and are rounded off to prevent tongue irritation.

narrowing exists posteriorly, expansion may be placed in the lingual wire. The buccal slit is spot welded and the appliance is ready for cementation.

As with the finger habit appliance, the open bite is actually increased temporarily because of the interposed crowns in the first molar area. This localized condition is eliminated within a week. The patient no longer can thrust the tongue through the incisal space. The dorsum is forced against the palate and the tip of the tongue soon finds that the most comfortable position during deglutition is against the rugae.

Depending on the severity of the open bite problem, four to nine months may be required for the autonomous correction of the malocclusion. Not all appliances are successful by themselves, and full orthodontic procedures are essential in many cases (Fig. 14–15). If the dentist has been careful in his case selection and has studied the problem thoroughly to ascertain that he is dealing primarily with a tongue thrust habit and not a basal and total malocclusion, if he places the appliance early enough so that he can expect the teeth to erupt and the alveolar bone to be laid down, his efforts should meet with routine success (Fig. 14–16). Extraoral reinforcement is frequently necessary. This contingency can be provided for by placing horizontal buccal tubes on the crowns. An arch wire or labial bow may be employed later, if indicated. The optimum age for placement of this type of appliance is between five and ten years. If placed after this age it is more likely that full orthodontic appliances and the services of an orthodontic specialist will be required.

Not all tongue thrust habits cause malocclusions in the anterior segments. Posterior open bite may exist (Fig. 14–17). Though not frequent, these habits do

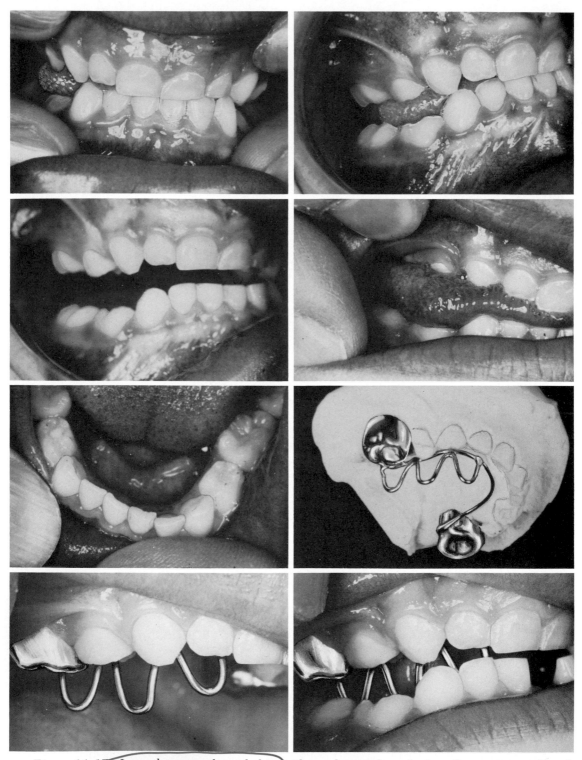

Figure 14-17. Lateral tongue thrust habit, with resultant infraocclusion of posterior teeth and an open bite. Modified tongue crib is used to prevent tongue thrust habit. Normal eruption of teeth then eliminates open bite problem. Full metal crowns are recommended over orthodontic bands for abutment teeth.

occur, creating infraocclusion of upper and lower buccal segments, possible functional problems and speech defects. A higher incidence of such habits is seen in Class II, Division 2 malocclusions and supports the hypothesis that tongue function is a factor in creating or at least perpetuating the undereruption seen in the posterior segments of patients with this category of malocclusion. A modified habit crib may be constructed to eliminate lateral tongue thrust and to allow eruption of the affected teeth.

LIP BITING AND SUCKING

While many cases of tongue thrust habit are attributed to a retention of the infantile suckle-swallow instinct, this is not true for the lip biting or sucking habits. In many instances the lip sucking habit is a compensatory activity that results from an excessive overjet and the relative difficulty of closing the lips properly during deglutition. It is much easier for the child to cushion the lip to the lingual side of the maxillary incisors. To achieve this position, he calls on the mentalis muscle which, in effect, extends the lower lip upward. It is easy to discern the abnormal mentalis activity by noting the puckering up of the chin during swallowing. Even as the tongue can deform the dental arches, so can an abnormal lip habit. When the habit has become pernicious, a marked flattening and crowding occurs in the lower anterior segment (see Chap. 6). The maxillary incisors are forced upward and forward into a protrusive relationship. In severe cases the lip itself shows the effects of the abnormal habit. The vermilion border becomes hypertrophic and redundant during rest. The mentolabial sulcus or suprasymphyseal cleft becomes accentuated. In some instances a chronic herpes with areas of irritation and cracking of the lip appears. Occasionally the lip sucking habit becomes a compulsive and gratificational activity, particularly during the sleeping hours. The telltale redness and irritation extending from the mucosa onto the skin below the lower lip can be seen by an observant dentist, even though the parent is unaware of the habit. There should be no difficulty in seeing the abnormal swallowing habit and associated hyperactive mentalis muscle activity. Here again, the dentist must be interested in the dynamic considerations of the stomatognathic system. The functional test is just as important as the habitual occlusal relationship check itself.

DIFFERENTIAL DIAGNOSIS. An important consideration here is the necessity for making a differential diagnosis before attempting to break the lip habit. If there is a Class II, Division 1 malocclusion or an excessive overjet problem, the abnormal lip activity may be purely compensatory or adaptive to the dentoalveolar morphology. To attempt to change the lip function without changing tooth position is to invite failure. The first service to be rendered in these cases is the establishment of normal occlusion. Generally, this requires the services of an orthodontic specialist and full orthodontic therapy. Placing only a lip appliance would merely be treating a symptom and would do little or nothing for the major problem. But if the posterior occlusion is normal or has been corrected by prior orthodontic therapy and there is still a lip sucking tendency, a lip appliance may be necessary. The number of cases in which there is need for a lip appliance are few. Abnormal lip activity is almost always associated with Class II, Division 1 malocclusions and open bite problems, and the elimination of the malocclusion usually restores normal muscle function.

In those instances in which the habit is primarily a neuromuscular tic or, as the mother says, "a nervous habit," the lip habit appliance can be quite effective. Minor malrelationships of the incisor teeth are eliminated by self-adjustment, and tooth-moving appliances are seldom needed. It is most gratifying to watch the tongue align the mandibular incisors as the lip appliance keeps the abnormal mentalis activity from forcing them lingually (Fig. 14–18).

FABRICATION OF APPLIANCES.   There are several possible ways to construct the lip habit appliance. The method described is one that has worked well for the author. Maxillary and mandibular alginate impressions are taken and poured up in plaster. For ease in handling, the casts can be mounted on a hinge type or straight line articulator. The mandibular first permanent molar teeth or second deciduous molar teeth are trimmed down as outlined for the fixed functional space maintainer and the finger sucking appliance. The dentist should be sure to carry the carving far enough gingivally. Full metal crowns or properly made orthodontic bands may be used on the abutment teeth (Fig. 14–19). If the appliance is going to be left in place for any appreciable time, full metal crowns are more likely to hold up under the pounding of the occlusal stresses. A 0.040 inch nichrome or stainless-steel base wire is then adapted, running anteriorly from the abutment tooth past the deciduous molars to the canine-first deciduous molar or canine-lateral incisor embrasure. Either interproximal area may be chosen to cross the base wire over to the labial depending on the clearance present as determined from an analysis of the articulated casts. After crossing the embrasure the base wire is bent to the level of the incisor labiogingival margin and carried across to the corresponding embrasure on the opposite side. The wire is then brought through the embrasure and carried back to the abutment attachment, contacting the lingual surfaces of the premolars lightly (Fig. 14–20). A careful check must be made that the anterior portion of the wire (the labial portion) does not contact the lingual surfaces of the maxillary incisors as the upper cast is brought into occlusion. If this happens, the base wire should be bent to assume a position further to the gingival. The wire should stand away from the labial surfaces of the mandibular incisors 2 to 3 mm. to allow them to move forward. A 0.036 or 0.040 inch nickel-chromium or stainless-steel auxiliary wire may then be added by soldering one end at the crossover embrasure and carrying the wire gingivally approximately 6 to 8 mm. This wire is then bent and carried across the mandibular incisor gingiva parallel with the base wire, bent again in the area of the opposite crossover embrasure, and soldered to the base wire. (See Figs. 14–19, 14–20.) The parallel portion of the wire should be approximately 3 mm. away from the gingival tissue. The base wire is then soldered to the crown or band attachments, and the wire assemblage is rechecked for possible occlusal or incisal interference. After cleaning and polishing, the appliance may be cemented to place on the teeth. If metal crowns have been used, it is desirable to make a buccal slit to allow the establishment of the correct gingival circumference of the crown and subsequent spot welding or soldering at this point, as outlined for the finger sucking appliance. The labial "plumper" may be modified by adding acrylic between the base and auxiliary wire portions (Fig. 14–21). This tends to reduce the irritation of the mucosa of the lower lip. Most of the appliances are worn approximately the same length of time as the tongue thrusting appliance. As with the finger sucking appliance, the lip appliance is reduced gradually before being removed. The auxiliary wires are removed first and the remainder of the appliance several weeks later. Particularly where there has been some crowding and retropositioning of the mandibular incisors, there need be no hurry to remove the appliance. A period of eight to nine months of wear is quite acceptable.

There is no question that the lip appliance permits the tongue to move the mandibular incisors labially. This not only improves their axial inclination, but

(Text continued on page 699)

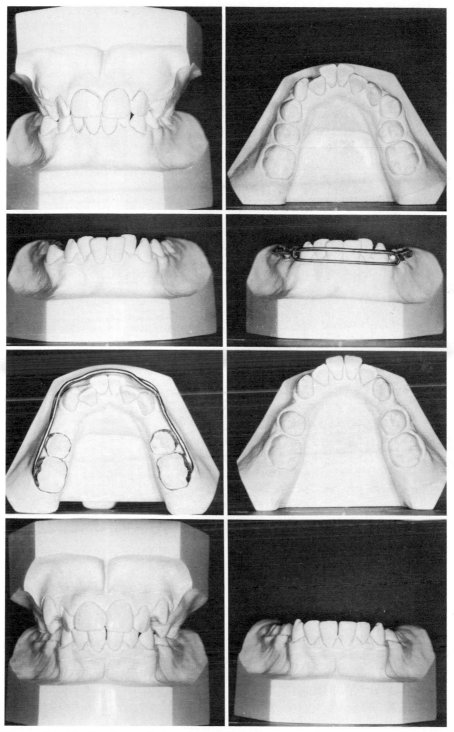

Figure 14–18 In this arch length problem first premolars have been removed by the orthodontist, and an appliance has been placed to hold the lower lip away because of its perverted activity. During the seven months of appliance wear, the canines have dropped distally into the extraction space, permitting the tongue to mold the anterior segment and eliminate irregularities. (Courtesy R. V. Winders.)

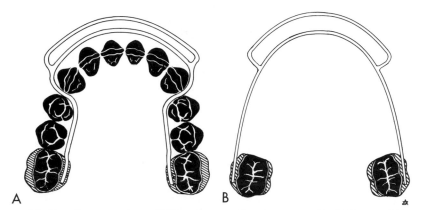

A   B

Figure 14–19   Construction of "lip plumper" to intercept lip biting and lip sucking habits. Full metal crowns may be used instead of orthodontic bands if appliance is to be worn for any length of time. *A,* Lingual arch, crossing over at canine first premolar (or canine lateral incisor) embrasure. *B,* Labial bow type (see Fig. 14–18).

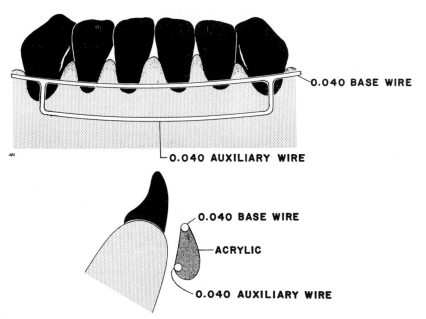

Figure 14–20   Labial detail of lip appliance showing wire skeleton (above) and acrylic overlay incorporating wires (below).

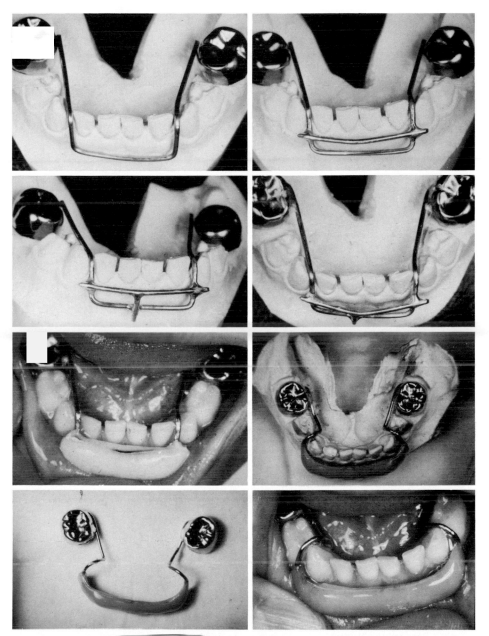

Figure 14–21. Lip habit appliance. A 0.040 inch bar is soldered to full metal crowns on second deciduous or first permanent molars. Bar may cross from lingual to labial either mesial or distal to canine, depending on occlusion and anterior spacing. The operator should be sure that labial assemblage is 2 to 3 mm. anterior to the labial aspect of lower incisors. Model is foiled first before endothermic acrylic is adapted to wire framework. Appliance is cemented in place for a period of three to six months, depending on severity of lip habit and amount of overjet. (From Graber, T. M.: The "three M's": muscles, malformation, and malocclusion. Am. J. Orthodont., 49:418–450, 1963.)

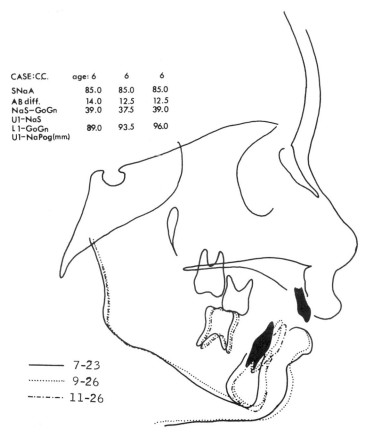

CASE:C.C.	age: 6	6	6
SNaA	85.0	85.0	85.0
AB diff.	14.0	12.5	12.5
NaS—GoGn	39.0	37.5	39.0
U1—NaS			
L1—GoGn	89.0	93.5	96.0
U1—NaPog(mm)			

———— 7-23
·········· 9-26
—·—·— 11-26

Figure 14–22   Lower lip sucking habit, associated with Class II, Division 1 maloc-clusion. Orthodontist placed lip appliance as the first assault on the problem. Mandibu-lar incisors have moved 6 degrees labially in four months. An unexpected phenomenon was the elimination of a functional mandibular retrusion, as the mandible itself came forward during this time.

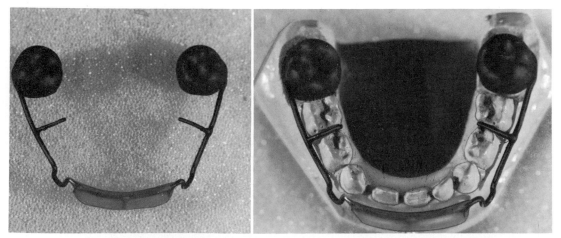

Figure 14–23   Lip sucking habit crib. Metal portion has been made black to better illustrate adaptation to model. Acrylic "plumper" on labial side of lower incisors is 3 to 4 mm. away from labial surfaces to allow tongue to move these teeth forward. Rests at deciduous molar embrasure prevent the appliance from being displaced gingivally by functional forces.

frequently the overbite is reduced. In some instances where there seems to be an actual functional mandibular retrusion, as a result of aberrant lip and associated muscle activity, the placing of a lip appliance at this time allows the incisors to come forward, and the mandible may also do the same (Figs. 14–22, 14–23). This is the same effect as seen in the Frankel type appliance (Fig. 14–27).

REMOVABLE ABNORMAL HABIT APPLIANCES

FOR CHEEK BITING. It was pointed out in Chapter 6 that abnormal muscle habits may also cause open bites or individual tooth malpositions in the buccal segments, even though the usual area of greatest deformation is in the anterior segment.[11] Where a persistent cheek biting habit exists, a removable crib may be constructed to break the habit or a vestibular or oral screen may be used (Figs. 14–24 to 14–28).

FOR ABNORMAL FINGER, LIP AND TONGUE HABITS. An effective means of controlling abnormal muscle habits and at the same time utilizing the musculature to effect a correction of the developing malocclusion is the vestibular or oral screen, or a combination of both. These removable appliances have been developed to a high degree of efficiency by Frantisek Kraus of Czechoslovakia.[12] The simple vestibular screen is an aid in restoring normal lip function and in retracting incisor teeth (Fig. 14–25). It may also be used to intercept finger sucking habits, but has the disadvantage of being readily removable by the patient if he so desires. Complete patient cooperation is absolutely essential.

The oral screen is a modified acrylic palate and is similar to the activator in appearance but much less bulky (Fig. 14–26). Either an acrylic or wire loop barrier may be constructed to prevent tongue thrust and finger sucking. Clasps may be added on the molars if added retention is needed. The combined oral and

(Text continued on page 703)

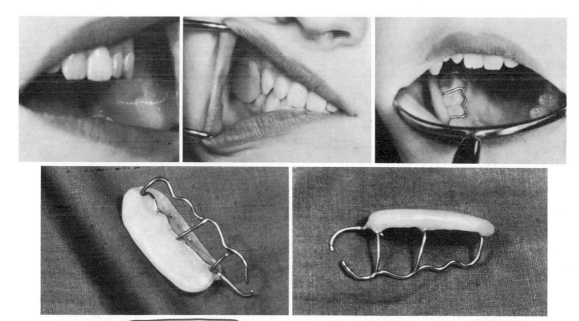

Figure 14–24 Cheek biting habit causing a posterior open bite in a young adult. A weltlike horizontal swelling (upper left picture) has formed as a result of constant irritation. The removable wire and acrylic crib breaks up the biting habit, allowing the teeth to erupt. For a posterior tongue thrust habit, the acrylic mass would be on the lingual instead of the buccal side.

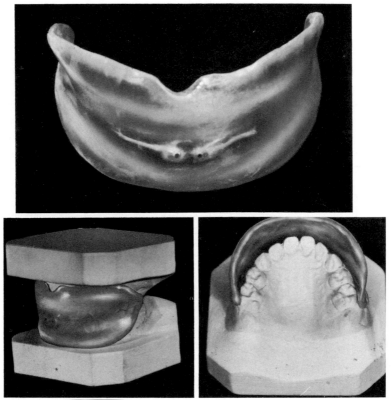

Figure 14–25 Vestibular screen. Note small air holes for breathing and relationship to teeth and supporting tissues. This type of appliance, if worn conscientiously, is an excellent deterrent for tongue thrust and finger sucking. Considerable attention to obtaining a proper fitting is necessary to ensure patient cooperation. (Courtesy F. Kraus.)

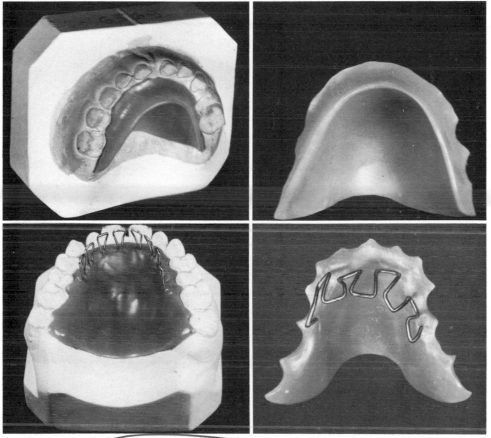

Figure 14-26. Oral screen appliances. These appliances may be made solely of acrylic (upper pictures) or of acrylic combined with wire loops (lower pictures). Their primary objective is to control tongue function. Ball clasps may be added in the molar area to increase the retention of the appliance and reduce the tendency for the posterior end to drop when the tongue thrusts forward.

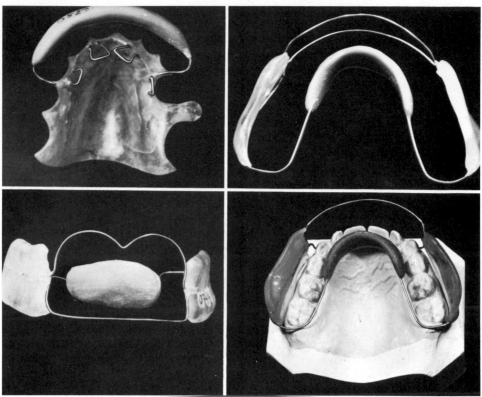

Figure 14–27 Combined oral and vestibular screens. Upper left picture shows modified acrylic palate and labial screen. The oral and buccal vestibular screen combination (upper right and lower left) aims at control of tongue thrust and excessive buccinator contraction. The appliance pictured (lower right) accomplishes much the same purpose. (Courtesy F. Kraus.)

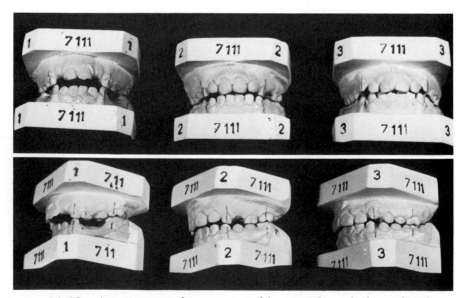

Figure 14–28.   Anterior open bite, corrected by use of vestibular and oral screens. This is an excellent example of channeling muscle forces into favorable directions to correct developing malocclusions. (Courtesy F. Kraus.)

vestibular screen is fabricated to control muscle forces both inside and outside the dental arches (Fig. 14–27). If used assiduously and constructed properly, the abnormal muscle forces can be intercepted and channeled into beneficial activity, reducing the developing malocclusion. Used alone, these appliances are limited in their scope of correction and should be employed as interceptive adjuncts for frank muscle perversion problems only. A careful diagnosis of the problem should be made before attempting correction with the vestibular or oral screen. If patient cooperation is not assured, fixed appliances are indicated. The vestibular and oral screens may also be used with fixed appliances to considerable advantage. In most instances their use should be under the guidance of an orthodontic specialist.

MUSCLE EXERCISES

It is a rather common occurence for a child of 7 or 8 years of age to have mildly protruding and spaced maxillary incisor teeth. The normal processes of growth and development usually take care of this temporary prominence. To aid in the autonomous correction, and to prevent the establishment of abnormal lip and tongue habits that might accentuate the deformity, simple lip exercises should be recommended. Hypotonicity and flaccidity of the upper lip are the most obvious characteristics of this kind of problem.[13] The child is instructed to extend the upper lip as far as possible, curving the vermilion border under and behind the maxillary incisors. This exercise should be done 15 to 30 minutes a day for a period of four to five months when a child has a short upper lip.

Where protrusion of the maxillary incisors is also a factor, the lower lip can be used to augment the upper lip exercise. The upper lip is first extended into the previously described position (Fig. 14–30). The vermilion border of the lower lip is then placed against the outside of the extended upper lip and pressed as hard as possible against the upper lip. This type of exercise exerts a strong retracting influence on the maxillary incisors while increasing the tonicity of both upper and lower lips. The exercise is particularly valuable for children who breathe through their mouths and seldom approximate their lips during rest. A minimum of 30 minutes a day is necessary to achieve any results. Where there is a frank Class II, Division 1 malocclusion with excessive overbite and overjet and abnormal perioral muscle function, these exercises are valuable before and during orthodontic therapy. As pointed out in Chapter 13, there is a sensual component in lip massage, and such an exercise may well serve as a substitute for finger and tongue habits, by virtue of similar gratificational response. While the exercise is not unpleasant and patient cooperation is easy to obtain, the skin immediately contiguous to the lip may become irritated. A mild emollient or plain petroleum jelly controls the problem.

Many times the child is seen before he is ready for tooth-moving appliances. A routine of daily lip exercise of the type described will tend to offset the deforming influence of the compensatory abnormal perioral muscle function associated with the malocclusion and increase the tonicity and the restraining influence of the lips. The exercise will call the child's attention to the protrusion of the maxillary incisors. Being aware of his problem, he may be more careful about engaging in activities that are likely to cause fracture of these accident-prone teeth.

For children with a developing Class II, Division 1 malocclusion, the playing of a wind instrument actually may be an interceptive orthodontic procedure.

The increased demands for intensive lip activity serve much the same purpose as the lip exercises. Some orthodontists prescribe blowing exercises to increase lip tonicity. It is probable that all exercises of this type are beneficial. Whatever the exercise used, however, it must be of sufficient frequency, intensity and duration each day over a considerable period of time for the beneficial effects to be achieved.

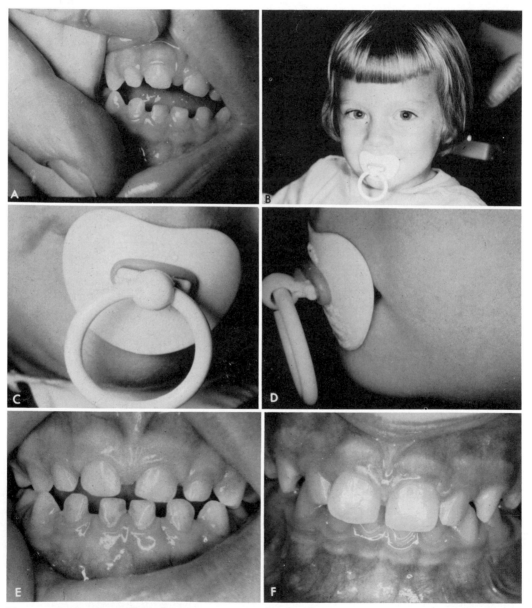

Figure 14–29   Open bite due to retained infantile deglutitional pattern. Use of properly designed pacifier closed down bite from (A) to (E) in six weeks. F shows same patient, five years later.

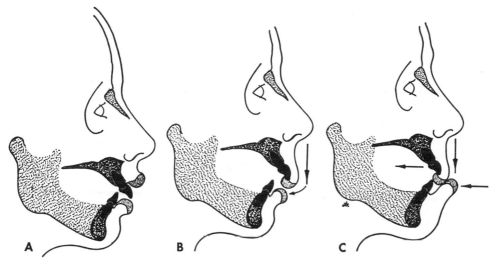

Figure 14–30 Lip exercises for prominent and spaced maxillary incisors and for short, hypotonic upper lips. A, Habitual posture with prominent incisors and short lip. B, Extending upper lip to increase tonicity and, when combined with a strongly contracted lower lip as in (C), to retract incisors.

DEVELOPING MANDIBULAR PROGNATHISM

While extraoral force, in conjunction with conventional intraoral appliances, is discussed in Chapters 11 and 18, the use of this form of therapy as an interceptive or at least palliative procedure without intraoral appliances is to be recommended in many cases[14] (Fig. 14–31).

It was pointed out previously that Class II and Class III malocclusions are similar in one respect; they are both largely maxillomandibular basal malrelationships. The mandible is protruded in Class III instead of being retruded as it is in Class II, Division 1 malocclusion. If it seems reasonable to retard the horizontal vector of the maxillary alveolodental complex in Class II malocclusions to permit an anteroposterior basal adjustment with the use of extraoral force, as described in Chapter 11, it would seem to make equally good sense to apply force against the mandibular arch and strive for a similar basal adjustment for mandibular prognathism. Unfortunately, considerable clinical experience does not validate this premise completely. Success of extraoral force against the mandibular dental arch in Class III malocclusions is limited in some cases. Results are unpredictable and spotty, with many patients responding dramatically while others show little apparent effect of extraoral force against the lower arch. Of course, there is no sure way of knowing what the problems would have been if nothing was done. How much worse would the prognathism have been? How much retardation was there? We can't say for sure.

Orthopedic therapy of extremities and the spine shows the potential for growth guidance of craniofacial structures. If a Milwaukee brace can straighten the spine of a growing child with scoliosis, why not a brace to straighten the jaws?[19] If primitive peoples could bind the calvarium, producing bizarre shapes of the skull, why not channel this growth guiding force to correct jaw and teeth relationships? The answer is that it can be done.[22] Moyers, Joho and others have demonstrated the use of orthopedic force on the orofacial complex in monkeys.[20,21] For Class III malocclusions, the author has placed quite a number of chincaps and jaw orthopedic extraoral appliances that deliver a retruding force against the

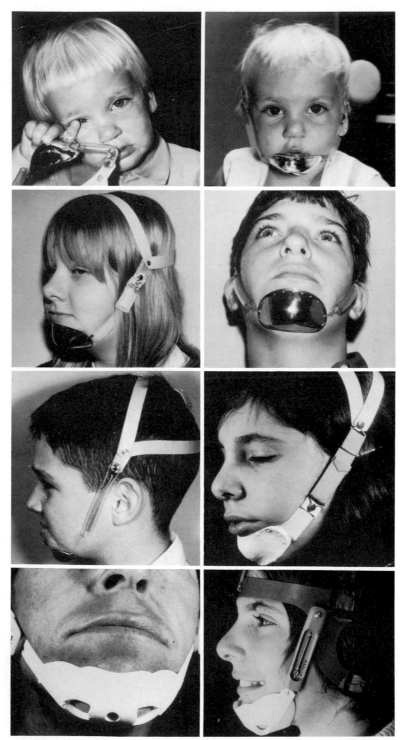

Figure 14–31 Chincap extraoral appliance, with headcap and elastics to exert upward and backward force on mandible. Metal cap is lined with soft tissue or talcum powder each night. The high pull headcap is preferred and is used in a similar manner to
correct anterior open bite, as well as Class III malocclusions.

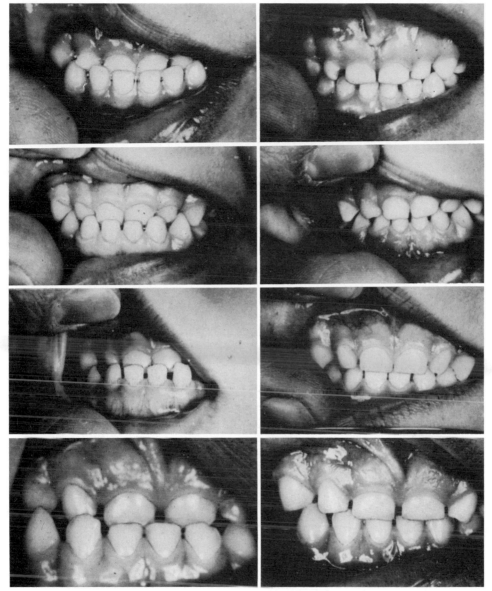

Figure 14–32 Class III malocclusions corrected only by means of chincap. All cases responded in less than eight months, and most responded in three to four months. No intraoral appliances were used. No temporomandibular joint disturbances occurred.

mandible proper. These have been placed early, and in the deciduous dentition, is possible. Most of the cases have responded well, with elimination of the Class III relationship and anterior cross-bite (Fig. 14–32). No intraoral appliances were used. In not a single case has a temporomandibular joint disturbance been observed, the claims to the contrary notwithstanding. Discomfort is minimal or nonexistent.

Even in those cases in which a Class III tendency still remains, probably requiring conventional therapy later, it is felt that the improvement has been worth the trouble. Minor problems such as chin irritation clear up under local medication. No other deleterious effects have been noted.

Since Class III malocclusions are among the most difficult to treat by the specialist and since surgical intervention is contemplated more frequently for this type of problem than any other malocclusion, it just makes good common sense that at least a chincap should be tried early to intercept the developing malocclusion and basal malrelationship. Thus, extraoral force is a valuable therapeutic adjunct in both mandibular prognathism and open bite problems, and with some modification, in Class II maxillary protrusion cases, to reduce the anteroposterior discrepancy. At the very least, it may serve to prevent a worsening malocclusion. Early prevention is the theme! (See Chap. 18 of this text and Chap. 10 of *Current Orthodontic Concepts and Techniques* by the author.[14])

As Weber[15-17] has pointed out repeatedly in the literature, these limited orthodontic procedures, properly chosen, with adequate specialty consultation and guidance, should play a part of everyday dental practice.

REFERENCES

1. Worms, F. W., Meskin, L. H., and Isaacson, R. J.: Open bite. Am. J. Orthodont., 59:589–595, 1971.
2. Tulley, W. J.: A critical appraisal of tongue thrusting. Am. J. Orthodont., 55:640–650, 1969.
3. Winders, R. V.: Tongue thrust-abnormal swallowing myometric research. J. Wisconsin Dent. Soc., 44:259–262, 1968.
4. Weiss, C. E.: Orofacial musculature imbalance and associated symptoms. Brit. J. Disord. Commun., 4:140–145, 1969.
5. Bosma, J. F.: Evaluation of oral function of the orthodontic patient. Am. J. Orthodont., 55:578–584, 1969.
6. Proffit, W. R., and Norton, L. A.: The tongue and oral morphology. A.S.H.A. Reports, No. 5, 107–115, 1971.
7. Hanson, M. L., Logan, W. B., and Case, J. L.: Tongue thrust in pre-school children. Am. J. Orthodont., 57:15–22, 1970.
8. Büttner, M.: Does thumbsucking cause an increase in the incidence of cases of mandibular retroposition? Sweisz. Monatschrift Zahnheilk., 80:32–36, 1970.
9. Popovitch, F.: The prevalence of sucking habit and its relation to malocclusion. Oral Health, 57:498–499, 1967.
10. Haryett, R. D., Sandilands, M., and Davidson, P. O.: Relative effectiveness of various methods of arresting thumbsucking. J. Canad. Dent. Ass., 34:5–10, 1968.
11. Graber, T. M.: The three "M's": muscles, malformation and malocclusion. Am. J. Orthodont., 49:418–450, 1963.
12. Kraus, F.: Prevence a Naprava Vyvojovych vad Orofacialni Soustavy. Prague Statni Zdravotnicke Nakladatelstvi., 1956.
13. Garliner, D.: Some ancillary results of the correction of abnormal swallowing habits. New York. Dent. J. 39:158–164, 1969.
14. Graber, T. M.: Current Orthodontic Concepts and Techniques. Philadelphia, W. B. Saunders Co., 1969.
15. Weber, F. N.: Orthorehabilitative procedures. D. Clin. North America, July, 1959, pp. 419–434.
16. Weber, F. N.: Orthodontic education for the nonorthodontist: why, where, and how. Am. J. Orthodont., 48:436–443, 1962.
17. Weber, F. N.: Symposium on orthodontics for the general practitioner (Foreword). D. Clin. North America, July, 1964.
18. Mathews, J. R.: Translational movement of first deciduous molars into second molar positions. Am. J. Orthodont., 55:276–285, 1969.
19. Stöckli, P., and Gisler, G.: Ergebnisse kieferorthopädischer Begleitbehandlung bei Skoliosepatienten. Deutsch. Zahn, Mund. Kieferheilk., 52:1–8, 1969.
20. Elgoyhen, J. C., Riolo, M. L., Graber, L. W., Moyers, R. E. and McNamara, J. A.: Craniofacial growth in juvenile Macaca Mulatta, Am. J. Phys. Anthropol., May, 1972.
21. Joho, J. P.: Die Reaction der Zahne und Kiefer auf Veränderung der Bisslage. University of Zurich, Zurich, Juris Druck Verlag., 1968.
22. Cutler, B. S., Hassig, F. H., and Turpin, D. L.: Dentofacial changes produced during and after use of a modified Milwaukee brace on Macaca mulatta. Am. J. Orthodont., 61:115–137, 1972.

chapter 15

SURGICAL ORTHODONTICS

In Chapter 6, cleft lip and palate were discussed as etiologic factors in mal-occlusion. The early attempts at surgical closure of these defects actually produced more severe dentofacial deformities. It was only through *team effort* that the multifaceted problems have been successfully controlled. It would be hard to find the facial cripples today that were so common as recently as 25 years ago. There are other areas of common concern among the specialties that profit equally from combined service and interspecialty care. Too many people think of orthodontics as dealing only with appliances and their manipulation. Nothing could be further from the truth. Closely allied in rendering the ultimate in orthodontic service are the orthodontist and the oral surgeon. Over and above care of cysts, supernumerary teeth, ankylosed teeth and the routine extraction of premolars in a large portion of orthodontic problems (Class I cases, particularly) are other examples of orthosurgical teamwork. These will be discussed and illustrated in this chapter.

1. Serial extraction
2. Surgical uncovering of impactions, positioning and transpositioning of teeth
3. Frenectomies and soft tissue control
4. Resections and ostectomies
5. Cosmetic surgery

SERIAL EXTRACTION

HISTORICAL DEVELOPMENT

Serial extraction is not new. An excellent study by Palsson[1] points out that throughout the history of orthodontics it has been recognized that the removal of one or more irregular teeth would improve the appearance of the remainder. Apparently Bunon, in his *Essay on Diseases of the Teeth*, published in 1743, made the first reference to the removal of deciduous teeth to achieve a better alignment of the permanent teeth. The names that stand out particularly for the modern development of the serial extraction concept are Kjellgren[2] of Sweden, Hotz[3, 4] of Switzerland, Heath[5, 6] of Australia, and Nance, Lloyd, Dewel and Mayne of the United States.[7-15] Nance[7] presented clinics on his technique of "progressive extraction" a number of times in the 1940's and has been called the "father" of serial extraction philosophy in the United States. The technique that is described in the following pages is based largely on Nance's recommendations and subsequent writings by Dewel, Mayne, Ringenberg, Hinrichsen, Fanning, Moorrees, et al.[16–22]

GROWTH AND DEVELOPMENT

It is in Class I cases that serial extraction finds its most successful application. How great a factor is growth in the alveolar arches? When and where does this happen? Is the timing sex-linked?

Longitudinal studies on arch length increase and increments of growth have been done.[22, 36] Figure 15–1 shows that by the end of the ninth year in girls and the tenth year in boys, the mandibular intercanine arch width dimension is essentially complete. In the maxilla, there is little further maxillary arch width increase in girls, after 12 years of age. In boys, the bar graph shows that the maxillary intercanine dimension may continue to increase until 18 years of age. As discussed in Chapter 2, this difference in increase of maxillary dimensions is due to the fact that the pubertal growth spurt in girls is from 10½ to 12 years of age, while in boys it is from 12 to 18 years of age.[36] The maxillary intercanine arch width increase serves as a "safety valve" for the dominant horizontal basal mandibular growth spurts. This terminal, horizontal, incremental mandibular growth is particularly a male sex-linked character and may be demonstrated routinely

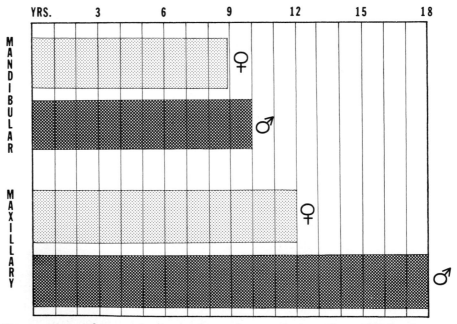

INTERCANINE ARCH GROWTH

Figure 15–1 This graph shows the early completion of mandibular intercanine growth, both in girls and in boys. In the maxilla, however, a significant sex-linked difference is seen. This is because the maxillary intercanine dimension serves as a "safety valve" for the puberty-linked horizontal basal mandibular growth increments. The later and continuing pubertal growth spurt in boys (12 to 18 years) accounts for the continuing intercanine increase in the maxillary arch. (Adapted from Moorrees, C. F. A., et al.: The consideration of dental development in serial extraction. Angle Orthodont., 33:44–59, 1963.)

with cephalometric radiographs. It would be inconsistent with the present knowledge of growth and development to expect *any* appliances to increase mandibular intercanine arch width after 10 to 11 years of age. The maxillary intercanine increase is a result of the need for adjustment for basal mandibular growth and must be left for this purpose.[31, 35, 36]

Thus, if there is a Class I malocclusion with generalized crowding, the clinician would be most unwise to resort to expansion of the maxillary and mandibular arches with fixed or removable appliances, hoping for growth to "bail him out." The creation of an abnormal muscle activity, with increased muscle tissue system pressures on the expanded dental arches, and the production of inharmonious relationship of the tooth system to the basal bone system (in other words the creation of two abnormal tissue systems from what was originally a normal relationship) merely to satisfy the demands of alignment of teeth are hardly calculated to enhance the longevity of the stomatognathic system. This is an iatrogenic malocclusion and the damaging effects are clearly evident to the periodontist at a later date.

DEVELOPMENTAL SPACING AND DENTITIONAL ADJUSTMENT

Although we can describe the broad growth trends for groups, growth prediction for the individual patient is still relatively inaccurate. Timing and precise increments for specific areas are clinically important in arch length as well as basal malrelationship problems, but the most sophisticated methodology still does not give us a reliable clinical tool. Fortunately, certain aspects of dentitional adjustment are amenable to measurement, as the deciduous-succedaneous developmental cycle proceeds. There are measurements we can make in both the anterior and posterior segments in both arches, which facilitate a program of guided or progressive extraction in discrepancy cases.

ANTERIOR SEGMENTS.   The fact that the permanent incisors are larger than the deciduous counterparts is quite obvious, even to the patient. But what is the exact size differential? Does it vary from patient to patient, from jaw to jaw? Direct measurement of this *incisor liability*, as it is termed by Mayne, is possible and recommended.[31] Long cone technique radiographs and plaster study model measurements accurately portray the size relationship of unerupted and erupted teeth. The deciduous-permanent tooth size differential averages 6 to 7 mm., even when there is no crowding. How is this discrepancy reconciled? Mayne lists the mechanisms of incisor liability adjustment.

1. Intercanine arch growth—3 to 4 mm.
2. Interdental (developmental) spacing—2 to 3 mm.
3. More anterior position of permanent incisors as they erupt—1 to 2 mm.

The actual size differential of the teeth establishes the magnitude of the challenge for these three developmental adjustments. Precise measurement must be made to determine the incisor liability. Mean values are not to be used here. The space situation is even more critical in the lower arch, since it is the contained arch. In addition, a transient developmental deep bite may well interfere with the attainment of optimal intercanine growth and labial positioning of the lower incisors.[20, 24] Late pubertal horizontal growth increments in the mandible, particularly in boys, can only exacerbate the crowding tendency. Any appreciable incisor liability, which would make demands on the adjustment mechanisms beyond the probable contributions listed above points strongly to a program of guided extraction in the mixed dentition period.

POSTERIOR SEGMENTS.   What about the possibility of making up for anterior crowding by using deciduous molar space? As pointed out in Chapter 2, the combined widths of the mandibular deciduous canine, first molar and second molar average 1.7 mm. more than the combined widths of the three permanent successors (Fig. 2–71). As Nance indicated, there is less width differential in the maxillary arch (average width difference 1 mm.). This "leeway space" exists on both sides, so it would average 3.4 mm. in the mandibular arch and about 2 mm. in the maxillary arch.[7] Can it be used for incisor crowding?

First of all, the "leeway space" varies considerably, depending on tooth size and the proportionate relationship of deciduous and permanent teeth. In addition, there is what Moyers calls the "flush terminal plane relationship" with the first permanent molars in an end-to-end cuspal contact[33] (Fig. 15–2). The orthodontist would call this a Class II tendency. This is a normal, transient developmental phenomenon and is seen in a large percentage of cases. With exchange of the deciduous for the permanent teeth, there is a mesial drift of the mandibular first molar, taking up the "leeway" space and allowing the mesial buccal cusp of the maxillary first molar to lock into the mesial buccal groove of the mandibular first permanent molar. The "leeway space," then, is usually a reserved bit of arch length to allow for the adjustment of maxillary and mandibular dental arches during the critical tooth exchange period.[7] Use of this space, holding back the mandibular molars to gain arch length anteriorly, may very well take a Class II tendency problem and make it a full Class II, Division I malocclusion. Prevention of the settling-in of the cusps and grooves may produce premature contacts,

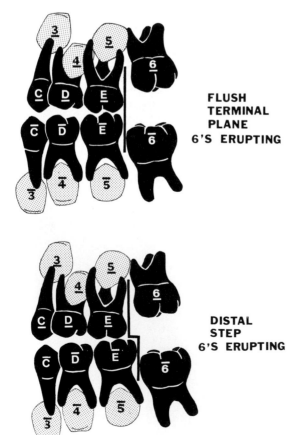

**FLUSH
TERMINAL
PLANE
6'S ERUPTING**

**DISTAL
STEP
6'S ERUPTING**

Figure 15–2 Moyers has reported that at least 50 per cent of normal developing dentitions have a flush terminal plane relationship that corrects itself only with the loss of the deciduous molars at the end of the mixed dentition period with the utilization of the leeway space. This Class II tendency may be accentuated with a distal step, if there is a morphogenetic Class II pattern or an excessively deep overbite and resultant functional retrusion. (From Moyers, R. E.: Development of occlusion. D. Clin. North America, pp. 523–536, 1969.)

enhancing bruxism and functional problems. To satisfy the demands of arch length, using the "leeway space," would be to obvert the developmental and physiologic phenomena that would normally occur.

ROLE OF EXPANSION

It was not until the early 1940's that expansion of the dental arches as a means of eliminating irregularities was pretty well-recognized by orthodontists as a "two-edged sword." In Class I malocclusions, it was possible to eliminate the irregularities, but teeth were moved into abnormal stress positions and into muscle forces. Thus, in a challenge which essentially involved harmonizing teeth with basal bone, with normal muscle and jaw relationships, an imbalance was established. Such measures provided a temporary correction at best.[24, 26]

In Class II malocclusions, expansion was and *still is* a valid treatment objective, because there is concomitant change in muscle function and jaw relationship with successful Class II therapy. Indeed, restoration of normal function is a prime treatment objective. However, in Class I malocclusions, where there is a lack of harmony between the amount of tooth material and the available basal bone and where the patient already has normal muscle activity, the movement of teeth off of basal bone into functional forces is not likely to produce a stable orthodontic result. The retainers splint the teeth, holding them outward in a sufficiently large enough arc to allow the alignment of individual units, but the muscle forces are constantly exerting greater than normal forces from the outside. As soon as the retainers are removed or the wearing is reduced sufficiently to allow the muscles to play a dominant role, there is a relapse and also resultant irregularity that may not be much different from the original problem. Considerable research in electromyography and telemetry, with sophisticated electronic equipment has validated the clinician's concern about expansion procedures in orthodontics in Class I malocclusions.[36]

The limitations of expansion techniques in the treatment of Class I malocclusion must be recognized. To ignore the interrelationship of the four tissue systems the tooth, nerve, muscle and bone systems—is to invite ultimate relapse. The problem, succinctly, is a five-room house on a four-room foundation. In Class I, the neuromuscular and bone systems are already harmonious in the interrelationships and it is the job of the orthodontist to bring the tooth system into balance by judicious, guided extraction procedures. As Dewel[13] says,

By this procedure, serial extraction avoids one form of orthodontic negligence; teeth in marked discrepancy cases are not first required to assume positions of extreme irregularity and then subjected to extensive orthodontic movement with extraction to establish acceptable occlusal relations. They are, instead, permitted to take these positions in the first place.

SELECTION OF TEETH FOR EXTRACTION

After recognizing the importance of harmonizing the amount of tooth material with the available bony support, the next obvious question is: What teeth should be extracted? Since most Class I malocclusions involve irregularities of the canines and incisors, with space deficiency appearing most critical in this area, the layman may ask, "Why not take out a tooth here?" It is not hard for the dentist to answer this question. The importance from an esthetic and functional standpoint of maintaining bilateral symmetry rules out the choice in all but a few exceptional cases (for example, cases involving unilateral congenital absence, anomalous teeth, cleft lip and palate and severe caries).

Historically, as extraction became more prevalent in orthodontics, the first premolars became the usual teeth of choice to be removed. But the mere removal of four teeth was no "open sesame" to success. The orthodontist soon found that unless he controlled the remaining teeth effectively with efficient multiband appliances, only part of the original malocclusion would be corrected. He might even face additional characteristics of malocclusion produced by tipping of teeth to poor stress-reception positions, or by his inept handling of the situation.

Orthodontic therapy in extraction cases requires a degree of orthodontic skill and training well beyond the level of general practice.[11] The need for control of individual teeth is paramount. An iatrogenic malocclusion with deep overbite, spaces, improper contacts, teeth in abnormal axial inclination and functional aberrations could well be worse than the untreated original crowding characteristics of the patient.[12, 16, 23] Thus, the pervading theme is that serial extraction is a valuable adjunct in treatment of Class I malocclusion, but it is an orthodontic decision and requires the knowledge, ability and clinical experience of the specialist who ultimately must complete the therapy in almost all cases. Much irresponsible tooth movement has been seen in pedodontic circles where there has not been the benefit of expertise in changing diagnostic decisions and appliance manipulation.[24]

As more and more orthodontists prescribe removal of teeth during orthodontic therapy, they find that the first premolar is not always the best tooth to be sacrificed. Sometimes it is the second premolar or the second premolars in one arch and the first premolars in the other arch.[38] Caries may necessitate the removal of a first permanent molar, or the choice may be maxillary second molars only. The decision depends on an exhaustive study of all available diagnostic criteria and a thorough understanding of orthodontic principles and mechanotherapy. At best, diagnosis is a tentative decision and re-evaluation of the patient's status at each examination with periodic radiographic survey is essential. There is no cookbook for guided or progressive extraction procedures. While the dentist in general practice cannot be expected to know all these things, he should at least be aware of what the orthodontist is doing and some of the general reasons behind his decisions.

The removal of certain teeth to establish a stable orthodontic result in harmony with the investing tissues has given rise to an additional question; When should the teeth of choice be removed? Taking a clue from nature, which exfoliates the deciduous canines early in arch length deficiency problems, is it advisable to remove the deciduous canines and deciduous molars early to allow the permanent teeth to align themselves better as they erupt?[24] Will this prevent the permanent incisors and canines from assuming positions of extreme irregularity which require extensive orthodontic therapy and extraction of premolars to achieve the desired result? Instead of waiting for all the permanent teeth to erupt into a full-blown malocclusion, why not intercept in the early mixed dentition by relieving the crowding to give nature a chance to adapt with adequate space? The answer is conditionally affirmative, but before embarking on this "robbing Peter to pay Paul" procedure the orthodontist must ask himself a number of questions (Fig. 15–3).

First, is the discrepancy between tooth size and available supporting bone such that the teeth will not be able to find sufficient room for proper alignment on their own?[19, 25] It must be remembered that the teeth have achieved their ultimate size when they erupt, but the dental arches have not. The parent's occlusion or the hereditary pattern may provide information of value at this

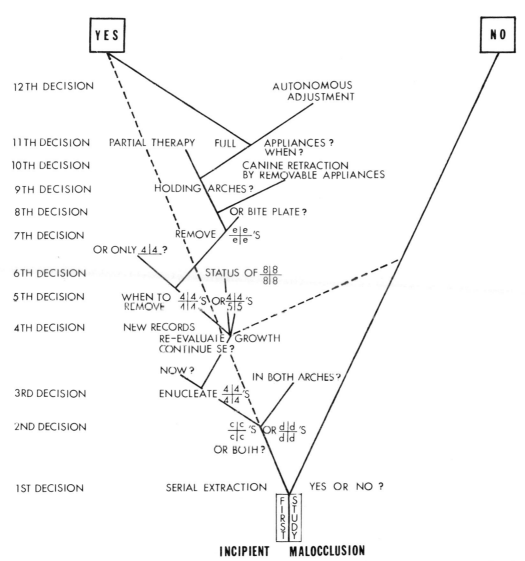

Figure 15-3 Which road shall it be? After a diagnostic study of an incipient malocclusion, a conditional affirmative or negative decision is made. But this tentative opinion is subject to constant assessment during the program of guided extraction. A "yes" decision for guided extraction means that at least a dozen decisions will have to be made over a period of two to four years of orthodontic pre-appliance guidance. Unless the dentist is prepared to travel the road and make the numerous decisions, based on periodic diagnostic criteria, he should not undertake the "trip" in the first place. (After Mayne, W. R.: *in* Graber, T. M. (ed.): Current Orthodontic Concepts and Techniques. W. B. Saunders Co., 1969.)

point. Detailed study and precise measurements of deciduous teeth and their permanent successors must be made before arriving at any decision.

Second, are both the patient and the parents aware that serial extraction is a continuing program of orthodontic guidance over a period of four or five years? Unless it is made clear to the parents that the child must be observed at periodic intervals over a prolonged period of time, that teeth will have to be removed during this period as directed by the orthodontist and that the orthodontic guidance will likely culminate in a period of actual mechanotherapy, then nothing should be started. A *poorly guided serial extraction program may be worse than nothing at all*, making the appliance problems more difficult or making complete correction impossible.[26]

Third, the orthodontist must be fully aware that serial extraction is not a pat "one, two, three" procedure. He may have to alter his tentative program one or more times during the period of observation, depending on the degree of self-adjustment, on other sequelae of malocclusion, on the speed and order of the eruption of permanent teeth and similar factors. What appears as a serial extraction case at 7 or 8 years of age may not seem so at 10 or 10½ years of age, as a result of developmental changes that could not be predicted. The orthodontist must be prepared to reverse his decision on the basis of current diagnostic records. He may have to institute mechanotherapy earlier than planned, or he may have to place appliances more than once if he is to achieve the total correction possible from an intelligently guided orthodontic management.

If the general practitioner wishes to undertake a serial extraction program, he must ask himself whether or not he has the skill and training required to cope with the problems of overbite, axial inclination, space closure, torque, rotations, paralleling and the complexities of the appliance necessary to achieve the best possible result for the patient. This is a rhetorical question, for very few general practitioners or pedodontists, indeed, have the training and experience necessary.[31] So-called orthodontic appliances, fabricated by self-styled orthodontic laboratories are most certainly not the answer. Yet, with proper orthodontic guidance and the recognition that appliance therapy must be expected and is required for almost all patients, serial extraction will become a valuable adjunct in practice, greatly reducing the amount of appliance therapy needed for the correction of Class I malocclusions. It will reduce the length of time that appliances will have to be worn and minimize untoward sequelae such as root resorption, decalcification and soft tissue proliferation that so often accompany protracted periods of appliance therapy. Possibly, too, financial investment for the patient may be decreased.

INDICATIONS FOR SERIAL EXTRACTION

When an orthodontist sees a child of five or six years of age with all the deciduous teeth present in a slightly crowded state or with no spaces between them, he can predict with a fair degree of certainty that there will not be enough space in the jaws to accommodate all the permanent teeth in their proper alignment.[25] As Dewel, Mayne and others have pointed out, after the eruption of the first permanent molars at six years of age, there is probably no increase in the distance from the mesial aspect of the first molar on one side around the arch to the mesial aspect of the first molar on the opposite side[7, 10, 22] (Fig. 15–4). If there is any change, it may be an actual reduction of the molar-to-molar arch length, as the "leeway space" is lost through the mesial migration of the first permanent molars during the tooth exchange process and correction of the flush terminal plane relationship[33] (Fig. 15–2).

There are other cardinal clues that point to the possibility of serial extraction (Figs. 15–5 to 15–8). The following is a list of possible clinical clues for serial extraction, occurring singly or in combination:

1. Premature loss
2. Arch length deficiency and tooth size discrepancies
3. Lingual eruption of lateral incisors
4. Unilateral deciduous canine loss and shift to the same side
5. Canines erupting mesially over lateral incisors
6. Mesial drift of buccal segments
7. Abnormal eruption direction and eruption sequence
8. Flaring
9. Ectopic eruption
10. Abnormal resorption
11. Ankylosis
12. Labial stripping, or gingival recession, usually of a lower incisor

If gingival recession and alveolar destruction are present on the labial of one or several mandibular incisors in a child eight or nine years of age, complete records should be taken to make a positive diagnosis and to outline a plan of management. If a child of this age has premature loss of one or both mandibular deciduous canines, this may well have been due to pressure against the deciduous canine roots by the crowns of the erupting permanent lateral incisors. This condition is a significant hint to a wise clinician. Very often only one mandibular deciduous canine is lost. As soon as one is exfoliated, the incisor teeth shift into the space created, relieving the pressure on the remaining canine. A check of the midline of the mandibular arch shows this quickly. Prompt removal of the remaining deciduous canines may be indicated (Figs. 15–7, 15–8).

Clues also are seen in the posterior segments. Rotated and tipped permanent molars in either arch are usually a sign of mesial drift of the buccal teeth, and the first molars in particular. Sometimes the teeth on both sides of the eden-

Figure 15–4 As Moorrees shows, total arch length, or clinical arch length from permanent first molar to its counterpart on the opposite side, maxilla and mandible, male and female, does not increase . . . it decreases. Mesial drift of the mandibular molar is greater, utilizing the larger leeway space provided by the mandibular second deciduous molar, to eliminate the flush terminal plane relationship. (Solid line = male; dotted = female.) (From Moorrees, C. F. A., et al.: The consideration of dental development in serial extraction. Angle Orthodont., 33:44–59, 1963.)

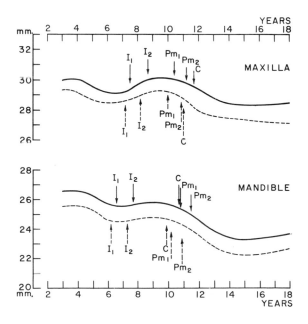

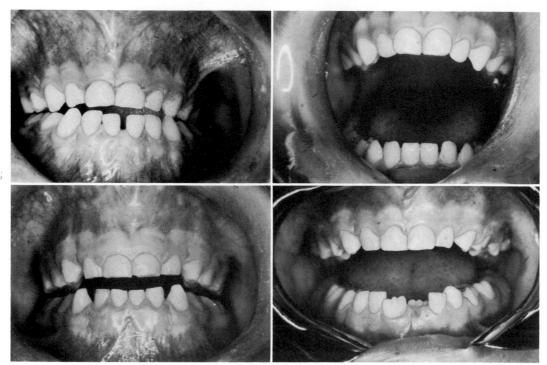

Figure 15–5 Clues for serial extraction. Deciduous dentitions with no "developmental" spacing, as illustrated, will have problems finding space for permanent successors, in all likelihood. When confronted with problems of this type, a complete radiographic survey should be made to determine the widths of unerupted teeth, and the magnitude of the potential discrepancy. (Courtesy W. R. Mayne.)

tulous areas tend to tip into the space. An orthodontic consultation becomes necessary, for the uprighting and distal tipping of these teeth to their normal positions may take the case out of the serial extraction category and make more extensive mechanotherapy necessary. Such a decision must be based on a thorough diagnostic discipline.

If the mixed dentition analysis, arch length measurements and the mesiodistal measurements of unerupted teeth substantiate the clinical impression of space inadequacy, the parent should be informed of the need for a long-range program of interceptive orthodontic guidance, with premature removal of deciduous teeth *in sequence* at times determined by the patient's own development. This is to allow improved alignment of the erupting permanent teeth by temporarily increasing the available space. Ultimately, permanent teeth usually have to be removed to eliminate the inherent arch length deficiency, and orthodontic appliances will be needed to establish the correct occlusion.

DEPENDENCE ON MAXILLOMANDIBULAR RELATIONSHIP.   It must be emphasized that any planned program of serial extraction is dependent on the maxillomandibular relationship. If it is normal, as evidenced by the correct interdigitation of the buccal segments (Class I malocclusion), chances of success are relatively good, with proper guidance and patient cooperation. If the maxillomandibular relationship is abnormal (Class II and Class III malocclusions), a serial extraction program must be approached with great caution, with considerable reservation and with the expectancy that the basal malrelationship must be adjusted by appliances prior to the completion of the permanent dentition. Dewel[13] writes, "Severe Class II discrepancy irregularities are treated primarily

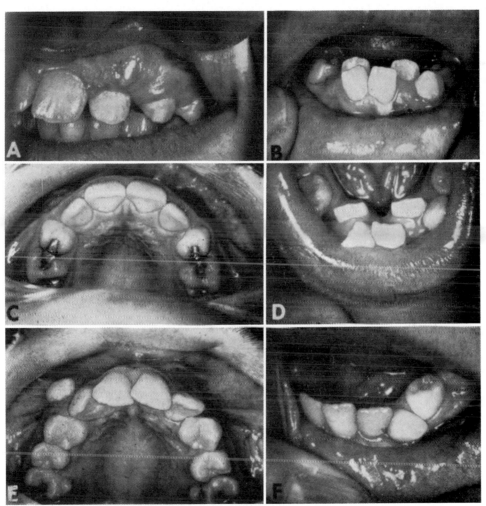

Figure 15–6 Clues for serial extraction. A, Maxillary canine mesial to normal, erupting labially to lateral incisor; B, arch deficiency, with laterals erupting lingually, canines labially, or mesially; C, mesial drift of buccal segments with totally inadequate space for canines; D, arch length deficiency; E, mesial drift, arch length deficiency, with canine erupting mesially over lateral incisor; F, deciduous canine being exfoliated prematurely due to crowding.

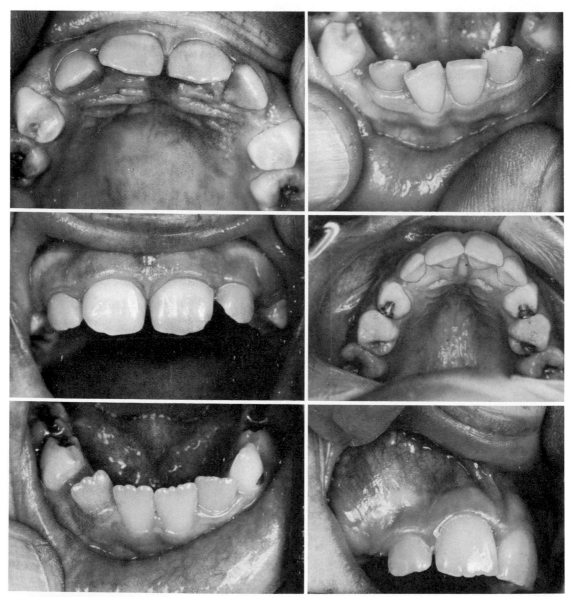

Figure 15–7 Clues for serial extraction for the observant dentist. Deciduous canines have been lost prematurely and autonomously as a result of nature's attempt to gain space. In picture at lower left, premature loss of lower right deciduous canine has allowed lateral incisor to erupt and drift distally, relieving the struggle for space momentarily, but with a probable shift of lower incisors, unless the deciduous lateral is lost on the other side. Note flaring of lateral incisors as unerupted canines are in contact with their apical portions. Beginning stripping of labial gingival tissue may be seen on incisors in picture at upper right. Canine bulges over lateral incisors (middle left and lower right pictures) are some of the most frequent sequelae of potential serial extraction cases.

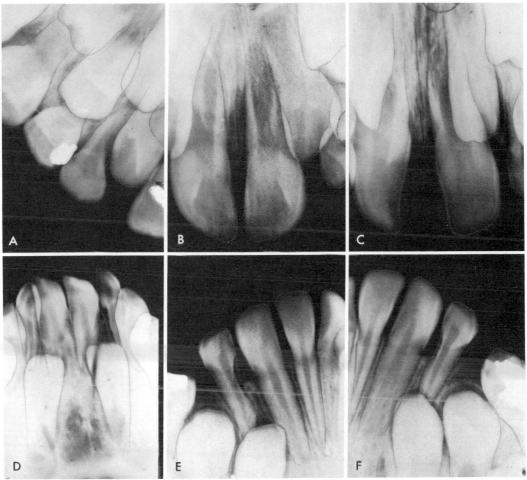

Figure 15–8 Intraoral periapical radiographs are excellent sources of serial extraction clues. A and B, Maxillary lateral incisors are blocked out of arch, with an abnormal resorption pattern. C, Lateral incisors are probably erupting lingually with arch length deficiency. D, E and F, Abnormal resorption patterns of deciduous teeth serve as a harbinger of future guided extraction procedures. Long-cone technique radiographs and careful measurement of unerupted teeth will assist in making a decision.

with Class II mechanics, with serial extraction more or less as an accessory to mechanical therapy." Only the orthodontist should make this decision.[31] The classic serial extraction technique must apply largely to Class I malocclusions. As Mayne[15] says,

In any discussion of serial extraction, we could quickly note reference to three systems of tissues: bone, muscle and teeth. Their interrelationship and significance is of the greatest importance to the successful application of serial extraction.

He points out that serial extraction should be limited largely to those cases that have good faces.[31]

. . . those that present harmony and balance of two tissue systems, bone and muscle, and varying degrees of disharmony in the third, tooth size. In these cases, the apical bases are located directly under one another and the incisor teeth are upright to these bases. They are reasonably well over the ridge and so related to facial anatomy as to produce the most complimentary facial esthetics.

TECHNIQUE OF SERIAL EXTRACTION

At the outset, it should be said that there is no one single technique for serial extraction. A tentative diagnostic decision is the best that can and should be made. Serial extraction is a long-range guidance program and it may be necessary to re-evaluate and change tentative decisions several times.

Although it is desirable to see a potential serial extraction case while all the deciduous teeth are still present and to make long-range plans at that time, all too frequently the orthodontist does not see the patient until he is seven or eight years of age, or even older (Figs. 15–6 to 15–8). At this time, the maxillary and mandibular central incisors are usually erupted, but there is inadequate space in the anterior segments to allow the normal eruption and positioning of the lateral incisors. In some instances, the mandibular lateral incisors have already erupted but are badly malposed, usually lingually. The maxillary lateral incisors may have erupted already, but they are usually lingually positioned and rotated. If they have not erupted, they may be palpated and located radiographically to the lingual side, in imminent danger of erupting into lingual cross-bite. Careful digital examination will disclose that the mandibular canines are bulging labially, deep in the oral vestibule. The maxillary canines may also be palpated low in the vestibular fornix, somewhat labial and medial to where they would normally be expected. There is often a slight diastema between the maxillary central incisors. But even if this space were closed, there would not be adequate space for the lateral incisors to assume their place in the dental arch. A laminagraphic radiographic examination is likely to reveal that all permanent teeth are present, but with totally inadequate space in the dental arch to receive them (Figs. 15–9, 15–10).

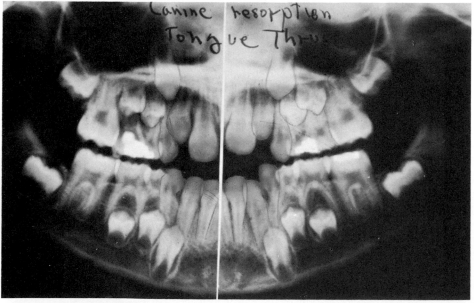

Figure 15–9 Seven-year-old girl with both tongue thrust habit and arch length deficiency. Lack of space for lateral incisors may mean rotation or eruption into lingual malposition, allowing canines to erupt abnormally mesially. The discerning dentist immediately suspects a potential case for guided extraction, merely by observing the abnormal mandibular deciduous canine resorption. He should obtain specialty consultation, even though the patient is only seven years old.

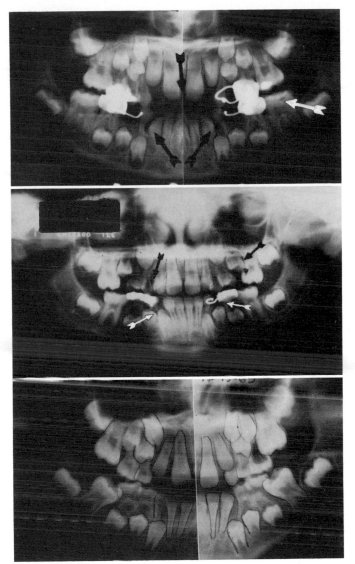

Figure 15–10   Three patients under pedodontic specialty care, but not referred for orthodontic consultation. Concern was parental, not pedodontic. In the top laminagraph, space maintainers have been placed despite abnormal resorption, premature loss, crowding, rotations—all clues for possible serial extraction. In center view, despite ectopic eruption of maxillary first molars, premature loss of deciduous second molars and arch deficiency, space maintainers were placed. No arch length determination had been made. In bottom view, multiple clues for serial extraction—ectopic eruption, premature loss, abnormal resorption, unilateral loss and shift, tipping, rotations, etc.—were not sufficient for the attending dentist to suggest an orthodontic consultation.

DIAGNOSTIC DISCIPLINE

Complete diagnostic records should be made and studied. This means study models, undistorted periapical radiographs, panoramic radiographs and cephalometric radiographs[29] (Chap. 8). The orthodontist uses a caliper or a fine line divider and measures the combined widths of the teeth present in each segment (Fig. 15–11). The circumferential measurement is made on the plaster cast from the mesial aspect of the first molar on one side to the mesial aspect of the first

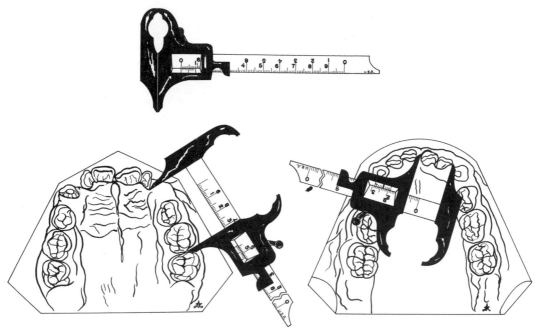

Figure 15–11. A Boley gauge, or a pair of fine line dividers, should be used to measure existing arch length from plaster study casts. These recorded measurements should be compared with those taken of unerupted teeth, from long cone technique intraoral radiographs, to determine incisor liability and posterior segment leeway space.

molar on the opposite side, and this measurement is recorded (Fig. 15–12). We have already mentioned the fact that the arch length from the mesial aspect of the molar on one side to the mesial aspect of the molar on the opposite side does not increase after these teeth have erupted and that it actually decreases with the elimination of the flush terminal plane relationship.[33] Thus, it becomes a simple matter of mathematics to add the combined widths of the permanent teeth as taken from the long cone technique intraoral radiographs and to compare this figure with the available arch length. It is not uncommon to find as much as a

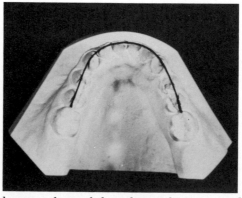

Figure 15–12 Molar-to-molar arch length may be measured by adapting soft brass separating wire around the arch from the mesial side of one first molar to the other, as illustrated. Wire is then straightened out and measured with a millimetric rule.

centimeter deficiency in either the maxillary or mandibular arch. To gain sufficient arch length at this time, the orthodontist may turn to expansion to create sufficient space for the eruption of lateral incisors, but we know his dubious chances for success if he sits back and waits for "growth and development."[35] If he has learned his lessons well in oral physiology, he knows he cannot disturb the balance of teeth and bone with that of the nerve and muscle systems. Any victory would be temporary, indeed. Thus, to provide a stable and healthy occlusion he must turn to guided tooth removal.

THREE STAGES IN SERIAL EXTRACTION THERAPY

Having established by careful diagnostic study that there is a significant deficiency, the orthodontist can embark on his planned program of guided extraction. This is usually done in three stages. Each stage accomplishes a specific purpose.

1. REMOVAL OF DECIDUOUS CANINES.   With deciduous canine exfoliation or removal, the immediate purpose is to permit the eruption and optimal alignment of the lateral incisors. Improvement in the position of the central incisors may reasonably be expected. Prevention of the eruption of the maxillary lateral incisors in lingual cross-bite or the mandibular incisors in lingual malposition is a primary consideration. But this improvement is gained at the expense of space for the permanent canines. Vitally important is the fact that correct lateral incisor position prevents the mesial migration of the canines into severe malpositions that will require concerted mechanotherapy later.

In the maxillary arch, the first premolars erupt uniformly ahead of the canines. In the mandibular arch, it is statistically less predictable. Sometimes, the orthodontist will try to maintain the mandibular deciduous canines somewhat longer hoping to retard the eruption of the permanent canines, while the first premolars take advantage of the edentulous area created by premature removal of the mandibular first deciduous molars. It is desired by most orthodontists embarking on a serial extraction procedure that the first premolars will erupt as soon as possible and ahead of the canines so the premolars may be removed, if necessary. This frequently does not happen (Fig. 15–13). As the experienced clinician knows, there is little evidence that the eruption sequence can be changed, anyway. The too early removal of mandibular deciduous first molars may very well delay the eruption of the first premolars, as a dense layer of bone fills in over them after the deciduous tooth removal. The question of deciduous canine versus deciduous first molar is largely academic, since nature usually eliminates the deciduous canines autonomously and early in the frank serial extraction case—often before the patient is even seen by the orthodontist.

It is important to expedite the normal eruption of the maxillary lateral incisors. Belated eruption and lingual malposition of these teeth permit the maxillary canines to migrate mesially and labially into the space that nature has reserved for the lateral incisors. These "high cuspids," as the orthodontist often calls them, make lingual cross-bite of the maxillary lateral incisors more certain, make orthodontic therapy more difficult and practically ensure that the first premolars will ultimately have to be removed. Remember, not *all* properly managed serial extraction cases inevitably require permanent tooth sacrifice.

Generally speaking, if nature has not already spontaneously exfoliated the deciduous canines or has exfoliated only one or two of them, these teeth are removed between eight and nine years of age in patients with an average developmental pattern.

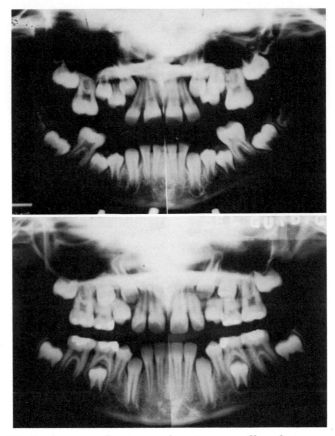

Figure 15–13   In the upper laminagraphic view, maxillary first premolars are clearly ahead of canines, but lower sequence is less clear—ahead on one side, about even on the other. In bottom view, the sequence is most desirable, with all four premolars erupting ahead of canines.

2. REMOVAL OF THE FIRST DECIDUOUS MOLARS.   By this procedure, the orthodontist hopes to accelerate the eruption of the first premolar teeth ahead of the canines, if at all possible. This is particularly "touch and go" in the mandibular arch where the normal sequence so often is for the canine to erupt ahead of the first premolar. The maneuver is seldom successful in the lower arch as has been indicated already. In Class I malocclusions especially, the first premolar may be partially impacted between the permanent canine and the still present second deciduous molar. Hence, the dentist may vary the first procedure of removing all four deciduous canines, as outlined above, and remove the first deciduous molars in the lower arch to tip the eruption scales in the direction of the first premolar. The need for another decision at this point emphasizes the strong necessity for a thorough understanding of the problem, a considered study of the patient's diagnostic records, clinical experience in similar cases and the *ability to assist with effective mechanotherapy at the proper time.*

There are times when the orthodontist, while removing first deciduous molars, must consider the possibility of enucleating the unerupted first premolars (usually in the lower arch) to achieve the optimal benefits of the serial extraction procedure. This is a most hazardous step and obviously requires keen diagnostic acumen. Yet in the properly chosen case, the autonomous adjustment and marked improvement in alignment following this step can be most gratifying to both the patient and the orthodontist (Fig. 15–14, A and B). Where the canines have erupted prior to the first premolars in the mandibular arch, the convex mesial coronal portion of the second deciduous molar may interfere with first premolar eruption. In such cases, it is necessary to remove the second deciduous molars. No firm rule can be developed here, and each case is judged on its merits with proper diagnostic criteria.

Generally speaking, the first deciduous molars are removed approximately 12 months after the deciduous canines. Thus, first deciduous molar removal would be between 9 and 10 years of age in the average developmental pattern. It would vary from child to child and might sometimes be done earlier in the mandible than in the maxilla, to enhance the early eruption of the first premolars.[16, 24] Timing is really not so critical for the removal of the first deciduous molars. There are those who might prefer to remove the remaining deciduous canines and first deciduous molars at the same time, somewhere between 8½ and 10 years of age. No obvious deleterious sequelae need be expected.

3. REMOVAL OF THE ERUPTING FIRST PREMOLARS. Before this is done, all diagnostic criteria must again be evaluated. The status of the developing third molars must be determined. It can be a serious mistake to remove four first premolars, only to find that the third molars are congenitally missing and there would have been enough space without premolar removal. If the diagnostic study confirms the inherent arch length deficiency, the purpose of this step is to permit the canine to drop distally into the space created by the extraction. If the procedure has been carried out correctly and the timing has been right, it is a most rewarding experience after the removal of the first premolars to observe the bulging canine eminences move distally on their own into the premolar extraction sites (Fig. 15–15). Clinical experience indicates that this happens more frequently in the maxillary than in the mandibular arch. The reason is the eruption sequence which so often permits the maxillary premolar to enter the oral cavity ahead of the lower first premolar. It is here that the timely removal of the unerupted mandibular first premolar may prevent the abnormal mesial eruption of the mandibular canine, which would increase the appliance challenge later.

As indicated previously, sometimes it becomes necessary to remove the mandibular second deciduous molars to permit the first premolars to erupt. This is a more conservative step and is usually preferable to enucleation. But it increases the chances for need of a holding arch to prevent undue loss of space and excessive mesial drift of the first permanent molar (Fig. 15–16). A series of decisions must be made throughout the period of serial removal of teeth. This is why observation appointments at three-month intervals are advisable.

There is considerable variability in the eruption of the individual first premolars and it is often necessary to remove them one or two at a time as they erupt. Close observation and team work among the general practitioner, the oral surgeon and the orthodontist are particularly important at this time. If a premolar is just beneath the surface and appears to be held up by a mucosal barrier, the general practitioner or oral surgeon may expedite the serial extraction procedure by incising the tissue and removing the unerupted premolar. Generally speaking, if the decision has definitely been made that it is necessary to remove the first premolar teeth, the sooner this is done the better the self-adjustment. It serves no purpose to wait for full eruption of the premolar teeth. From the psychological point of view, the fewer surgical experiences, the better.

(Text continued on page 731)

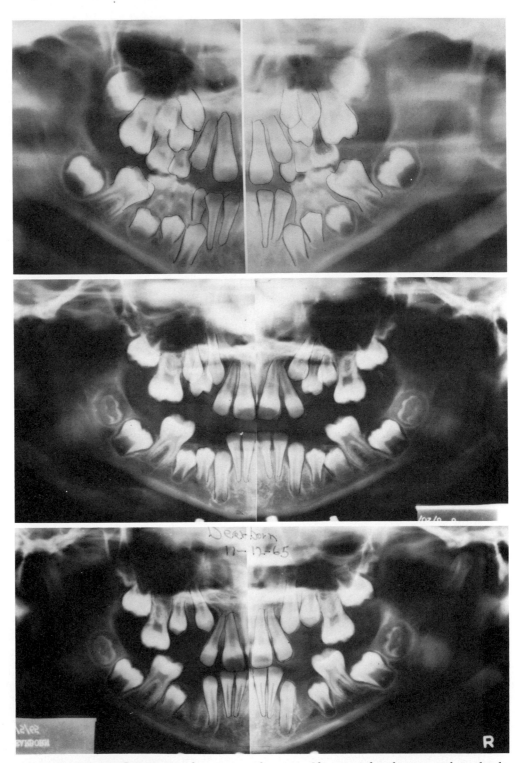

Figure 15–14 Laminagraphic views of severe Class I malocclusion with multiple serial extraction clues (ectopic eruption, drift, premature loss, shift to one side, flaring, etc). Deciduous teeth have been removed in middle left picture, and four first premolars are now out in the bottom left view, enucleated because of the "log-jam" seen in middle left view. In the three right-hand views, eruption is proceeding, with significant autonomous improvement. The partially impacted lower second molar in the middle right view was surgically uprighted (see Figs. 15–30 and 15–33). The lower right view shows complete adjustment.

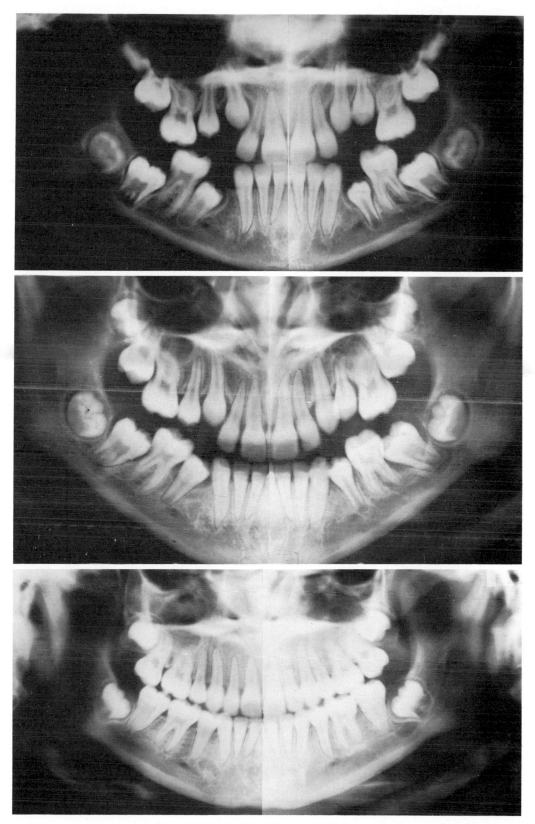

Figure 15–14 (continued)

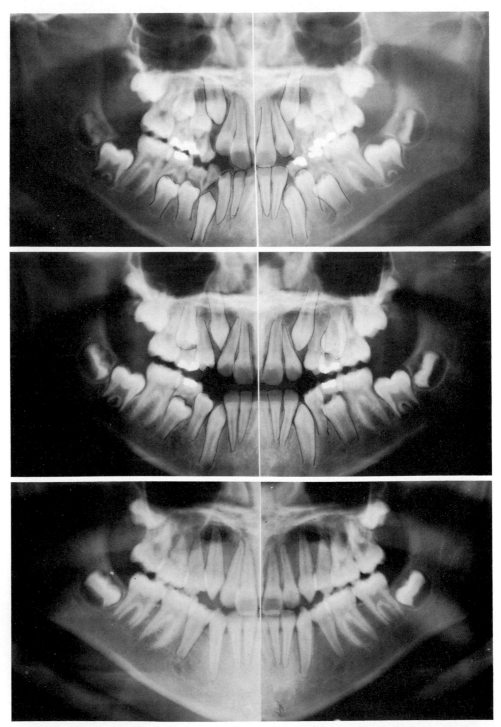

Figure 15–15 A series of laminagraphic views, showing autonomous adjustment possible with properly guided serial extraction procedures. Note significant uprighting of canines as they move back into space created in first premolar area.

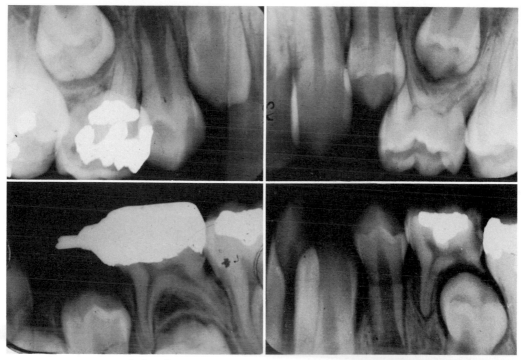

Figure 15–16 Second deciduous molars may interfere with first and second premolar eruption and should be removed if this is the case. Holding arches are seldom necessary.

VARIATIONS IN SERIAL EXTRACTION PROCEDURE

Since there are a number of variables that contribute to the decision on "what" to remove and "when" in serial extraction, it is not possible to develop hard and fast rules that apply in all cases. In most instances the serial extraction procedures are instituted when the patient is about 8 years of age. There is an interval of about 6 to 12 months between each step, as dictated by clinical and radiographic evidence of growth and development, sequence of eruption and self-adjustment initiated by the serial extraction procedure.

Not all changes are favorable. Careful, continuous observation is necessary. There is often an increased inclination of the teeth on either side of the first premolar extraction site. As we know, the long axes of the teeth converge in the maxillary arch[34] (Fig. 15–17). The compensating curve and the occlusal surfaces of the mandibular arch form a concave arc, so the long axes in the mandibular buccal segments diverge. Thus, there is automatic paralleling of the roots with the removal of the first premolar in the maxillary arch. On the contrary, the removal of the mandibular first premolar allows the tipping together of the crowns, accentuating the "V" or "ditch," as it is called in some orthodontic quarters. Seldom does the distance between the apex of the mandibular canine and the apex of the mandibular second premolar decrease on its own. Uprighting requires fixed banded appliances.

The "bite" tends to close at least temporarily during the extraction supervision period in most instances, particularly in cases with a Class II tendency. A. Martin Schwarz showed that there are three periods of physiologic raising of the bite: the eruption of the 6-year molar, the eruption of the 12-year molar and the 18-year molar.[37] This does not happen all the time, but ample evidence

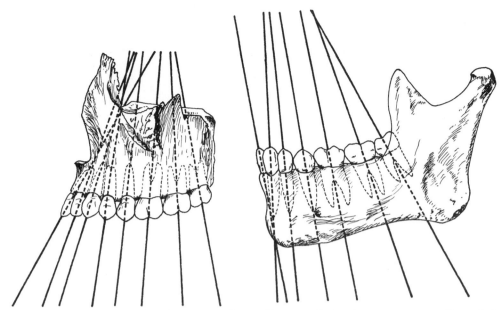

Figure 15–17 Axial inclinations of maxillary teeth (top) converge apically, while they diverge apically in the mandibular arch (bottom). This permits self-paralleling of maxillary canines and second premolars, but interferes with root parallelism in the mandibular arch, creating what the orthodontist calls "the ditch." Thus, appliances are almost always required to upright mandibular teeth, regardless of the high level of self-improvement in other malocclusion details.

exists to show that even in serial extraction cases, there is an autonomous reduction of the overbite with the eruption of the second and third molar teeth. This bite opening, together with the horizontal growth increments to the mandible in the terminal phases of development, should improve the overbite. However, there is no harm in placing an acrylic bite plate in the mixed dentition. It certainly may help and can do little harm. Preventing overclosure, stimulating eruption of posterior segments and eliminating functional retrusion are worthwhile objectives. In addition, if anchorage is a problem at all in the maxillary arch (this would be especially true in Class II cases), a removable palatal appliance is valuable in retracting the canines before the placing of fixed appliances to complete the arch consolidation.[11]

Sometimes there is a further reduction in arch length during the period of guidance. The lower incisors, while aligning themselves, may also become more upright (lingually inclined), which increases the overbite tendency. In our experience, mandibular lingual or maxillary holding arches are required only in extreme arch length deficiency cases (Fig. 15–18). In the lower arch, particularly, holding arches may interfere with optimal adjustment and prevent closure of the space in the extraction site. Continuous observation of the occlusal relationship of the first molars is advisable because of the occasional forward rotation of the maxillary first molars, with the mesiobuccal cusp turning lingually. To prevent this tendency and the creation of a Class II relationship, a maxillary holding arch may be advisable in some cases.[28] These problems constitute a minority of the cases, but they point out the need for continuing guidance by the orthodontic specialist.

There are times, though very few, when with proper guidance and optimal self-adjustment, the teeth will align themselves and, under the influence of function and balancing muscle forces, assume near normal positions over basal bone, making mechanotherapy unnecessary. Such a case is shown in Figure 15–19. Since this gratifying response unfortunately is too rare, the wise dentist will continue to rely on the "team," getting orthodontic and surgical consultation before he embarks on a path strewn with indiscriminately removed deciduous canines, molars and first premolars.

Occasionally, it is advisable to remove the second premolars instead of the first premolars.[38] Such a decision may mean the removal of second premolars in one arch and first premolars in another. Canine position, arch length needed, restorative status of premolar segments, tooth shape, amount of overbite and overjet are just some of the factors that influence such a decision. If there is an open bite tendency, sometimes the removal of second premolars in the mandibular arch will be preferable. This reduces the tendency to relapsing open bite and lingually inclined incisors that are seen sometimes with lower first premolar removal. Where there is congenital absence of mandibular second premolars, the first premolars may drift distally into the space if the second deciduous molars are removed on time (Fig. 15–20).

Class II, Division 1 and Division 2 malocclusions, with arch length deficiency characteristics, pose different problems. Serial extraction is still a valuable treatment adjunct but must be closely coordinated with several periods of mechanotherapy (Figs. 15–21 to 15–28). Basal discrepancy and overbite constantly mitigate the achievement of optimal self-adjustment so often seen in Class I cases where serial extraction has also been employed. Careful study of all available diagnostic records must precede any decision on tooth sacrifice, and full diagnostic records should be obtained at least at yearly intervals. Particularly important in assessing the changing situation are study models and panoramic and cephalometric radiographs.

(Text continued on page 744)

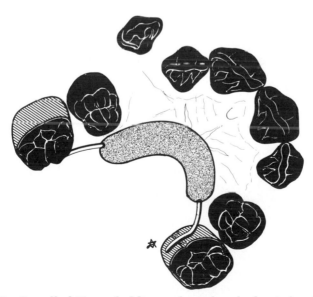

Figure 15–18 So-called Nance holding arch, with orthodontic bands on first permanent molars, and heavy (0.040 inch) lingual wire, approximating vertical portion of the palate. Acrylic "button" has been added to prevent the wire from becoming embedded in the palatal tissue. As drawing shows, first premolars have been removed, permitting canine teeth to drop distally into the spaces created. The holding arch prevents mesial migration of molars in severe discrepancy cases.

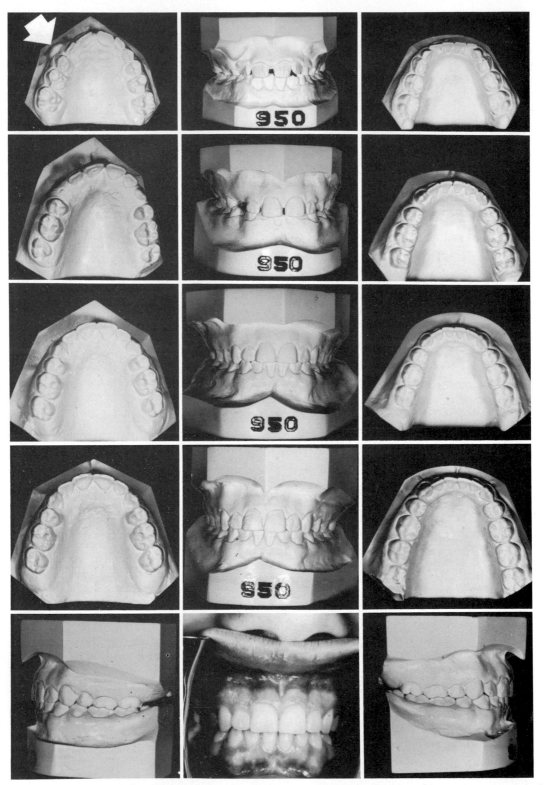

Figure 15–19. Serial extraction guidance with no appliances used at any time. Upper right canine had been completely blocked out of the arch. Large permanent teeth (seen from radiographs) and a 9 mm. discrepancy in the mandibular arch lead to serial extraction decision. Second and third rows show autonomous adjustment at yearly intervals. Note that the overbite is deepest in the second row and decreases spontaneously thereafter. There is a five-year interval between the third and the fourth and fifth rows. Laminagraph showed normal third molar eruption.

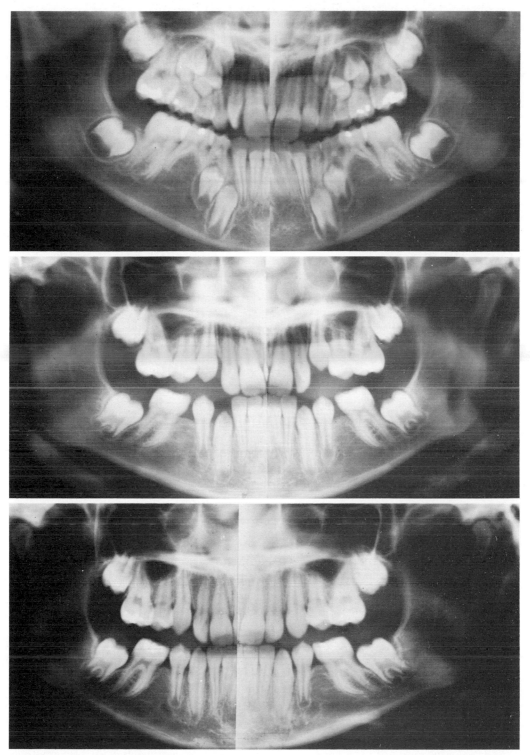

Figure 15–20 Congenital absence of mandibular second premolars in serial extraction case. First premolars were removed in maxillary arch; second deciduous molars in mandibular arch. Note particularly the distal drift of the mandibular first premolar teeth, as well as canines. Relatively little mesial drift of mandibular molars is seen. Third molars are congenitally missing.

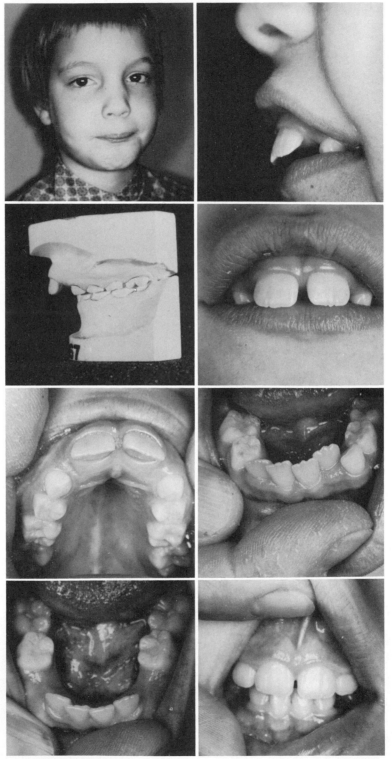

Figure 15–21   Class II, Division 1 malocclusion with severe arch length deficiency (see Fig. 15–24 for laminagraphs), abnormal tooth, muscle and basal bone system relationships. These are multiple serial extraction clues. Extraoral force and bite plate were used during serial extraction program to eliminate horizontal and vertical discrepancy problems.

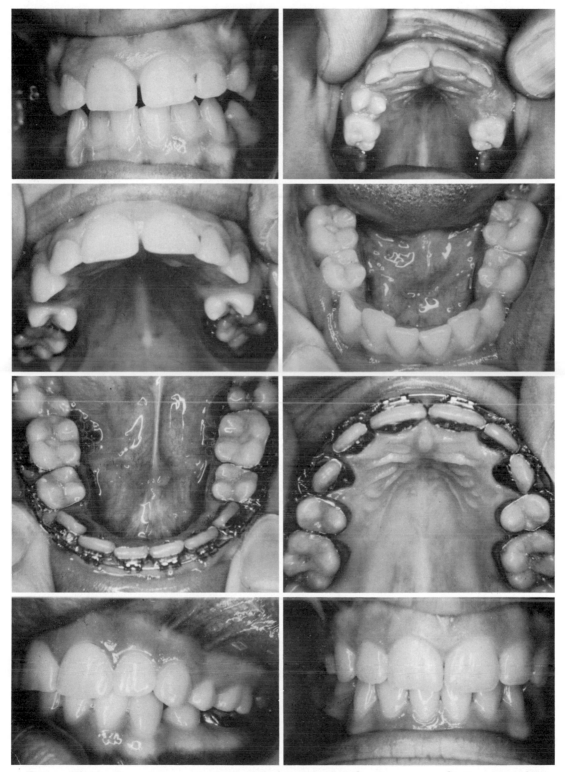

Figure 15–22   Same case as in Figure 15–21. Continued autonomous adjustment, making a Class I problem from a Class II problem because of extraoral orthopedic force guidance, as serial extraction procedes. Full appliances are placed to accomplish objectives of leveling, uprighting, paralleling, rotation correction, overbite control, etc. Appliances were placed for seven months.

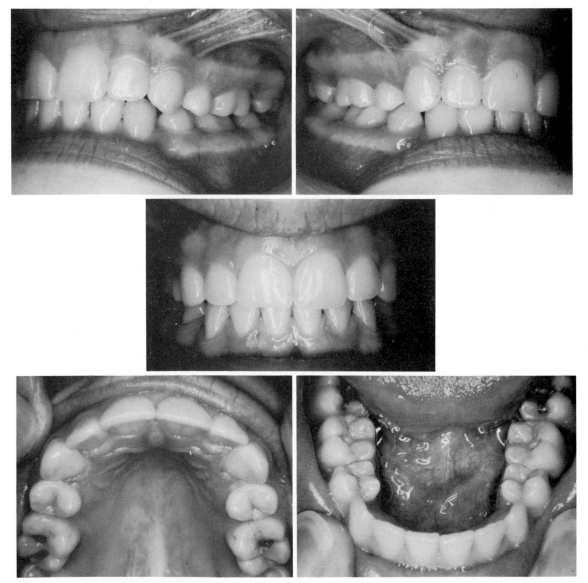

Figure 15–23   Completed case, same as in Figure 15–21.

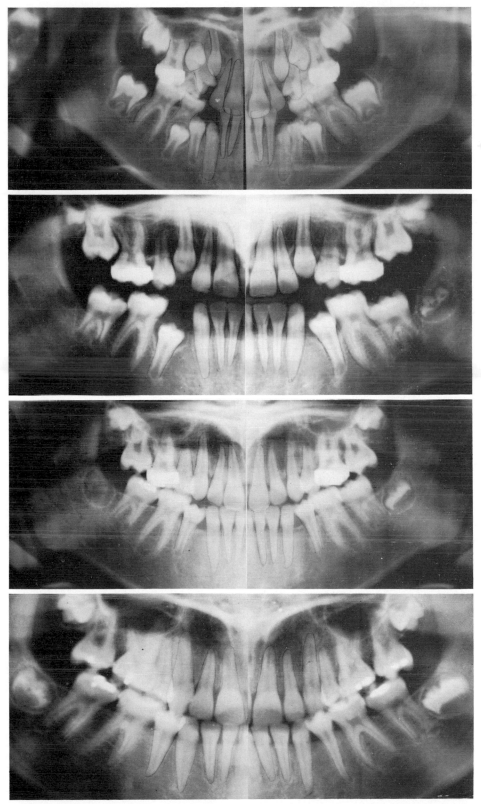

Figure 15–24   Serial laminagraphs to show autonomous improvement. Bands on maxillary first permanent molars are for extraoral appliance used for elimination of Class II relationships.

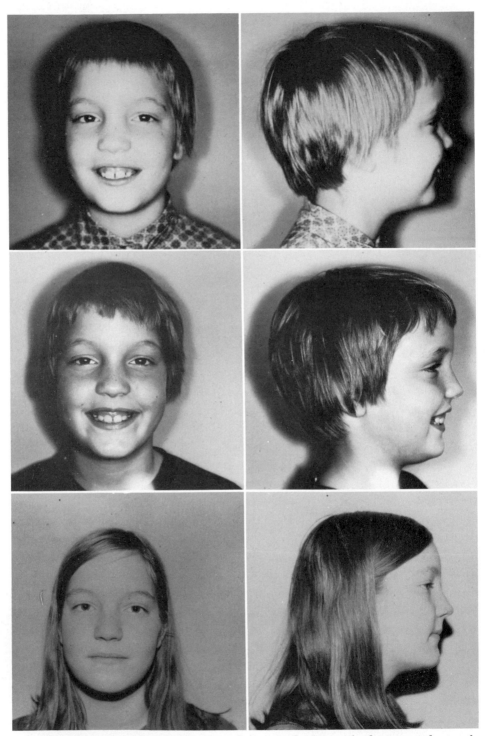

Figure 15–25 Facial views before, during and after orthodontic guidance show significant facial improvement.

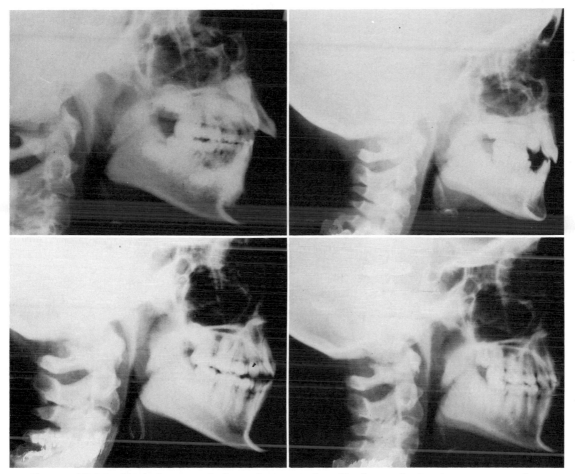

Figure 15–26 Cephalograms before, during and well after orthodontic treatment, showing basal adjustment achieved.

Case: L.H. age:	7	8	9	10	12	13	14	16
SNaA	76.5	75.5	75.0	74.0	76.0	74.0	74.0	75.0
AB Diff.	5.5	3.0	3.0	2.0	3.0	1.0	0.0	0.0
NaS-GoGn	36.0	36.0	37.0	36.0	35.0	33.0	33.5	29.0
U1-NaS	102.0	83.5	83.5	91.5	97.0	97.5	92.0	95.0
L1-GoGn	89.0	91.5	90.0	90.0	87.0	89.5	92.0	89.5
U1-NaPog(mm)	11.5	4.0	4.0	4.0	5.0	2.0	0.0	1.5

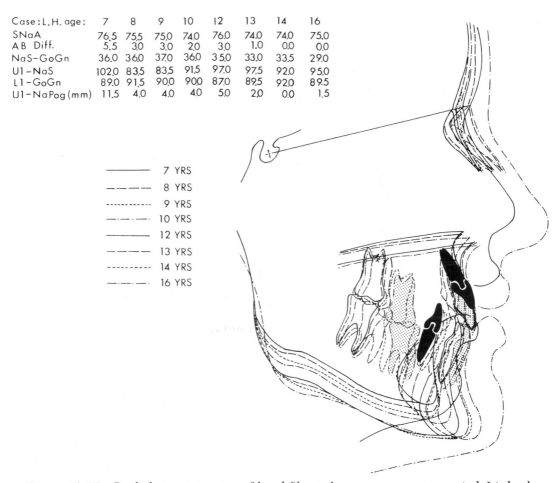

————— 7 YRS

— — — 8 YRS

············· 9 YRS

—·—·— 10 YRS

————— 12 YRS

— — — 13 YRS

············· 14 YRS

—·—·— 16 YRS

Figure 15–27   Cephalometric tracing of head films taken over a ten-year period. Little change in incisor axial inclination is observed. But counterclockwise growth has resulted in a reduction of the mandibular plane inclination, as well as a 5.5 degree reduction in the apical base difference. Note the significant direction change of mandibular growth, with a swing from primarily vertical to a horizontal direction during prepubertal and pubertal growth periods. Without this type of growth, the problem would have been much more difficult to correct.

Figure 15–28   A Class II, Division 1 serial extraction case, again requiring a basal adjustment, concurrent with serial extraction procedures. Top row of casts were taken when therapy was started. Second row of casts were taken at end of appliance guidance. Occlusal views before serial extraction and at end of mechanotherapy are in third row. Intraoral sequence was taken after removal of lower fixed lingual retainer. Serial extraction alone, without concomitant appliance guidance, would have resulted in a Class II malocclusion, with four less teeth.

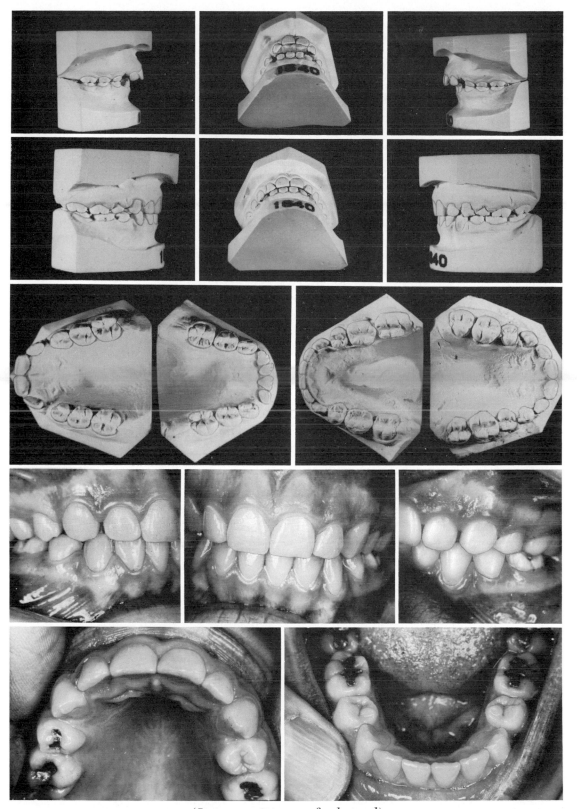

(See opposite page for legend)

PROBLEMS IN SERIAL EXTRACTION

There is no form of therapy that does not have its contraindications and limitations. It has already been emphasized that there is no "cookbook" for serial extraction. The timing of tooth removal may be important. It is not always possible to see the patient when we want to or to remove specific teeth at the optimal time for the greatest improvement. The orthodontist must be prepared to change his treatment plan continually and the word "tentative" is essential for any serial extraction guidance program. Many potential serial extraction cases turn out ultimately as conventional orthodontic therapy with no teeth being removed. Or, because third molars are congenitally missing, arch length was gained on the posterior end of the alveolar trough; or, the orthodontist had the oral surgeon remove the third molar teeth to gain this space. In some instances where mandibular arch length is almost adequate, the orthodontist is willing to accept minor irregularities of the lower incisors and remove only the maxillary first premolars. Orthodontic clinicians will testify to the fact that it is much easier to close spaces in the maxillary arch in the first premolar area than in the mandibular arch.

More frequently, the serial extraction patient comes in with better adjustment in the maxillary than in the mandibular arch. Almost always, there is the "ditch" between the permanent canine and the second premolar in the mandibular arch. Whereas the roots of the maxillary canine and maxillary second premolar parallel themselves fairly well with autonomous adjustment, this is almost never true in the mandibular arch.[34] It is necessary for the orthodontist to resort to stringent appliance guidance to close the space and upright the teeth. This is within the realm of conventional therapy and can be accomplished uniformly with a high level of success. Treatment procedures usually do not exceed 6 to 12 months of mechanotherapy. In other words, in the average serial extraction case, mechanotherapy is reduced at least 50 per cent in terms of time and effort, when compared with the conventional four premolar extraction case that has not had the benefit of guided extraction procedures.

Occasionally, the removal of premolars does not stimulate the distal migration of canines. Figure 15–29 shows a case in which one maxillary canine remained impacted in a horizontal position. In such instances, the change in treatment plan requires uncovering the canine surgically, placing some sort of guiding appliance and literally pulling the tooth down into normal position. Experience with hundreds of serial extraction cases demonstrates the fact that few patients follow a "normal" schedule. Eruption in one quadrant often precedes eruption in the other three. The experienced clinician learns to wait for nature to provide all self-help before rushing in with appliances as the teeth peek through the tissue — an all too common error for the neophyte. Thus, appliance placement frequently is postponed until the patient is 13 to 14 years of age, particularly for male patients.

Large restorations or caries in second premolar teeth may indicate the removal of one or more second premolars instead of a first premolar.[38] A discretionary decision should be made on the basis of the restorative status, as well as the morphology of the teeth which may be highly variable. As mentioned previously, congenital absence of one or more premolars may also serve to create a problem and will require a change in the conventional serial extraction procedures (Fig. 15–20).

The removal of premolars in the mandibular arch may enhance the overbite tendency. The mandibular incisors align themselves but also tend to move lingually, increasing the overbite. This may signal the need for holding arches, or a

(Text continued on page 748)

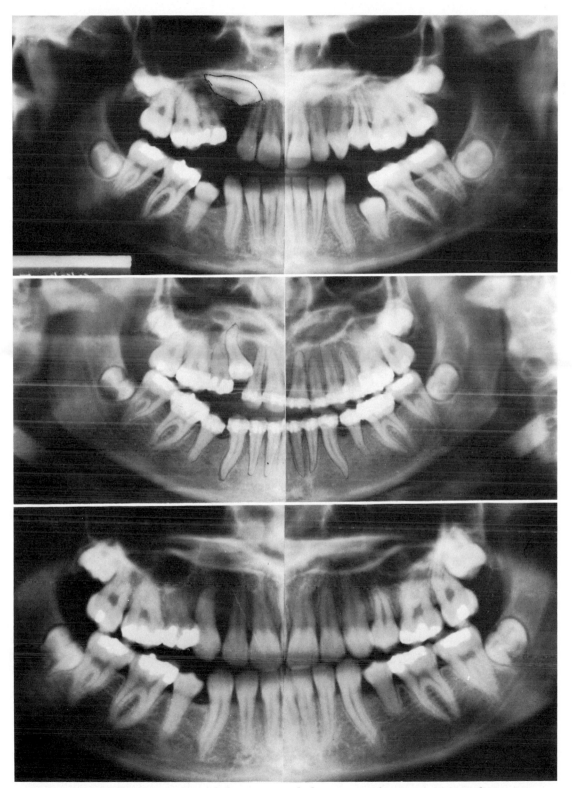

Figure 15–29   Canine on upper left is impacted, despite serial extraction procedures. Stringent and protracted mechanotherapy was required to achieve results shown in bottom view.

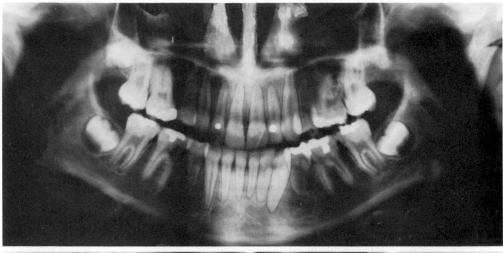

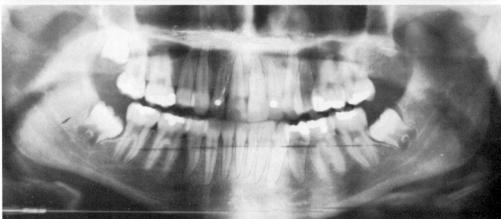

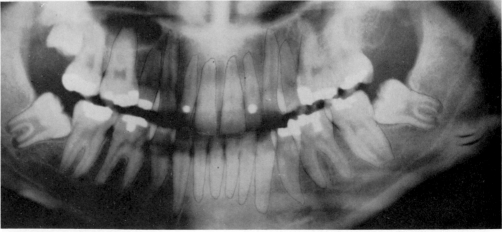

Figure 15–30   This series of six laminagraphs is important because it illustrates a common phenomenon. An apparently successful four first premolar serial extraction case (top left) is shown with seemingly normal eruption of mandibular third molars at 14 years of age. The middle left view shows beginning tipping of these teeth, and the bottom left view shows obvious impaction at 18 years of age. The lower right third molar was removed because of congenital absence of its opponent. The lower left third molar was surgically uprighted. The right middle picture is after an interval of one month; the lower right after an 8-month interval. This orthosurgical-general practitioner teamwork is frequently needed for similar problems.

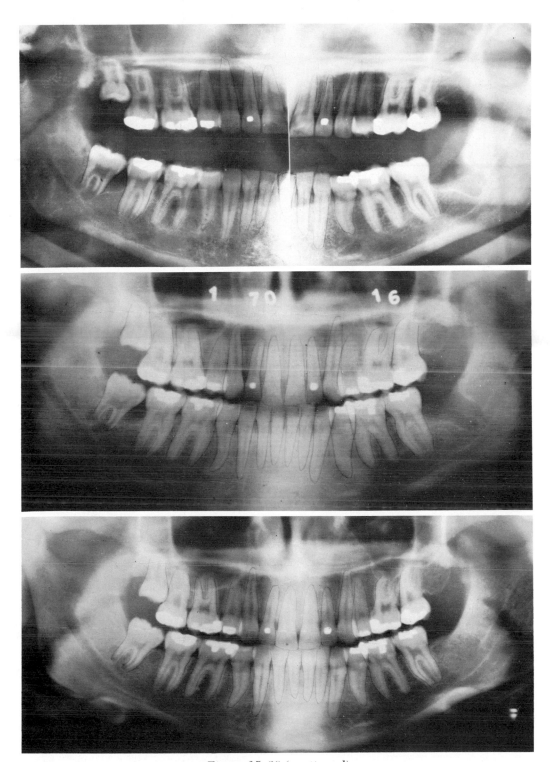

Figure 15–30 (continued)

bite plate. The orthodontist has the appliances to control this tendency adequately, but it should be recognized. This emphasizes again the need for mechanotherapy at the end of the guided extraction period.

In four first premolar extraction cases, whether serial guidance has been used or not, the ultimate status of the third molars should be considered.[30, 39, 40] Parents are often told that the easy removal of the first premolars will enhance the likelihood of the normal eruption of the third molars later and prevent the traumatic removal of impacted teeth. While this may be true in some cases, a substantial number of records taken by the author now indicate that first premolar removal may actually enhance the impaction and forward tipping of the mandibular third molars, as Figure 15–30 shows. It is important that the orthodontist continue to observe the erupting third molars, following the completion of mechanotherapy, and even during the retention phase of guidance. If it appears that the third molars are imminently impacted, then they may be surgically uprighted with uniformly good results.[30] Failure to do so means the loss of all four third molars, making this an eight-tooth extraction case. The orthodontist's responsibility is not over when he removes the appliances. G. P.-orthosurgical teamwork continues until the completion of the dentition.[41]

SURGICAL UNCOVERING OF IMPACTIONS, POSITIONING AND TRANSPOSITIONING

NONERUPTION AND IMPACTIONS

In unerupted incisors, where there is no supernumerary tooth to serve as a cause for impaction, a mucosal or bony barrier may be upsetting the timetable of normal eruption. Proper surgical intervention may prevent the need for future orthodontic mechanotherapy. As pointed out in the section on serial extraction, noneruption may be due to arch length deficiency. Therefore, a differential diagnosis must be made, which may require cross-consultation between general practitioner, surgeon and orthodontist.

Canine impaction is a complex subject.[41-44] The maxillary or mandibular canines may be labial, lingual or in varying positions. There is often an arch length deficiency — again a clue for serial extraction. All too frequently, the timing of interceptive procedures has been poor, and the impaction is a *fait accompli*. Proper guidance, with early diagnostic records and orthodontic consultation, can prevent many of these impactions from assuming the degree of severity they demonstrate in many cases. Merely removing tissue from an impacted canine is not the whole answer. The total occlusion problem should be studied. Perhaps it means creating a pathway toward normal occlusion; perhaps it means creating arch length so that the tooth may assume normal position; perhaps it means surgical positioning of the coronal portion; perhaps it means a combined surgical-orthodontic endeavor.

There are a number of attachments being used to bring impacted teeth into place. Figure 15–31 shows celluloid crown forms that have been placed after surgical uncovering. Bands were cemented later to guide teeth into place (A to C). If celluloid crowns are used on premolars, they should be left on until the tooth has erupted sufficiently to place epoxy bonded plastic brackets or bands for final positioning (D). Sometimes cast gold overlays may be used after surgical uncovering (E and F). These are then ligated by steel ligature of elastic thread to move the tooth toward its normal position. Final positioning is again done with an orthodontic bracket attached to a band or to the tooth directly. Alternate means of guiding impacted teeth into position are illustrated in Figure 15–32. A wire "snare" (or a chain) may be wrapped around the crown of the unerupted tooth to help guide toward normal position.

Surgical uncovering and the placement of a full plastic or metal crown is the most frequently used and most successful technique.[44] Most canine impactions are palatal. With proper removal of bone around the coronal portion of the canine to permit the cementation of the metal crown, eruption into the mouth can be expected almost routinely. The metal crown usually extends through the mucosa, preventing it from healing over the unerupted tooth. Clinical experience gives the impression of more rapid eruption due to constriction of the scarred mucosa around the crown. A recent report of 2000 cases treated in this manner states that without exception, the teeth erupted into the oral cavity, permitting the subsequent orthodontic movement into optimal position.[44] In this manner, the length of appliance wear is greatly reduced, and the need for actually pulling the canine down from its original position is eliminated except in exceptional cases. The exceptions seem to include labially or buccally malposed canines, which show much less tendency to erupt toward normal position after surgical uncovering.

With premolar impactions (which may also be handled with the full metal crown technique), space adequacy should be determined. Lack of space may require removal of the impacted tooth or a contiguous unit. Subsequent mechanotherapy is almost always required.

Molar impactions are seen more frequently now with the routine use of laminagraphy. Despite apparently successful orthodontic mechanotherapy, even with the removal of first premolars (as in a serial extraction case), problems arise. The ultimate status of second and third molar position and occlusion is often assumed to be normal for many 13- to 14-year-old patients, when their orthodontic appliances are removed. But 3 to 6 years later, well out of retention and orthodontic guidance, the patient may be confronted with yet another extraction decision, this time involving third molar teeth. The extraction of four more functional units then makes a total of eight lost teeth, which may lead to unfavorable sequelae of deepening bite, adverse profile changes and premature aging of the dentition. Surgical positioning may be the right answer.[30] Autogenous transplantation also offers a possibility.

The author has had considerable opportunity to make use of the surgical-orthodontic teamwork in these repositioning cases. There has been a very high level of success in the uprighting process for both second and third molar teeth[30] (Figs. 15–30, 15–33). Generally speaking, the teeth are tipped, keeping apical movement to a minimum, disturbing the "umbilical" cord, or entering vessels and nerves as little as possible. The optimal time for uprighting seems to be right after two thirds of the roots are formed, though it can be done later. If it is carried out too early, root formation does not continue to completion. The technique is used most frequently on mandibular molars, which seldom require splinting. The uprighted tooth is usually wedged between the mesial tooth and the distal alveolar bone. Occlusal equilibration is often required, and relief of mucosal tissue may be necessary to prevent occlusal impingement and postoperative soreness and infection. Contraindications are teeth with extreme horizontal impactions or widely divergent roots. Teeth that are fully formed, with vertical alveolar bone growth completed offer a lesser chance for success. Autotransplantation is becoming an increasingly frequent, and successful, ortho-

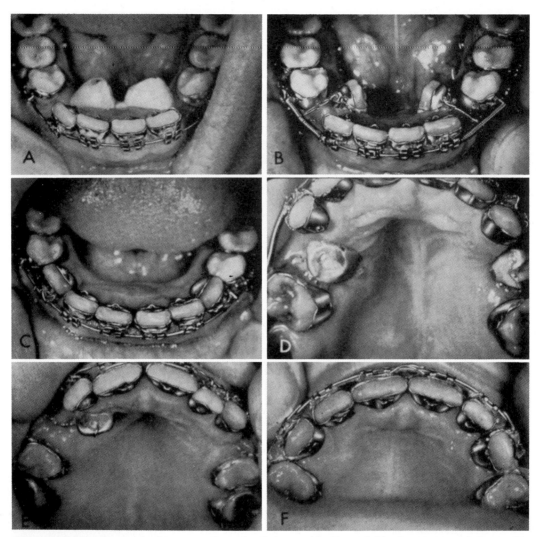

Figure 15–31   Control of impacted teeth. Pictures (A, B, and C) of patient with lingually impacted mandibular canines. Celluloid crowns placed after surgical exposure and subsequent eruption (A) replaced by orthodontic bands and guided into position as space is created (B and C). Celluloid crowns placed on palatally impacted second premolars (D) until sufficient eruption permits banding. Palatally impacted canine (E) uncovered and cast gold overlay cemented. Tooth is guided into position and conventional band is placed (F). (Graber, T. M.: J. Oral Surg., 25:201, 1967.)

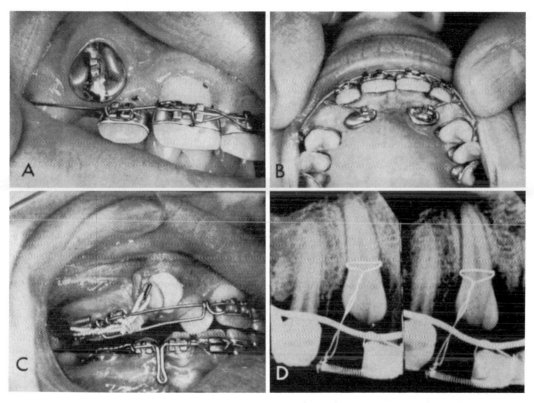

Figure 15–32   Control of impacted canines. Cast gold overlays (A and B) have brackets soldered for positive control. Hook cemented in place on exposed canine (C) is less satisfactory but adequate for initial stages. Steel ligature wire "snare" (D) guides unerupted canine toward normal position so band may be placed. (View C, courtesy of H. Vanoucek; view D, courtesy of E. Johnson) (Graber, T. M.: J. Oral Surg., 25:201, 1967.)

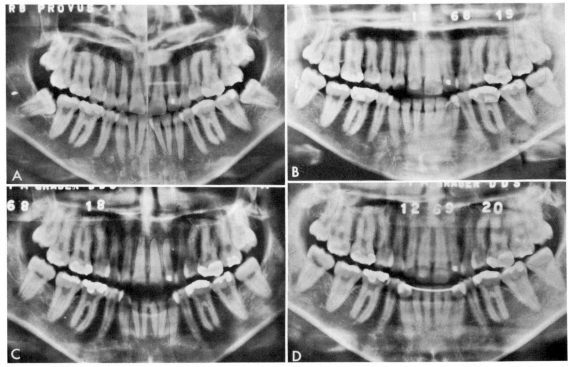

Figure 15–33   Serial extraction case at 18 years of age, with impacted mandibular third molars and incisor crowding (there was a strong horizontal mandibular growth change subsequent to mechanotherapy). The third molars were surgically uprighted, and views are shown at yearly intervals in B, C and D. The lower canine-to-canine lingual retainer is worn after re-alignment of mandibular incisors. Orthodontic responsibility of any problem should extend through the teen years, until the status of third molar teeth has been determined.

surgical procedure, particularly in the molar segments (Fig. 15–34). As with the surgical uprighting described previously, root filling may not be necessary.

Slagsvold and Bjercke have experimented with autotransplantation of premolars for missing anterior teeth since 1959.[52] The main steps of their operation are as follows:

(1) Tooth to be transplanted is uncovered, loosened, slightly lifted out of its crypt and put back again. Although the coronal part of the follicle may be injured, care is taken not to injure the apical part with its epithelial sheath. Mucoperiosteal flaps are sutured back for temporary protection until the tooth can be transplanted.

(2) The alveolar process is exposed and a cavity is prepared in the bone in the desired edentulous area.

(3) The premolar is taken out of its crypt and placed directly in the bony cavity.

(4) The mucoperiosteal flaps are sutured over the transplanted tooth, if possible for protection.

In a report on 26 cases, all teeth are still in place.[53] The transplanted premolars erupted rather quickly. Root formation continued on all transplanted teeth to a satisfactory length. Periodontal conditions were normal, with a normal alveolar crest height (Figs. 15–35 to 15–37). On the debit side, enamel anomalies, characterized by a somewhat white appearance, were observed in teeth transplanted at a stage when root formation had just started. Roentgenograms showed progressive pulp closure for the part formed before and immediately after the

(Text continued on page 757)

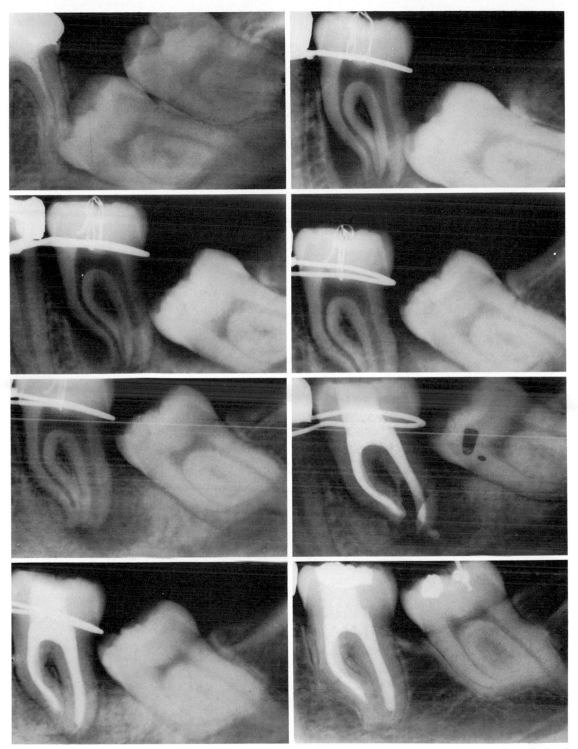

Figure 15–34 An excellent example of surgical orthodontics. Impacted second and third molar teeth, with a badly broken down first molar. Eighteen year old patient. Surgeon removed the defective first molar and transplanted the third molar in its place, upper right. Second row left is seven months lateral second row, right, six months later. In third row, after an interval of nine months more, a periapical involvement is seen. A root-filling was done on the transplanted third molar, third row, right. Second molar is beginning to upright and erupt. In bottom row, six months after root fill, second molar eruption continues. In lower right view, two and a half years later, transplanted tooth is stable and healthy, with a PDM. Second molar has erupted and now has occlusal restorations. (Courtesy Robert Jans.)

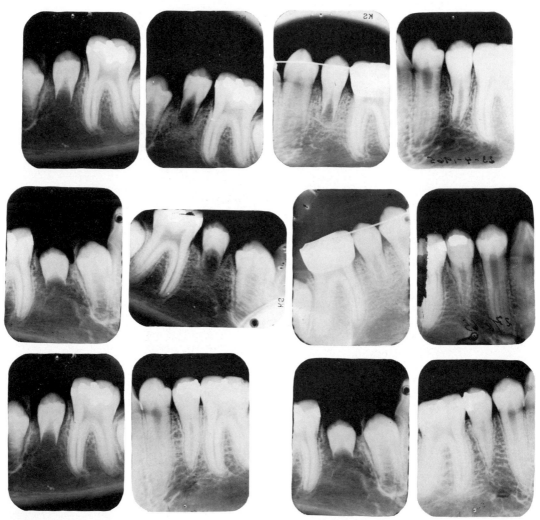

Figure 15–35   Autotransplantation of premolars. Radiograph series (top row) showing post-operative development of upper left second premolar which was transplanted to the site of the lower left second premolar. Middle row is of same patient, showing progressive changes in development of an upper right second premolar which was transplanted in lower right second premolar space. The bottom views shows a comparison of both transplanted teeth over an approximate five-year period. Note periodontal membrane, bone texture, amount of root growth, etc. (Courtesy O. Slagsvold.)

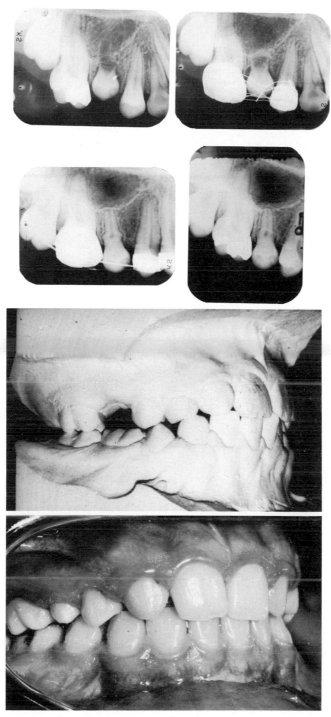

Figure 15–36   A girl, 11 years, 10 months of age. Upper right second premolar and lateral incisors are congenitally missing. A lower second premolar was transplanted to the edentulous area. The radiographic series was taken also over an approximate five-year period. Root morphology is not quite normal, but the tooth is healthy and functional. Bottom views show before and after orthodontic treatment. Lower spaces were closed and canines were moved into lateral incisor position in maxillary arch. (Courtesy O. Slagsvold.)

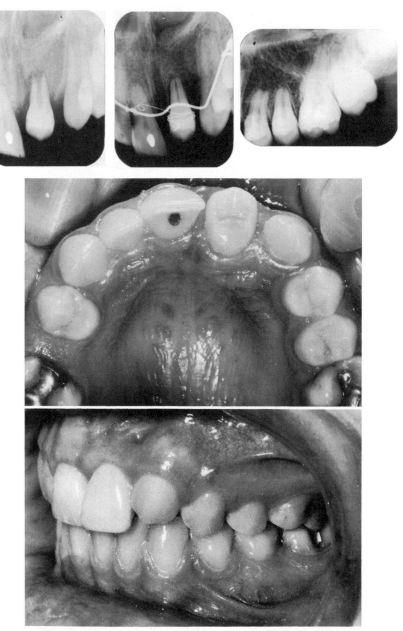

Figure 15–37   Central and lateral incisors of a girl 9 years, 6 months lost due to an accident. A decision was made to substitute the second premolar from the right side for the left central incisor. The radiographs show relatively little increase in root length. But, when compared to the homologous tooth (upper right), the shape and size of the roots are nearly the same. The tooth is clinically healthy (middle row) and serves as a base for a jacket crown restoration (bottom). (Courtesy O. Slagsvold.)

operation. Vitality tests showed minimal or no response. This was interpreted as a greater difficulty of the stimulus to reach the remaining normal pulp. In cases where it is indicated to transplant one premolar from one jaw to the other, in congenital absence cases, for example, Slagsvold and Bjercke have had similar success. Lemoine, Petrovic and Stutzmann substantiate the continuation of periodontal membrane in their study of autotransplantation in the white rat, although they found calcification in the radicular canals, not seen radiographically in the human by Slagsvold.[54]

FRENUMS AND LABIAL STRIPPING

The controversy over the cause-and-effect relationship of frenums and diastemas is a graphic illustration of the need of orthosurgical teamwork. Many a frenum has been "clipped" surgically when it was not necessary. As described in Chapter 2, the transient "ugly duckling" stage, with its flared lateral incisors and space between the maxillary incisors is hardly due to the tissue attachment. The adjustment will be autonomous, if left alone.[28] Also, we know that an incisor diastema may be a hereditary characteristic, and regardless of whether or not we clip the frenum, the space may persist. We may also find heavy fibrous frenums, but no diastemas. Cross-consultation is desirable to prevent loss of patient confidence in dental service. Often the frenum is removed and the space remains, despite the surgical assist. So often, it requires both resection and orthodontic therapy. Even then, it is better to first close the space orthodontically, then carefully resect the fibrous attachment and ligate the teeth together immediately afterward. Scarring then assists closure. If surgery is done before space closure, scar tissue may form and will hinder elimination of the diastema.

The confounding problem of a labial cleft or stripping in conjunction with crowding of the lower incisors has no easy solution. Perhaps primary consideration is periodontal. The orthodontist sees this condition frequently and does not know how to handle it. The establishment of normal occlusion does not usually eliminate the labial cleft and hyperemic gingival tissue. Massage, conservative medication, excision of muscle attachments, surgical flaps may all be indicated at one time or another. Teamwork G.P.-ortho-perio-surgical cross-consultation is recommended.

The frequent gingival hypertrophy during orthodontic therapy offers another opportunity for teamwork. Part of the problem is likely to be hormonal, and is tied to pubertal growth phenomena. Usually the hypertrophic tissue disappears after removal of appliances. All too frequently, however, the character of the tissue becomes fibrous, and a residual bulbous interdental papilla is the result. Here again, conservative medication, proper prophylaxis and massage are indicated (or possible surgical removal). The surgeon, periodontist, orthodontist and general practitioner should work in concert to maintain the best possible health during orthodontic treatment.

RESECTIONS

Since two thirds of orthodontically treated cases are anteroposterior basal malrelationships, with the teeth reflecting this discrepancy, both surgeons and orthodontists are interested in correction.[42-51] While the more conservative or-

(Text continued on page 765)

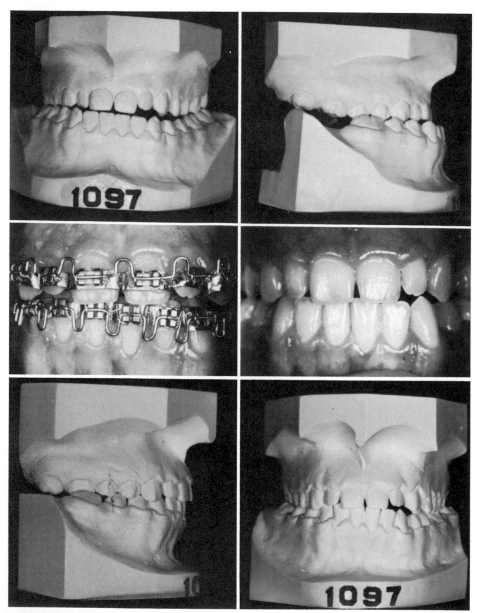

Figure 15–38 Class III mandibular resection in young female adult. Before and after plaster casts show change effected. Appliances are multilooped to allow intermaxillary elastic traction during fixation. No fragment fixation or muscle re-attachment was done. Cephalometric tracings show partial relapse over a seven-year period (Fig. 15–39).

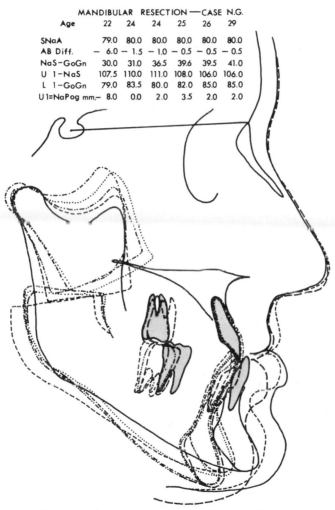

MANDIBULAR RESECTION—CASE N.G.						
Age	22	24	24	25	26	29
SNaA	79.0	80.0	80.0	80.0	80.0	80.0
AB Diff.	−6.0	−1.5	−1.0	−0.5	−0.5	−0.5
NaS−GoGn	30.0	31.0	36.5	39.6	39.5	41.0
U 1−NaS	107.5	110.0	111.0	108.0	106.0	106.0
L 1−GoGn	79.0	83.5	80.0	82.0	85.0	85.0
U1=NaPog mm.	−8.0	0.0	2.0	3.5	2.0	2.0

Figure 15–39 Same case as in Figure 15–38. Note dramatic initial change, with subsequent opening of "V" in ramus cut, due to lack of fixation of fragments and change of muscle pull and attachments. Open bite may occur due to temporalis and pterygomasseteric sling action in this type of resection.

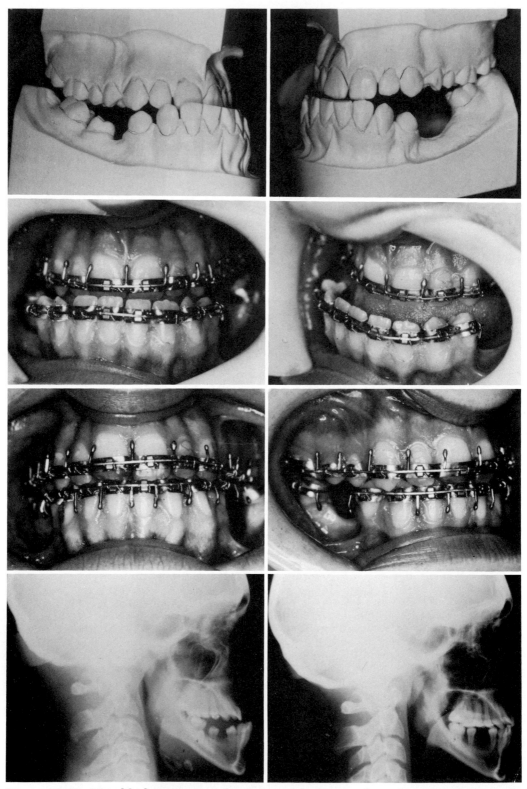

Figure 15–40   Mandibular resection, showing casts before, appliances in place before and after resection, and lateral cephalograms which depict the marked reduction into a normal anteroposterior relationship. Vertical spurs on arch wires are for intermaxillary elastic traction immediately following the surgical reduction. (Courtesy D. Laskin and S. Peskin.)

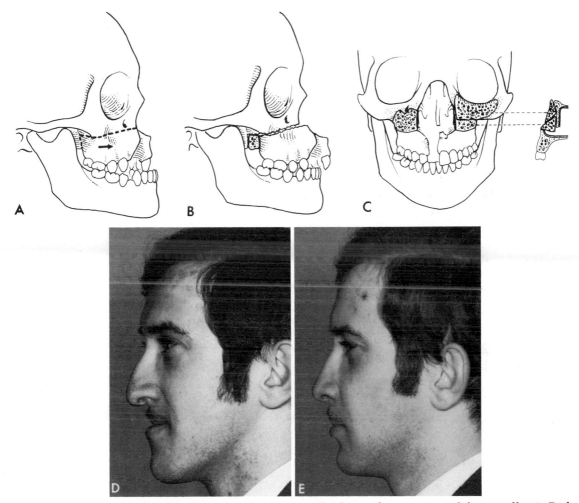

Figure 15–41   High Le Fort I type of osteotomy for forward movement of the maxilla. A, Path of bone cuts (dashed line). B, Repositioned maxilla with bone implanted behind tuberosity to stabilize maxilla. C, Postoperative anterior view; a bone implantation was necessary to prevent scar tissue contraction which would pull the maxilla back. D & E, Preoperative and postoperative profiles. Correction of profile was achieved through forward movement of the maxilla only. There was no supplemental correction of the nose. (Courtesy Obwegeser. H.: Surgical correction of maxillary deformities *in* Grabb, W. C., et al. (eds.): Cleft Lip and Palate. Little, Brown and Co., 1971.)

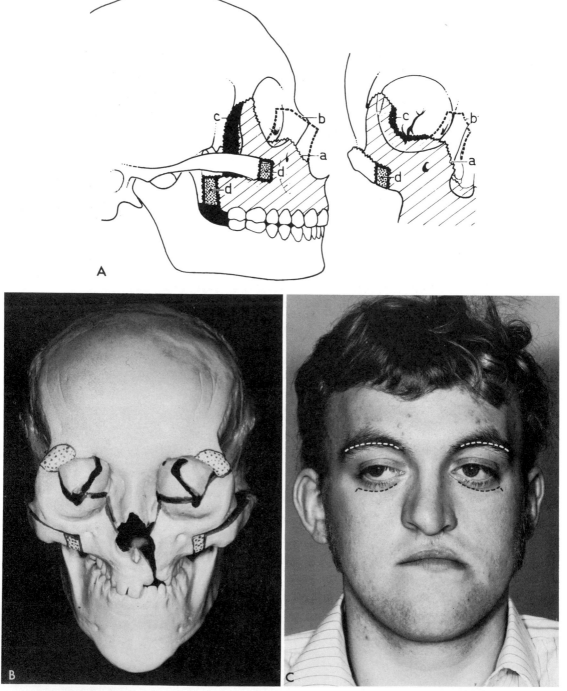

Figure 15–42   Forward advancement of middle third of the face via a Le Fort III type of oste-otomy. A, Schematic drawing of cuts on facial bones: lacrimal sac and lacrimal canal may be ex-cluded (a) or included (b); defects in orbital walls (c) may not need bone implantation (d) to stabilize and to secure the bony union. B, Bone implantation at zygomaticofrontal suture area. C, Skin incision outline used in this case. Notice pseudo-exophthalmos. D and E, Preoperative and postoperative profile views. F, Cephalograms taken before operation, after operation during intermaxillary fixation with craniofacial suspension to pins in frontal bone, and after postoperative fixation. (Courtesy Obwegeser, H.: Surgical correction of maxillary deformities *in* Grabb, W. C., et al. (eds.): Cleft Lip and Palate. Little, Brown and Co., 1971.)

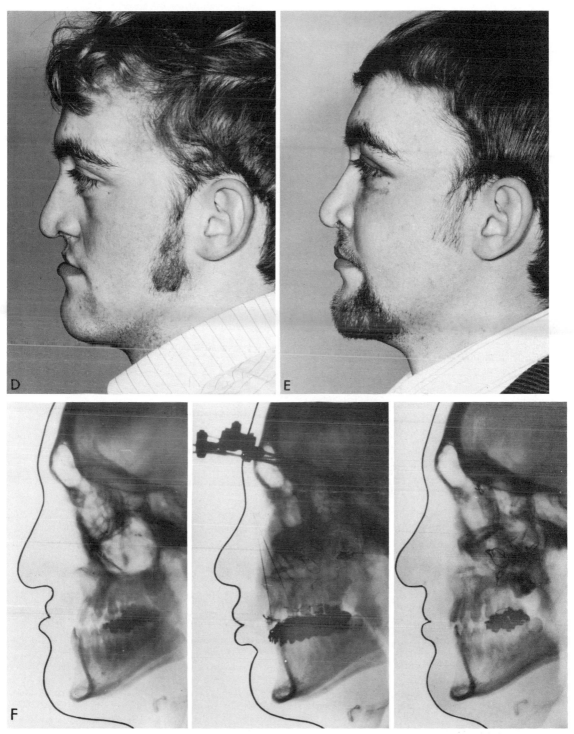

Figure 15–42 (continued)

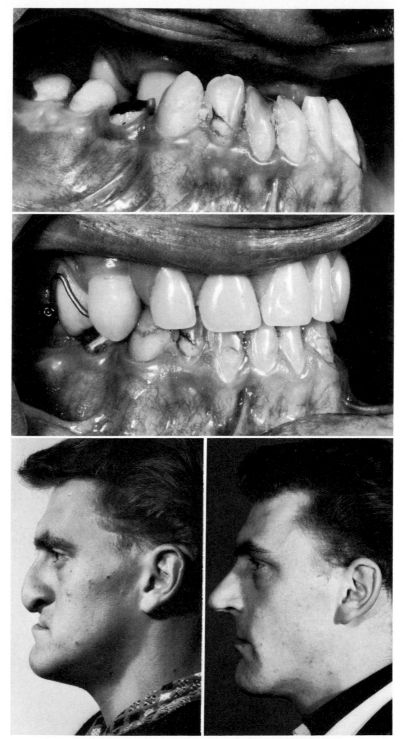

Figure 15–43 Extreme pseudoprognathism with complete nonocclusion in a case of bilateral cleft, corrected by repositioning the three maxillary segments and moving the mandible backward via the intraoral sagittal-splitting procedure. Top and middle views are preoperative and postoperative occlusion (a provisional partial denture is inserted in middle view). Bottom row is patient's profile before and after treatment. Several operations were needed for osteotomies and cleft closure. A final operation was performed for reconstruction of the lip and columella. (Courtesy Obwegeser, H.: Surgical correction of maxillary deformities *in* Grabb, W. C., et al. (eds.): Cleft Lip and Palate. Little, Brown and Co., 1971.)

thodontic growth guidance approach may be preferable, often the decision cannot be made in this direction because of severity of the malrelationship, age of the patient, amount of growth left, socio-economic and time factors. Mandibular resections were used for a long time, with indifferent results until adequate diagnosis and muscle control as well as bone control became the order of the day. Surgery has developed excellent jaw-positioning techniques which involve a minimum of trauma and adverse iatrogenic sequelae. Today, maxillary ostectomies for protrusion are done almost as frequently as mandibular procedures, particularly in young adults beyond growing age. Even with modern surgical techniques, orthodontics is still needed as part of the correction. Excellent results can be obtained by this orthodontic-surgical "team approach" (Figs. 15–38 to 15–43).[56]

COSMETIC SURGERY

Closely allied to resection is the question of cosmetic revision. After all, "looks" are a major motivation for orthodontic treatment, too. After mechanotherapy, enlarged noses and receding chins often remain to plague the patient. Chaconas, in his study of nasal growth, indicated that Class II patients showed more pronounced elevation of the bridge of the nose.[55] The configuration of the dorsum of the nose followed the general convexity of the Class II face. Class III cases actually showed a concave dorsum tendency, paralleling the face. Stopping short with malocclusion correction only, particularly when removal of four first premolars may have accentuated the midface prominence, is not in the best interests of the patient. Surgical consultation is indicated; many patients would

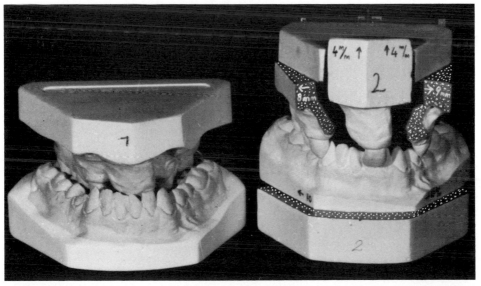

Figure 15–44 Plaster casts of case in Figure 15–43, showing the displacement of the three maxillary segments and the retropositioning of the mandibular dentition. The approximate distances moved are shown in millimeters on the right-hand model. (From Obwegeser, H.: Surgical correction of maxillary deformities *in* Grabb, W. C., et al. (eds.): Cleft Lip and Palate. Little, Brown and Co., 1971.)

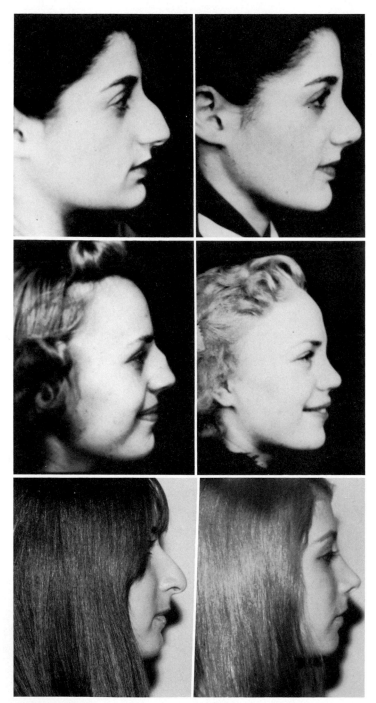

Figure 15–45 Before and after profile photos of rhinoplasty operations. Convex profiles and Class II malocclusions are more likely to need this correction. (Top and middle views, courtesy W. Slaughter.)

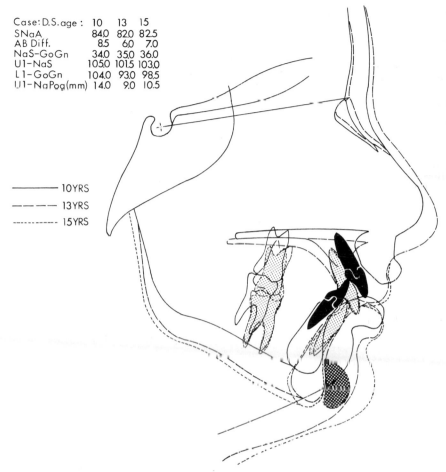

Case: D.S. age :	10	13	15
SNaA	84.0	82.0	82.5
AB Diff.	8.5	6.0	7.0
NaS-GoGn	34.0	35.0	36.0
U1-NaS	105.0	101.5	103.0
L1-GoGn	104.0	93.0	98.5
L1-NaPog (mm)	14.0	9.0	10.5

———— 10YRS

– – – – 13YRS

- - - - - 15YRS

Figure 15–46 Class II, Division 1 malocclusion with vertical (clockwise) growing face. Correction of occlusion still left the appearance of a retrusive mandible. A genioplasty was performed. The implant insertion (some surgeons prefer cartilage, some polyurethane foam or Silastic) improved the chin button contour.

benefit. Parents should be informed of the possible surgical service and its attendant rewards at the time orthodontic treatment is begun. If not, both the general practitioner and orthodontist may be blamed for the lack of guidance.

Genioplastics, as well as rhinoplasties, make dramatic profile changes. Either bone removal and shaping for prominent chin buttons, or cartilage or plastic implants for "chinless wonders" are desirable both orthodontically and psychologically (Figs. 15–45, 15–46). Teamwork is again the order of the day.

REFERENCES

1. Palsson, F.: Foregangare til den S. K. Serieextraktionen. Odont. Rev., 7:118–135, 1956.
2. Kjellgren, B.: Serial extraction as a corrective procedure in dental orthopedic therapy, Trans. Eur. Orthodont. Soc., 134–160, 1947–48.
3. Hotz, R.: Active supervision of the eruption of teeth by extraction. Trans. Eur. Orthodont. Soc., 134–160, 1947–48.
4. Hotz, R.: Orthodontics in Daily Practice. Berne, Hans Huber, 1962.

5. Heath, J.: The interception of malocclusion by planned serial extraction. New Zealand Dent. J., 49:77–88, 1953.
6. Heath, J.: Serial Extraction and Mechanically Guided Development. Melbourne, Verona Press, 1958.
7. Nance, H.: Serial extraction procedures. Personal communication. 1946.
8. Lloyd, Z. B.: Serial extraction. Am. J. Orthodont., 39:262–267, 1953.
9. Lloyd, Z. B.: Serial extraction as a treatment procedure. Am. J. Orthodont., 42:728–739, 1956.
10. Dewel, B. F.: Serial extraction in orthodontics: indications, objectives and treatment procedures. Am. J. Orthodont., 40:906–926, 1954.
11. Dewel, B. F.: The indications and technique of the edgewise appliance in serial extraction procedures. Trans. Eur. Orthodont. Soc., 3–26, 1956.
12. Dewel, B. F.: Serial extraction: procedures and limitations. Am. J. Orthodont., 43:685–687, 1957.
13. Dewel, B. F.: Serial extraction. Presentation at 21st Annual Denver Summer Meeting, Denver, Colorado, August 4 to 8, 1958.
14. Dewel, B. F.: A critical analysis of serial extraction in orthodontic treatment. Am. J. Orthodont., 45:424–455, 1959.
15. Mayne, W. R.: Serial Extraction as an Adjunct to Orthodontic Treatment. Audio-Visual Sequence. St. Louis, American Association of Orthodontists, 1965.
16. Ringenberg, Q.: Serial extraction: stop, look and be certain. Am. J. Orthodont., 50:327–336, 1964.
17. Hinrichsen, C. F. L.: Serial extraction in mixed dentition orthodontics. Aust. Dent. J., 6:201–209, 1961.
18. Neumann, B.: Planned serial extraction in orthodontic treatment. Dent. Abstr., 6:489–490, 1961.
19. Fanning, E. A.: Effect of extraction of deciduous molars on the formation and eruption of their successors. Angle Orthodont., 32:44–53, 1962.
20. Norman, F.: Serial extraction. Angle Orthodont., 35:149–157, 1965.
21. Seward, F. S.: Natural closure of deciduous molar extraction spaces. Angle Orthodont., 35:85–94, 1965.
22. Moorrees, C. F. A., Fanning, E. A., and Grøn, A. M.: The consideration of dental development in serial extraction. Angle Orthodont., 33:44–59, 1963.
23. Owen, D. G.: Incidence and nature of space closure following premature extraction of deciduous teeth. Am. J. Orthodont., 59:37–49, 1971.
24. Graber, T. M.: Serial extraction: a continuing diagnostic and decisional process. Am. J. Orthodont., 60:541–575, 1971.
25. Lysell, L.: Relationship between mesiodistal crown diameters in the deciduous and permanent lateral teeth. Acta Odont. Scand., 18:1–11, 1960.
26. Graber, T. M.: Postmortems in post-treatment adjustment. Am. J. Orthodont., 52:331–352, 1966.
27. Ringenberg, Q. M.: Influence of serial extraction on growth and development of the maxilla and mandible. Am. J. Orthodont., 53:19–26, 1967.
28. Graber, T. M.: Orthodontics: Principles and Practice. 2nd ed. Philadelphia, W. B. Saunders Co., pp. 714–739, 1966.
29. Graber, T. M.: Diagnosis and panoramic radiography. Am. J. Orthodont., 53:799–821, 1967.
30. Peskin, S., and Graber, T. M.: Surgical repositioning of the teeth. J.A.D.A., 80:1320–1326, 1970.
31. Mayne, W. R.: Serial extraction in, Graber, T. M. (ed.): Current Orthodontic Concepts and Techniques, Philadelphia, W. B. Saunders Co., vol. 1, pp. 179–274, 1969.
32. Hotz, R. P.: Guidance of eruption versus serial extraction. Am. J. Orthodont., 58:1–20, 1970.
33. Moyers, R. E.: Development of occlusion. D. Clin. North America, Philadelphia, W. B. Saunders Co., pp. 523–536, 1969.
34. Dempster, W. T., Adams, W. J., and Duddles, R. A.: Arrangement in the jaws of the roots of the teeth. J.A.D.A., 67:779–797, 1963.
35. Enlow, D. H., and Moyers, R. E.: Growth and architecture of the face. J.A.D.A., 82:763–774, 1971.
36. Moorrees, C. F. A., Burstone, C. J., Christiansen, R. L., Hixon, E. H., and Weinstein, S.: Research related to malocclusion. Am. J. Orthodont., 59:1–18, 1971.
37. Schwarz, A. M.: Lehrgang der Gebissregelung. Vienna, Verlag Urban & Schwarzenberg, 1961.
38. Dewel, B. F.: Second premolar extraction in orthodontics: principles, procedures and case analysis. Am. J. Orthodont., 41:107–120, 1955.
39. Laskin, D. M.: Evaluation of the third molar problem. J.A.D.A., 82:824–828, 1971.
40. Weinstein, S.: Third molar implications in orthodontics. J.A.D.A., 82:819–823, 1971.
41. Graber, T. M.: Team effort: oral surgery and orthodontics, J. Oral Surg., 25:201–224, 1967.
42. MacIntosh, R. B.: The surgical approach to Class II, Division I malocclusion. J.A.D.A., 82:796–804, 1971.
43. Byrd, D. L., and Murphey, P. J.: The surgical approach to Class III malocclusion. J.A.D.A., 82:813–818, 1971.
44. Clark, D.: The management of impacted canines; free physiologic eruption. J.A.D.A., 836–840, 1971.
45. Walker, R. V.: Delayed occlusal and maxillofacial deformities after trauma. J.A.D.A., 82:858–861, 1971.
46. Rosenstein, S. W.: Pathological and congenital disturbances: the orthodontic viewpoint. J.A.D.A., 82:871–875, 1971.

47. Sarnat, B. G.: Clinical and experimental considerations in facial bone biology; growth, re-modelling and repair. J.A.D.A., 82:876–889, 1971.
48. Obwegeser, H. L.: Surgical correction of maxillary deformities *in*, Grabb, W. C., Rosenstein, S. W., and Bzoch, K. R. (eds.): Cleft Lip and Palate. Boston, Little, Brown & Co., 1971.
49. Obwegeser, H. L.: Surgical correction of the small or retro-displaced maxillae. The "dish-face" deformity. Plast. Reconst.: Surg., 43:351–370, 1969.
50. Obwegeser, H. L.: Der offene Biss in chirurgischer Sicht. Sweizt. Monat. Schrft. Zahnheilk., 74:668–79, 1964.
51. Köle, H.: Chirurgische Kieferorthopädie. Leipzig, Barth, 1965.
52. Slagsvold, O., and Bjercke, B.: Autotransplantasjon av premolarer. Gøteb. Tandläk. Sällsk. Årsbok. 45–85, 1967.
53. Slagsvold, O.: Autotransplantation of premolars in cases of missing anterior teeth. Trans. Eur. Orthodont. Soc., 473–486, 1970.
54. Lemoine, C., Petrovic, A., and Stutzmann, J.: Inflammatory process of the rat maxilla after molar autotransplantation. J. Dent. Res., 49:1175, 1970.
55. Chaconas, S. J.: A statistical evaluation of nasal growth. Am. J. Orthodont., 56:403–414, 1969.
56. Salzmann, J. A.: An appraisal of surgical orthodontics. Am. H. Orthodont., 61:105–114, 1972.

chapter 16

LIMITED CORRECTIVE ORTHODONTICS: REMOVABLE APPLIANCES

Although it is preferable to prevent or intercept a developing malocclusion, it is frequently not possible. Even when the dentist sees the patient early enough, the preventive and interceptive procedures discussed in Chapters 13 and 14 may not be sufficient to cope with the problem. If the situation confronting the dentist gives all indications of being a total or full-fledged malocclusion, corrective procedures are beyond the scope of general dental practice and require the services of a trained specialist. *It is a moral and professional obligation of the dentist to see that the patient is guided into the proper hands so that this service can be rendered.* Most patients with full-fledged malocclusions should see an orthodontist by eight years of age. Actual corrective procedures may not be instituted at this time, but the judicious removal of deciduous teeth to ameliorate the malocclusion may be recommended (serial extraction). (See Chap. 15.) In any event, the orthodontist then assumes the responsibility for the long-range orthodontic guidance, though the dentist continues to oversee the total dental service, coordinating all aspects. However, timing of orthodontic treatment is so important that it is better to let the man who is going to render the corrective services make the decisions. (See Chap. 11, Orthodontic Appliances and Treatment Philosophy.)

Many of the orthodontic problems that the dentist sees in his everyday practice are not full-fledged malocclusions. Corrective procedures for these problems do not require the same specialized level of technical proficiency and training demanded by routine orthodontic service. Along with the ability to render preventive and interceptive orthodontic assistance, the recognition and correction of the orthodontic problems described in the following pages will help the dentist to perform a more complete and satisfying professional service.

These limited corrective measures are divided into three groups for the sake of organization of the material presented. Chapter 16 is devoted to a discussion of removable appliances; Chapter 17 covers certain specific procedures employing limited fixed appliances; and Chapter 18 describes more complex limited fixed appliances, primarily for the general dentist who has had some previous orthodontic training or who is working in conjunction with an orthodontist, that sees the patient periodically and assists the dentist. There is a significant increase in the amount of these cases, as the specialist finds his practice devoted to full-fledged malocclusions, with little time for anything else. Particularly in areas where there is no specialty service at all, such a consultative-treatment relationship broadens the scope of dental care. Surely the image of dentistry benefits, also.

If the dentist follows the directions outlined under each heading and if he seeks frequent consultation with a competent orthodontic specialist if problems arise or when there is a question about advisability and timing of orthodontic therapy, he should have no considerable difficulty. For the neophyte, it is most prudent to seek orthodontic consultation *before* each limited case is started until a reliable clinical judgment can be developed. Many a deceptively simple orthodontic problem has turned out to be only a local manifestation of a broader and more complex malocclusion. Emulating our medical confrères in this teamwork service will benefit both the patients and the dental team.

In this chapter are discussed the problems of excessive overbite, opening and closing spaces, retracting prominent incisors and ligation.

PROBLEMS OF EXCESSIVE OVERBITE

It was pointed out in Chapter 9, Unfavorable Sequelae of Malocclusion, that excessive overbite predisposes a patient to periodontal involvement. Abnormal function, improper mastication, excessive stresses, trauma, functional problems, bruxism and clenching, and temporomandibular joint disturbances make geriatric dental service a losing battle unless overbite can be controlled. Constriction of the mandibular anterior segment and progressive crowding and irregularity of the teeth in this area are inevitable sequelae. Although overbite correction remains a continuing problem for even the most competent orthodontist, considerable benefit may be realized from the use of the bite plate.

BITE PLATE THERAPY

Teeth out of occlusal contact with the opposing arch continue to erupt to a certain degree. The PVD-OVD (postural-occlusal vertical dimension) relationship is best served by a 2 to 4 mm. interocclusal clearance. Normally, eruption of posterior teeth that encroach on this space will not hold unless there is re-education of the perioral musculature—a most unlikely prospect. But if there is an excessive interocclusal clearance in which the occlusal vertical dimension is not in harmony with the postural resting vertical dimension, or in which the patient closes from postural resting position 3 or 4 mm. and keeps on closing because the posterior teeth have not erupted sufficiently (Fig. 16–1), the bite plate can stimulate eruption that will hold (Fig. 16–2). Although this applies primarily to the young and growing patient, eruption is still possible in the young adult, albeit to a lesser degree and over a longer period of time. (See Chap. 3, Physiology of the Stomatognathic System.)

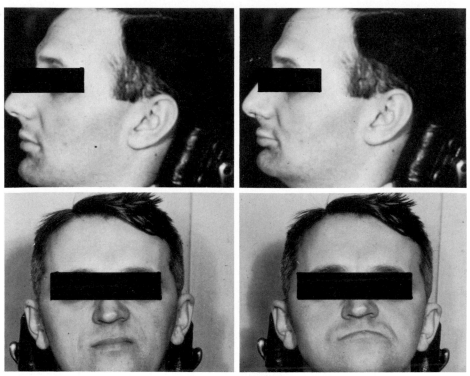

Figure 16–1   Excessive overbite in adult. (Top) class II malocclusion and (bottom) Class III malocclusion. Postural position is on left and habitual occlusal position on right. A very large interocclusal space permits overclosure and a deep bite. Normally, there should be little or no change in lip contour between postural resting position and habitual occlusal position. A marked decrease in facial height and pursing of the lips on closure indicate lack of harmony of the two vertical dimensions.

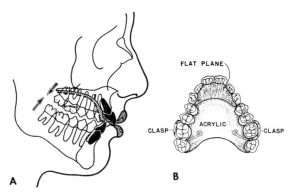

Figure 16–2   The maxillary bite plate. The flat plate behind the maxillary incisors is made so that an occlusal vertical dimension harmonious with the postural rest vertical dimension is established when the mandibular incisors close into contact with the plane. Posterior teeth in infraocclusion are allowed to erupt to the proper occlusal plane level, reducing the excessive interocclusal space or clearance. Eruption of posterior teeth is considerably slower in the adult than in the child. For the adult, the appliance serves primarily as a "crutch" to prevent damaging consequences of overbite.

Clinical experience has shown that the maxillary bite plate is effective in fostering more favorable development of the mandibular arch in deciduous Class I closed bite cases and in many deciduous Class II cases.[1-3, 14] Most encouraging is the observation of increase of intercanine width as a result of bite plate therapy (Figs. 16–3 to 16–5). The removal of the restricting influence of the maxillary arch on the contained mandibular arch seems a plausible explanation. Vertical and horizontal changes are most likely in the mixed and early permanent dentition when growth and developmental increments are significant. Intensive appliance wear, during both day and night, is a prerequisite, however.

In the adult, as it has been pointed out, eruption takes place but at a much slower rate. There is a strong tendency toward the return of the original vertical occlusal relationship if bite plate therapy is discontinued. This does not mean

AVERAGE INCREASE IN DECIDUOUS MANDIBULAR INTERCANINE WIDTH
(Measurement in millimeters enlarged 10 times)

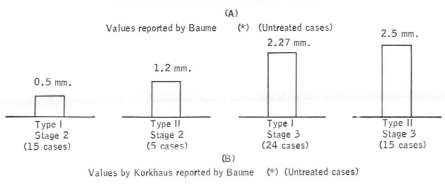

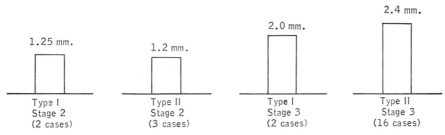

Type I: Interdental mandibular spacing present
Type II: No interdental mandibular spacing
Stage 1: Deciduous dentition is completed
Stage 2: First permanent incisors have erupted
Stage 3: All permanent incisors have erupted

Baume reports no spontaneous spacing of the mandibular incisors after complete eruption of the deciduous teeth (Stage 1). Classification of occlusion not reported.

Figure 16–3   Chart 1; compiled by Mathews from material by Baume (upper half of chart) and Korkhaus and Neuman (lower half of chart). There is an increase of 0.5 mm. shown by Baume from completion of deciduous dentition to eruption of mandibular central incisors in patients with interdental spacing, as opposed to 1.2 mm. in patients with no interdental spacing. In the period from completion of the deciduous dentition until eruption of all four incisors, Baume shows an increase of 2.27 mm. in Type I cases (spacing present) and 2.50 mm. in Type II cases (no spacing present). There is general agreement in the data of Baume, Korkhaus and Neuman. These average values represent changes without orthodontic appliances.[1, 2]

that the bite plate is any less needed. Indeed, a bite plate may serve as a valuable "crutch" and may have to be used indefinitely, at least at night, to prevent deteriorating periodontal conditions, trauma and abnormal tooth guidance of the mandible during mastication, temporomandibular joint disturbances and clenching or bruxism (Fig. 16–6). Elimination of dominent posterior temporalis muscle activity with its attendant functional retrusion effects, which at times may mean exacerbation of a Class II anteroposterior tendency, is a good example of applied biology. (See Fig. 3–22.) By restoring stress to the mandibular incisors so that the force is transmitted primarily through the long axis of these teeth, by stimulating eruption of posterior teeth and thus reducing the severe canine interference so often seen, by preventing overclosure, tooth guidance and

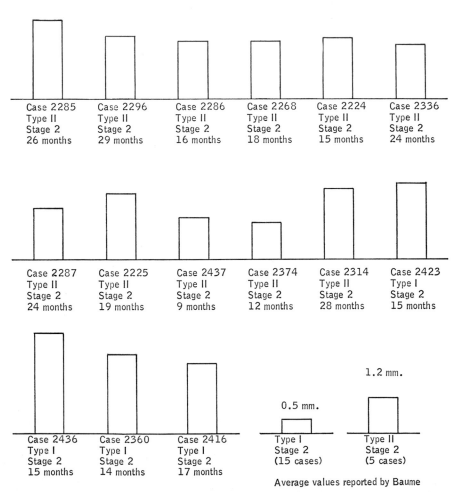

INCREASE IN DECIDUOUS MANDIBULAR CUSPID WIDTH IN CLASS I
CASES TREATED WITH HAWLEY BITE PLANES
(measurement in millimeters enlarged 10 times)

Figure 16–4 Chart 2; marked increases in mandibular intercanine width in 15 Type I and Type II cases under bite plate treatment for an average of 19 months. The dimensional increases from complete deciduous dentition to eruption of central incisors ranges from 1.2 to 3.5 mm. Compare the individual changes with the mean values reported by Baume[1, 2] in the lower right hand part of the chart; also, see Chart 1.

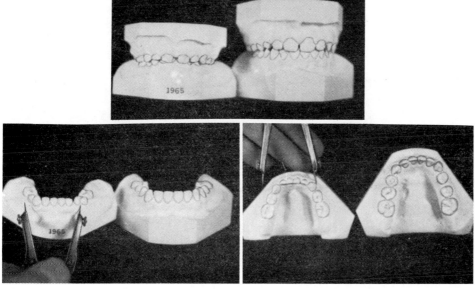

Figure 16–5   Developmental progress from late deciduous to early permanent dentition with intermittent use of a bite plate for over five years. Note the significant intercanine width increase and reduction in overbite.[1,2]

temporomandibular joint aberrations, the bite plate broadens the horizons of preventive dental service (Fig. 16–7).

In addition to actual correction of abnormal overbite in younger patients, frequent use as a dental "crutch" and as a periodontal treatment adjunct, the bite plate may also serve as a valuable diagnostic tool. When used as a splint, the bite plate assists in diagnosing and alleviating temporomandibular joint complaints.

A high degree of success has been achieved in diagnosis and treatment of temporomandibular joint disturbances with bite plate therapy together with heat, massage and muscle relaxants. Because of the psychogenic and tension release (neuromuscular) aspects of TMJ problems, something must be done to eliminate the triggering effect of occlusal contact and overclosure.[4] The "splint," "brace" or "crutch" concept is emulated in various general orthopedic problems as a conservative adjunct to treatment. Clinical experience indicates significantly more favorable patient response than that from cortisone or sclerosing injections, or extirpation of the articular disk, so often resorted to by an orthopedic surgeon, unaware of the therapeutic potential of the bite plate.[16]

In problems of full mouth reconstruction, a bite plate is invaluable in establishing the proper and most comfortable occlusal vertical dimension before the teeth themselves are modified with permanent fixed restorations.[5] Many a dentist has found to his chagrin that a patient cannot tolerate a bite-opening reconstructive procedure after the last crown has been cemented. (See *Diagnostic Splints.*) Harmonizing occlusal vertical dimension with postural vertical dimension is a top priority objective.

Where bruxism is present, a bite plate may show that excessive overbite is a causal factor, and its elimination may mean the cessation of the grinding and clenching that has plagued the patient for years. No longer can the intelligent dentist ignore the vertical dimension in dentistry if he desires to establish a healthy, stable and properly functioning occlusion for his patients.[8]

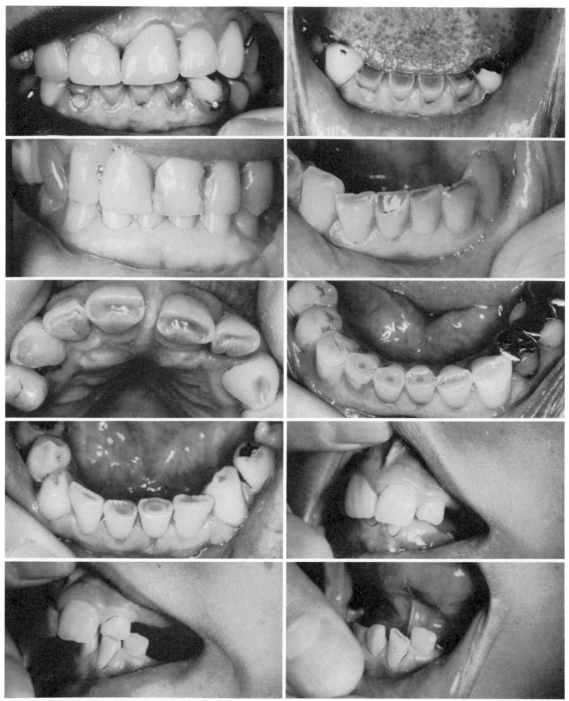

Figure 16–6 Bruxism—often a consequence of excessive overbite, exacerbated by neurogenic or tensional release factors. Although the greatest amount of destruction is usually in the anterior teeth, the trigger area is frequently in the posterior segments. Bruxism is common in the deciduous dentition. An example of damage in the mixed dentition is seen in pictures in the fourth row, right, and in the bottom row. Excursive bruxing has grooved the maxillary incisal margin and worn away the distal incisal angle of the mandibular left central incisor. Note the receding gingival margin in this area. Orthodontic correction, a bite plate, or both are indicated. (See Figure 6–86.)

Figure 16–7 Posterosuperior displacement, or functional retrusion, frequently associated with excessive overbite. A bite plate that is constructed to prevent mandibular overclosure past the point of initial tooth contact will also eliminate the abnormal translatory condylar movement from 2 to 3 that may serve as a precursor of temporomandibular joint problems.

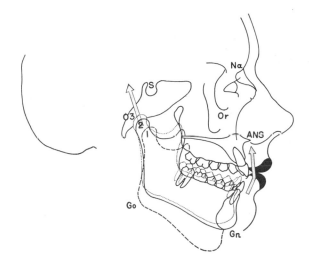

CONSTRUCTION OF BITE PLATES

The construction of the maxillary bite plate is relatively simple. After study models and other diagnostic criteria have been obtained, a separate maxillary impression is made. A stone model is poured and made ready for the fabrication of the bite plate. It is recommended that clasps be made for the last molar

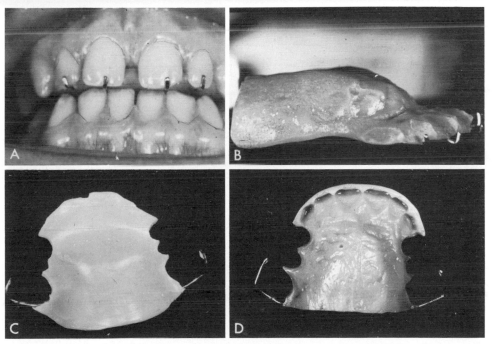

Figure 16–8 A and B, Use of metal incisal hooks in cases where overjet permits, to prevent labial movement of incisors and to transmit some of the force of occlusion down the long axis of these teeth. Hooks also assist in retention of the appliance. C, A bite plate with molar clasps, but no labial wire or incisal hooks. This type is almost exclusively used in conjunction with fixed orthodontic appliances. D, Overjet is sufficient to permit the acrylic to be carried over to the labial surfaces of the incisors, as recommended by Sved.

tooth to assist in retention. These may be the usual circumferential type, the Adams clasp or ball clasps (Figs. 16–15, 16–21.) If the maxillary bite plate is to be worn for any length of time, it is advisable to incorporate a labial wire (Fig. 16–11). Prolonged wear of the bite plate without any restraining force exerts a labial thrust tendency on the incisors, increases the overjet and may stimulate incisor spacing and flaring. The use of a labial wire prevents this labial displacement of the incisors and improves retention. An alternate method is the use of metal incisal hooks or, if there is sufficient overjet, the acrylic itself may be carried up over the incisal margin to the labial as in the Sved type bite plate (Figs. 16–8 to 16–10). Incisal hooks are less desirable, since they may cause notching of the incisors. Unlike the labial wire, they permit little adjustment.

After the clasps and labial wire have been adapted, the palatal portion may be waxed up and cured by flasking, packing, and so forth, which provides a more accurate and less porous reproduction. Alternately, endothermic acrylic may be used, and powder and monomer may be mixed directly on the cast after it has been painted with separating medium. To provide the necessary bite opening, a flat plane starting approximately 1 mm. from the incisal margin and carried posteriorly about 1 cm. is constructed behind the maxillary incisors. One need not be concerned at this point about the correct vertical dimension since this can be taken care of by removing the excess acrylic on the plane during the adjusting of the appliance in the mouth.

After the bite plate has been polished it is placed in the patient's mouth, and the fit of the clasps and the adaptation of the acrylic are checked. All sharp

(*Text continued on page 784*)

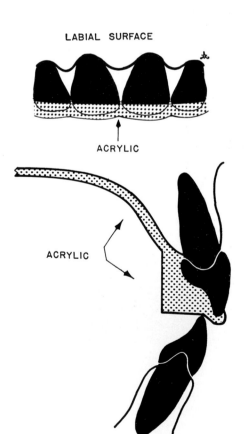

LABIAL SURFACE

ACRYLIC

ACRYLIC

Figure 16–9 Sved type acrylic bite plate which prevents incisor movement and transmits part of the forces of occlusion to the long axes of the incisor teeth.

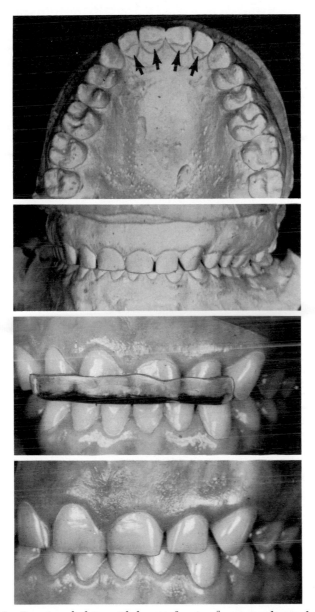

Figure 16–10 Bruxism habit, with heavy facets of wear on lingual side of maxillary incisors (arrows), and excessive overbite. Bite plate was designed with acrylic labial flange to protect maxillary incisors. Even though the patient was an adult, sufficient eruption of posterior segments occurred to decrease overbite and to reduce damaging effects from bruxism.

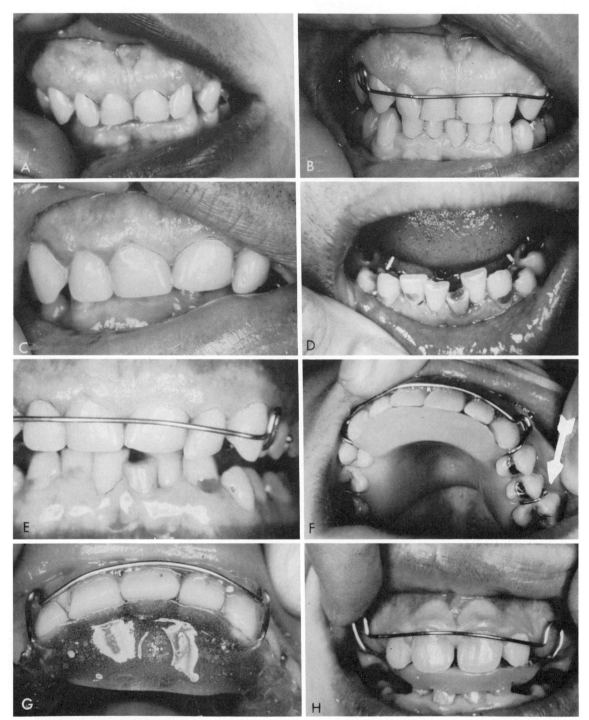

Figure 16–11 Deep overbite and the bite plate. (A and B) The use of the "crutch concept" in adult dentitions eliminates temporomandibular joint (TMJ) problems, bruxism and clenching and retards tissue breakdown. In C, D and E, crowded lower incisors receive more physiologic stress with bite plate wear, improving soft and hard tissue health in 28-year-old male. F illustrates bite plate wear with added retention from ball clasps at molar-premolar embrasure. Occasionally, in TMJ problems, an inclined plane must be added (G) to guide the mandible anteriorly, as well as to "open the bite." Elimination of functional retrusion is desirable. In H, a conventional bite plate has been modified by carrying acrylic over lower incisors to splint them against labial movement during the wearing of a Milwaukee scoliosis brace. Care must be taken not to exceed the postural resting position.

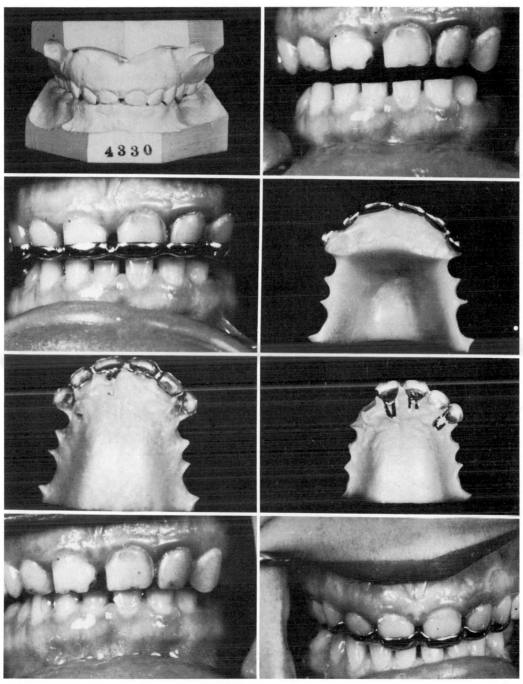

Figure 16–12   Young adult with deep overbite and severe bruxism habit. Temporomandibular joint complaints were constant; maxillary lateral incisor jacket crowns kept breaking. Deep overbite, bruxism and TMJ symptoms were eliminated, but only after a Vitallium cast was made to cover the incisal portions which were being chipped away by nocturnal gnashing. Even then, the Vitallium cast was fractured once and had to be replaced. Correction took three years. Bite plate must be worn indefinitely at night to prevent relapse to overbite and clicking, crepitus and pain in the temporomandibular joints.

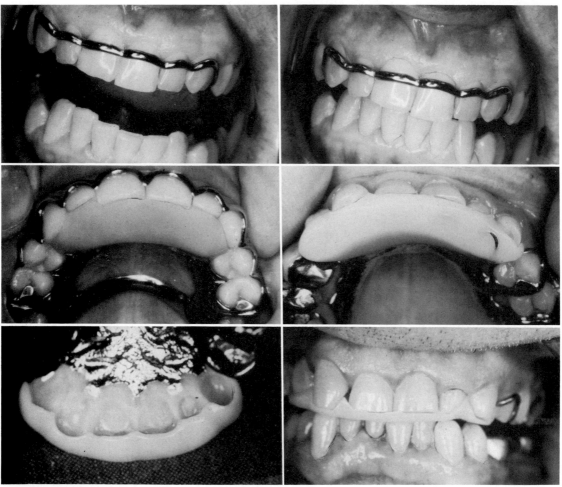

Figure 16–13A   Cast chrome-cobalt alloy framework, combined with acrylic for semipermanent stabilizing "crutch." Unfavorable sequelae of bruxism and deep overbite are reduced with nighttime wear. Labial casting should not impinge on gingival margin. As shown in top row, casting should be just above labial convexity. Alternately, acrylic may be used as a Sved type addition to the metal framework, where overjet and overbite permit (second row, right, and bottom row). The labial metal scallop is usually more satisfactory, however.

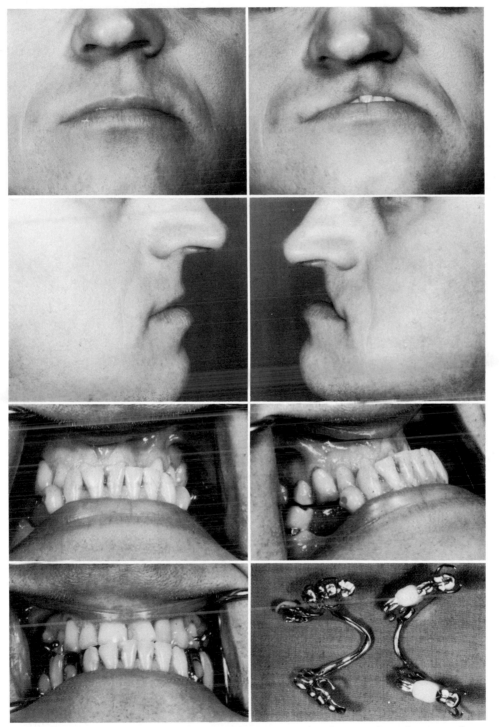

Figure 16–13B Severe lack of harmony of occlusal vertical with postural resting vertical dimension. Large interocclusal clearance permits overclosure into Class III relationship. Note marked facial changes on frontal and profile views. Metal castings reduce the interocclusal clearance from 15 mm. to 3 mm. Horizontal discrepancy is largely eliminated, and facial harmony is restored. (Bottom row, left, shows castings in place.)

projections of the acrylic into the interdental spaces should be removed. Clasps should contact the molar teeth lightly but passively. If a labial wire has been used, it should contact the incisors at about the apical third. The postural resting position of the patient should first be established with the bite plate out of the mouth. Then the bite plate is placed in the mouth and, with the aid of articulating paper, reduced to a level 1 to 2 mm. less than the postural resting vertical dimension. Under no circumstances should the vertical dimension established with the lower incisors in contact with the bite plate exceed the postural resting dimension.

Whenever the bite plate is used as a treatment adjunct, it should be worn at all times, with the possible exception of meal time. After the correct occlusal vertical dimension has been achieved through the eruption of the posterior teeth, the length of time that the bite plate must be worn may be reduced by half, but its use as a retaining appliance should continue for 6 to 12 months or longer on this basis, depending on the amount of eruption that has been achieved, the age of the patient, the type of occlusion and the individual relapse tendency.

If the bite plate is used as a dental "crutch" and there is no reasonable likelihood of permanent correction, it must be worn indefinitely (Fig. 16–11). In most instances it is sufficient to wear it only at night for this purpose. In cases of bruxism, where it is used to prevent occlusal sensory stimuli from triggering the grinding phenomenon, it must also be worn indefinitely. The majority of patients learn to rely on the bite plate and feel they actually cannot go to sleep without it. If it is likely that the patient will wear the bite plate for quite some time, particularly in cases of clenching or bruxism, it must be made sturdily to withstand considerable stress. A restraining labial wire, or a labial acrylic incisal extension should be incorporated to prevent labial movement of maxillary incisors. Ordinary bite plates may not hold up under severe grinding assaults in some bruxism patients. The patient in Figure 16–12 broke an all-acrylic bite plate within three nights, snapped off metal incisal hooks and chipped the enamel of her maxillary incisors in a week, and actually fractured a vitallium casting that was made subsequently, before breaking the habit. In any case, the acrylic portion of the plane must be rebuilt at periodic intervals as it is worn down. A cast metal lingual and labial skeleton makes a good base for long-term adult use (Figs. 16–13, 16–29).

DIAGNOSTIC SPLINTS

If the bite plate is to be used as a diagnostic splint in temporomandibular joint disturbances and mandibular displacements, or in the establishment of a correct vertical dimension before the full mouth reconstruction, the labial wire may not be necessary. A mandibular diagnostic splint serves equally well and is less bulky in instances in which a prereconstructive occlusal vertical dimension determination is being made. In the case of either maxillary or mandibular splint, it is wise to carry the acrylic over the occlusal surfaces to the buccal occlusal margins (Figs. 16–14, 16–28). The amount of acrylic on the occlusal surface should be little more than the thickness of one sheet of base-plate-wax—only enough to eliminate tooth guidance through premature contacts if a functional problem is present. The diagnostic splint is "ground in" with the help of articulating paper so that the teeth in the opposing arch all contact at the same time and all have freedom of movement. Another reason for "grinding in" is so that newly established occlusal vertical dimension with the diagnostic

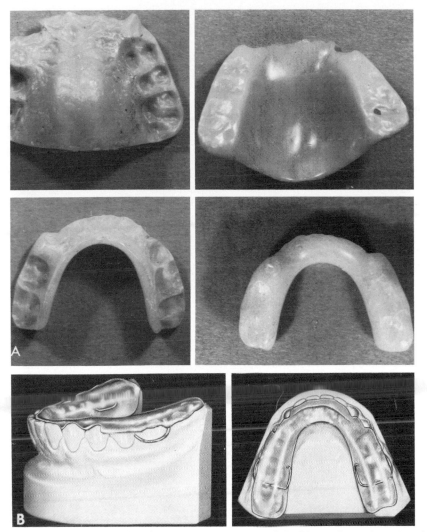

Figure 16–14   A, Palatal and occlusal views of modified bite plate (above) and tooth-side and occlusal views of mandibular splint (below). Both may be used as diagnostic splints for temporomandibular joint disturbances, or to determine correct occlusal verti-cal dimension, before permanent reconstruction procedures. B, Mandibular occlusal splint in space on cast, showing amount of tooth coverage. (From Fischer, B.: Clinical Orthodontics. A Guide to the Sectional Method. W. B. Saunders Co., 1957.)

splint in place will be in centric relation, and the relations of condyle, articular disk and eminence will be harmonious. If the problem is one of an excessive overbite, and the aim is to establish the correct occlusal vertical dimension in harmony with the postural resting vertical dimension, the occlusal surfaces of the splint may be altered by adding or removing endothermic acrylic. Such splints should be worn for at least four to six weeks in complete comfort by the patient before the dentist can be reasonably sure that his permanent recon-struction may safely duplicate this occlusal vertical dimension as determined by the diagnostic splint.

For temporomandibular joint disturbances, it is preferable not to carry the acrylic over the occlusal surfaces of the posterior teeth at first. Rather, the initial diagnostic splint should be a simple flat plane bite plate, maintaining mandibular incisal contact within the limits of the postural resting vertical dimension. If this does not alleviate the symptoms of pain and crepitus, additional acrylic may be added to convert the anterior portion to an inclined plane, which guides the mandible forward, eliminating excessive overjet as well as overbite. The condyle is moved anteriorly within the functional range. Crepitus is eliminated in most cases after the initial unlocking "pop." Postarticular connective tissue cannot then be traumatized by abnormal functional retrusion.

Where teeth have been lost in the molar area, there is a tendency at times for the condyle to move distally and superiorly. Posterior temporalis activity appears to adjust, but becomes dominant over middle and anterior temporalis fibers. In such TMJ problems, adding acrylic occlusal blocks on the bite plate posteriorly may be indicated to restore a normal condyle-articular disk-eminence relationship. A differential diagnosis must be made from a careful perusal of all diagnostic criteria. When in doubt, start with the simple, flat plane bite plate. Add the anterior inclined plane or posterior occlusal acrylic only if pain has not been eliminated.

OPENING AND CLOSING OF SPACES AND RETRACTION OF INCISORS WITH REMOVABLE APPLIANCES

Minor problems of space are within the realm of limited corrective orthodontic procedures. Although success is possible in local disturbances only, and not in general malocclusions, valuable service may be rendered to the patient. The broad expanse of the palate permits a tissue borne appliance to distribute the stresses created and provides adequate retention possibilities at the same time. Since these appliances are under the direct control of the patient, it is imperative that the dentist have reasonable assurance of patient cooperation; otherwise, he will fail or do actual harm. If the Hawley type appliance is constructed properly and used properly, it is the most useful tool available to the dentist for palliative or interceptive procedures (Figs. 16–15, 16–16).

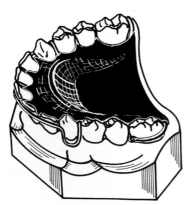 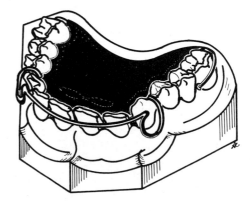

Figure 16–15   Maxillary removable appliance utilizing palatal surface for anchorage. Clasps around molars may be circumferential, ball type or arrow type to assist in retention. To close anterior spaces, acrylic is cut away on the lingual side of incisors and vertical loops are closed slightly, increasing labial wire pressure on incisors. To assist in incisor retraction, hooks may be bent in labial wire at each vertical loop to receive elastics (right). (See Figs. 16–29 and 16–30.)

Figure 16–16 Cross section of palatal appliance with labial wire. To retract incisors, acrylic is cut away at lingual-gingival margin of incisors (arrow) and labial vertical loops constricted so that contacting round-wire labial bow exerts pressure toward the lingual aspect. If less tipping is desired, the labial wire must approximate the gingival margin.

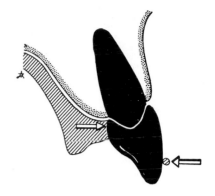

A common situation confronting the dentist is the spacing of the maxillary incisors. In many instances the spacing may be attributable to a longactive finger habit and to abnormal function of the perioral musculature. As was pointed out in Chapter 6, Etiology of Malocclusion: General Factors, the continuation of such habits can increase the severity of the orthodontic problem. The use of a removable orthodontic appliance to eliminate the abnormal morphology that enhances the deforming muscular forces is truly an example of interceptive orthodontics.

A typical example of a case in which the use of removable orthodontic appliances is of value would be that of an 8-year-old child with a normal molar relationship but with protruding and spaced maxillary incisors (Fig. 16–17). Often, because of the finger and lip habit, there may be a significant open bite tendency. There is no contact between maxillary and mandibular incisors during function. In this case, the patient must bring his food around to the side of the mouth to tear it off. During swallowing, the lower lip cushions to the

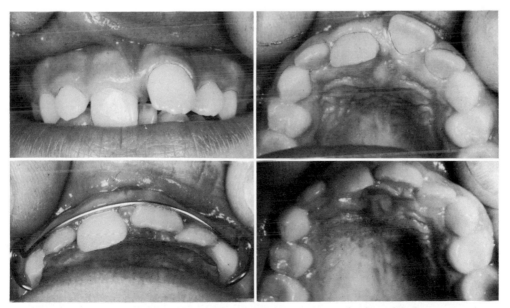

Figure 16–17 Labially malposed maxillary incisor, which is likely to remain in an abnormal position because of a bad lip habit. Since there is adequate space, a removable appliance may be used to retract the incisor to a position within normal limits, at least eliminating the deforming lip habit.

lingual side of the upper incisors, and at the same time the tongue can be seen intruding through the interdental space between the maxillary and mandibular incisors. If left unattended, the problem may get worse because of the deforming muscle forces. The child cannot close his lips without conscious effort and without the recruitment of muscle fibers that are not ordinarily involved in tonal or resting activity. There is the added hazard of possible fracture of the maxillary incisors because of their prominent and vulnerable position. It is very likely that the apices of the incisors are still wide open, making any fixed orthodontic appliance therapy premature and potentially hazardous.

FABRICATION OF APPLIANCE

As with any orthodontic problem, complete diagnostic records should be taken before any therapy is instituted. If the apices are wide open, it is better to postpone treatment until they close over partially. Generally speaking, all four maxillary incisor teeth should be clinically present for at least six months. Clinical examination may reveal that a heavy, fibrous frenum contributes to the spacing between the maxillary incisors. If a removable appliance is to be used, the frenum may be dissected out later in conjunction with appliance therapy. Other possible factors may cause or perpetuate the diastema, as listed in the chapters on etiology, and these must be checked. If a thorough study of all diagnostic records indicates that the normal complement of teeth is present, that there are no supernumerary teeth and that root formation is sufficiently advanced, an impression may be made for the appliance.

FIRST APPOINTMENT.   An accurate alginate impression should be taken of the maxillary arch including the tuberosity, if possible. No bubbles should be present in the palatal area. The impression should then be poured up in stone and separated in a manner similar to the technique used for the construction of the maxillary bite plate. (See also Chap. 8 on Diagnostic Procedures, Aids, and Their Interpretation.)

Next, the wire framework is fabricated. No. 139 wire-bending pliers are recommended, although clasp-bending pliers can be made to work. A Bernard type wire cutter is most serviceable for all gauges of orthodontic wire (Fig. 16–18). Actual bends are made by holding the round wire firmly with the beaks of the pliers and using the thumb assisted by the forefinger of the other hand to make the desired bends. The student is advised to practice making bends in random lengths of wire to develop a proficiency in making even-flowing and symmetrical bends (Fig. 16–19). In most cases 0.032 inch round (20 gauge) or 0.036 inch (19 gauge) nichrome or stainless-steel wire is used. The heavier gauge wire is used for the clasps and longer labial bow spans. Retention clasps may be of the circumferential, ball or arrow-crib type and are placed on the permanent first molars whenever possible (Figs. 16–15, 16–20, 16–21). The palatal projection of the clasp should be carefully adapted to the tissue and should be one half to three quarters of an inch long. A flat circular loop or sharp bend on the palatal end will provide added retention in the acrylic. Unless appliances are fabricated by an experienced orthodontic technician, complicated construction should be avoided. Seldom is it possible to make the arrow type clasp completely passive. Frequently the patient distorts the clasp, and retention is reduced while unwanted tooth movement is enhanced. Generally speaking, the simple circumferential or ball type clasps offer the best retention with a reduced likelihood of problems during therapy. After clasps are made for the first permanent molars, the labial wire is constructed

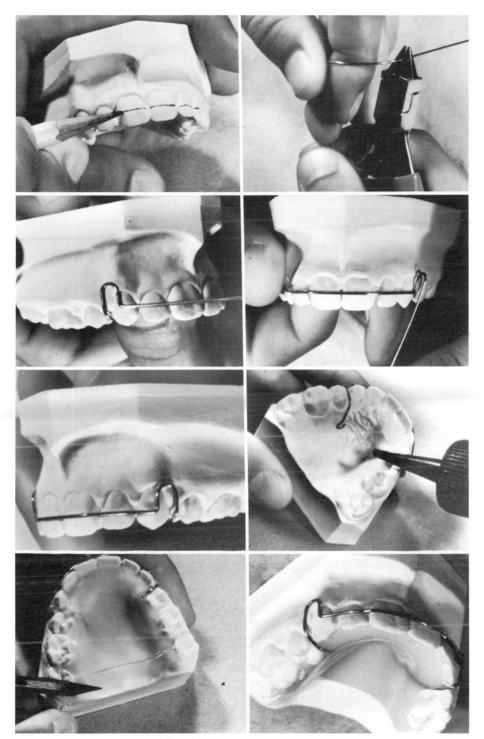

Figure 16–18. Fabrication of Hawley-type removable appliance. Pencilled line shows level of labial wire placement. #139 plier is used to make bends and vertical loops, after .030 nichrome or stainless steel bow is shaped by drawing it gently between thumb and forefinger. After bow is fitted passively, endothermic acrylic powder and monomer are added to model that has been painted with separating medium. Cutting off excess, appliance is polished in usual manner. (Courtesy, James McNamara, Jr.)

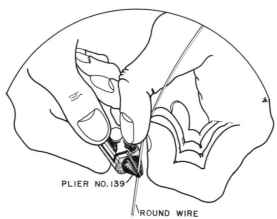

PLIER NO. 139

ROUND WIRE

Figure 16–19   An acceptable wire-bending procedure. The No. 139 pliers are held firmly in one hand; the round wire is grasped at a right angle. The wire is held between the thumb and forefinger of the other hand, and the bend is made over the round beak of the plier with thumb pressure. The remaining fingers contact each other lightly as a stabilizing "rest" during the bending procedure.

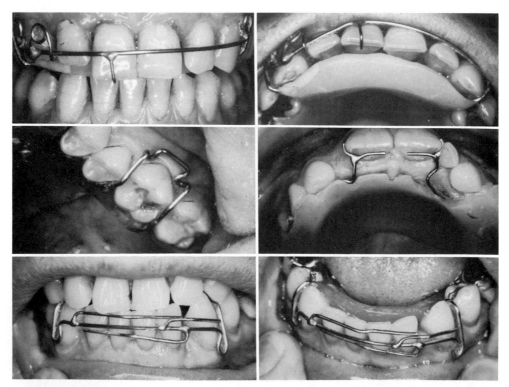

Figure 16–20.   Modifications of removable appliances. To prevent incisor elongation, where there is bone loss (top row), a metal spur with gentle pressure on incisal margin may depress the tooth slightly. Arrow clasps (middle row, left) may be used instead of ball or circumferential clasps for improved retention. Finger springs from palatal acrylic (middle row, right) are often indicated for labial tooth movement. By carrying acrylic over posterior teeth, added retention is achieved. In the bottom row, three additional finger springs have been added to a labial wire of a lower removable appliance to provide greater selectivity of tooth movement than the labial wire alone gives. The acrylic must be cut away on lingual to permit any lingual movement of the teeth, however.

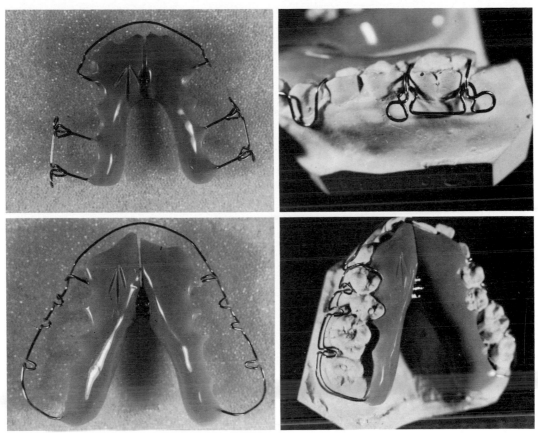

Figure 16–21 Variations of arrow type clasps. Labial wire may be separate (top) or continuous with posterior clasp wire. An expansion screw may be incorporated in the split palate, or a continuous coverage over the whole palate may be made. Generally speaking, the continuous clasp is more difficult to make and easier to distort. Ball clasps are almost as effective and may be adjusted to maintain retention. (Bottom) Acrylic is cut away from molars to permit buccal movement of lingually malposed premolars as expansion screw is opened. Thus, selective expansion is possible and desirable occasionally. (See Chap. 11, Removable Appliances.)

(Fig. 16–20). One should start first by forming a flat circular retention loop that extends well into the palate. The 0.032 or 0.036 inch wire is adapted to the palatal tissue and carried over the embrasure between the deciduous canine and first deciduous molar (between the canine and first premolar in an older patient) to the labial side. A sharp but well-rounded bend is made gingivally here to start the fabrication of the vertical loop. The loop should be 10 to 12 mm. long and should approximate but not contact the gingival tissue. Care must be taken not to carry the loop too high, lest it impinge on muscle attachments and irritate the mucosa. The mesial arm of the loop should make a horizontal bend at the canine-lateral incisor embrasure and should traverse the incisor segment in the middle third of the incisor crowns. The wire should contact the labial surface of each incisor but should not be adapted to the individual irregularities of the malocclusion. This means a relatively straight labial wire. At the opposite lateral incisor-deciduous canine embrasure, a vertical loop of the same size is formed and the remaining wire is adapted over the contact of the deciduous canine-first deciduous molar embrasure and carried on through to the lingual aspect to form the flat circular retention loop approximating the palate. The vertical loops should be approximately 5 mm. wide. This allows sufficient room for their constricting adjustments in the retracting process.

The neophyte often makes numerous small compensatory bends as he carries the wire across the labial surface. This is not only unnecessary but usually undesirable. After it has been determined that both the clasps and labial wire are properly adapted and passive, they may be affixed to the casts by the generous use of sticky wax on the labial and buccal surfaces. As with a bite plate, the acrylic portion may be fabricated by waxing, flasking, boiling out and curing under pressure; or it may be made directly by the use of endo-thermic techniques which permit the application of powder and monomer directly to the model surface after it has been painted with a separating medium (Fig. 16–18). The flasking and pressure-cure procedure is more desirable because there is less distortion and porosity and probably less likelihood of breakage. Great care must be exercised in the polishing of the acrylic. It is quite easy to catch the labial wire clasps on the polishing brush or wheel and distort them.

SECOND APPOINTMENT.   The removable Hawley type appliance is placed at the time of the second visit. Since this is usually a "mouthful" for the young patient, it is wise to allow a period of two to three weeks for him to become accustomed to wearing and speaking with the appliance before a tooth-moving adjustment is made. It is also a good idea to prescribe the use of a denture adhesive powder for the first couple of days while the tissue adapts, the appli-ance settles and muscle control improves. The child is instructed to wear the appliance at all times except when eating and even then if possible. The proper oral hygiene is demonstrated and the patient is instructed in keeping the appliance itself clean. Since the appliance has a bad tase for a couple of days, caused by the free monomer, it is a good practice to have the patient soak the appliance in a sweet-tasting mouth wash when it is not in his mouth. It must be made quite clear that the appliance is not to be inserted or removed by touch-ing the labial wire. After the first couple of days, insertion and removal are primarily under the control of the patient's tongue. If a plastic retainer case is furnished at the time that the appliance is given to the patient, there will be less likelihood of breakage or loss when it is removed at meal time.

THIRD APPOINTMENT.   At the third visit the acrylic is cut back 5 to 6 mm. from the lingual surface of the maxillary incisors (Fig. 16–22). This step is impor-tant, since the tissue tends to pile up and becomes quite sore if sufficient acrylic is not removed. Hypertrophy of tissue also interferes with lingual tooth move-ment. The 5 mm. minimum distance should be maintained between the plastic and the lingual surfaces of the incisors during treatment. At the third visit the vertical loops are closed slightly by pinching the vertical arms together with No. 139 pliers or office pliers. Check the vertical position of the labial wire after constricting the vertical loops. Constant wear, or the routine adjustments, may change the height of the labial wire unfavorably. If too much of an adjustment is made, the posterior end of the retainer will drop down into the floor of the mouth. This self-limiting feature prevents the use of excessive force.

FOLLOW-UP APPOINTMENTS.   Subsequent adjustment appointments should be at 3- or 4-week intervals. As the maxillary incisors are retracted, the spaces between them close. If a heavy, fibrous frenum is present, it may be necessary to excise the lingual and interdental attachment. This should be done, however, as the incisors themselves approximate each other. In this manner the healing and scar tissue contraction tends to bring the incisors together. If the frenum is removed prior to the closure of the diastema, the scar tissue may serve as a barrier.

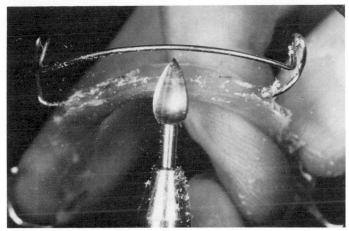

Figure 16–22   Trimming the acrylic away from the lingual aspect of the incisors with a pear-shaped vulcanite type bur.

As the incisors move lingually under the influence of the retracting labial wire of the removable appliance, the patient finds it easier to bring the lips together without conscious effort (Fig. 16–23). In the terminal phase of treatment, the perverting forces of the perioral musculature are no longer actively forcing the maxillary incisors labially. Indeed, normal function assists the orthodontic appliance in the retraction process.

Not only may abnormal lip and tongue habits be eliminated by the retraction of the maxillary incisors, but finger habits that are often associated with the protruding and spaced incisors may also disappear. There is less sensory

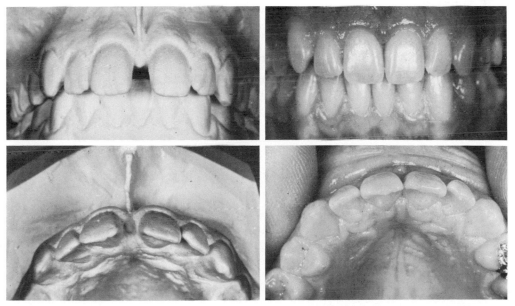

Figure 16–23   Diastema and protrusion in 12-year-old girl (left), corrected in 4 months with palatal removable appliance. Appliance is then worn as a retainer for an additional 6 to 12 months.

satisfaction gained from placing the finger in the mouth because the hard palate is covered with the acrylic. In many instances the removable appliance serves as a substitute for the finger during the waking hours. The tongue constantly works the appliance up and down in the mouth and this activity seems to provide the kinesthetic neuromuscular release that the patient previously obtained from the finger habit. This is not always desirable, but preferable to a confirmed finger-sucking habit.

Future orthodontic therapy may very likely be necessary in all cases of mixed dentition, such as the examples just described. Both the dentist and the parent should understand this. As with any type of medical or orthopedic therapy, a "one shot" assault on the problem may not be completely successful. Success is no more automatic and permanent in dentistry than in medicine.

Diastemas and protruding incisors are both esthetic disabilities and dental health hazards in adults. They may likewise be a serious psychological handicap. Patients with problems similar to those illustrated in Figures 16–24 to

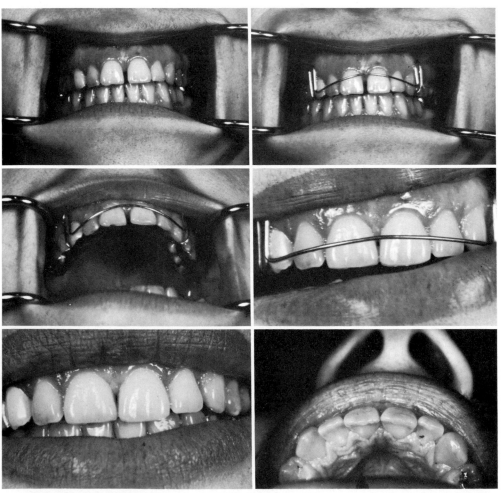

Figure 16–24 Diastema present, marring an otherwise normal occlusion for an 18-year-old girl. Entire removable appliance management was under control of a dental student. Therapy took 12 weeks. Appliance was then worn as a retainer at night for 6 months.

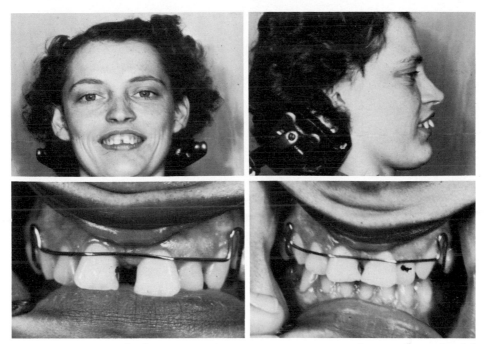

Figure 16-25 Wide diastema and incisor protrusion provide an esthetic disability that may be largely eliminated by a removable palatal appliance. Because of the partial tipping of the maxillary central incisors during the diastema closure, incisal leveling is indicated. Indefinite night-time wear of the appliance as a retainer is required.

16–26 frequently request the removal of disfiguring incisor teeth and replacement with dentures. Since teeth can be moved in adults, as well as in children, much can be done to cause an esthetic improvement and increase the longevity of the patient's own teeth – particularly if such limited orthodontic procedures are accomplished in conjunction with conservative periodontal therapy. The price that the patient has to pay is usually the indefinite wearing of the appliance as a retainer at night. Again, the concept of a "dental crutch" should not disturb a patient after the reason for its use is explained any more than an "eye crutch" (eyeglasses) should.

STRIPPING INCISORS

Occasionally there is a slight lack of arch length in the maxillary anterior segment, causing the arch to "buckle" and making an incisor move labially. The lip may get partially under this protruding tooth and increase its protrusion beyond the line of occlusion, creating an unsightly appearance. If the arch length deficiency is mild and if the problem is caught in its incipiency, judicious stripping of the contacts with a lightning strip in conjunction with the wearing of a Hawley type appliance may retract the offending tooth partly or completely, depending on the problem, the shape of the teeth, etc. (Fig. 16–27).

Although the greatest amount of the stripping is confined to the malposed tooth and the contiguous teeth, it is often necessary to strip the contacts of all four incisors to gain sufficient room to achieve any appreciable retraction. Such a procedure usually requires a series of a half dozen or so appointments, stripping a bit more each time and constricting the labial bow of the palatal appliance.

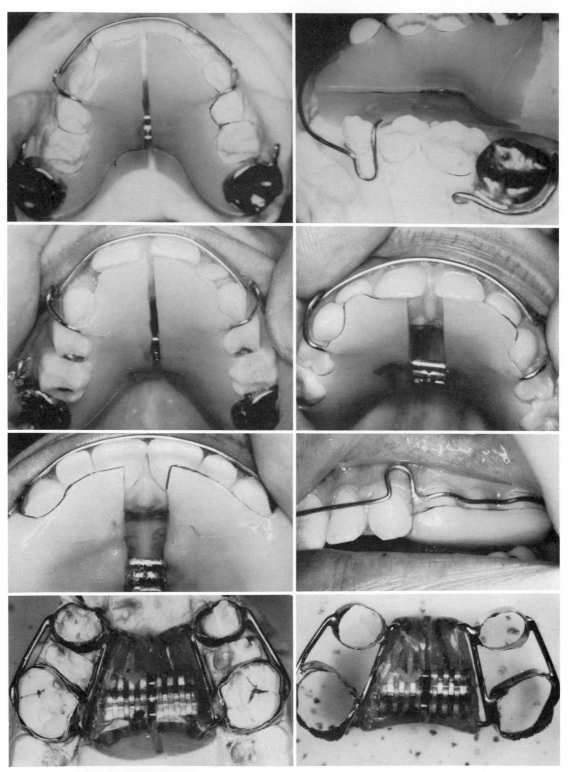

Figure 16–26 Palatal expansion appliances. Jackscrew provides bilateral expansion force. Full coverage metal crowns with buccal lugs to hold molar circumferential clasps enhance retention (top row and second row, left). Note amount of expansion that may be achieved by periodic opening of center jackscrew (second row, right and third row, left). Acrylic may be carried over occlusal for removable appliance (third row) to increase effectiveness and retention. Or bands may be made and cemented to buccal segment of teeth (bottom row). Removable appliances are for slow expansion; cemented appliance for rapid palatal expansion.

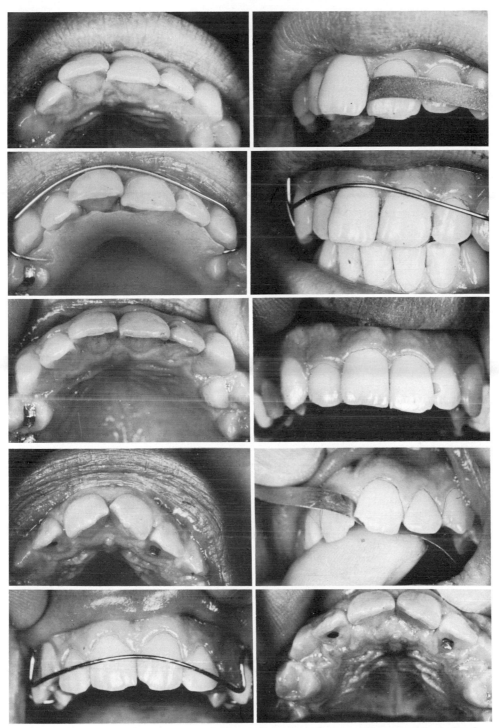

Figure 16–27 Stripping procedure combined with use of removable palatal appliance. In Case 1 (top 6 views), upper right central incisor is moved lingually as labially malposed tooth and contiguous contact points are stripped. In Case 2 (bottom 4 views), both central incisors are rotated back into normal arch form by stripping and constricting labial wire on removable appliance. Six to ten visits are usually required to achieve the desired results. Interval between adjustments should be approximately 4 weeks.

Grinding of the incisal margins of the opposing incisors is usually necessary to remove occlusal interference to the retraction. After optimal alignment has been achieved, the palatal appliance is worn at night as a retainer. Wearing time is reduced gradually as the relapse tendency diminishes. It is better to be *conservative* with a stripping procedure and accept a partial correction, than to remove too much tooth material and either expose the dentin, make the contact points broad surfaces that are more susceptible to caries or change the shape of the teeth so much that they look unnatural.

RETRACTING APPLIANCE WITH BITE PLATE

In some cases the maxillary incisors cannot be moved very far lingually before the cinguli of these teeth contact the incisal margins of the mandibular teeth. As the maxillary incisors are tipped lingually by the removable appliance, they tend to elongate, also increasing the overbite. If a bite plate is incorporated with the Hawley type appliance, further retraction can be accomplished in conjunction with eruption of posterior teeth, maintaining a normal overbite. Overbite correction is unpredictable both as to amount and time. Usually the combined problem requires considerably more time than mere space closure alone. The dentist must be careful not to retract the maxillary incisors too rapidly or ahead of eruption of the posterior teeth. Overly rapid retraction causes premature contact and a jiggling of the maxillary incisors, increased mobility and a greater sensory response. In some instances a functional mandibular retrusion is created. Eruption should be gained first in order to reduce the overbite, and then

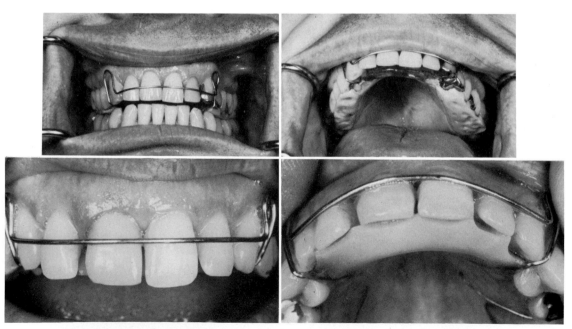

Figure 16-28 For certain tooth movements, it is advantageous to "block open the bite" by carrying the acrylic over the occlusal surface. This is done most frequently in cross-bite conditions, but it also is indicated in some temporomandibular joint disturbances. Acrylic is cut away from last tooth to allow it to erupt, and each tooth anterior to this is progressively exposed, when eruption is desired. Then anterior teeth may be retracted, by cutting away acrylic on lingual of these teeth, and constricting vertical loops on the labial bow. Note that acrylic also contacts lower incisors, to prevent their overerupting.

the incisor retraction should be attempted. Some lower incisor leveling may be required, on both an esthetic and a functional basis. When a bite plate is added to the Hawley type removable appliance, it is necessary to cut back on the acrylic directly behind the maxillary incisors at each adjustment. If there is not a minimum of 3 to 4 mm. clearance between the teeth and the acrylic, an adverse soft tissue response may occur.

An alternate means of gaining eruption of posterior teeth while retracting incisors is to carry the acrylic over the occlusal surfaces of the posterior teeth to block open the "bite." The occlusal portion is trimmed away for the last tooth first, to allow it to erupt; then the next tooth forward, and so forth, until a new occlusal level has been established for the entire buccal segment. Incisors may be retracted gradually during this process (Fig. 16–28).

MODIFICATIONS OF THE BASIC HAWLEY APPLIANCE

It has been shown that the basic palatal removable appliance with molar clasps and a labial bow, with or without a bite plate, is a versatile orthodontic adjunct that can be used at all ages. But the basic design can be modified to make the removable appliance much more useful. The simplest modification is to augment the labial wire with hooks for elastics (Fig. 16–29), or actually substitute hooks for elastics in place of the labial bow to retract maxillary incisors (Fig. 16–30). Elastics are very effective and cut down the number of observation visits, since the patient merely changes elastics to renew the desired tension on the teeth being moved. Greater care must be taken to prevent the "piling up" of tissue lingual to the maxillary incisors, however. This can be done by keeping the acrylic cut away, by interrupting the use of elastics, or by actual excision of excessive tissue.

Wide experience by European orthodontists has shown that removable appliances can be adapted to do much more than tip incisors lingually to close spaces.[17] (See Removable Appliances in Chap. 11.) Where there is congenital absence of maxillary lateral incisors, a tooth size discrepancy such as a peg lateral, or a missing incisor with drifting of contiguous teeth, auxiliary springs or loop springs may be added to the labial wire to assist in tooth alignment and space consolidation (Figs. 16–31 to 16–37). The added appurtenances give greater control of individual teeth but also are more difficult to manipulate and may cause untoward results. Used carefully, and with a little ingenuity, fixed orthodontic bands may be coupled with removable appliances to broaden the scope of service. Such combinations, if they are to be used by the dentist in general practice, however, must be simple and limited to such problems as cross-bite or occasional rotations (Fig. 16–37). It is recommended that the dentist seek orthodontic consultation *before* undertaking any procedure that seems at all complicated. This means consultation with the orthodontic specialist, not the so-called orthodontic laboratory.

Lower removable appliances are more difficult to tolerate by the patient, and are generally not as satisfactory for any appreciable movement. Tissue irritation is more likely, partly due to the fact that the total tissue borne area is considerably less. Lower incisors may be moved readily, however (Fig. 16–34). Where there is a traumatic end-to-end incisal relationship, mandibular incisors may be moved lingually, if there is adequate space. Indefinite retention may be necessary and the operator should make sure that incisor spacing is not a manifestation of a tongue thrust or tongue posture problem (Fig. 16–38).

(*Text continued on page 805*)

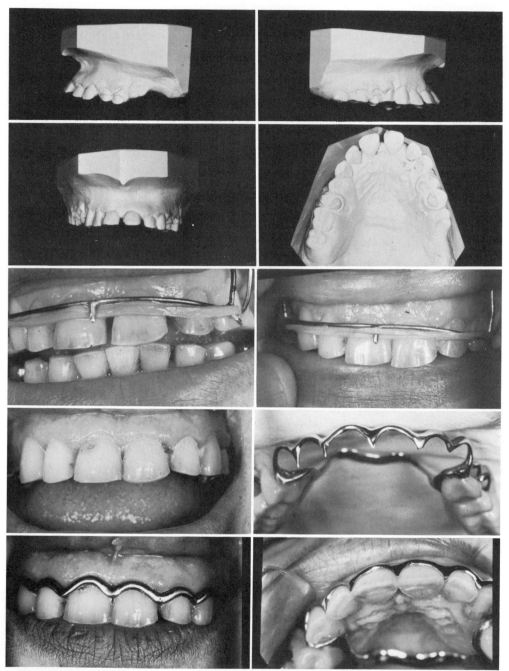

Figure 16–29   Limited adult orthodontics with palatal removable appliance. Dental radiographs showed bone loss and deep pockets around maxillary incisors. Patient complained of incisors "fanning out." Conventional Hawley type appliance modified with elastic hooks retracted incisors. Scaling, packs and rigorous massage restored tissue integrity. Partial denture incorporates a labial-gingival scallop to serve as a passive stabilizing adjunct. Continued conservative periodontal care is still required, but the patient has her own teeth and a new personality.

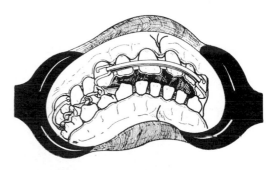

Figure 16–30 Modified removable palatal appliance with elastic hooks substituted for labial bow to retract maxillary incisors.

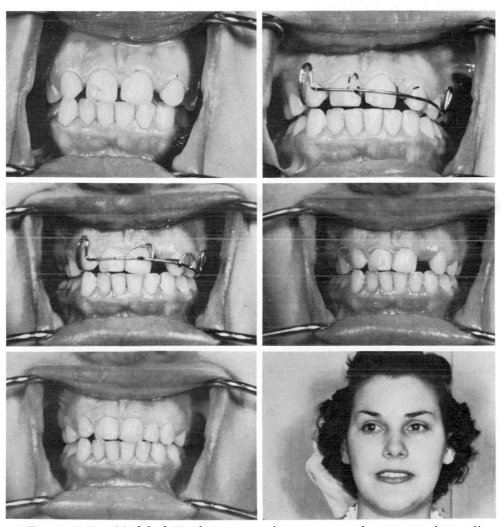

Figure 16–31 Modified Hawley type appliance was used to cope with maxillary incisor spacing as a result of congenital absence of the lateral incisors. Since there was not enough room to replace two teeth and since the midline deviated to the left, it was decided to move the central incisors to the right and close existing spaces on the right side. This was done with a loop spring soldered to the labial arch, with the help of finger springs from the lingual side. After the right central incisor had been moved into contact with the canine, the loop spring was moved along the labial wire to move the left central incisor into contact and to correct the midline. The problem of restoration was then simple but was made possible only through limited orthodontic procedures (lower views.)

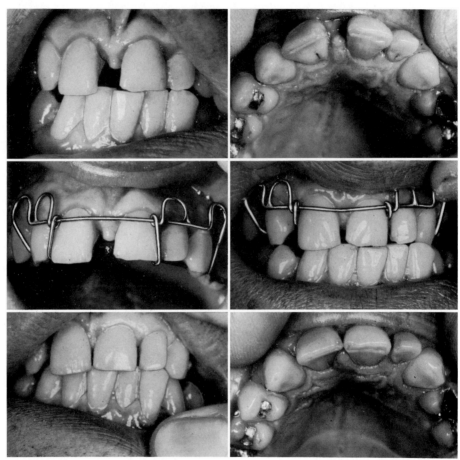

Figure 16–32 Diastema closure for a 45-year-old man. Conventional Hawley palatal appliance with vertical loop finger springs. Distal ends of loops are soldered; mesial ends wrapped around and extended incisally to engage distal surfaces of central incisors. Vertical loops are opened gradually to move central incisors together. With excessive overjet, acrylic is cut away on lingual side and the labial wire is constricted by pinching the labial bow vertical loops closer together. There is often a tendency for the interdental papilla lingual to the incisors to become inflamed, and conservative medication is necessary. After space closure, the appliance is worn indefinitely at night as a retainer.

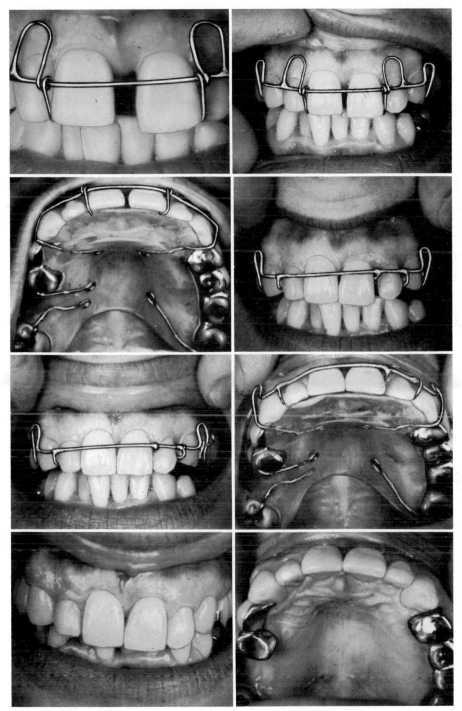

Figure 16–33 Diastema closure and retraction with vertical spring loops, finger springs and closing of labial base wire vertical loops. The auxiliary springs were first opened to move central incisors together (top row). Lateral incisors were then moved mesially with short spurs adjusted to bear on distal surface of lateral incisors. Spurs then act as retaining elements, while the base labial bow itself is retracted by pinching up vertical loops. Acrylic must be cut away on lingual aspect as incisors are retracted, but is not cut, except to free incisors for mesial movement as they are moved together by the auxiliary loop springs.

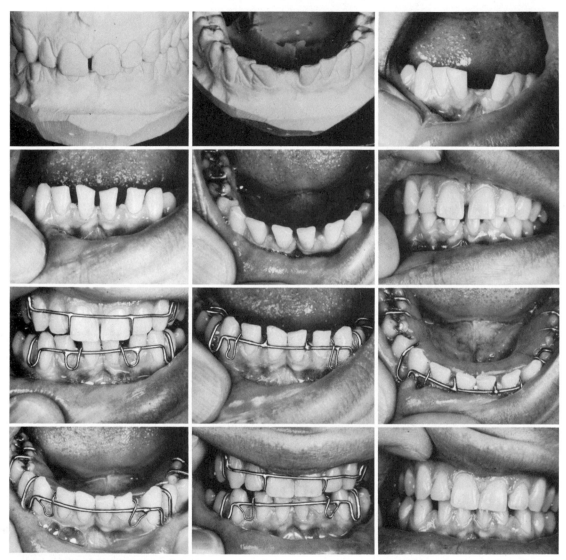

Figure 16–34   Upper and lower incisor diastemas. Lower incisor diastema was closed partly by elastics (second row), and then finger springs on the labial wire of the removable appliances moved the central incisors together. Spurs were placed to hold lower incisors (third row), and the vertical loop springs moved distally to move lateral incisors mesially. Patient continues to wear maxillary bite plate appliance to help eliminate overbite. Both appliances serve to hold diastema correction.

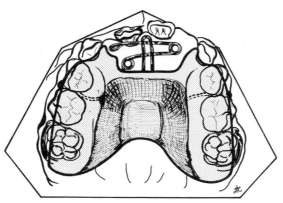

Figure 16–35 Modified removable palatal appliance to move central incisor labially. Finger spring is deeply anchored in acrylic and recurved twice by forming helical coil loops before it engages the malposed central incisor. In this manner, a light but continuous force is exerted on the tooth. A "spring guard" protects the spring from functional stress and prevents the spring from creeping up toward the incisal. Added retention is given to the palatal portion with circumferential clasps on the first permanent molars and by carrying the acrylic up over the occlusal. Anterior cross-bite may be corrected with this type of appliance. (See Chap. 17.)

Posterior teeth as well as anterior teeth may be moved with the removable appliance in the maxilla and mandible. Posterior tooth movement usually involves opening spaces rather than closing them. Most frequently, as the result of premature loss, teeth have drifted into edentulous spaces and must be moved back to their original position to allow eruption of the permanent teeth. Modified clasps or auxiliary springs can achieve the desired result, if the space closure is not a symptom of a general malocclusion and if the problem has not gone on so long that the eruption of permanent teeth on either side has also been abnormal. In the latter case complete orthodontic procedures are usually necessary, and the patient should be referred to a specialist. If these problems are recognized in time, many patients can be saved from having to undergo extensive fixed appliance mechanotherapy (Figs. 16–39 to 16–44). A word of caution about moving posterior teeth—occlusion is a more potent factor in these cases. The inclined plane action may be working at cross purposes to the orthodontic adjustment. The addition of a bite plate to the removable appliance may be beneficial. Also, judicious equilibration during therapy may make tooth movement easier.

Posterior occlusion may be improved considerably in the mixed dentition in properly selected cases, for example, using an activator in Class II, Division 1 problems (Fig. 16–45). The activator, or monobloc, and the propulsor, which work in similar ways, make use of muscle forces to retract the maxillary anterior teeth, eliminate functional retrusions and take advantage of whatever mandibular horizontal growth occurs during treatment.[6] Claims of growth stimulation remain to be proven, however. Since there is a distinct likelihood of the need for further treatment in permanent dentition, such treatment is most successful under the guidance of a trained specialist. (See Removable Appliances in Chap. 11.)

Another type of removable appliance that doubles as a retainer and mouthguard for contact sports is the polyethylene soft plastic positioner-like appliance. Fabricated from thermal sensitive blanks under pressure, these appliances have the advantage of no wirework to distort, and they are considerably less

(*Text continued on page 811*)

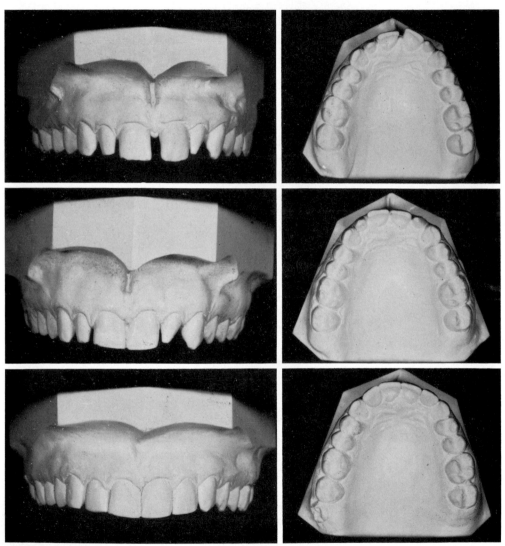

Figure 16–36   Diastema associated with "peg" lateral incisors. Central incisors are moved together with removable palatal appliance and jacket crowns are then made to restore proper size of lateral incisors and to act as retainers to keep central diastema closed.

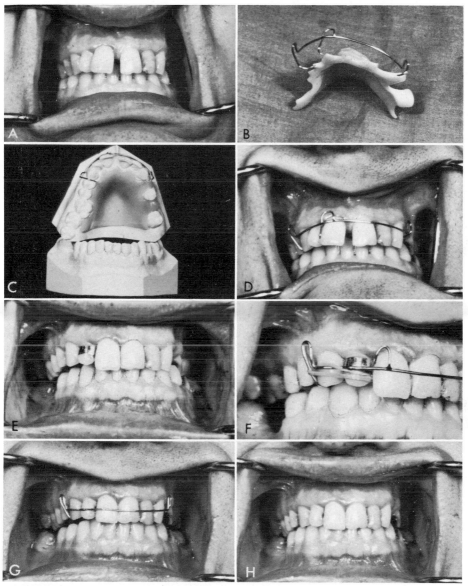

Figure 16–37 Advanced periodontal problem, with upper right central incisor excessively mobile and with pockets on the lingual side. Before replacing lost teeth, a modified palatal appliance was placed to move the malposed central incisor mesially and to retract it (A, B, C and D). A vertical loop finger spring assisted in the diastema closure. Since the right lateral incisor was still rotated, a band with a lingual spur was placed (E), and a small elastic worn from the band to the vertical loop of the labial bow to rotate the mesial angle labially (F). After correction, vertical loop finger spring was removed and endothermic acrylic added on lingual side of upper incisors to help stabilize new positions. Continued periodontal therapy is indicated.

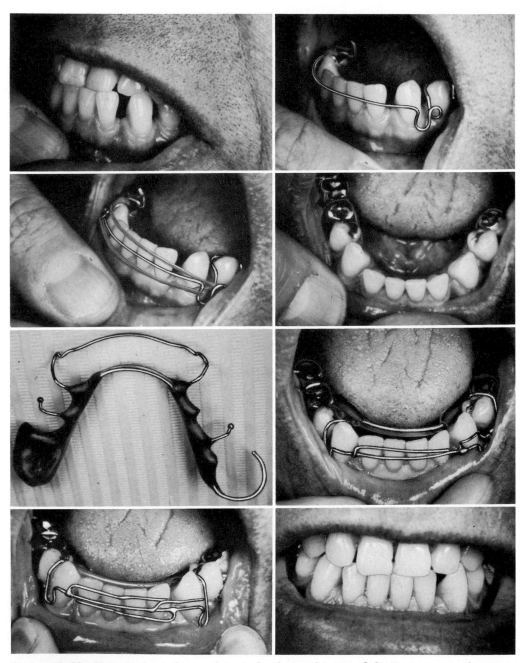

Figure 16–38 Traumatic end-to-end incisal relationship in adult. Posterior teeth are missing and there is spacing in the lower arch. A removable appliance, utilizing the edentulous area and ball clasps for retention, was used. Note the metal lingual bar behind the lower incisors. This reduces tissue irritation, since it is well away from the gingiva, is strong enough with minimum bulk and also serves to hold the tongue at least partially away during the retraction process. A metal bar behind the mandibular incisors is usually preferable to a full acrylic appliance. Elastics may be used in conjunction with wire assemblage (second row, left). Auxiliary finger springs may be soldered on labial wire for more detailed tooth movement (bottom row, left). Occlusal equilibration is usually necessary in the terminal phase of therapy.

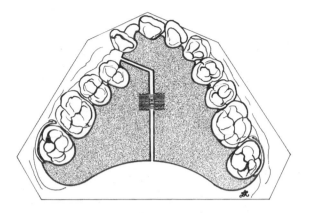

Figure 16–39 Split palate removable appliance used in cleft palate cases. Jackscrew type expansion screw is gradually opened up to spread buccal segments.

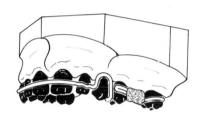

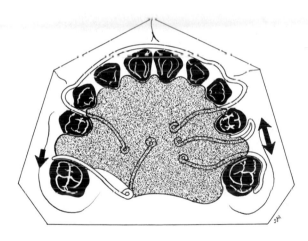

Figure 16 40 Modified removable palatal appliance, used to move first molars distally, to open space in upper left second premolar region by moving first premolar mesially and to correct incisor rotations. Acrylic is incorporated into edentulous areas to facilitate retention and function. It also prevents overeruption of opposing tooth.

Figure 16–41 Correct (A) and incorrect (B) methods of winding helical coil finger spring for use in removable palatal appliance. To activate spring, helical coil should always be closed—never opened—for optimal efficiency.

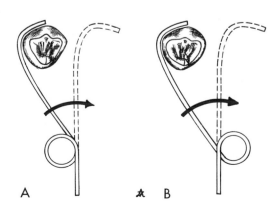

A   B

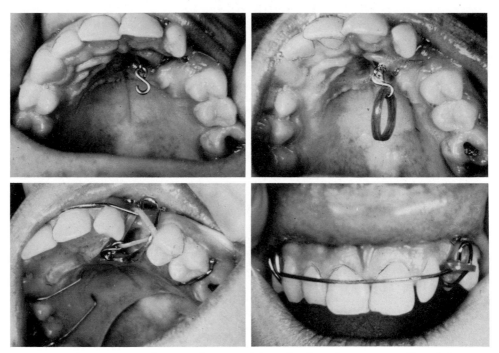

Figure 16–42 Versatile use of removable palatal appliance. Maxillary left canine is uncovered for a 14-year-old girl. There is adequate space in the arch. (Top) A hook is cemented on the exposed canine crown, and an elastic is attached. (Bottom) A plain Hawley type appliance is worn, with a cut-out portion for the impacted canine. The elastic is stretched from the hook to the labial bow and loop of the appliance. As the canine moves toward its correct position, a spur may be soldered on the labial bow loop to maintain tension on the elastic and to ensure proper direction of pull. Elastic is changed every day by the patient.

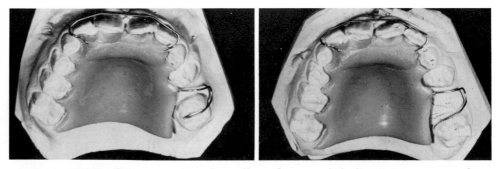

Figure 16–43 Premature loss has allowed upper left first permanent molar to drift mesially. The first molar was moved distally half its width, as shown by the placement of the removable appliance on the original and finished casts with the same adjustment in the spring.

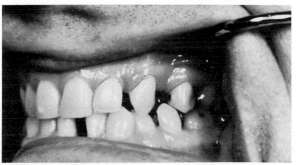

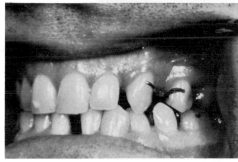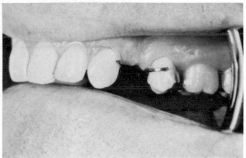

Figure 16–44 Loss of first premolar has allowed canine and second premolar to drift into edentulous area. A removable palatal appliance with finger springs in the space of the missing tooth can restore continuity of the arch, permitting the placement of a proper fixed bridge.

likely to be broken. As with the tooth positioner, minor tooth movement may be accomplished. The technique of re-setting teeth on the plaster model and fabricating is described in Figure 16–46. Although the illustration shows a maxillary appliance, minor tooth movements may also be accomplished in similar fashion for the mandibular arch. To serve as a retainer for both arches, a correlator has been developed (Fig. 16–47). This reduces the need for a separate lower retainer, as impressions of the cusps of the mandibular teeth are made in the maxillary appliance. The patient is required to bite into the appliance for a prescribed amount of time each day and to wear the modified orthobite appliance at night, as with any conventional retainer.

THE REMOVABLE HAWLEY APPLIANCE—THE DENTAL CRUTCH

Although the removable Hawley type appliance has shown itself to be a valuable adjunct in adult periodontal care and in achieving orthodontic corrections of a primarily esthetic nature, the results obtained are usually unstable. Semipermanent retention seems to be the order of the day. Hence the concept of the Hawley type appliance as being a "dental crutch." This same philosophy of use has been described for the bite plate, which is really nothing more than a modified Hawley appliance.

One of the fundamental concepts of periodontal therapy is to distribute stress equally to as many teeth as possible. Stress should be absorbed in a vertical manner or through the long axes of the teeth.[7] As bone is lost around the teeth, lateral stresses tend to jiggle the teeth unduly. This in turn accelerates the destructive processes and the teeth begin to shift. The maxillary incisors are

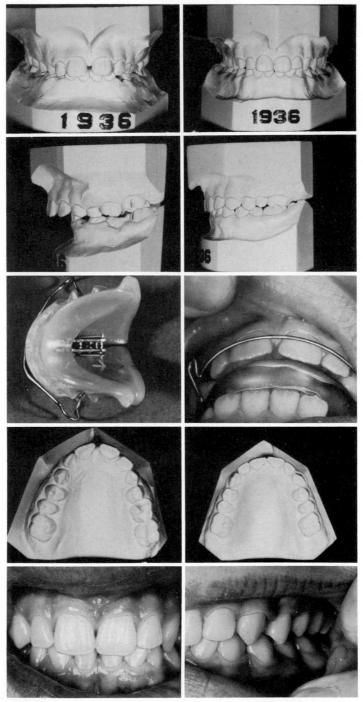

Figure 16–45 Correction of a Class II, Division 1 malocclusion with monobloc or activator therapy. Casts in two top rows show before (left) and after (right) treatment. (Third row) Appliance has split palate, jackscrew in center, labial wire and indentations of lower incisors to hold mandible forward. Retracting force of muscles is transmitted to maxillary arch. Together with growth and development, and elimination of any functional retrusion, proper interdigitation and elimination of excessive overjet are achieved. Guidance was under an orthodontist, who could step in at any time with fixed appliances, as indicated in most similar problems. (Fourth row) Occlusal views before and after show change in arch configuration. (Bottom row) Patient is shown one year after appliance removal.

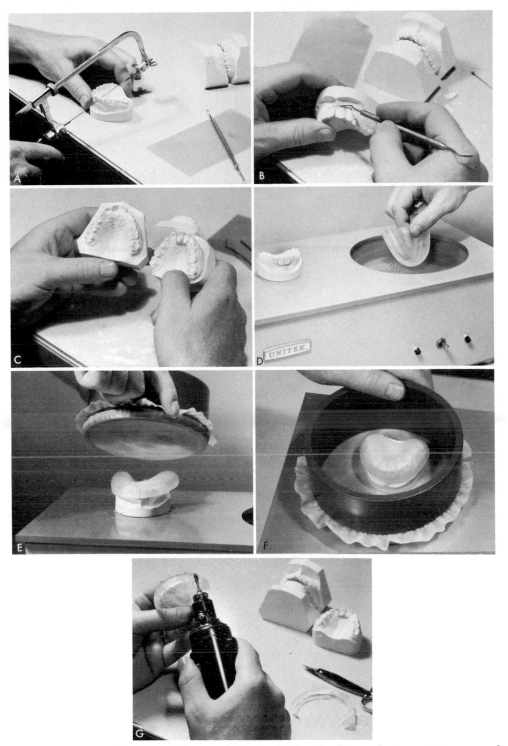

Figure 16–46 Crane orthobite technique. A, The duplicate plaster cast is prepared by cutting off teeth to be reset in wax, before fabricating the elastoplastic appliance. B, The cut off teeth are waxed in their new positions. C, The reset model is compared with the original. Check with opposing model, also. D, The thermal sensitive orthobite form is heated in thermostatically controlled water bath. E, The model is placed over vacuum hole, covered by softened thermoplastic blank and then diaphragm is placed on top. F, Vacuum is formed under elastoplastic form to adapt it to plaster model. Finger pressure may be used to assist, where needed. G, Periphery and palatal extension are trimmed, finished and polished. (Courtesy Unitek Corp.)

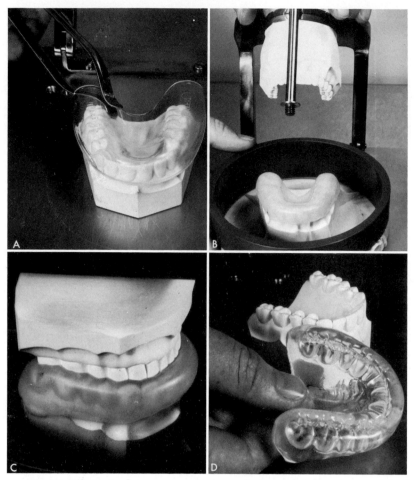

Figure 16–47   Klein-Anderson correlator technique for forming vinyl plastic retainers. A wax bite is used to relate the upper and lower casts on the correlator. The upper cast is keyed to the top plate of the Orthovac unit; then the lower cast is attached to the plate on the upper arm of the articulator by adding plaster. A, The vinyl plastic blank is softened as shown in the previous figure and placed on the maxillary cast. B, The vacuum forming of the upper cast detail is done and the plaster-mounted lower cast is being brought into position for making an impression of occlusal and incisal detail in the still soft vinyl plastic. C shows the lower cast locked into position with the upper and lower cast detail now impressed in the vinyl plastic. D, The plastic has been cooled, trimmed and polished, and is now ready for wear. A prescribed period of exercise by biting into the vinyl plastic retainer assures maintenance of interarch integrity. (Courtesy Unitek Corp.)

particularly susceptible to positional change. A progressive "fanning out" occurs along with an increase in the procumbency of the mandibular incisors and the tendency toward an excessive overbite. In some cases, as granulation tissue forms in the pockets, there is a pathologic "migration" of the incisors. The Hawley removable appliance, with or without the addition of a bite plate, is often able to stop the progressive destruction of the investing tissues and the ultimate loss of the teeth. The labial wire splints the maxillary incisors and greatly reduces the jiggling and traumatic effects of lateral stresses. The reward is a periodontal membrane reduced in thickness, a decelerated rate of bone loss and a return of the health of the gingival tissues. Conservative periodontal therapy is instituted along with the wearing of the removable appliance.

This means a thorough scaling, polishing of the root surfaces, elimination of pockets, and a stark discipline of gingival massage and home care.

If the maxillary incisors have fanned out and no longer are in contact with with the mandibular incisors during habitual occlusion, they may be retracted to a more favorable inclination and the spaces may be closed (Fig. 16–37). The occlusal vertical dimension need not be opened at all in some cases to achieve this objective. In many cases, however, only a partial retraction can be obtained before the maxillary incisors are jammed against the incisal margins of the opposing mandibular teeth. A careful analysis of the amount of interocclusal clearance must then be made. The postural resting position vertical dimension is determined, as well as the habitual occlusal vertical dimension, and the difference between these two dimensions is precisely measured. If it is excessive (and such is often the case in this problem), then it is possible to incorporate a bite plate with the removable Hawley type appliance. Eruption of posterior teeth in adults is usually slow, but over a period of time it does occur. If the teeth and investing tissues are healthy, the gingival margin follows the teeth as they erupt. In other words, there is no increase in the length of the clinical crown.

As the posterior teeth erupt, the maxillary incisors may be retracted still further into better axial inclination and remaining spaces may be closed. These changes will not come overnight. The dentist must remember that the malocclusion was also a long time in the making, and reversal of the process cannot be expected to lead to a leap back to normalcy.[8] If the dentist continues his conservative periodontal guidance and if the patient follows the home care routine, there should be continued improvement in the health of the investing tissues. It is not unreasonable to expect complete cessation of bone loss, and some dentists claim that there is actual restoration of part of the lost alveolar crest in selected cases. Periodic occlusal equilibration is also indicated during this extended program. This cannot be stressed too strongly. Appliance wear alone is inadequate and may cause actual harm. Judicious removal of prematurities and distribution of functional stresses are recommended, whether an appliance is worn or not. It is frequently necessary to add new acrylic to the bite plate portion of the appliance, since acrylic is softer than the teeth and wears down readily under the onslaught of occlusion. Little hope should be given to the patient that he can discontinue the use of the removable appliance. Indefinite nocturnal wear is a likely prospect. After the optimal result has been achieved, however, some dentists prefer to substitute a completely passive retaining appliance. A labial bar, following the gingival scalloping, is cast in gold or in a chrome-cobalt alloy, and the ends are brought through the lateral incisor canine or the canine-first bicuspid embrasure to the lingual surface to anchor in the acrylic palatal portion (Fig. 16–13). Cast clasps are usually made for the first molar teeth, if present. In an advanced problem the appliance is worn all the time. If the situation is caught early enough and is completely under control, the patient should get by with wearing the appliance just at night (Fig. 16–29).

LIGATING TEETH IN CONJUNCTION WITH PERIODONTAL THERAPY

While the removable appliance can be used to splint teeth during periodontal therapy, it must be remembered that it is under the control of the

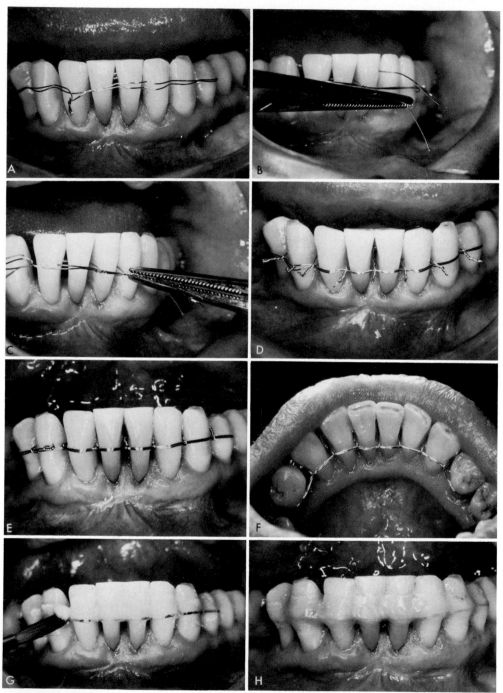

Figure 16–48 Construction of temporary wire ligature splint. A, Horizontal loop loosely aligned in position incisal to the cingula. B, Interdental loops are inserted. C, Interdental loops tightened. D, All the interdental loops and the horizontal loops are tightened. E, Splint in position with interdental loops bent inward to avoid tissue irritation. F, Lingual view showing position of splint in relation to cingula. G, Acrylic is brushed onto the wire to stabilize splint, to minimize food accumulation and protect the tissues from irritation. H, Acrylic polished. *Notice that the acrylic tapers toward the incisal edges and does not encroach upon the gingival embrasure.* (Glickman, I.: Clinical Periodontology. Philadelphia, W. B. Saunders Co., 1972.)

patient. Lack of cooperation means failure, no matter how strenuous the efforts of the dentist. For this reason some dentists prefer the use of a fixed ligating technique that does not depend on patient cooperation to the degree that the removable appliance does (Fig. 16–48). As with the removable appliance, the primary aim is to stabilize the teeth and prevent excessive jiggling and traumatic deterioration of the investing tissues.

USE OF LIGATURES ALONE

The simplest ligation procedure requires only an ample supply of soft stainless-steel ligature wire.[9] The greatest stability seems to come from a wire approximately 0.012 inch in diameter. It is most frequently used for the maxillary and mandibular incisors. One end of the ligature wire is passed from the labial to the lingual surface through the canine-first bicuspid or canine-lateral incisor embrasure. It is brought back across the lingual and through the next embrasure to the mesial and then to the labial surface. The other free end of the ligature wire that has remained on the labial surface is brought across the labial surface of the canine (or lateral incisor), and a single twist is made with the wire brought through from the lingual surface to pull the wire tightly against the labial, lingual and proximal surfaces of the tooth. The labial wire is then passed through the same embrasure and the twist is pulled into the interproximal area to prevent any irritation of the lip. The same procedure is repeated for each tooth to be included in the ligation process. It is not advisable to include more than six teeth on one strand of wire. As the lingual wire is brought through the embrasure to the labial surface for the last tooth, it is twisted up tightly with the labial wire for six or more turns. Ordinary office pliers may be used. Excess ligature wire is cut off with a crown-and-collar-shears, leaving a quarter inch twisted pigtail. The pigtail is then tucked carefully into the interproximal space.

Some ligation techniques involve the use of brass wire. This works equally well, but because it is a softer wire it tends to hold debris more readily. Since one of the greatest drawbacks of the ligation technique is the tendency for the wire to trap debris and cause decalcification or caries, anything that can be done to reduce this problem is recommended.[10] Rigorous oral hygiene is a "must," or the wire should be removed immediately. In any event, a new wire should be placed every four to six weeks. The dentist must be careful that the wire does not impinge on the gingival tissue because this will become an irritant for the patient. Rotations may be accentuated by ligating, and this tendency should be checked carefully. In advanced cases of bone loss, ligation may cause exfoliation of incisors as the wire creeps to the narrower root portion. It is obviously contraindicated in such cases.[12] Periodontal consultation is recommended, in any event.

LIGATION TO STABILIZING ARCH

An alternate but perhaps more satisfactory approach for the patient with advanced periodontal involvement is the use of the stabilizing arch. Orthodontic bands are made for the first molar teeth. (See Chap. 17 for details of fabrication.) Horizontal buccal tubes are soldered on the first molar bands to receive a 0.020 inch stainless arch wire. A circular loop or vertical loop is bent into the arch wire just mesial to the anterior ends of the buccal tubes. The arch wire is then inserted and the loops are tied back against the buccal tubes with stainless-steel ligature wire. Occlusion must be checked carefully to see that the opposing teeth do not impinge on the arch wire at any point if the appliance has been placed in the lower arch. The stabilizing arch should have point contact on the buccal surfaces and surface contact on the labial of the incisors. The teeth to be splinted are then ligated directly to the arch, using 0.012 stainless-steel ligature wire. Both wires are passed to the lingual of the first embrasure, one over and one under the arch wire. The two ends are carried across the lingual surface and through the next embrasure, one over and one under the arch wire. Each wire is carried around the arch wire and back into the same embrasure to the lingual. The two ends are carried across the lingual surface of the next tooth and through the embrasure in the same manner as just outlined. Because of the greater stability afforded by the arch wire, it is not necessary to incorporate all the teeth with one length of ligature wire.

If the six anterior teeth are to be splinted, it is usually better to use two ligature wires. The ends of the first ligature wire are twisted together on the labial surface at the midline embrasure and the pigtail tucked under the wire and between the teeth as previously described. The second ligature is passed around the arch wire and to the lingual surface at the same embrasure and brought through the central incisor-lateral incisor embrasure, lateral incisor-canine embrasure and canine-first premolar embrasure before being twisted over the arch wire on the buccal surface. The quarter inch pigtail is then tucked into the interproximal area. As with the plain ligature wire, the patient must keep his teeth scrupulously clean at all times. The diet should not include foods that are too rough for fear of distorting the arch wire. Care must be taken not to impinge on the gingival tissue and cause an irritation that will be magnified by the patient's home care routine. The ligature wires should be changed every six weeks, at which time it may be necessary to remove and reform the arch wire if the occlusion has caused a "bowing" in the buccal segments.

In no instance should ligation be considered as a semipermanent procedure. Although it works well during an intensive period of periodontal therapy, prolonged use may actually hinder progress and pose a constant threat of decalcification and caries.[13, 14] After the periodontal therapy is completed and the dentist feels further need for stabilization, he must turn to the removable Hawley type appliance, the cast labial bar appliance previously described or full mouth rehabilitation. If teeth are missing in the buccal segments, the cast labial bar may be incorporated on a partial denture.

REFERENCES

1. Mathews, J. R.: Maxillary bite plane application in Class I deciduous occlusion. Am. J. Orthodont., 45:721–737, 1959.
2. Mathews, J. R.: Functional considerations of the temporomandibular articulation and orthodontic implications. Angle Orthodont., 37:81–94, 1967.
3. King, A. T.: A simpler treatment of Class I with deep overbite. Int. J. Orthodont., 7:86–88, 1969.
4. Graber, T. M.: Overbite—the dentist's challenge. J.A.D.A., 79:1135–1145, 1969.
5. Posselt, U.: The Physiology of Occlusion and Rehabilitation. 2nd ed., Philadelphia, F. A. Davis Co., 1968.
6. Hotz, R.: Orthodontie in der Täglichen Praxis. 4th ed., Berne: Hans Huber, 1970.
7. Berliner, A.: Ligatures, Splints, Bite Planes, and Pyramids. Philadelphia, J. B. Lippincott Co., 1964.
8. Mayne, W. R.: Limitations in preventive orthodontics in Controversies in Dentistry, D.C.N.A., 15:919–937, 1971.
9. Glickman, I.: Clinical Periodontology. Philadelphia, W. B. Saunders Co., 1971.

10. Sassouni, V., and Forrest, E. J.: Orthodontics in Dental Practice. St. Louis, C. V. Mosby Co., 1971.
11. Fleming, J., and Prasad, A. R.: Periodontal status of the incisor teeth in normal and deep overbite cases. J. Indian. Orth. Soc., 1:14–22, 1969.
12. Rateitschak, K. H.: Orthodontics and periodontology. Int. Dent. J., 18:108–120, 1968.
13. Schmuth, G. P. F.: The importance of orthodontic therapy for prevention of periodontal diseases. Oest. Z. Stomat., 66:6–10, 1969.
14. Straub, W. J., and Peterson, L. N.: Combined periodontic and adult orthodontic therapy. Academy Rev., 6:90–92, 1958.
15. Cousins, A. J. P., Brown, W. A. B., and Harkness, E. M.: An investigation into the effect of the maxillary biteplate on the height of the lower incisor teeth. Dent. Pract., 20:107–111, 1969.
16. Greene, C. S., Laskin, D. M.: Splint therapy for the myofascial pain-dysfunction (MPD) syndrome: a comparative study. J.A.D.A., 84:624–628, 1972.
17. Adams, C. P.: Removable appliances yesterday and today. Am. J. Orthodont., 55:748–764, 1969.

chapter 17

LIMITED CORRECTIVE ORTHODONTICS: FIXED APPLIANCES

It is the author's opinion that fixed orthodontic appliances should usually be employed only by an orthodontic specialist. Yet even some of the simplest orthodontic problems demand tooth control beyond that conferred by removable appliances. It has been pointed out in the section dealing with the closure of anterior spaces, for example, that removable appliances work by retracting the maxillary incisors to a smaller arc. In a number of instances, the occlusion prevents complete space closure; or the crowns of the incisors tip toward each other, but the roots remain separated. The bodily movement of the incisor teeth that is so necessary to close some diastemas properly is not possible with removable appliances.

Where there is congenital absence of one or more teeth or loss of a tooth due to caries or an accident, fixed orthodontic appliances are almost always preferable because of the more precise control of the teeth and their axial inclination. Adjustments are more positive; there is less dependence on patient cooperation. Because of the inherent advantage of fixed over removable appliances for certain limited orthodontic problems, their use will be described for specific circumscribed conditions. At the same time, the warning is given to the dentist who has had no training in fixed appliance construction and manipulation that he may get into trouble and render a disservice to the patient. Hence this section is primarily for the dentist who has had some previous orthodontic training, or for the dentist who will undertake these techniques in conjunction with an orthodontist. Such "team" effort is to be recommended and should be encouraged by the orthodontic specialist, the pedodontist and the general dentist.

Although the description of techniques in this chapter is fairly detailed, it is not possible to impart adequate clinical judgment for their use. Only through actual experience under competent guidance may this all-important requirement be satisfied.

In this chapter, molar band fabrication and cementation, the orthodontic arch wire, attachment band fabrication and placement, anterior cross-bite correction and posterior cross-bite correction are discussed.

MOLAR BANDS

With a little experience the operator will find that he can fabricate bands quite satisfactorily directly in the mouth. If he thinks of each band as a possible food trap for cariogenic debris and if he demands of himself the same degree of performance in making a band that he attains in making a proximal inlay, it will not take him long to reach clinical proficiency. The band fitting must conform to the most exacting requisite of proximity of band and tooth in all areas. Do not depend on the cement for retention.

FABRICATION

Molar bands may be made either by the direct or indirect technique. The indirect technique of fabricating metal crowns and bands for habit appliances and space maintainers has already been described in Chapters 13 and 14. If the dentist has a good technician available, the indirect technique is quite satisfactory. Each band must be adapted and burnished directly on the tooth before cementing, however, because the indirect technique is seldom accurate enough to allow this on the stone model. If total time consumed in band fabrication is a major consideration and if the bands have to be made by the dentist himself anyway, the direct band-forming procedure is the answer, eliminating the time-consuming steps of impression-taking, pouring up, separating and trimming the model or die for each tooth. Preformed bands of all sizes are available from the major orthodontic supply houses (Fig. 17–3). The technique of their use is described in the brochures available with the purchase of these bands and in several specialty-oriented textbooks.[1,2] Initial unit cost of preformed bands is higher, though they undoubtedly make up for this in chair time saved for the operator after he has developed his technique of fitting preformed bands properly.

For the dentist who wishes to form bands directly, band material is available in rolls. Either precious metal or stainless-steel material may be used, depending on the preference of the operator, his previous training and the availability of a good welder, passivator and orthodontic blowpipe (Fig. 17–1). In addition to the No. 139 wire-bending pliers and the Bernard type wire-cutting pliers (Fig. 16–18), and any office pliers or clasp-forming pliers he may already have, the dentist would do well to obtain pliers similar to those illustrated in Figure 17–2. At the very least, he should have regular How pliers, universal type band-forming pliers and ligature-cutting pliers.

In the forming and fitting of all bands, the band material must pass through the proximal contacts readily. If either the band material or the preformed bands have to be forced past the contact points, the chances are good that it will not be possible to obtain a well-fitting band by working and contouring the band material past the contact point or contact surface bind (Fig. 17–3). Separating wires should be used, following the technique illustrated in Figures 14–6 to 14–9. The separating wires should be left in for about a week before removing. It is then quite easy to slip the proper thickness band material between the contacts. For the molar bands, 0.005 by 0.180 inch stainless-steel strip band material is easy to adapt and strong enough to withstand the stresses of occlusion. A strip of material approximately two and a half inches long is wrapped around the first molar tooth and drawn to the lingual side with a pair of office pliers (or band-forming pliers) (Fig. 17–4). With an amalgam plugger, one must carefully adapt the band material on the buccal surface, maintaining pressure from the

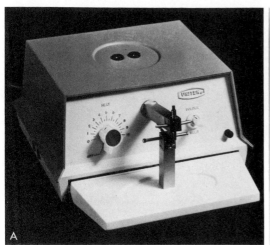
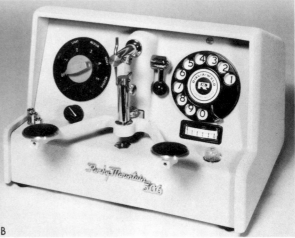
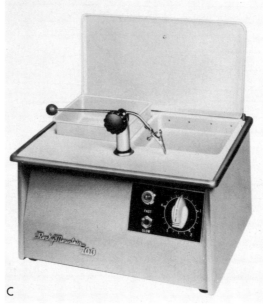

Figure 17–1   Welding, heat-treating and passivating equipment. Welders (A and B) are combined resistance and capacitor type. Passivator (C) is a combined heat-treating passivator and electric soldering unit. (A, courtesy Unitek Corp.; B and C, courtesy of Rocky Mountain Dental Products Co.)

lingual surface by pulling continuously on the office pliers. This works the excess material around to the lingual surface. The gingival tissue must cover the gingival peripheral margin of the band material. For most molars, 0.180 inch width band material is sufficient to extend just below the margin and yet requires little or no occlusal trimming at the mesial and distal marginal ridges.

After the buccal surface of the band has been thoroughly adapted and all the excess material has been worked to the lingual side, the amalgam plugger is placed firmly in the buccal groove to hold the band material in place and the band-forming or office pliers are placed with the beaks against the lingual band material surface. With considerable but controlled pressure, the beaks are moved slowly together, maintaining continuous pressure against the lingual surface. Holding the pliers with the beaks tightly together and pressed against

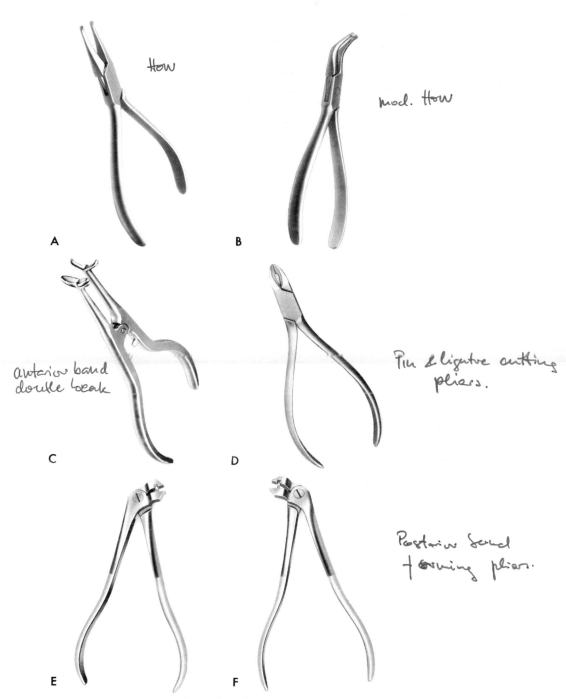

Figure 17–2   A, Regular How pliers for placing and removing arch wires, tying ligatures and for utility procedures. B, Modified How pliers for lower arch primarily and for assisting in band forming. C, Double beak anterior band-forming pliers. D, Pin- and ligature-cutting pliers. E and F, Peak posterior band-forming pliers. (Courtesy Rocky Mountain Dental Products Co.)

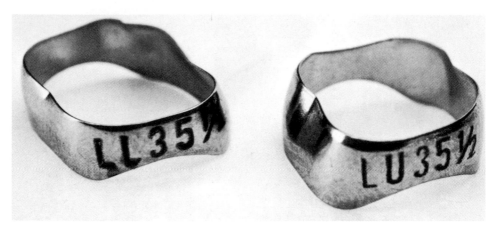

Figure 17–3 Preformed seamless lower and upper molar bands. (Courtesy Unitek Corp.)

the lingual contour, the band material is readapted to the tooth on both the buccal and lingual surfaces.

The band is then removed and examined. If it was formed properly, the buccal groove should be clearly registered in the band material and the shape of the molar should be clearly evident. When the lingual legs of the band material are brought together in the relationship established by the plier beaks, they should be at the same level, not one higher or one lower. It is important to keep the joint vertical and as parallel with the long axis of the tooth as possible. The band should have been seated far enough down on the tooth so that there is no overlapping of the band material on the mesial and distal aspect at the marginal ridge. Scribing of the gingival-proximal periphery is seldom necessary. Excessive proximal gingival contour and cutting is the mistake made by the neophyte. The proximal scribing should be minimal to ensure maximal band retention. The two lingual legs are then approximated carefully in their correct relationship and carried to the spot welder. The legs are welded together right at the joint. Though not essential if the band is properly made, it is a good technique to reinforce the welded joint. An "insert" of the same band material is laid parallel with the joint and welded to place on either side of the seam (Fig. 17–4). Next, the lingual legs are cut off with a crown and collar shears and the surface smoothly polished. The band is replaced on the molar and readapted with the flat amalgam plugger or by driving it to place with a mallet and orangewood stick, an Eby type band driver (Fig. 17–5), or a Swinehart band driver. A tighter and more desirable fit is thus obtained.

After the bands have been properly fitted to the molar teeth, horizontal buccal tubes of the desired size are chosen, depending on the problem to be corrected. If only the molars are to be banded and a heavy arch wire used, the tube is likely to be 0.040 or 0.045 inch round. If anterior edgewise attachment bands are used by the orthodontist, the tube will probably be a rectangular or edgewise tube. Buccal tubes, like other appurtenances, may either be welded or soldered. Because of the strong stress at this point, particularly with a heavy arch wire, some operators prefer to solder the tubes, feeling that the bulk of solder around the tube gives greater strength (Fig. 17–6). If the flanges of a welded tube are adapted properly first, however, reinforcement is seldom necessary. In any case, the tubes should parallel the occlusal surface of the band and be in such position with respect to the remaining buccal segment teeth that

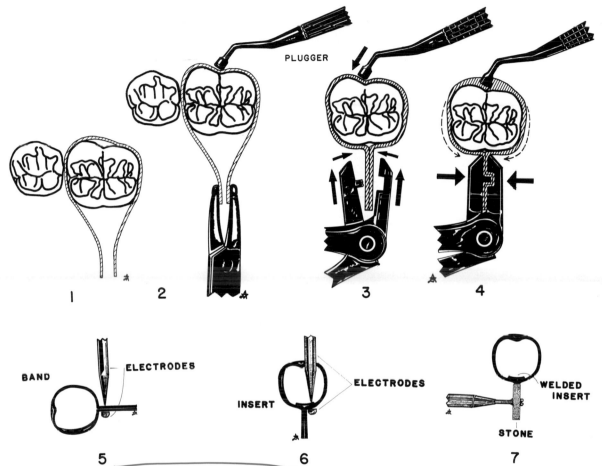

Figure 17–4. Direct band-forming procedure. 1, Band material is brought through mesial and distal embrasures after separating wires have been removed. 2, While holding the free ends together with How or office pliers, the buccal surface is adapted to the tooth with a round amalgam plugger, working the excess lingually, as a slight constant pull is maintained by the holding pliers. 3 and 4, The band material is pinched together with How pliers, and then grasped with Peak pliers. While holding the adapted band firmly in place with the amalgam plugger on the buccal aspect, close the Peak pliers with a firm and continuous grasp, working all excess material into the beaks of the pliers. 5, Spot welding of band at lingual joint. Both legs should be directly superimposed and the joint vertical to the occlusal surface of the band if formed properly. 6, Small stainless-steel insert of 0.004 or 0.005 inch band material, laid directly over joint and spot welded to place after adapting. 7, Lingual extensions cut off and polished with a carborundum stone and pumice-impregnated rubber disk.

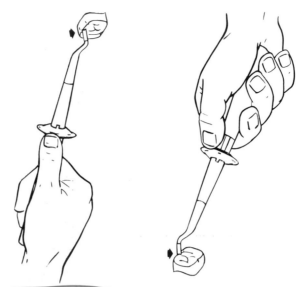

Figure 17–5 Use of band driver to seat molar bands firmly with a "drive fit." Place point on lingual occlusal aspect of upper molar band (left) and buccal occlusal of lower molar band (right). (Courtesy Rocky Mountain Dental Products Co.)

a straight wire or arch wire will lie in close proximity to the premolars and canines and yet have both ends insert and withdraw freely from right and left molar bands (Figs. 17–7, 17–8). This assumes molars are in normal position. If they are rotated (Fig. 17–8B), the tube should parallel the buccal surface, and the arch wire will then exert a correcting influence on the malposition. (See discussion on arch wires.)

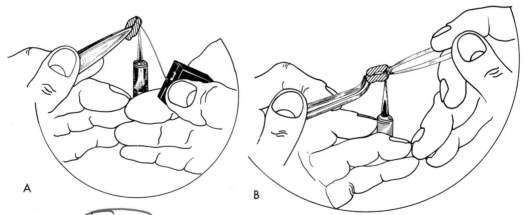

Figure 17–6 Soldering of buccal tube on molar band. A, Solder is allowed to flow lightly over fluoride-fluxed buccal surface at point where tube is to be placed. Flame is primarily on band. B, Fluxed tube is held in place with tweezers or soldering needle, and flame is directed primarily on tube to "pull" solder onto tube surface contiguous to the band. Note the use of finger rests during soldering procedure. The tube may also be held in its proper position by a soldering needle inserted in the tube lumen. This requires less heat to make the solder flow and allows precise tube positioning on the band.

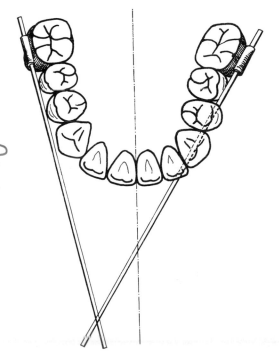

Figure 17–7 Placing of straight diagnostic wires in horizontal buccal tubes of molars before cementing the bands. This is to check the proper tube position on the band and the parallelism to permit easy insertion and withdrawal of the arch wire.

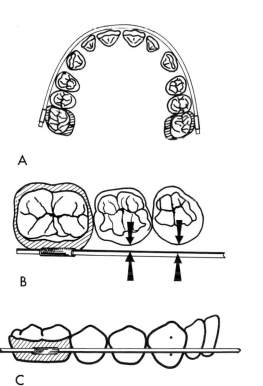

A

B

C

Figure 17–8 Proper tube positioning, so that arch wire may be formed readily to assume proper relationship to buccal and labial surfaces of the teeth anterior to the molar bands (A and B) and parallel with the occlusal surfaces (C), with a minimum of compensating bends.

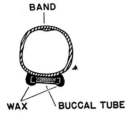

BAND

WAX   BUCCAL TUBE

Figure 17–9 Molar band with buccal tube filled with wax before cementation. Band should be clean and dry. One must make sure that there is no wax on the inside of the band when placing it in the buccal tube.

CEMENTATION

Before cementing any band, each tooth should be cleaned thoroughly, pumiced, and all debris rinsed away. While the cement is being mixed, the cheeks should be blocked away with cotton rolls and the tooth to be banded should be isolated. Some dentists wipe each tooth with alcohol to remove the mucin and then dry the tooth with a blast of warm air.

Although the same cement is usually used as for cementing inlays or full crowns (zinc oxyphosphate), the mixing procedure is slightly different. An average mix should take approximately two minutes to make. A small portion of powder is incorporated each time and thoroughly spatulated over a wide area before taking in the next amount of powder. In this manner the heat may be dissipated over the surface of the glass slab slowing down the setting time materially. Also, a thicker, more putty-like mix may be used. Such a consistency provides greater strength and reduces the tendency of the free acid to etch the tooth surface. After the cement has reached the proper consistency, the clean and dried band is placed on the ball of the index finger. If the band has an attachment or tube, this should be filled with wax (Fig. 17–9). The thumb is placed on the periphery of the band to steady it and the band is filled with cement by drawing the spatula over the inverted gingival margin at several places along the periphery (Fig. 17–10). The band is carried to the isolated and dried tooth and pressed in place using the index finger or ball of the middle finger as a plunger to squeeze the cement from beneath the gingival periphery as the band slides into place. The use of an orangewood stick and mallet or a

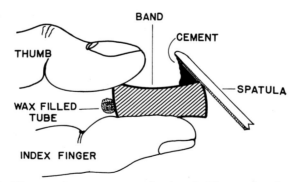

BAND

CEMENT

THUMB

SPATULA

WAX FILLED
TUBE

INDEX FINGER

Figure 17–10 Placing the cement in the band. The occlusal surface of the band should rest on the ball of the forefinger or middle finger, which will serve as a plunger to force the cement out the gingival portion of the band when the band is pushed to place on the tooth. It is wise to fill the band and to see that the entire periphery is covered with cement. Excess cement will be forced out of the band anyway and ensures that the cement bond is complete to prevent decalcification of the tooth or peeling away of the band.

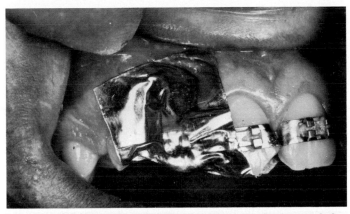

Figure 17–11   Covering a cemented band with tin or aluminum foil to isolate it from the saliva and to prevent the patient from tasting the cement. The foil is peeled away after the cement is dry and the excess cement may be removed with a universal type scaler.

band driver is recommended (Fig. 17–5). A heavy round amalgam plugger serves as an effective seating instrument also. A beaver-tail burnisher helps adapt the occlusal margin at this time. A small square of aluminum or tinfoil should then be adapted over the cemented band, isolating it from the saliva and permitting the patient to close his mouth and swallow (Fig. 17–11). After the cement is thoroughly set, the foil is removed and the excess cement carefully chipped away. The dentist should remove the cement by moving a universal type scaler *parallel* with the margin of the band, not *perpendicular* to it.

Spurs or sharp attachments are likely to irritate the contacting mucous membrane of the cheeks and tongue. A supply of utility wax helps the patient for three or four days until the epithelium adapts to the irritation. In an emergency, chewing gum, preferably sugarless, may be used to cover sharp edges.

THE ARCH WIRE

For a long time, molar bands were called "anchor" bands because they served to hold the arch wire, which did the actual moving of the desired teeth. It became apparent to observant clinicians that the so-called anchor teeth moved too; but since their resistance was so much greater than that of the incisor teeth (the teeth usually being moved) the molar bands have continued to be referred to as anchor bands. Each molar band thus carries a horizontal buccal tube to hold the arch wire and partially control arch wire activity.

Arch wires may be made in a number of sizes. In multibanded techniques, under the control of an orthodontist, these wires vary from 0.011 to 0.022 inch in round wire and from 0.012 to 0.028 inch in square or rectangular arch wires. The dimension of the wire chosen depends on the appliance used, therapeutic objectives, training of the orthodontist, etc. (See Chap. 11.)

In limited orthodontic procedures, where a minimum number of bands is used or where the span of distance between bands is greater, a heavier arch wire is likely to be used. Unlike the smaller gauge arch wires, which may be deformed a good deal to move teeth, the heavier arch wires are relatively rigid and serve as a base for tying ligatures, as in ligation techniques used in conjunction with periodontal therapy (see Chap. 16), or as a receptor of extraoral force that must be delivered to the molar teeth alone or to the entire dental arch (Fig. 17–8). The heavy arch wire depends on itself for the strength to resist deformation, not on a number of attachments to individual teeth. The use and fabrication of this type of arch wire is described in this chapter under Anterior Cross-bite, in Chapter 18 in retraction of anterior teeth and in extraoral force techniques.

ATTACHMENT BANDS

For the precise control of individual teeth, orthodontic bands must be placed. For the dentist interested in limited orthodontic procedures, this usually means one or more incisor bands in addition to the molar bands just described. Or, it may mean the fabrication of maxillary and mandibular premolar bands to correct cross-bite of specific teeth.

Attachment bands may be made by both the direct and indirect techniques, but direct band formation is considered more desirable if the dentist plans to make the bands himself. There are orthodontic laboratories which do a good job of fabricating attachment bands as well as molar bands if they are given a model specifically prepared for the indirect technique. A discussion of these methods is beyond the scope of this book.

POSITIONING OF BANDS

Any orthodontic band should be made to fit as accurately as possible because of the heavy pounding by functional forces. A number of attachments are available. The edgewise attachment is one of the most universally used by orthodontists and is quite versatile. (See Chap. 11.) It will serve quite well for limited orthodontic problems. There are a number of variations of the original edgewise bracket. The twin edgewise bracket has a wider bearing surface on the arch wire and thus has better rotation control. (See Chap. 11.) A single edgewise bracket can be used, if rotating eyelets or spurs are placed on the mesial and distal sides of each band (Figs. 11–8, 11–9). Preformed bands are available in many sizes with the brackets already attached to the band. Or, the bands may be formed directly, using band material strips with or without the brackets attached. In either case it is imperative that each band be accurately positioned on each tooth. The bracket should be at the middle third of the tooth mesiodistally and incisivogingivally (Figs. 11–32, 11–57). The slot in the bracket that receives the arch wire should be perpendicular to the long axis of the tooth.

Every band should go to its proper place with a "drive fit." One of the biggest criticisms of orthodontic appliances made by improperly trained operators or some laboratories is that the teeth, in many instances look like the proverbial island in a sea of cement. This happens if the band is too large. If preformed bands are used, a band stretcher is needed since it is wise to select a band a trifle on the small side. If band material is to be used, or 0.003 by 0.125 inch band material strips with brackets prewelded on them, band-forming pliers make it easier to position the band properly on the tooth (Figs. 17–2C, 17–12). Rounded beak office pliers or How pliers may be used, however. The

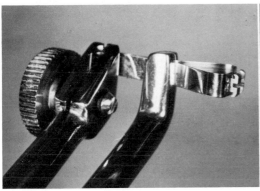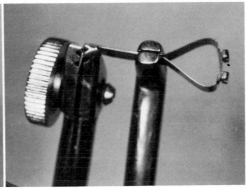

Figure 17–12 "Pinching" an attachment band with band-forming pliers. The two free ends of the band strip are approximated and both folded at right angles with office pliers to form a ¼ inch tab. The tab is inserted in the vise-grip of one beak of the pliers and the double thickness of band material slid into a slot on the other beak. The knurled nut of the vise-grip is tightened securely. Gentle pressure on the plier handles moves the slotted beak along the band loop. The loop is placed over the desired tooth and adapted with a round amalgam plugger as the handles are firmly pressed together. This draws the constricted and adapted band loop tightly around the tooth. The band is now ready to weld and place the insert. (See Fig. 17–4.)

technique is similar to molar band forming. The band is placed with the bracket in its proper position on the labial surface of the incisor and the 0.003 by 0.125 band material burnished around toward the proximal and lingual surfaces. With one thumb nail in the bracket slot, to hold the desired position on the tooth, the two ends of the band strip are pinched together in the middle of the lingual surface. (See Fig. 17–12.) The joint should be parallel with the long axis of the tooth and both legs should meet at the same level. The projections are then spot welded as close to the tooth and band itself as possible. The excess is cut off from the lingual projections, leaving a tab of about a quarter of an inch (Fig. 17–13). A piece of 0.003 by 0.125 inch band material is laid inside the band, directly over the joint and parallel with the seam. The insert is then spot welded to place on either side of the seam. Next, the tab is trimmed closely to the band with a crown and collar shears and polished down with a mounted stone and pumice-impregnated rubber disk (Fig. 17–4). The band is placed on the tooth and pushed firmly to its correct position with a No. 1 round amalgam plugger or a band driver. The plugger or a beaver-tail burnisher may then be used to adapt the margins on the labial, lingual and proximal surfaces. By driving the band with a band driver or an orangewood stick and mallet placed on the lingual surface, any slight excess on the proximal surfaces may be taken up.

If the band is being made for a lateral incisor or canine where there is a strong distal proximal convexity, it is difficult to fit the band without having it stand away at the distal-incisal angle. This may be corrected by cutting the band very carefully at this point with a crown and collar shears to a depth of about a sixteenth of an inch. The free ends are then overlapped at this slit to follow the tooth contour and spot welded. The band should be checked to make sure that there are no sharp projections as a result of the welding of the insert or the clipping and overlapping of the distal-incisal margin. A pumice-impregnated rubber disk is used to polish down these areas.

0,15 cm

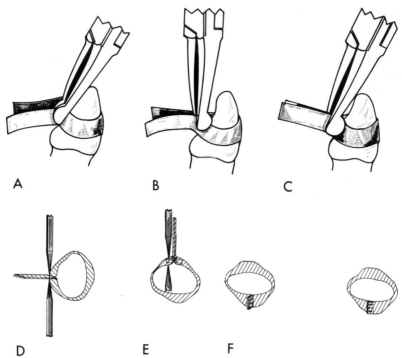

Figure 17–13   Forming a canine band by the direct method, using How pliers. A, Initial "pinching up" of contoured canine blank on the lingual side. Labial surface is burnished down and excess worked lingually. B and C, Reproducing surface detail in lingual contour of band by using narrow beaks of How pliers. D, Welding pinched up joint together. Seam should be parallel with the long axis of the canine. E, Welding of lingual insert inside joint. F, Lingual tab has been cut down to 1/8 inch and is folded over while band is on tooth and burnished to place. Tab is spot welded and smoothed down, adding greater resistance to masticatory stress.

SPECIAL PROBLEMS AND TECHNIQUES WITH CANINE BANDS

Canine bands often pose a special problem because of their shape and marked convexity on the labial surface. If possible, contoured canine blanks should be used, with the bracket being placed after the band has been formed so as to be more precise in getting the bracket in its proper position with respect to the long axis of the tooth. Satisfactory bands may be made using ordinary How pliers. The canine contoured blank is wrapped around the canine, with the free ends being pulled lingually by the How pliers. By holding the labial surface steady with the finger or a round plugger, the lingual surface is "pinched up" with the flat portion of the How beak against the tooth to form a sharp joint (Fig. 17–13A). By reversing the How pliers, the concavity of the lingual contour above the cingulum may be reproduced in the band (Fig. 17–13B). By moving the narrow plier beaks gingivally over the convex cingulum, all the lingual morphologic detail may be closely approximated by the band material (Fig. 17–13C). The band is then spot welded at the lingual joint as with the molar and incisor bands and an "insert" welded to place over the joint on the inside of the lingual surface (Fig. 17–13D, E). The quarter inch lingual tab may either be polished off or folded over and welded to the lingual band surface and then smoothed off. The canine takes heavy functional stress, and the extra thickness of band material reduces the chance of breakage or of breaking the cement seal (Fig. 17–13F). The band is ready to weld or solder on the bracket, after it has been taken back to the tooth and all the margins burnished. An Eby band driver should be used with the tip on the lingual surface at the seam to take up any slack and ensure a snug fit. Rotating eyelets on the mesial and distal sides of canines are usually a wise procedure and ensure better tooth control for the orthodontist.

After the attachment band has been formed and carefully readapted to ensure the best possible fit, it may be cleaned by dipping it into hydrochloric acid and rinsing it, by putting it in a passivator for a couple of minutes or by dipping it in alcohol and drying it with a blast of warm air. As with molar band appurtenances, soft utility wax should be adapted under the wings and in the slot of the bracket to prevent the cement from entering these areas during the cementation procedure. The tooth to be banded is then pumiced, rinsed, wiped with alcohol, isolated with cotton rolls and dried with a blast of warm air preparatory to the actual cementing. (See discussion on Cementation.) The band should we well filled with cement of the proper consistency. It should be pushed to place by using the thumb, middle finger or index finger as a plunger to force the excess cement from the gingival portion of the band (Fig. 17–10). Some dentists deem it advisable to wipe a thin layer of cement over the tooth first before cementing the band to make sure that the entire surface is covered. The band should be driven to place or pushed strongly with the amalgam plugger. The bracket position should be checked to make sure that it is in the middle third of the tooth and that the slot is indeed perpendicular to the long axis. The tooth may then be covered with foil, as outlined earlier, until the cement sets (Fig. 17–11). In removing the excess cement, one must take care not to peel away the attachment band periphery.

ANTERIOR CROSS-BITE

Periodic observation, correlation of facial pattern, information on direction of tooth eruption, timing of eruption, prevention of prolonged retention and a certain amount of patient education during the critical exchange period, i.e., instructing the patient what to look for, will permit the interception of some developing cross-bites (Fig. 17–14). This was discussed in Chapter 14, Interceptive Orthodontics. The use of the tongue blade and finger pressure were described. Because the timing of this procedure is so critical, however, in most instances the dentist is confronted with a *fait accompli*, and is faced with the problem of full correction of the incisor cross-bite.

Before the dentist undertakes correction of an anterior cross-bite he must determine whether the cross-bite is a symptom of a more generalized malocclusion or purely a localized irregularity. If he has taken a good set of study models, complete periapical radiographs or a panoramic radiograph and facial photographs, and has the patient in the chair for examination, he should find answers to the following questions. How many teeth are involved? From a study of each cast—maxillary and mandibular—which incisor teeth seem to show greater malposition and abnormal arch position, upper or lower? Does the cross-bite involve only the teeth, or do the teeth reflect the anteroposterior jaw relationship or an apical base dyplasia? Is the path of closure normal from postural resting position to occlusion, or is there a convenience swing or ante-

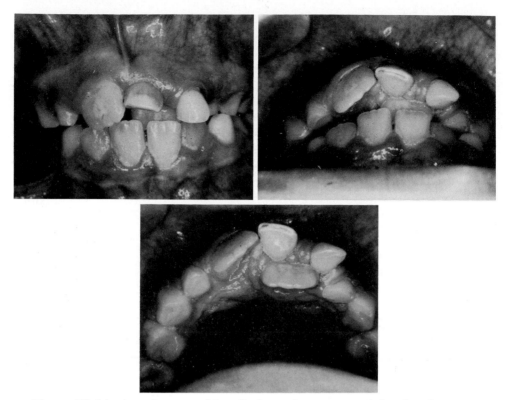

Figure 17–14   Anterior cross-bite. Prolonged retention of the deciduous central incisor created the present problem. Interceptive guidance with a tongue blade would have helped at the right time. Now, with the severe locking on occlusion, a guide plane is necessary. Time is important, since the maxillary left lateral incisor will tend to drift mesially and block the forward movement of the central incisor.

rior displacement, with translatory condylar movement from rest to habitual occlusion—in other words, a functional cross-bite? Is there adequate room to correct the tooth or teeth in cross-bite? If the diagnostic information indicates with a fair degree of certainty that the problem is not a symptom of a general malocclusion (a basal malrelationship, a generalized arch length deficiency or both) and if the localized aberration is such that there is sufficient room at the desired site, simple corrective procedures are then possible. If there is any question at all, have a consultation with an orthodontist. Or, as happens in so many cases, if the cross-bite is only one facet of the total malocclusion, the patient should be referred immediately for specialist therapy. Even the best corrective procedures are not always able to recover the damaging effects of cross-bite (Fig. 17–15).

INCLINED PLANE APPLIANCE OPPOSING TOOTH IN CROSS-BITE

One of the simplest and most effective means of correcting the lingual cross-bite of a maxillary incisor is the use of an acrylic or cast metal inclined plane that is cemented to the mandibular incisors opposing the tooth in cross-bite (Fig. 17–16). This type of appliance, if properly constructed, can correct a cross-bite in a matter of days. In no instance should it be left on longer than six weeks. A prerequisite for the inclined plane is a normal or excessive overbite

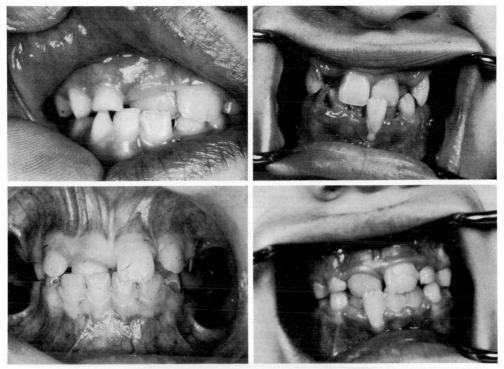

Figure 17–15 Anterior cross-bite—a damaging malocclusion.

and adequate space in the arch to bring the incisor into correct anteroposterior relationship with the opposing mandibular incisors. If there is an end-to-end overbite relationship or an open bite tendency, the use of a guide plane is contraindicated.

A careful examination of the cross-bite area should be made with the teeth in full occlusion. If it is apparent that the maxillary incisor is causing the difficulty, as is usually the case, with the opposing mandibular incisor labially displaced as a consequence, the choice of the guide plane as a corrective adjunct is proper. If the mandibular incisor is primarily displaced labially with the maxillary incisor in relatively normal position, corrective measures should be directed toward the mandibular incisor segment. In the latter instance, the cross-bite is usually a symptom of a broader malocclusion and there is seldom sufficient arch length to retract the labially malposed incisor into a correct anteroposterior relationship with the maxillary incisor. In such instances, full corrective meas-

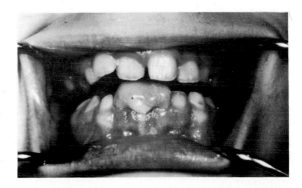

Figure 17–16 Acrylic inclined plane to "jump the bite" for a lingually locked maxillary incisor.

ures are required (Fig. 17–15, upper right). A slight adaptive labial malposition of a mandibular incisor, however, resulting from a significant lingual version of the opposing maxillary incisor, will show considerable autonomous correction as soon as the correct overjet is established, if space is adequate. The labial stripping and tissue damage so often seen around the labially displaced mandibular incisor will largely disappear after the correction of the cross-bite (Fig. 17–15). This is not true in all cases.

A complete radiographic examination should be made before placing a corrective appliance. Sometimes the lingual version of a maxillary incisor may be due to a supernumerary tooth, and this possibility should be checked. Also, the relative state of development of the apices of the incisors must be determined before the teeth are moved. Appliances placed too early may cause a foreshortening of the root. It must be stressed again that adequate space in the area of cross-bite for correction of the incisor malposition is an essential prerequisite.

The following steps are to be followed in the fabrication, placement and control of a cemented acrylic inclined plane:

First Appointment. 1. Alginate impressions are taken of the maxillary and mandibular dental arches. Both impressions are poured up in plaster or stone. The mandibular impression is poured up twice, with the first model to serve as a working model for the construction of the appliance, the second as a study model.

2. With a soft lead pencil, a line is drawn on the working model to indicate the approximate coverage of the mandibular incisors by the acrylic. The inclined plane ordinarily should incorporate a tooth and a half on either side of the cross-bite area. Four mandibular incisors are sufficient to give stability to the inclined plane (Fig. 17–17).

3. The working model is carefully foiled in the area outlined by pencil or painted with a separating medium.

4. The inclined plane is then waxed up on the foiled working model. The wax should not impinge on the gingival tissue (Fig. 17–18). The inclined plane angle should be at approximately 45 degrees to the occlusal plane and should extend sufficiently posteriorly so that the patient cannot readily drop behind

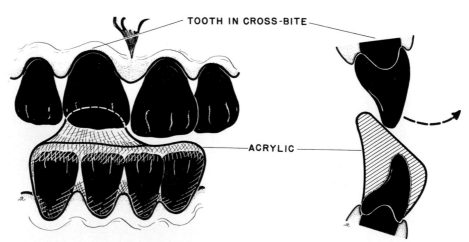

Figure 17–17 Relationship of tooth in cross-bite to inclined plane and the coverage of the mandibular incisors by the acrylic. Only the tooth in cross-bite contacts the guide plane.

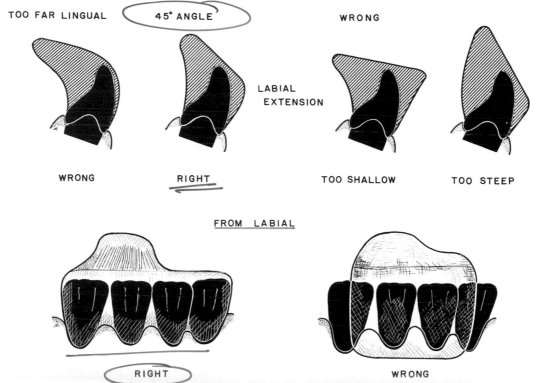

TOO FAR LINGUAL   45° ANGLE   WRONG

LABIAL EXTENSION

WRONG   RIGHT   TOO SHALLOW   TOO STEEP

FROM LABIAL

RIGHT   WRONG

Figure 17–18   Acrylic guide plane. Design, coverage and inclination of plane are important. A plane that is too shallow is as likely to cause failure as a plane that is too steep. If soft tissue is covered, considerable irritation may occur.

the appliance and dislodge it. The waxed guide plane is checked with the opposing maxillary cast to make sure that *only* the tooth in cross-bite is contacting the plane.

5. The guide plane is invested and processed in regular acrylic. This is more satisfactory than fabricating the guide plane with endothermic acrylic that has not been cured under pressure. The harder the surface of the inclined plane, the less likelihood there is of a catch or groove being formed by the incisor in cross-bite. The guide plane is then polished and is ready for cementation.

SECOND APPOINTMENT. 1. On the second visit, one tries the guide plane in the patient's mouth. If it does not go completely into place, the inside portion should be checked to make sure that there are no particles left from the working model or any undercuts. Interferences are removed as needed and the patient is made to bite in centric relationship. One must make sure that the tooth in cross-bite is the only one contacting. It is wise not to "open the bite" more than 4 or 5 mm. Too large an opening may cause muscle fatigue because of the increase of the vertical dimension beyond the rest or postural position of the mandible. A slight opening beyond postural resting position is to be desired, to utilize muscle force for the cross-bite correction. The inclined plane should be smoothly polished again if any adjustments have been made.

2. The mandibular incisor teeth are isolated with cotton rolls, cleaned and dried carefully, and the inclined plane is cemented (a *thin* mix of zinc oxyphosphate cement is recommended). Firm pressure is needed to seat the appliance, because of the hydraulic effect of the contained cement. An "escape" hole may

be made with a fine fissure bur at the lingual-incisal margin, if desired, to further ensure complete seating of the guide plane. The excess cement is wiped off and the appliance is allowed to set for 10 to 15 minutes before any pressure is placed on it. One must check again to make sure that the maxillary incisor in cross-bite is the only tooth in contact with the guide plane.

3) It is essential to warn both the parent and the patient of the diet limitations during the wearing of the cemented appliance. Food should be kept soft and the emphasis should be on liquids for the first several days. There is usually a strong sibilant speech defect during the correction. The patient should be admonished against digital manipulation of the appliance so as not to loosen it. In any event, occlusal stress sometimes breaks the cement seal and the patient must come back to have the appliance re-cemented. Normally, provided that there is adequate room and that the dentist makes sure that no groove or "catch" develops on the inclined plane to restrict forward movement of the malposed tooth, the correction is usually effected in 7 to 14 days. An appointment should be made for one week following the cementation.

THIRD APPOINTMENT. At the third visit the patient is carefully examined. The mandible is guided into a retruded position during closure, and the antero-posterior relationship carefully checked in the cross-bite region. If it appears that the patient is now able to bite behind the upper incisors, the guide plane is removed with an orangewood stick and mallet. Two or three sharp blows in an upward direction are usually sufficient to dislodge the appliance. If this does not work, the acrylic on the labial surface may be cut through to the labial surface of one of the covered incisors and the cement seal broken by wedging a heavy universal type scaler in the slot. The orangewood stick and mallet routine is then used again.

With the appliance removed, the teeth should then be checked in full occlusion. If it appears that the tooth has not been brought "over the fence," the appliance is re-cemented. One must be sure to polish the inclined plane again if this is the case. Usually, however, the tooth will be sufficiently forward to permit the normal overjet relationship. Under no circumstances should the dentist try to gain *full* alignment of the tooth in cross-bite. All he should aim for is to eliminate the cross-bite. Autonomous adjustment usually takes care of the balance (Fig. 17–19). The *great danger of getting over-eruption of the posterior teeth with prolonged wearing of the guide plane should not be ignored*. Under no circumstances should the appliance remain in the mouth for longer than six weeks. If for some reason this approach has not succeeded, one of the following methods may have to be employed.

After the removal of the inclined plane, the patient is instructed in the intense use of a tongue blade to maintain the cross-bite correction and to bring about the normal alignment of the malposed tooth (Fig. 17–20). An hour or two a day for 10 to 14 days following the removal of the guide plane is usually recommended. A Barton bandage or vertical pull chincap may assist in keeping the teeth in occlusion and will prevent relapse. An orthobite plastic retainer will do likewise, permitting further correction of the malposed teeth. (See Chap. 16.)

ADVANTAGES AND DISADVANTAGES OF INCLINED PLANE. The advantages of the guide plane are:

1. Ease of fabrication
2. Rapidity of correction using functional and muscle forces
3. Lack of soreness or looseness of the teeth during movement
4. Rarity of relapse

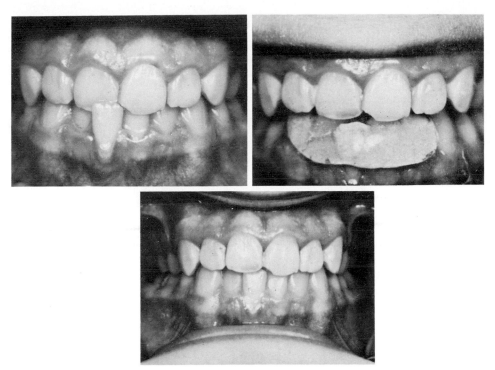

Figure 17–19 Correction of lingual cross-bite of maxillary central incisor by endothermic guide plane formed directly on lower incisors. Oblong mass of setting acrylic was forced over lower incisors, adapted with fingers to approximate contour desired and removed when it started getting hard and warm. After setting completely and cooling off, it was trimmed to proper size, polished, checked in the mouth for correct inclination and coverage, and cemented. The plane was worn for only six days and removed. The remaining adjustment was due to the forces of occlusion after the incisor had been brought across labially. This type of fabrication is less desirable than the indirect technique of making the guide plane on a plaster model, however.

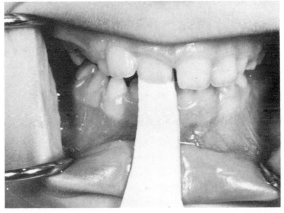

Figure 17–20 Using a tongue blade to complete alignment of a central incisor that has been "jumped" across the bite with a guide plane. One or two hours a day of biting on the wood incline is required for a period of two weeks following removal of acrylic guide plane.

The disadvantages of the inclined plane are:

1. Strong limitations on diet during the wearing of the appliance
2. Creation of a temporary speech defect
3. Tendency to create an anterior open bite if the appliance is left in place too long
4. Possibility of the appliance becoming loose and requiring recementation because of the strong occlusal stresses upon it
5. Imperfect alignment of the malposed tooth when the appliance is removed. The dentist must rely on autonomous adjustment for the balance of correction.

CAST, CROWN OR BANDED INCLINES APPLIED TO MALPOSED TOOTH

CAST INCLINE. An alternative method of utilizing the proprioceptive control of occlusion to move a lingually locked maxillary incisor into correct position is the placement of the incline on the lingually malposed tooth itself. This type of appliance is considerably less bulky. The simplest way to fabricate an inclined plane for the tooth in cross-bite is to carve up in inlay wax on the working model the pattern on the tooth in question. After that, the maxillary cast is articulated with the opposing mandibular cast to ensure a correct contact of the waxed up inclined plane with the mandibular incisors. If need be, the wax pattern may be placed in the patient's mouth and checked to make sure that the incisal contact is correct. No undercuts should be present (Fig. 17–21). The inclined plane angle should be at approximately 45 degrees to the occlusal plane. The pattern is invested, cast and finished, following the usual procedures for the conventional cast crown. Silver or a low-carat gold are all satisfactory and serviceable materials for the short time needed, and they are relatively inexpensive. Make sure the metal is not too soft, however.

INCLINED CROWN. Stainless-steel crowns for the incisor teeth are available in various sizes, much like the posterior crowns used in habit appliances and space maintainers. These crowns can be adapted for use as an inclined plane. A metal crown which is purposely too long gingivo-incisally is chosen for the tooth in lingual cross-bite. The crown is fitted, making sure that the *incisal* margin extends 1 or 2 mm. beyond the level of the contiguous teeth. A double thickness of 0.006 by 0.200 inch band material is spot welded or soldered to the lingual side of the crown. This strip of double-thickness material is carried over

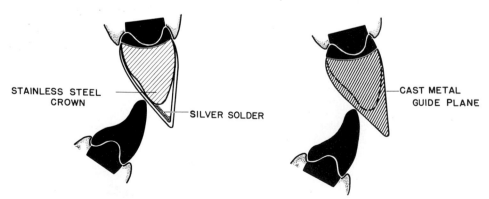

STAINLESS STEEL CROWN — SILVER SOLDER   CAST METAL GUIDE PLANE

Figure 17–21   Stainless-steel crown and cast metal guide planes for correcting cross-bite of individual teeth. One must be sure that no undercuts are present when cementing cast incline. Silver solder has been added in crown to reinforce the relatively thin crown as incisal stress is brought against it.

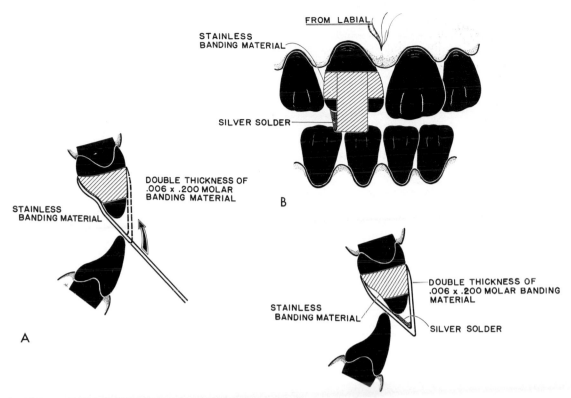

STAINLESS
BANDING MATERIAL

FROM LABIAL

SILVER SOLDER

B

DOUBLE THICKNESS OF
.006 x .200 MOLAR
BANDING MATERIAL

STAINLESS
BANDING MATERIAL

A

DOUBLE THICKNESS OF
.006 x .200 MOLAR BANDING
MATERIAL

STAINLESS
BANDING MATERIAL

SILVER SOLDER

Figure 17–22 Banded incline for anterior cross-bite correction. Note that double thickness of molar band material is used for incline portion. The operator should be sure to check extension of incline toward the labial side by having the patient close his mouth against the incline, before bending the strip of band material back to the labial surface of the band. A, The strip of band material should be adapted to the lingual contours of the tooth. After the incisor tooth has been brought labially across the bite, the banded incline may be cut off and removed easily. Greater care must be taken in oral hygiene with this type of guide plane.

the incisal margin to form an inclined plane at about 45 degrees to the occlusal plane. The crown is placed on the malposed tooth, and the patient closes gently in centric relation to establish the anterior extension of the inclined plane (Fig. 17–21). The crown is then removed, and the plane construction is completed by making a sharp bend in the double-thickness band material so that it turns back toward the labial surface of the crown. One should spot weld and solder at this point. The crown is tried again in the patient's mouth. The labial-incisal margin of the double-thickness plane may then be reinforced by the addition of the silver solder on the inside of the plane.

BANDED INCLINE. A variation of the inclined crown is the banded incline. A regular orthodontic band is fabricated for the maxillary incisor in lingual cross-bite. This may be either a preformed band or one made out of stainless banding material. A double thickness of 0.006 by 0.200 inch molar banding material is welded on the lingual surface and brought up over the labial-incisal margin, forming the inclined plane in the same manner as described above for the full crown (Fig. 17–22). The band may then be tried on the tooth of the patient and checked by having the mandible close in centric relation. A mark should be made on the band material at the point of contact of the opposing mandibular incisor. The band is then removed and the double layer of band material bent back toward the labial surface of the band at a point approximately 2 mm. beyond the lower incisor mark. The material is welded or soldered to the labial surface of the band. As with the construction for the full steel crown, it is wise to reinforce the inclined plane portion and the incisal angle with silver solder.

THERAPY WITH SINGLE INCLINED PLANE.   Therapy and patient instructions are the same for all three variations of the single inclined plane—the cast, the crown and the band. Before the appliance is cemented, it is checked carefully to make sure that the mouth is not open too far beyond postural resting position. The patient should not be able to protrude or retrude the mandible too readily beyond the inclined plane, or this will defeat the purpose of the appliance.

After the cementation of the appliance, the patient is instructed to be very careful with his diet. If he bites too hard he may make both the tooth in cross-bite and the opposing incisor quite sore. It is here that the proprioceptive sense comes into play. Since the inclined plane opens the mouth beyond postural resting position, the inclined plane will be in contact with the opposing mandibular incisors most of the time when the mandible is not in active function. It is this constant pressure more than the momentary contact during mastication and deglutition that really serves to move the lingually malposed incisor labially.

Because the lingually locked incisor is covered with the appliance, it is more difficult to check the actual progress than with the acrylic guide plane that is cemented on the mandibular anterior teeth. For this reason the dentist should check very carefully the relationship of the tooth with the plane cemented. One method is to take a wax or modeling compound "core" right after the cementation and to use this as a guide for movement on subsequent observation visits.

REMOVAL OF SINGLE INCLINED PLANE.   Whereas it is relatively easy to remove the acrylic guide plane to check the occlusion and to re-cement the plane, this becomes much more difficult when the cast, crown or banded inclined plane appliance is used. The latter must usually be cut off the tooth, which may destroy the appliance. Since the stress of constant incisal contact is limited to the malposed tooth and one or two mandibular teeth at the most, when the maxillary cast or banded incline is used, it is possible for a lower incisor to become mobile and painful. If there is adequate space, this tooth may move lingually. In most instances such a response is favorable. Even though the maxillary incisor may be the primary offender in the cross-bite situation, there is usually a secondary labial malposition of the opposing mandibular incisor. The acrylic inclined plane prevents the mandibular incisor from moving, but the single unit plane on the opposing tooth stimulates movement. The combined reciprocal action of labial movement of the upper incisor and lingual movement of the lower incisor often results in an even quicker reduction of the cross-bite. For this reason, this type of appliance is seldom left in place more than three weeks. In most instances the operator is safe to remove the plane after two weeks. As with correction of anterior cross-bite using the acrylic guide plane, adequate space and sufficient overbite are essential prerequisites. Also, no grooves or "catches" should be allowed to develop to prevent free movement of the desired teeth.

USE OF ARCH WIRE AND MOLAR BANDS

In some instances there is so little overbite that the placing of the guide plane would serve to allow eruption of the posterior teeth and the creation of an anterior open bite before the cross-bite is corrected. The guide plane is contraindicated in such cases. The use of a palatal removable appliance, with a lingual finger spring and guard for this purpose is illustrated in Chapter 16 (Fig. 16–35). Another appliance that may be used is the simple labial arch wire and two maxillary first molar bands (Fig. 17–23).

FABRICATION. The first molar bands may be made directly in the mouth or indirectly on the model. For the direct technique, preformed molar bands of assorted sizes are available. Stainless-steel crowns also serve quite satisfactorily, and are fitted in the manner described in Chapters 13 and 14.

After molar bands have been cemented with 0.040 inch horizontal buccal tubes attached, the arch wire is formed. This wire may be 0.040 inch nichrome or stainless steel. To prevent the incorporation of sharp bends, as much as possible of the initial forming into a paraboloid arch shape is done with the fingers. To secure the right arch length, a steel or brass ligature wire is run around the dental arch from the distal end of one molar tube to the other. A quarter of an inch extra is allowed on each side. Working from a properly sized paraboloid arch wire, slight compensating bends are made so that the arch wire approximates all the teeth in the anterior and buccal segments and yet the ends withdraw and insert freely in the horizontal molar buccal tubes. The arch wire should contact or approximate the middle third of the buccal and labial surfaces of the molars and incisors. The posterior ends of the arch wire should be exactly parallel with the buccal tubes on the molars, if they are to withdraw and insert with minimum effort (Figs. 17–7, 17–8, 17–23).

VERTICAL SPRING LOOP. Some means of controlling the forward and backward movement of the arch wire is necessary in most orthodontic problems. A simple spur may be used at the mesial end of the molar tube, soldered directly to the arch wire. This is not versatile and requires removal of the arch and resoldering the spur each time a new position is desired. An equally simple but more practical and adjustable mechanism is a vertical spring loop, soldered

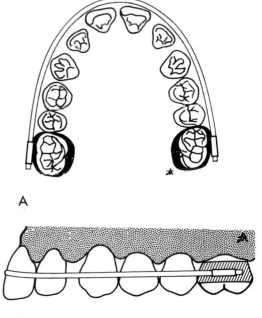

Figure 17–23 Molar bands with 0.040 inch round horizontal buccal tubes and a 0.040 inch diameter round stainless-steel or nichrome arch wire. Either spurs on the arch wire at the mesial ends of the buccal tubes or vertical loops must be placed to control arch wire anteroposterior movement in tubes. A, Occlusal view to show proper arch relationship to buccal and labial surfaces. B, Lateral view illustrates parallel relationship of buccal tube and arch wire with occlusal plane.

A

B

on the mesial end and wrapped around the arch wire on the distal end of the loop approximating the horizontal buccal tube.

The technique for soldering and fabricating the vertical spring loop is illustrated in Figures 17–24 to 17–27. A 0.030 inch nichrome round wire is soldered to the arch wire top surface a centimeter to the mesial side of where it enters the buccal tube. To establish this point on each side, the arch wire is fitted properly and then inserted in the buccal tubes on the cemented molar bands (Fig. 17–23). Not more than one sixteenth inch of the arch wire should project from the distal ends of the tubes; these ends should be rounded and polished. The exact position for placement of the soldered end of the vertical loop may then be scratched directly on the arch wire at the desired position with a marking file. The arch wire is removed and the smaller gauge loop wire soldered to the heavier arch wire. Solder may be placed at the scratch mark first and then allowed to flow to the smaller wire by directing the heat primarily on the fluxed loop end. Optionally, the solder may be applied to the end of the loop wire first. The end is placed against the fluxed scratch mark on the arch, then the blowpipe flame is directed primarily on the heavier wire. One must be sure to use the proper heat zone of the flame to reduce oxidation (Fig. 17–24); the flame is kept as small as possible to do the job. The biggest mistake made in soldering is to use too much heat. Excessive heat destroys much of the spring quality of stainless steel, softening the wire. Heat hardens nichrome wire but will make it quite brittle and easy to break if too much heat is applied for too long.

The auxiliary spring wire is formed into a vertical loop by wrapping it around the round beak of the No. 139 pliers. Since the beak is fairly small, the largest diameter of the beak may be used for the wrap-around. The operator must be consistent and use the same size loops on both sides of the arch wire. The free end of the loop is then wrapped around the arch wire completely and the excess cut off. The end is polished to prevent any irritation of the tissue. This procedure is repeated on the opposite side of the arch. To prevent gingival impingement, the vertical loops slope upward and outward at approximately 15 degrees away from vertical. The arch wire is then placed in the buccal tubes

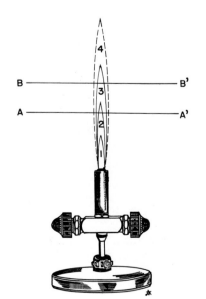

Figure 17–24 Zones of heat in an orthodontic blowpipe flame. For the greatest heat and least oxidation, the zone between the lines A-A' and B-B' is recommended. Keep flame small and maintain proper air-gas ratio. For soldering stainless steel where lower temperatures are required, the tip of zone 4 is more desirable. Fluxing must be ample to prevent oxidation.

Figure 17–25 Soldering wires of different gauges. When soldering a smaller wire to a larger one (for example, an auxiliary loop spring to an arch wire), it is better to flux the end of the small wire and then place ample solder on the fluxed end to the small wire first. Reflux this end and then carry it to the fluxed scratch mark of the larger wire, where union is desired.

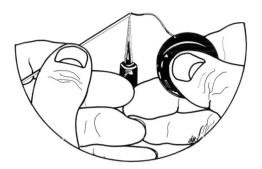

and the loops closed or opened by sliding the free end mesially or distally along the arch. To close the loop, the two legs are merely "pinched" together with How or office pliers. To open the loop, the top portion of the loop is grasped with the flat beaks of the office pliers and flattened. The distal end of the loop will automatically move away from the mesial leg. Control of the vertical loop permits the advancing or retracting of the arch wire. The same technique of arch fabrication may be used for an arch wire to receive extraoral force or intermaxillary elastics. Loops are easily soldered to the inferior surface of the arch wire at the canine-lateral incisor embrasure to receive the extraoral force appliance arm, or the intermaxillary elastic (Fig. 17–28). (See Chap. 18.)

When the arch wire is first placed, the distal ends of the vertical loops just touch the mesial ends of the buccal tubes. To tie the arch wire into place, a steel or brass ligature wire is passed through the vertical loop and around the distal end of the buccal tube, and the two ends of the ligature wire are twisted tightly. The excess ligature wire is cut off leaving a "pigtail" about an eighth of an inch in length. This is tucked under the arch wire so that it will not irritate the buccal mucosa.

LIGATION OF MAXILLARY INCISOR TO ARCH WIRE. In the anterior cross-bite situation previously described, where there is a maxillary incisor in lingual cross-bite with adequate space in the arch but with insufficient overbite to allow

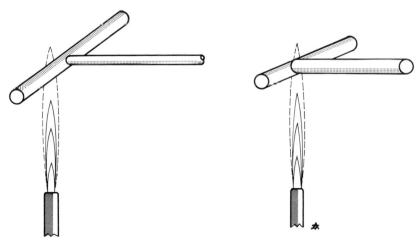

Figure 17–26 Soldering wires of different gauges. Smaller wire end that has already been covered with solder and refluxed is approximated with scratch mark on larger wire. Heat of flame is directed primarily on larger wire to allow solder to flow to it (left). If both wires were the same gauge, the heat would be directed precisely at the point of union (right).

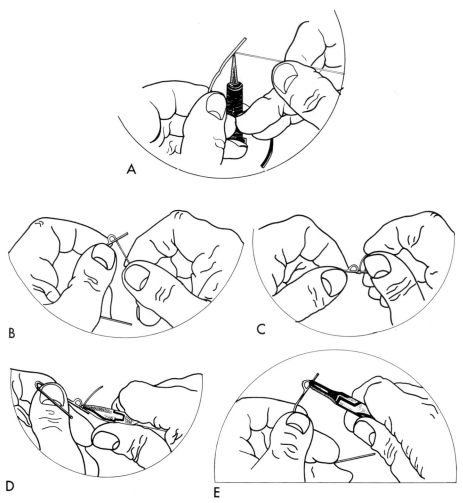

Figure 17–27 Soldering and fabricating a vertical spring loop. A, Attaching the mesial end of the 0.030 inch nichrome auxiliary wire to the arch wire (see Fig. 17–26). B, Loop has been formed over round beak of No. 139 pliers and distal end is ready to wrap around the facial surface of the arch wire. C, Distal end of loop has been wrapped around arch wire, using strong thumb and forefinger pressure. D, Excess wire is removed with wire cutting pliers. E, Cut end is polished and firmly pressed against arch wire with office or How type pliers.

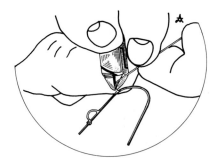

Figure 17–28 Fabricating an extraoral loop or intermaxillary elastic hook. A 0.030 inch nichrome auxiliary wire is soldered to arch wire as outlined in Figures 17–24, 17–25. Scratch mark on arch is usually at the canine-lateral incisor embrasure. Loop or hook is bent mesially over the round beak of No. 139 pliers. When extraoral force arms only are to be used, the mesial end of the loop is often soldered also, to give added strength to the attachment since this is an area of great stress. The procedure is repeated for the opposite side.

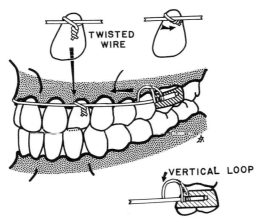

Figure 17–29   Use of labial arch with vertical spring loops to correct incisor lingual cross-bite in case where guide plane is contraindicated. The lingually malposed incisor is ligated to the arch wire as illustrated and the ligature pigtail tucked under the arch. The vertical spring loops at the molar tubes are opened to "advance" the arch wire. (See dotted outline at molar tube.) This exerts a labial vector of force on the ligated tooth, with the reciprocal force being directed against the molars. The same appliance can be used to retract incisors by closing the vertical spring loops and ligating the free distal end of the loop to the buccal tube. In this instance there is a forward reciprocal vector against the molars as the incisors are being moved lingually, which may have to be offset by extraoral force or intermaxillary elastics. (See Chaps. 11 and 18.)

the use of a guide plane, this tooth may be ligated directly to the labial arch wire (Fig. 17–29). A steel ligature is passed through the mesial embrasure, around the lingual and back through the distal embrasure. One end of the ligature wire passes beneath the arch wire, the other above it. The dentist then places the ball of the index finger on the lingual surface of the tooth in cross-bite and the thumb of the same hand against the arch wire directly labial to the tooth. Pressing the two together until the tissue blanches between them, he then twists the "pigtail" of the ligature wire until it is pulled up tightly. The excess is cut off as previously described and the pigtail tucked under the arch wire out of harm's way. This is usually quite adequate pressure, although additional force may be gained by opening the vertical loops at the molar buccal tube and advancing the arch wire to the labial.

At least a 2-week period should elapse before another corrective adjustment. Three or four such adjustments are usually required. The malposed tooth, however, can be moved completely into correct alignment, in contrast with the guide plane, where the tooth is moved only across the bite and the balance of the movement relies on autonomous adjustment. The correction thus takes eight to ten weeks to complete. The patient can be expected to complain more of looseness and soreness of the malposed tooth than if the same problem had been corrected by means of the guide plane.

The use of this labial arch wire to close or open spaces or to retract or advance incisors is described later.

POSTERIOR CROSS-BITE

Accidents of eruption also occur in the buccal segments, and the cross-bite of a maxillary or mandibular premolar may result. Posterior cross-bite, however, seldom occurs if there is adequate space in the arch to accommodate the teeth. The dentist will usually observe an arch length deficiency when he sees a premolar in cross-bite. This problem requires the services of a specialist.

In some instances the prolonged retention of a deciduous molar deflects the erupting premolar to the buccal or lingual side. Even though the retained deciduous molar is removed, the premolar may not move into normal position because of occlusal interference. Despite adequate space, the inclined plane action prevents autonomous adjustment. In a case of this type, the dentist may render invaluable limited corrective assistance with simple appliances over a relatively short time. Using the hypothetical case of a child 12 years of age with a maxillary first premolar in buccal cross-bite, the following procedure may be employed.

Orthodontic bands must be made for the malposed tooth and for the opposing mandibular premolar (Figs. 17–4, 17–5, 17–12, 17–13). If there is sufficient arch length in the maxillary arch to accommodate the buccally locked premolar, separating wires are usually not necessary to permit the forming and cementing of the premolar bands. In the opposing arch, however, it may be necessary to place separating wires for a week to create the desired space. Often there is a tendency for the mandibular premolar to be moderately displaced lingually as a result of the primary cross-bite malposition of the opposing premolar. This is favorable if there is adequate space in the dental arch to allow restoration of normal position so that the force employed for the correction is of a reciprocal nature.

The bands for both premolars may be formed directly in the mouth, as outlined earlier in this chapter. The material should be 0.004 inch thick and 0.150 inch wide. The band material is wrapped around the tooth, adapted with an amalgam plugger and pulled up tightly either on the buccal or lingual side with office pliers. (Of course, band-forming pliers may be used if available.) Properly sized preformed and contoured bands may be used. As with the molar bands, the gingival periphery of the bands should terminate in the gingival crevice on the proximal end, though it may be above the gingival margin on the buccal and lingual sides. The band is spot welded and an insert placed at the joint, as described previously for attachment bands. After the band has been polished, it is replaced on the tooth and readapted with an amalgam plugger and the margins are carefully burnished. Assuming that the maxillary premolar is in buccal cross-bite and the mandibular premolar in lingual cross-bite, a spur of 0.030 inch steel or nichrome is soldered on the buccal surface of the maxillary premolar and another spur is soldered on the lingual surface of the mandibular premolar. These spurs are placed obliquely so as to serve as hooks for intermaxillary elastics (Fig. 17–30). The ends of the spurs are carefully polished to prevent irritation to the contiguous soft tissue. The bands may then be cemented in place. (See Cementation and Figs. 17–10, 17–11.)

After the cement has set and the excess has been removed, an intermaxillary "through-the-bite" elastic is placed. Wait 12 hours before routine elastic use to allow complete setting of the cement. To provide the correct tension, it should be the one that is stretched roughly twice its length when in place (Figs. 17–31, 17–32). The elastic is worn by the patient at all times except during meals. Each time an elastic is removed, it is discarded and a new one put in place after the meal. Elastics are worn while asleep and awake. The reciprocal action of the elastic tends to move the mandibular premolar buccally and the maxillary premolar lingually.

Care must be exercised to prevent the mandibular premolar from moving

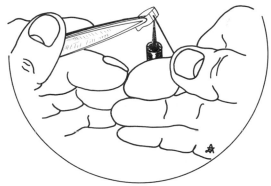

Figure 17–30   Soldering cross-bite spur on attachment band at an oblique angle. Solder is first placed on end of wire. Band and solder-tipped wire are fluxed and held over blowpipe flame with heat directed primarily on band. Solder will flow from wire to band. Excess wire is cut off and free end polished to prevent irritation. Spur is now ready to receive intermaxillary elastic.

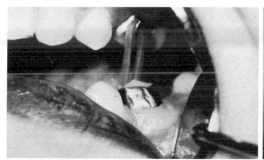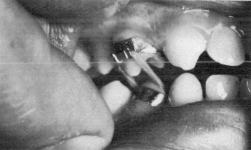

Figure 17–31   Posterior cross-bite correction. Maxillary premolar in buccal cross-bite with sufficient arch length to permit it to be moved lingually. Either soldered wire spurs (left), welded or soldered hooks (right) or prefabricated buttons may be used to hold the "through-the-bite" intermaxillary elastic.

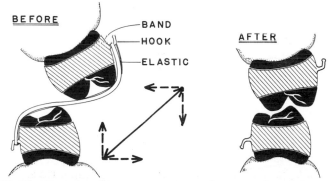

Figure 17–32   Drawing illustrates reciprocal action of cross-bite elastics.

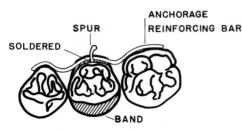

SOLDERED — SPUR — ANCHORAGE REINFORCING BAR

BAND

VIEW FROM OCCLUSAL

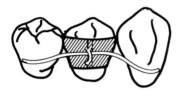

VIEW FROM LINGUAL

Figure 17–33 Bolstering anchorage in cross-bite correction to prevent mandibular second premolar from moving too far buccally under influence of criss-cross elastics. Reinforcing bar utilizes resistance of first premolar and first permanent molar. This arrangement may also be placed in upper arch, or on buccal aspect if needed.

too far to the buccal. If the dentist expects that this might be the case, he may bolster his mandibular anchorage by placing a horizontal bar on the lingual side of the mandibular band so that the ends of this bar engage the tooth on either side (Fig. 17–33). This, in effect, pits the resistance of three teeth against that of one—the maxillary premolar in cross-bite.

If the patient cooperates and if room is adequate, cross-bite correction in the premolar area takes 8 to 15 weeks. Tissue reaction is variable and correction may take as long as 16 weeks. Even though cross-bite correction is usually self-retaining, it is advisable to leave the bands in place after the correction and to have the patient wear elastics over a short period of time for a few hours a day just to assure the stability of the result.

A frequent form of posterior cross-bite is that of the maxillary second molar. The mandibular molar is forced lingually as it erupts, with the occlusal surface

CROSS BITES   MOLAR

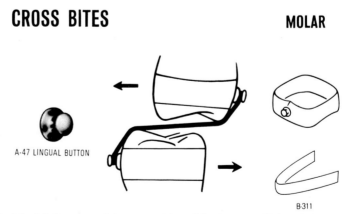

A-47 LINGUAL BUTTON

B-311

Figure 17–34 Molar cross-bite correction. Maximum efficiency is attained by using preformed bands and welding lingual buttons on the buccal and lingual sides of the bands, as indicated. Patient comfort is greater than with spurs or hooks. (Courtesy Rocky Mountain Dental Products Co.)

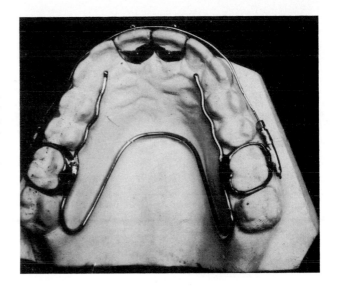

Figure 17–35 Bilateral expansion appliance designed by H. C. Pollock. The fixed removable lingual arch could be removed for adjustment and replaced or could be activated directly in the mouth. Buccal tubes on the molar bands allowed correction of individual tooth malpositions and incisor retraction, as indicated.

contacting the tongue. Cross-bite correction is similar to the technique just described (Fig. 17–34). Molar bands may be made directly or indirectly. There is usually greater sensitivity to the elastic hooks or spurs and likely discomfort for three or four days, particularly on the lingual side of the lower band, with irritation of the tongue. It usually takes 16 to 20 weeks to eliminate the second molar cross-bite. In stubborn cases, some occlusal adjustment is necessary to "jump" the bite by reducing the large maxillary lingual cusp. If this condition is not intercepted before eruption of third molars, cross-bite correction may require third molar removal. As with so many interceptive and limited orthodontic procedures, consultation with an orthodontist may be beneficial before instituting appliance therapy.

It was pointed out in Chapter 6 that finger and tongue habits often create a narrow maxillary arch. As the patient closes from postural resting position to occlusion, there is a premature contact caused by the narrowed maxillary buccal segments. Frequently there is a convenience swing to the right or left, from the point of initial contact. Generally, the swing is to the side opposite the side at which the finger is being sucked. For example, if the patient sucks his left thumb (placing it on the left side of arch), the mandible will probably swing to the right, creating what is apparently a right mandibular cross-bite. This does not mean that only the right maxillary buccal segment is collapsed, as some clinicians assume. The narrowing is bilateral and the correction must be bilateral. Such a problem is shown in Figure 17–36. A removable appliance with a mid-sagittal jackscrew may also be used to correct the bilateral narrowing. (See Fig. 16–26.)

One of the first fixed-removable appliances developed for treatment problems was the Pollock appliance (Fig. 17–35). Expansion was placed in the lingual wire assemblage. The appliance was constricted to fit into the lingual attachments on the molars. As the wire attempted to return to its original expanded conformity, the lingual extensions on each side exerted a buccal force vector. Usually buccal molar tubes are placed and a labial arch is used, if needed for individual tooth position change or incisor retraction (Figs. 17–35, 17–36). The lingual assemblage is placed away from the palate if a finger or tongue habit is still present; otherwise, it more closely follows the palatal contour.

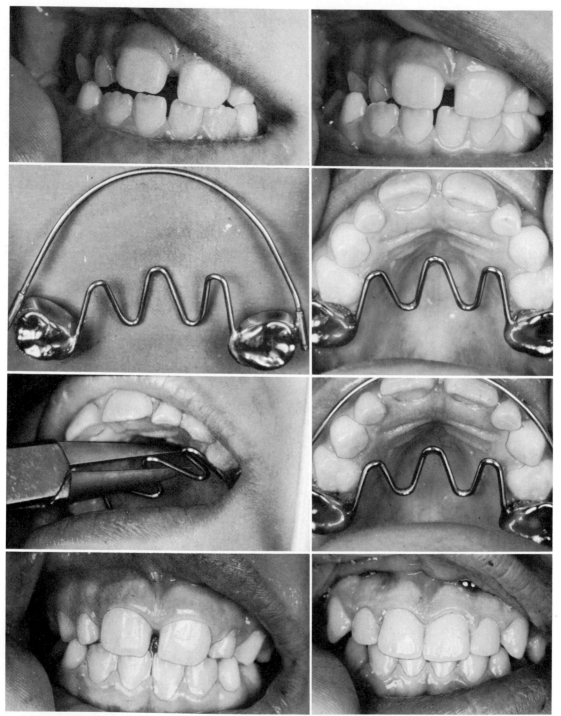

Figure 17-36   Tongue thrust habit, narrow maxillary arch and convenience shift to patient's right. Top row, left, shows point of initial contact with midlines in correct relationship. Full occlusion (top row, right) shows shift and cross-bite on patient's right. (Second row) Appliance with labial wire in buccal tubes on full metal crowns. Appliance is cemented on second deciduous molars. Third row shows pliers opening palatal "V" loops to enhance expansion. (Third row, right) Both lingual and labial wires are in place. Upper right deciduous canine may be ligated to arch wire, if necessary. (Bottom row, left) Immediately after appliance removal. (Bottom row, right) One year later with self-closure of diastema.

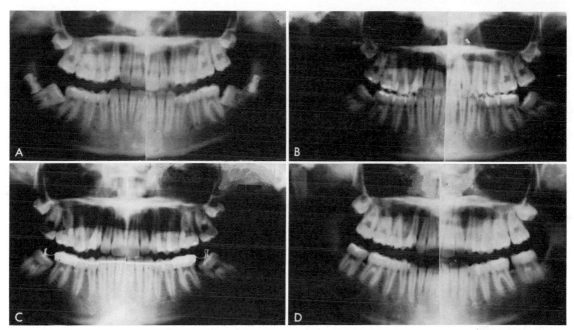

Figure 17–37 Impacted second and third molars in a 12-year-old boy. Mandibular third molars were removed. After a year of "watchful waiting" for eruption, lower molar bands and a lingual arch were fabricated. Finger springs were soldered to the lingual arch, engaging the central fossae of the partially erupted second molars. Progress of the correction was constant and uneventful.

A simple lingual arch may be used at times to effect tooth movement. Labial or buccal tipping of individual teeth is accomplished readily. Individual finger springs may be soldered to the arch wire, even as with the removable appliances, as described in Chapter 16. Figure 17–37 illustrates the use of a lingual arch and finger spring combination to tip upward mandibular second molar teeth that were impacted. An alternate method would have been surgical uprighting (see chap. 15).

REFERENCES

1. Moyers, R. E.: Handbook of Orthodontics. 3rd ed. Chicago, Year Book Medical Publishers, Inc., 1972.
2. Graber, T. M. (ed.): Current Orthodontic Principles and Techniques. Philadelphia, W. B. Saunders Co., 1969.
3. Gianelly, A. A., and Goldman, H. M.: Biologic Basis of Orthodontics. Philadelphia, Lea & Febiger, 1971.
4. Hemley, S.: A Textbook on Orthodontics. Washington, D.C., Coiner Publications, 1971.
5. Fogel, M. S., and Magill, J. M.: The Combination Technique in Orthodontic Practice. Philadelphia, J. B. Lippincott, 1972.

chapter 18

LIMITED CORRECTIVE ORTHODONTICS: ORTHOREHABILITATIVE PROCEDURES AND EXTRAORAL FORCE

ANTERIOR SPACING PROBLEMS

The dentist frequently sees patients with normal occlusion except for the maxillary anterior segment. The incisors may be flared labially and spaced; this condition may respond to a removable appliance (Chap. 16). Wherever possible, use of a removable appliance rather than fixed appliances is encouraged for the dentist in general practice. If one assumes that the removable appliance will accomplish the therapeutic objective, then the dentist who uses it is less likely to face tissue damage or an iatrogenic malocclusion. The choice of the proper appliance should be made after consultation with an orthodontic specialist. Frequent cross-consultation is strongly encouraged. Both the patient and the dentist will benefit.

In some cases one or more teeth may have been lost through an accident or caries, or there may be a peg-shaped or abnormally shaped lateral incisor, or actual congenital absence, with drifting and tipping of contiguous teeth. Before making an artificial replacement that is esthetically and functionally proper, orthodontic procedures are indicated to align the anterior teeth. For effective control of individual teeth, orthodontic bands must usually be placed. There are many variations of anterior spacing problems. In some instances it is possible to close the space of a congenitally missing tooth; in others, it is necessary to open space for an artificial replacement. Overbite and overjet are important conditioning factors.

EXAMPLE OF ANTERIOR SPACING PROBLEM—ANTERIOR DIASTEMA

Since it is not possible to describe all different anterior spacing problems and the orthorehabilitative therapy employed in each instance, a hypothetical anterior diastema problem is used to illustrate limited orthodontic treatment procedures. The procedures can be modified for other anterior spacing problems.

A 9-year-old boy comes into the dentist's office for the first time, and a large space between his upper front teeth is immediately noticed. The parent is concerned and asks what should be done. There may or may not be a heavy frenum attachment, but the incisors are upright, mesiodistally, so that the teeth are apparently bodily displaced from their normal position of proximal contact. There is a slightly excessive overjet because of the increase in anterior arch length, but the occlusion of the posterior teeth is normal. This type of patient is not an unusual one. Lip activity may actually be accentuating the malocclusion, and is of concern to the dentist.

INITIAL CONSIDERATIONS

To close the space with a removable appliance means tipping the crowns together, since there is relatively little control possible for the movement of the apices. With bands on the central incisors and hooks for elastics or contractile thread, the teeth may be moved together quickly, but this is a tipping and possibly rotational movement; the apices may still remain separated, with the diastema opening up again when restraining appliances are removed (Fig. 18–1A). To ensure bodily movement of apices as well as crowns, both central incisors

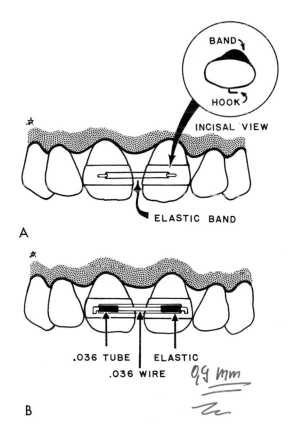

Figure 18–1 Closing central incisor diastema with simple fixed appliances. A, Use of hooks on labial side of band in conjunction with elastic for motivating force. This seldom produces desired positioning of teeth because of tipping and lack of rotational control. B, Bodily movement of incisors is effected by elastic because horizontal tube attachments on bands prevent tipping and rotation of teeth. Orthodontic brackets can produce the same movement with similar control and more versatility in placing and removing the arch wire.

may be banded and horizontal tubes placed in the middle third of their labial surfaces. A short segment of arch wire the same size as the inside diameter of the tubes is slid into place and the ends bent down to reduce irritation and to prevent the segment from coming out (Fig. 18–1B). A rubber elastic, contractile thread or a stainless-steel figure-of-eight ligature is then placed over the projecting arch segment ends so as to move the central incisors together. Since the tube must slide mesially in maintaining a constantly parallel relationship to the arch segment, as in a sleeve and arm situation, the whole tooth moves mesially as a unit, root as well as crown. This is truly a reciprocal anchorage setup, with stationary or bodily resistance of each incisor. The correct axial inclination is maintained as the diastema is closed, and there is less chance for relapse than with the "tipping" of a removable appliance.

If lateral incisors are already in good position and merely diminutive or peg-shaped, all that has to be done to ensure space closure at the midline is to place jacket crowns on the lateral incisors, restoring normal shape and size to these teeth (Fig. 16–36). But, unfortunately, when central incisors are displaced bodily the lateral incisors are usually also displaced. Overjet becomes excessive because of the increase in arch length. Two bands alone are inadquate, regardless of the type of attachment.

In most problems where there is an anterior diastema the fixed appliances required must move the teeth in all planes of space—vertically, labially, lingually, mesially and distally. This means bands for at least the four incisors and possibly the canines, and molar bands for the first permanent molars to receive the motivating arch wire.

If intraoral radiographs show that the apices of the incisors are sufficiently formed; if a study of other diagnostic records indicates clearly that the spacing is purely a local problem, with normal arch relationship in the buccal segment; if the dentist knows how to make attachment bands and molar bands properly, has had some previous experience with moving teeth and has a healthy regard for potency of fixed appliances, he may try the following fixed banding approach for correcting the spacing—*provided he has an orthodontist with whom he may consult over any problems that may arise.* An even better arrangement in fixed appliance cases is to make definite arrangements for periodic checks of the patient's progress by the orthodontist to make sure treatment is progressing satisfactorily. (Some sort of per-visit financial remuneration can be established to compensate the orthodontist for his time and advice, as is done so frequently in medicine.)

THERAPEUTIC PROCEDURE

The four maxillary incisor teeth are banded and attachments placed on the labial surfaces to accommodate an orthodontic arch wire. Twin edgewise brackets, single edgewise brackets with rotation eyelets at the mesial and distal surfaces or twin-wire brackets may be used (Fig. 18–2). Great care must be taken that the bands are made properly and that the brackets occupy the middle third of the teeth, gingivo-incisally and mesiodistally. The first permanent molars are banded, using rectangular buccal tubes. (See discussion on molar band fabrication in Chap. 17.) A 0.016 inch stainless-steel arch wire is carefully shaped to follow the contour of the maxillary arch, and the arch ends are inserted in each molar buccal tube. The arch wire should fit into the bracket slot with only very slight pressure. If the lateral incisors are either set back lingually a bit or not as far erupted, with the corresponding coronal portions higher than for the central

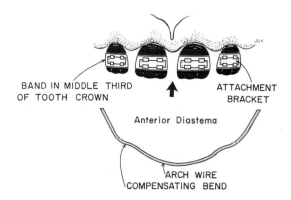

Figure 18–2 Incisor teeth banded and ready for placement of 0.014 or 0.016 inch stainless-steel arch wire. Because of different heights of central and lateral incisors, offset and compensating bends would be necessary to permit arch wire to lie passively in all brackets. Twin edgewise brackets are used to give rotational control. This eliminates the need for rotating eyelets in most instances.

incisors, compensating or offset bends should be made between the central and lateral incisors to permit the arch wire to lie relatively passively in the attachment bracket slots (Fig. 18–2). The posterior ends of the arch wire should project approximately a quarter of an inch distal to the buccal tubes when the arch wire is in place. These ends must be turned sharply to the lingual side with a How or office pliers to prevent laceration of the mucosa of the cheek, after the arch wire has been tied into the brackets. The dentist should always check these ends with his index finger before dismissing the patient (Fig. 18–3).

After it has been determined that the arch wire is passive, or that the deformation of the arch is of a very slight degree as it is inserted in the bracket slots, stainless-steel ligature wire is used to "tie in" the arch to place. The ligature is passed beneath the upper and lower wings of the bracket, passing over the arch wire on the mesial and distal ends (Fig. 18–4). The two ends are twisted to form a "pigtail." All but an eighth of an inch of this pigtail is cut off, and the remainder is tucked securely under the arch wire with a flat amalgam plugger to prevent irritation of the lip (see Fig. 12–9).

Appointments should be at approximately 3-week intervals. One or two adjustments are usually sufficient to iron out the offset bends and to level the incisors. At each visit the arch wire is removed by clipping the ligature ties with ligature-cutting pliers and straightening the bent in ends of the arch before grasping the arch firmly just mesial to the buccal tubes and pulling sharply in an anterior direction.

After one or two visits to permit the leveling of the incisors, an 0.018 inch

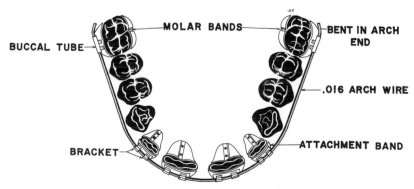

Figure 18–3 Occlusal view to show relation of arch wire to teeth in the buccal segment. Note that the distal ends of the arch wire are bent sharply to the lingual aspect after the arch has been inserted, to prevent irritation of the buccal mucosa.

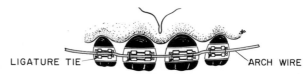

LIGATURE TIE   ARCH WIRE

Figure 18–4   Arch wire tied in place and ligature pigtails tucked under arch wire to prevent irritation of lip.

stainless-steel arch wire is placed in the same manner as the 0.016 inch arch wire. The arch should be a smooth-flowing paraboloid arc with as few compensating bends as possible. Again, the index finger should be run all around the arch from one end to the other to make sure no sharp projections are there to irritate the cheek and lips.

After a 3-week period, a 0.020 inch stainless-steel arch wire may be made. Two circular or vertical loops are bent in the arch wire just mesial to the molar tubes to permit the tying back or retracting of the maxillary arch wire (Fig. 18–5). The loops are carefully bent with a round-nose pliers (No. 139, for example), avoiding a sharp bend which might predispose the wire to a break at this point. Spurs may be soldered to the arch wire instead of using the circular loops bent into the arch, but they are less satisfactory because the heat needed for soldering reduces the spring tension of the wire. The incisor bands are then ligated to the arch wire, but instead of ligating each tooth separately, a figure-of-eight ligature is used between the maxillary central incisors to bring them together (Figs. 18–6, 18–7).

If the dentist prefers, contractile elastic thread may be used to ligate the central incisors together.[2] The elastic thread, by true reciprocal force, moves the incisors together bodily. Any tendency for the teeth to tip as they move toward the midline is resisted by the sleeve-like relationship of the bracket to the arch wire. After two or three adjustments, the maxillary incisors are in contact and are then tied in this position with a steel ligature wire. The lateral incisors may then be brought toward the midline in a similar manner. At the same time, the arch wire is being tied strongly to the distal by steel ligatures wrapped around the circular or vertical loops and over the wire protruding from the end of the buccal tubes. Thus, the space between the incisors is closed by combined mesial move-

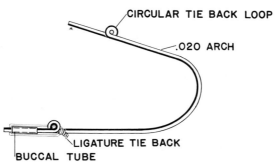

CIRCULAR TIE BACK LOOP

.020 ARCH

LIGATURE TIE BACK

BUCCAL TUBE

Figure 18–5   Circular tie-back loops, just mesial to horizontal molar buccal tubes. Ligating these distally exerts a lingual pressure on the incisor teeth. If contractile thread is used to do the ligating, more force is exerted; and if small rubber elastics are hooked over the circular loop and distal end of the arch wire, even more retracting force is applied. Circular or vertical closing loops may be bent in the arch wire to provide even greater efficiency.

Figure 18–6 A, Space closure using figure-of-eight steel ligatures to move incisors bodily along arch wire toward each other. This is reciprocal anchorage, but the force is dissipated by the incisors moving toward each other. B, The use of compressed coil spring in a case with congenital absence of maxillary lateral incisors. Canines are moved distally into contact at the same time that the central incisor diastema is closed. The arch wire is tied back at the molar tubes (Fig. 18–5) to prevent the incisors from moving labially.

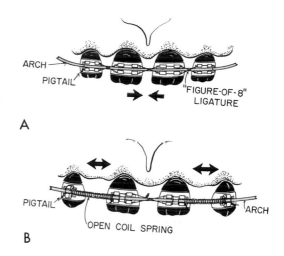

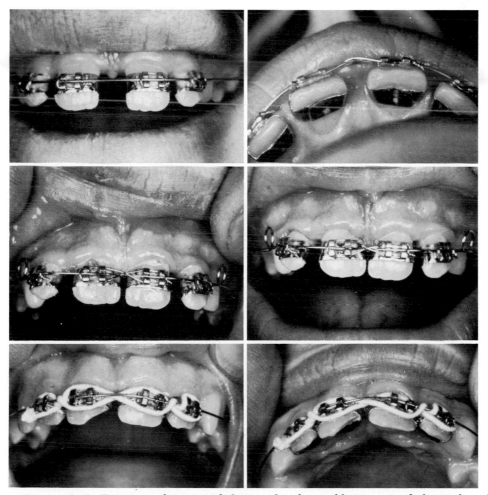

Figure 18–7 Diastema closure with figure-of-eight steel ligatures and elastic thread. Note circular closing loops bent in arch wire (middle views) to aid in space closure through retraction of incisors. Tie-back loops at molar tubes cannot be seen.

ment of the incisor teeth and retraction of these teeth to a more favorable overjet relationship. With any excessive overbite, the use of mild tip backs of the wire at the molar tubes (accentuated curve of Spee) will exert a corresponding depressing vector on the maxillary incisor segment, as the horizontal malrelationships are being eliminated. Conversely, a reverse curve of Spee in the arch will help, if there is an open bite tendency.

Orthodontic consultation is recommended repeatedly because of possible unfavorable response, such as mesial movement of the buccal segments, or at the very least, a disturbance of posterior occlusion, requiring more extensive corrective measures. Since problems arise for the specialist, with all his training and experience, this may happen more frequently for the general practitioner.

THERAPEUTIC ADJUNCTS

PALATAL BITE PLATE. If an excessive overbite is present, it is often necessary to use a palatal bite plate in conjunction with the fixed appliance. This may be constructed in the manner described in Chapter 16. If there has been a heavy frenum attachment that has been determined to be a primary etiologic factor, the incisors are moved into contact first, the frenum is carefully dissected out, and the arch wire is replaced to hold the teeth together while the tissue heals. It may take anywhere from three to nine months to achieve the correct contact relationship, overjet and overbite, depending on the nature of the original malocclusion.

COIL SPRING. An excellent adjunct in space control is a finely wound coil spring. This comes in the "open or push" or "closed or pull" coil variety. If used properly, the coil spring delivers a light, continuous force (Fig. 18–6B). Adjustments need be made less frequently because of the longer-acting characteristics for the appurtenance. Coil springs used in conjunction with anterior bands are particularly valuable where there are missing teeth and the dentist wants to consolidate space for a prosthesis and align the remaining teeth by bodily movement.

In Figure 18–8 the use of a "push" coil spring is illustrated. The force is of a reciprocal nature, moving the canines distally and the maxillary incisors mesially. In Figure 18–9 a "pull" coil spring is being used to move the maxillary central incisors bodily toward each other. Teeth moved in this manner tend to "spin" or rotate; therefore, the operator must be careful to make antirotation ligature ties to counteract the tendency. Also, prophylaxis is more of a problem for the patient.

RUBBER DAM ELASTIC. Another method of closing spaces is the use of the light rubber dam elastic. If there is a diastema between the maxillary central incisors, these teeth may be banded and either brackets or horizontal tubes may be soldered on the labial surface (Fig. 18–1B). A short section of arch wire is inserted in the brackets or tubes and an elastic attached to the distal ends of the tubes. If the teeth move, they have to move bodily as the tubes slide along the arch wire segment. The use of a horizontal tube also prevents the teeth from rotating as they migrate toward the midline. Instead of the rubber dam elastic, elastic thread may be used to effect the same movement (Fig. 18–7). In the past, contractile silk ligature has been used for the same purpose, but its slower action and tendency to trap food make it less satisfactory.

PLACEMENT OF HAWLEY TYPE RETAINER

After the malocclusion is corrected, appliances are removed, and a removable Hawley type retainer is placed and worn for an additional three to six

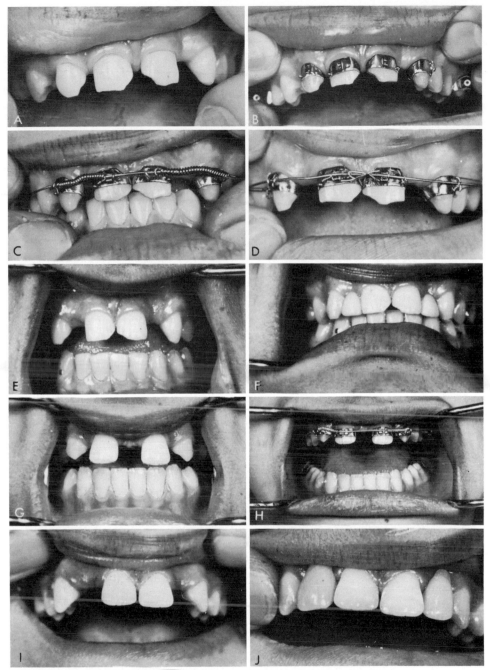

Figure 18–8 Use of "open coil" or "push coil" spring to consolidate space for prosthetic restoration of missing teeth. In the first case (A to F), normal-sized lateral incisor replacements are not possible without closing central diastema. Incisors and molars are banded (B) and an 0.018 inch steel arch placed with push coil springs compressed in edentulous spaces (C). After central incisors are moved together and canines moved into contact with first premolars, figure-of-eight ligature ties are used to hold them for about six weeks. Then appliances are removed and a retaining appliance is placed with the missing teeth until such time that permanent restoration is feasible. In the second case (G to J), the problem is similar but more severe. It was handled in the same manner. In both instances the arch wire was tied securely to the molar tubes to prevent the central incisors from moving labially as they moved together.

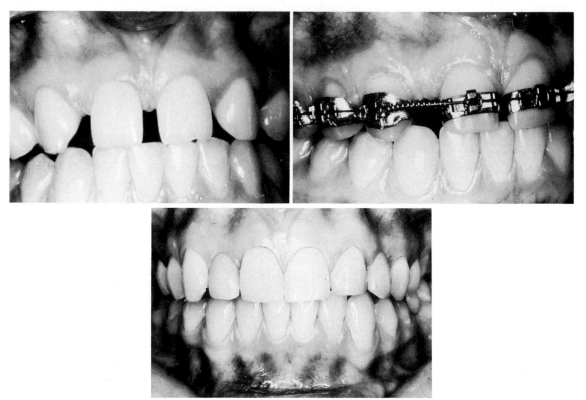

Figure 18–9   Congenital absence of maxillary lateral incisors. Spaces for missing teeth opened by push (compressed) coil springs. Rotations controlled by Steiner antirotation bracket. Prosthetic replacement may be temporary, using a removable palatal appliance, or permanent appliance, if the patient is old enough. (From Norton, L. A., and Parker, W. T.: Management of repositioned teeth in preparation for fixed partial dentures. J.A.D.A., 81:916–922, 1970.)

months to ensure the stability of the orthodontic result. (See section in Chapter 16 on The Removable Hawley Type Appliances — The Dental Crutch.) As described previously, minor movements and space control are possible with the Hawley type appliance. Such an appliance may even be modified if a fixed bridge is made, or may have teeth added to it to hold the spaces created until a permanent fixed or removable restoration is constructed (see Fig. 18–9). It may still be used indefinitely as a splint, or "crutch," if needed.

This basic appliance may be modified for use where there is congenital absence, a tooth missing due to caries or accident, or in certain types of cross-bite, where incisors are rotated (Fig. 18–6B).

The greatest danger the dentist faces, however, is to undertake correction of a problem beyond the scope of his training. This is particularly the case when he has been successful in completing treatment of a simple limited corrective problem of the type just outlined. As Figure 18–12 shows, the cross-bite has been corrected and the rotation of the upper right central incisor eliminated with a relatively simple appliance, but the "happy ending" has not been reached yet. There is still inadequate space for the lateral incisors to erupt, and further therapy is likely. Prior orthodontic consultation before undertaking deceptively "simple" problems will save many heartaches for both the patient and the dentist.

(*Text continued on page 866*)

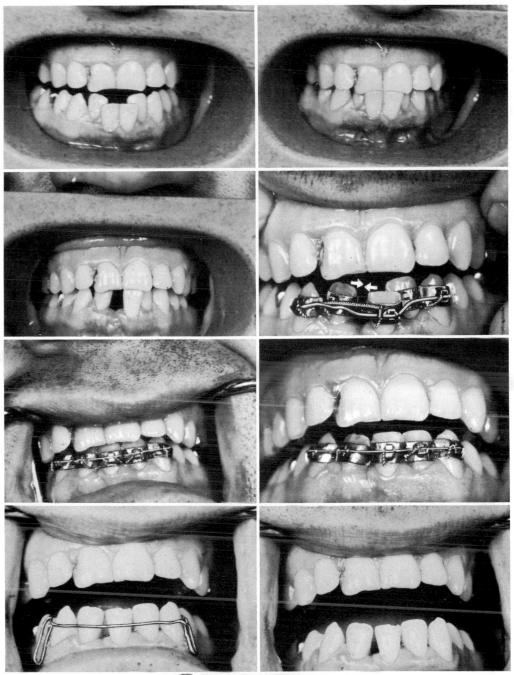

Figure 18–10 Use of "closed coil" or "pull coil" spring to move teeth together. Force application is reciprocal as with push coil, but dissipated only on teeth to which springs are attached as space is closed (see arrows). Traumatic occlusion is eliminated by removal of an incisor and alignment of remaining lower anterior teeth. No molar bands were used in this case, though they are generally advisable to give better control and to prevent "canine roll." A retainer is shown in place, but after the first six weeks after the band removal the result is largely self-sustaining. Even with fixed appliances, space control and uprighting of teeth adjacent to the extracted incisor are incomplete. As a result, the gingival tissue appears "punched-out" in this area. Further treatment to accomplish root paralleling would have been desirable.

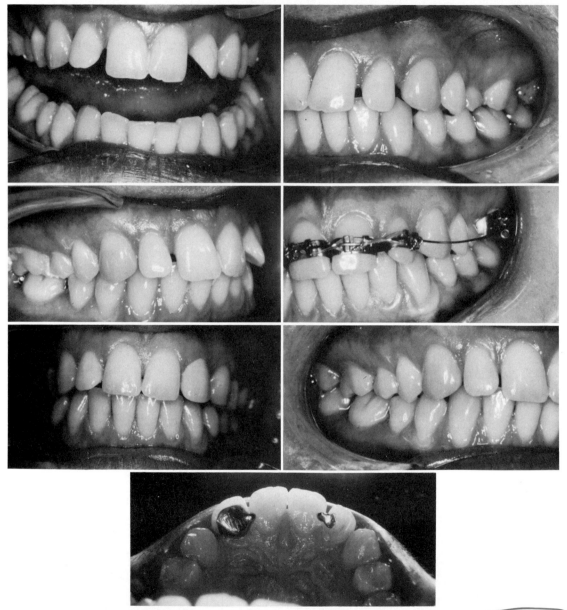

Figure 18–11   Space closure and rotation of maxillary lateral incisors. Use of twin edgewise anterior brackets for rotational control. Alastik unit joins all incisors to establish contacts. Lingual dovetail restorations with rests on central incisors prevent relapse to original malocclusion. (Courtesy George F. Andreasen.)

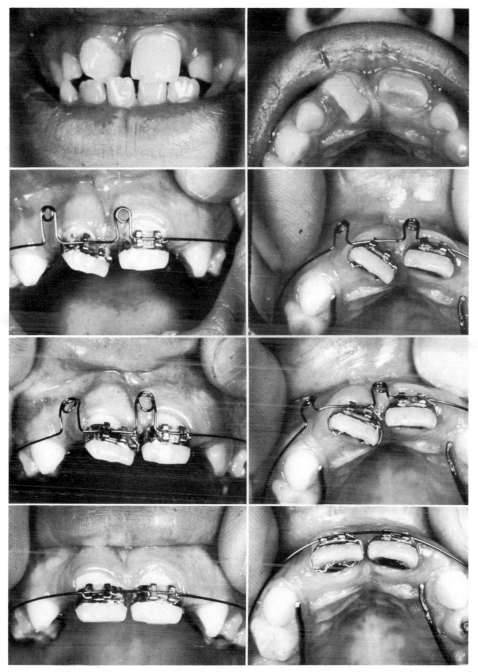

Figure 18–12   Correction of rotated incisor in lingual cross-bite. If left unattended, this kind of malocclusion may cause both lateral incisors and canines to erupt into abnormal positions and may permanently damage the investing tissues around the opposing incisors by virtue of the traumatic occlusion. Vertical helical coil springs in arch wire provide a lighter but longer-acting and effective force for correcting the rotation. Note how the arch is deformed when tied into the mesial rotation eyelet (third row). A plain round arch wire is placed after the incisors have been positioned.

UPRIGHTING MOLARS AND OPENING AND CLOSING SPACES IN PREPARATION FOR PROSTHESES (POSTERIOR SEGMENTS)

It has already been pointed out that the movement of posterior teeth is often quite difficult. Greater root surface is involved, increasing the tissue resistance to movement and making the anchorage needed to effect the desired movement a greater consideration. As many orthodontists know from bitter experience, for every force introduced there is an equal and opposite force that has to be dissipated somewhere. Even the most careful and skilled orthodontist must at times accept unwanted tooth movement to achieve his primary objective. Most of the time this unwanted tooth movement comes as he attempts to move posterior teeth. Because of the difficulties, the dentist must confine himself to the simplest of fixed orthodontic procedures in the posterior segments. Problems must be local, therapy of relatively short duration, appliances simple and adjustments easily controlled, with all responses being reasonably predictable. Finally, the dentist, like the orthodontist, must be willing to accept the fact that he cannot always achieve his therapeutic objective. A partial correction may be the optimal result obtainable. Generally speaking, the use of a removable appliance is less likely to get a dentist into real trouble—but also less likely to achieve the desired tooth movement. Here again, consultation between the general practitioner and the specialist is desirable.

CONSEQUENCES OF MOLAR LOSS

One limited orthodontic service that can be rendered with fixed appliances without becoming too involved is the uprighting and alignment of the posterior teeth where they have tipped and rotated into an edentulous area due to the removal of a first permanent molar. It is an unfortunate fact that many children lose their first molar teeth because of lack of caries control. The periodontist knows the broad implications of such loss. He sees the same people in later life with contiguous teeth drifting into the spaces, with excessive overbites, with tipped teeth receiving stress laterally instead of through their long axes, with traumatic interferences, premature contacts, tooth guidance problems (Fig. 18–22), functional retrusions and temporomandibular joint problems and, as a result of one or more of the conditions, soft tissue pathology and bone loss (Figs. 18–13, 18–14).

Edward H. Angle called the first molar the "key to occlusion" and as far as the stability of the denture is concerned this is no exaggeration.[1] If the first molar must be lost, strenuous efforts must be made either to control the space closure with fixed orthodontic appliances—or to maintain space and insert a suitable replacement to preserve the integrity of the surrounding teeth and investing tissues.

Space control is almost always a greater challenge in the mandibular first molar area. After early loss of a maxillary first molar, one may later find a relatively normally positioned second molar still in its place. This is not so in the lower arch, where the crown will tip forward only, while the apices remain "as is." Movement of the mandibular molars seems to be more difficult for the orthodontist and the presence, position and relative state of development of the third molar is a factor. Yet it is the lower molar loss that presents the greatest damage potential, and should be controlled. Space closure is seldom possible or desirable with limited therapy.

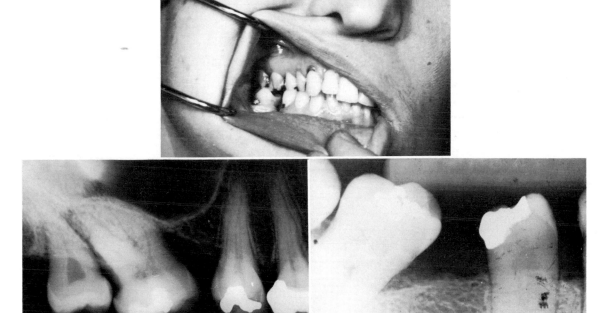

Figure 18-13   A lost first permanent molar, whether it is an upper or lower molar, means a developing malocclusion as the contiguous teeth drift, tip and elongate. Pocket formation is followed by bone loss, traumatic occlusion and ultimate loss of one or more teeth unless the dentist reverses this trend and restores stress to the long axis of the teeth by uprighting them and stabilizing them in their proper positions with a properly made fixed or removable bridge.

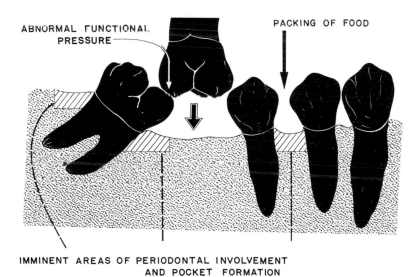

Figure 18-14   Areas in which damage is most likely to result from the loss of a mandibular first permanent molar. As the molar tips, stress is no longer transmitted to the lamina dura as tension but as pressure on the mesial surfaces of the alveoli.

If the space loss is only slight, a split acrylic spring type removable space regainer may be used to re-establish the proper space (Fig. 18–15). Or, a jackscrew arrangement can be built into the space maintainer, with the space being opened gradually as the jackscrew is opened (Fig. 18–16). Then the nut is crimped on the threaded end section to hold the space regained. An alternate type of space regainer that works well for opening small spaces for premolars and first permanent molars (where such space is available in the dental arch) is the cantilever spring-and-bar space regainer (Fig. 18–17). This type of appliance is less resistant to displacement by the forces of occlusion than the jackscrew two-unit appliance, and it is harder to deep clean (see space regainer, Fig. 13–15).

All too often the dentist sees the patient first "after the horse is practically out of the barn." The first molar may have been lost at 8 or 9 years of age; by the time the child is 12 to 15, the second molar has erupted into a mesially tipped position and the premolars have drifted distally, opening up contacts which allow the packing of food. The opposing teeth may already have elongated and created additional functional problems (Fig. 18–13). It is still not too late to recover the situation in many instances. Simple fixed orthodontic appliances may be used, and these, in conjunction with selective occlusal grinding, may achieve a relatively satisfactory result in a period of 4 to 8 months. The reward is a lifetime of stable occlusion if the situation is handled properly.

In the maxillary arch, as it has been pointed out already, the loss of a first permanent molar need not be disastrous. The second permanent molar may come forward in relatively untipped attitude. The long axes converge apically in the maxillary arch; they diverge apically in the mandibular arch. Premolars may or may not drift distally. Stresses are usually still delivered primarily through the long axes of these teeth. This is seldom true in the mandibular arch, however. The second molar, when it erupts, usually tips forward at an oblique angle, and the mandibular premolars usually move or tip distally. The second molar is particularly susceptible to abnormal stresses, with the alternate bone breakdown and deposition at the mesial and distal surfaces and with ultimate pocket formation (Figs. 18–13, 18–14). It is wise to correct such problems before the third molar erupts. If this is not possible, sometimes it is necessary to remove the third molar to upright the tipped second molar. The best age for correction is between 12 and 16 years. A limited fixed appliance technique is described here, using the loss of a mandibular first permanent molar as an example. In this hypothetical

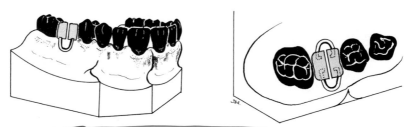

Figure 18–15. Split acrylic spring space regainer. A 0.032 inch stainless wire is soldered to form an ellipse. The ellipse is compressed about one third its diameter in the edentulous space that is to be increased. An acrylic mass is incorporated over it, either by waxing, flasking and curing or by using endothermic acrylic. Careful adaptation of the acrylic to the proximal surfaces of the contiguous teeth is necessary for maximal retention. After the acrylic has been polished and tried for fit, it is divided down the center with a safeside disk, restoring the stored spring action. Minor adjustments are made with flat beak pliers at lingual and labial loops.

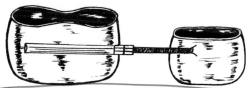

Figure 18–16. Jackscrew type space regainer-maintainer. This type of space regainer is more durable than the cantilever type, but less desirable if the teeth contiguous to the edentulous area are markedly tipped, since movement with this type of appliance is only along the long axis of the horizontal molar tube that houses the threaded end section. After the two nuts have been turned enough to open the desired space, they may be crimped to lock them and prevent unwinding.

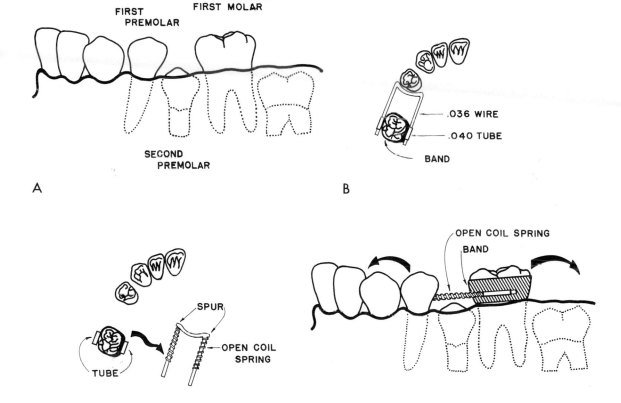

Figure 18–17. Cantilever type coil spring space regainer. A, Drift of contiguous teeth partially impacts an erupting second premolar. B, Molar is banded, 0.040 inch horizontal tubes are placed on buccal and lingual sides, and 0.036 inch crib fabricated and fitted so it glides freely in the tubes. C, Spurs are soldered at the mesial end of the U-shaped bar and open coil springs one third again as long as the space fitted on the U-crib. D, The U-crib with springs in place is slid into the buccal and lingual tubes, compressing the open coil spring. The resultant reciprocal force tips the molar distally and the first premolar mesially. (Courtesy H. P. Hitchcock.)

case, the patient is assumed to be 13 years of age, and the damaging effects of the loss will not have been felt yet.

THERAPEUTIC PROCEDURES

As with any limited orthodontic problem, complete diagnostic records should be made. Study models should be related properly and the facets of occlusal wear should be noted and recorded. Radiographic examination shows the position of the unerupted third molar and any tissue pathology. All caries should be eliminated before the fixed orthodontic appliance is placed.

BANDING OF TEETH.   In most cases it will be necessary to make orthodontic bands for the tipped second molar and for the two premolars. It is good practice to include the canine in this setup (Fig. 18–18).

The band for the second molar tooth may be made either indirectly from a stone model or directly in the mouth. (See Chap. 17.) As with the fixed appliance constructed for anterior space control, the molar band should have a horizontal rectangular (0.022 by 0.028) tube soldered or welded on the buccal surface. The tube should parallel the occlusal surface and be perpendicular to the long axis of the tooth (Fig. 18–18). It is likewise possible to construct the bands for the premolars and canines directly or indirectly since these teeth are usually spaced, and bands can be made easily in either instance without any special preparation. The mandibular premolars are the most difficult teeth to band. These bands tend

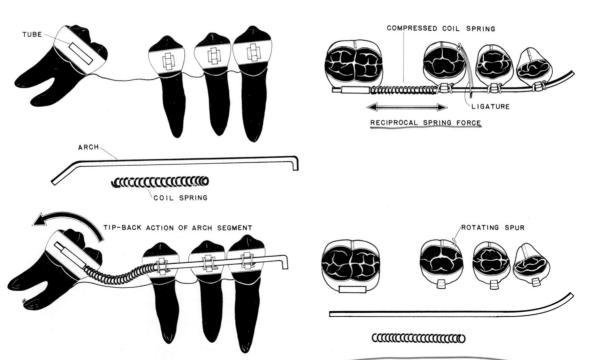

Figure 18–18 Diagram of appliance construction for uprighting mandibular molars and premolars where a first permanent molar has been lost. Band and bracket position is important. Molar tube should parallel occlusal surface. Rotating eyelet should be placed mesial to second premolar and mesial to first premolar if the latter has any appreciable distance to travel. Coil spring should be one fourth to one third again as long as the space between the molar tube and second premolar bracket. When compressed into the available space, it tips the molar back with the help of the arch segment action, and at the same time moves the second premolar mesially.

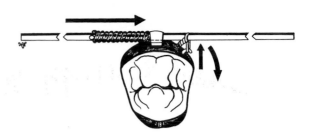

Figure 18–19 Detail of antirotation tie for second premolar in coil spring uprighting appliance illustrated in Figure 18–18. Coil spring tends to "spin" premolars unless precautions are taken.

to loosen under the pounding of occlusal forces more than for any other teeth. Hence the bands must be made carefully and must be well adapted to the teeth. Excellent preformed contoured bands may be procured commercially with or without the brackets already attached. Contoured 0.004 by 0.150 inch band material strips with or without the brackets attached are also available. The same situation prevails for the canines. Ordinary strip band material may be used and satisfactory bands can be fabricated, but they require more time and considerable contouring to achieve the desired fit. Preformed contoured bands are quite a time saver here, too.

As with the anterior teeth, the brackets should be placed as closely to the middle third of the premolar teeth as possible. The slot should be perpendicular to the long axis of the teeth. In some instances the bracket position must be altered by moving it gingivally because of the occlusal contact of the opposing premolar cusp. The occlusion should be checked as each band is being formed to make sure that the bracket is not being pounded, creating a prematurity. As with the anterior bands, the author prefers the use of a twin edgewise bracket because of its greater arch wire-bearing surface and greater resistance to rotational forces. In addition to the twin edgewise bracket a rotating eyelet or spur should be placed at the mesial surface of the second premolar band to counteract the strong rotating effect of the "push" coil spring that will be used to upright the second molar and close the spaces in the premolar area (Fig. 18–19). After all the bands have been made according to the techniques described in the previous chapter, they should be driven to place and checked carefully before cementation. If there is no occlusal interference endangering either the horizontal buccal tube or the brackets, the bands may then be cemented. The time-tested zinc phosphate cement is quite safe to use for bands, but some of the newer polyacrylic or epoxy compounds are superior for bands that are likely to be under severe stress.[3, 4] (See discussion in Chap. 17 on Cementation.)

FABRICATION OF ARCH WIRE. After the excess cement has been removed, the arch segment may be fabricated and placed. It is wise to start off with a 0.016 inch stainless-steel round wire. The wire is inserted in the horizontal buccal tube on the second molar and allowed to protrude on the distal approximately one eighth of an inch. The anterior portion is lifted up to the level of the bracket on the canine and clipped off approximately one quarter inch mesial to the canine bracket. As the arch wire is lifted to the level of the bracket slot, there is a "tipback" action on the molar and a strong reciprocal depressing force on the premolars and canine (Figs. 18–18 to 18–20). The 0.016 inch stainless-steel wire segment is removed, and the last quarter inch on the anterior end is bent down at a right angle to the segment itself.

A 0.007 or 0.008 inch thick "push" or open coil spring is then selected for the space between the mesial surface of the molar tube and the distal surface of the second premolar bracket. This spring should be approximately one fourth again

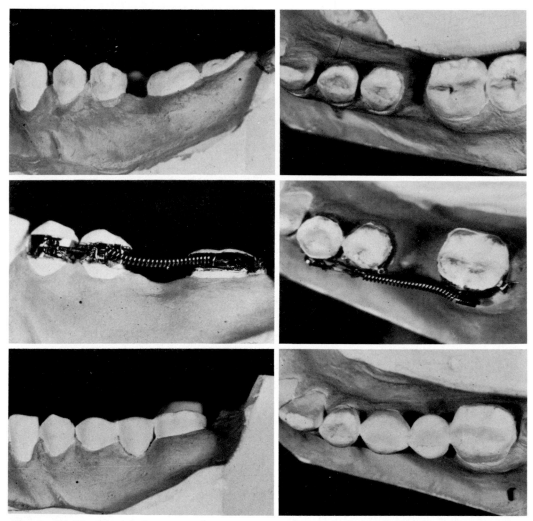

Figure 18-20 Uprighting second permanent molar and closing premolar and canine spaces. Third molar was removed. Although fixed bridge did not restore complete mesiodistal width of first permanent molar, it distributes stress physiologically to abutment teeth. (Courtesy Raleigh Williams.)

as long as the space. The coil spring is placed on the wire segment, and the segment is then inserted into the molar buccal tube with the anterior portion being lifted to the level of the brackets and inserted. The anterior bent-down vertical portion of the segment is approximated mesial to the canine bracket. The coil spring is compressed between the mesial side of the molar tube and the distal side of the premolar bracket (Figs. 18–18 to 18–20). Stainless-steel ligature wire is then used to ligate the 0.016 inch arch segment into place on the premolar and canine brackets. The pigtails are clipped and tucked in carefully beneath the arch wire segment.

It is good practice to turn in the distal end of the arch wire slightly toward the molar band to prevent the cheek from being irritated by it. The dentist should run his finger over the appliance to make sure that there are no sharp projections. It is wise to give the patient some soft utility or baseplate wax to adapt over the appliance in the event that there is some soft tissue irritation. Chewing gum may be used in an emergency. An analysis of the forces involved shows that there is a tipping upward and backward of the second molar. A mesial vector combined with a depressing force is exerted against the premolars and canine (Fig. 18–18).

FOLLOW-UP APPOINTMENTS AND ADJUSTMENTS.   After the appliances are placed, the patient is instructed about proper prophylaxis and diet limitations. He should be particularly admonished against eating sticky, chewy candy, popcorn and the like. The teeth will probably be sore for two to three days. If there has been some overeruption of the opposing first permanent molar, it also may be sore because of the creation of a traumatic occlusion. Frequently it is necessary to do some equilibration to expedite tooth movement and reduce the trauma. Adjustments should be made at approximately 3-week intervals. At the second or third visit, a 0.018 inch stainless-steel round wire is substituted for the initial 0.016 inch wire and a new length of 0.007 inch open coil spring one fourth again as long as the space between the mesial side of the molar buccal tube and the distal end of the second premolar bracket is placed on the arch segment. This is ligated to place again with the anterior end of the segment bent down at the mesial surface of the canine and the distal end of the segment is bent in slightly toward the band at the posterior end of the molar tube.

Three weeks later, at the third or fourth visit, a rectangular wire segment, 0.022 by 0.022 inch or 0.021 by 0.025 inch is substituted for the 0.018 inch round segment. The anterior end is bent down as previously and the push coil spring

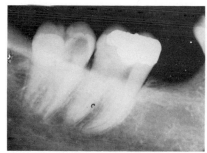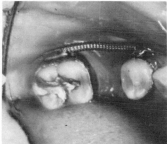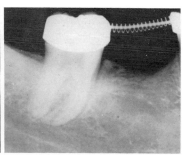

Figure 18–21   Uprighting second permanent molar. Mandibular third molar has been removed because of carious involvement. Interval between radiographs is four weeks.

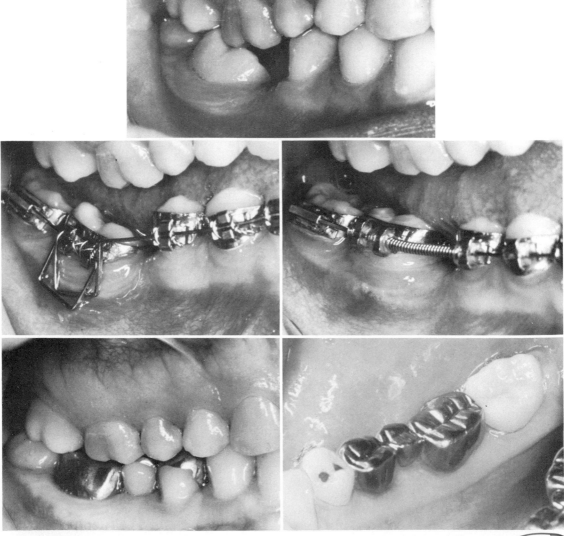

Figure 18–22   Loss of mandibular first molar with overeruption of opposing tooth. A Stoner boxloop helps to upright the mandibular second and third molar teeth, which have both been banded. A push coil spring completes tooth positioning and space consolidation. A three-tooth fixed partial denture re-establishes normal function. (From Norton, L. A., and Parker, W. T.: Management of repositioned teeth in preparation for fixed partial dentures. J.A.D.A., 81:916–922, 1970.)

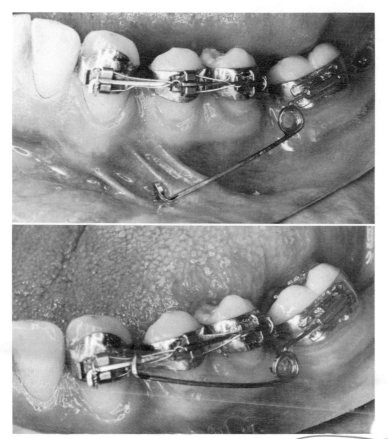

Figure 18–23   Uprighting of mandibular second molar by helical loop uprighting spring. Reciprocal depressing force is resisted by canine and premolar anchorage unit. (From Norton, L. A., and Proffit, W. R.: Molar uprighting as an adjunct to fixed prostheses. J.A.D.A., 76:312–315, 1968.)

either transferred or a new one of the same size added to the segment before tying it to place. The use of the rectangular arch segment provides better control of the teeth involved. Sometimes the round arch wire segments tend to rotate in the edgewise brackets. This is not possible with a rectangular wire. As the second permanent molar begins to upright, it is necessary to put a "tip back" bend in the arch segment (Fig. 18–18). The segment is then lifted up and snapped into the premolar and canine brackets.

In most instances, in a period of 12 to 16 weeks the second permanent molar is uprighted, sufficient space created, and the contact relationships established between the premolars and canine (Figs. 18–21 to 18–24). It is not always feasible to create the entire space of the missing lower first molar. Too long a treatment period may produce unwanted mesial movement of the premolars and canine. Rather, strive for an upright second molar and space closure in the premolar-canine region. A slightly smaller portion is not a major concern (Figs. 18–20, 18–22, 18–23). Since it is usually not advisable to place a fixed bridge until the patient is 16 or 17 years of age, the band and bar space maintainer of the type described in Chapter 13 may be used, modifying the second molar band and the second premolar band to accept the bar, or a removable Hawley appliance may be placed. Clasps can be made for the edentulous area to safeguard the

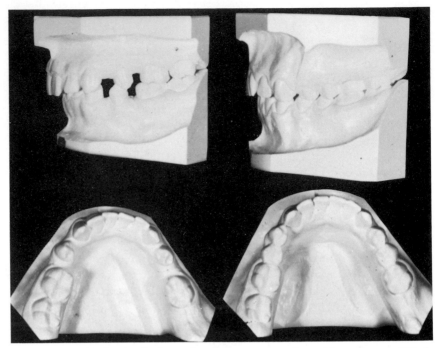

Figure 18–24   Multiple drifting due to premature loss. Use of a modified molar-uprighting appliance allowed space consolidation and normal eruption of second premolars, restoring the integrity of the dental arches. (Courtesy R. S. Freeman.)

space and contact relationship created by the orthodontic therapy. A tooth may be added to the retaining appliance, or acrylic can be extended into the space to restore function and to prevent the elongation of the opposing tooth.

EXTRAORAL FORCE

As more and more orthodontists have come to recognize that Class II and Class III malocclusions are maxillomandibular malrelationships primarily and that the teeth merely reflect these malrelationships, they have turned to the use of extraoral force to assist them in establishing a proper occlusion. Extraoral force itself is inadequate. Intraoral appliances are necessary to receive and direct this force, usually. *In the great majority of cases the control of mechanotherapy of this type should be in the hands of a competent orthodontist.* Growth and developmental timing are important factors in the success or failure of extraoral therapy. A careful diagnosis and case analysis is always essential. Sometimes it becomes necessary to determine the feasibility of tooth sacrifice in conjunction with extraoral force. The demands of the intraoral appliance setup in such instances are far beyond the training of the average dentist. But the dentist should be aware of the mechanics of extraoral force and the philosophy behind its use, and there are certain limited conditions where he may find it of great value in solving minor orthodontic problems. If he stays within the limits outlined herein he can anticipate a minimum of trouble. If he *always* has a specialist consultation first, both he and the patient will benefit; and there should be no hesitancy to seek further counsel during actual treatment. Problems arise even for the most competent clinician.

CONDITIONS FOR USE OF EXTRAORAL FORCE

The specific conditions over which the dentist in general practice may exert some control with the use of extraoral appliances are as follows:

1. Mild Class II, Division I malocclusions that have developed because of prolonged finger habits. In these cases, where there is an end-to-end molar relationship and where incisors must be retracted to a more normal overbite and overjet relationship, a short period of extraoral force serves to re-establish and hold the correct molar relationship and, at the same time, assist in the retraction of the maxillary incisors. Usually a period of 6 to 19 months of therapy in the mixed dentition is involved. The patient must always be told of a possible second period of therapy in the permanent dentition, depending on tissue response, growth and development and patient cooperation.

2. Where there has been mesial drift of the first permanent molars due to premature loss of the second deciduous molars in the maxillary arch. The use of extraoral force permits the restoration of normal first molar position, obviating the need for using teeth for anchorage. Anchor teeth anterior to the space in question might be disturbed and moved into positions of malocclusion with conventional intraoral appliances.

The concept of extraoral force, of using an area outside the mouth as a base for anchorage, is not new. There were Edward H. Angle's remarks[1] in 1887:

The value of the occipital bandage is, I believe, becoming more and more appreciated, and is especially applicable in this class of cases (maxillary protrusions). I am using the appliance in my sixteenth case, and I consider it much more satisfactory than any of the few devices described in our literature on the subject (Figures 11-50, 11-51.)

An infinite number of mechanical contrivances have been fabricated to employ the back of the head, the top of the head and the back of the neck. The method of execution may vary but the philosophy is the same. Intraoral appliances must depend at least partly on other teeth for anchorage or resistance to movement. This means unwanted movement of the so-called anchorage teeth in many instances as the orthodontist struggles to achieve his primary objective. In the correction of Class II, Division 1 malocclusions, this has meant dragging the mandibular teeth forward off their base as intermaxillary elastics were employed to retract the maxillary dentition. Certain appliances reduce this tendency; proper appliance manipulation also helps; extraction of certain teeth during orthodontic therapy may allow the orthodontist to maintain the mandibular incisors over basal bone, but the unwanted vector of force is still there. A source of anchorage outside the mouth can eliminate this problem and introduce other problems, as will be discussed later.

MILD CLASS II MALOCCLUSIONS OF PRIMARILY LOCAL NATURE AND HABIT SEQUELAE

As was pointed out in Chapter 6, thumb and finger sucking with concomitant and subsequently abnormal lip and tongue activity can produce morphologic changes that are particularly apparent in the maxillary arch. (See Chap. 6.) With the increase in overjet, the labial inclination of the maxillary incisors and the narrowing of the maxillary arch, there is frequently a Class II tendency in the buccal segments. Some authorities attribute this to the fact that the buccinator mechanism literally wraps around the end of the maxillary arch as it inserts into the pterygomandibular raphe (Chap. 3). Abnormal function would exert a forward-propelling force against the maxillary dentition, primarily, and thus could possibly cause the Class II tendency. If the dentist can eliminate the abnormal functional pattern, he can also do away with those forces which create the morphologic aberrations and problems of interdigitation of upper and lower teeth.

THERAPEUTIC PROCEDURES

There are a number of ways of employing extraoral force to retract maxillary incisors and to drive first molar teeth distally. One simple, temporizing adjunct to reduce severe protrusion and to move the incisors back from their advanced position of extreme vulnerability to damage is a combined elastoplastic "mouth guard" intraoral appliance and extraoral traction. No bands are required (Fig. 18–25). Conscientious use by the patient reduces incisor protrusion, spacing and excessive overjet, particularly in habit problems. When the elastoplastic portion is fabricated, the incisor teeth may be cut off the stone model and reset slightly as with the positioner and orthobite techniques (see Figs. 16–46, 16–47). This alone is inadequate to reduce the protrusion. An extraoral force arch of 0.040 inch stainless-steel must be embedded in the labial portion of the plastic to receive elastic traction from a conventional headcap, or the high pull type of headcap, depending on the direction of force desired (see Fig. 18–25).

Because of the future orthodontic treatment implications, consultation with an orthodontic specialist is strongly recommended. It should be made quite plain to the parents and the patient that this is only the first assault on the problem and is analogous to what the orthopedic surgeon and general physician often do for specific types of orthopedic problems.

If fixed appliances are to be used, and this is generally preferable, one of the simplest appliances is the combined labial bow and arch wire, which inserts into horizontal buccal tubes on the first molar teeth (Fig. 18–26). The molar bands are made directly or indirectly (Chap. 17). Next, 0.045 inch buccal tubes or double buccal tubes (Fig. 18–27) are soldered or welded at approximately the middle third of the buccal surface, gingivo-occlusally and lined up with straight wires so that the arch wire will approximate the buccal surfaces of the premolars and will insert and withdraw easily with no compensating bends (Figs. 17–7, 17–8). The arch wire-labial bow combination is available commercially but it can be fabricated readily. The size of the headgear arch may be determined by the Mayne headgear computer for choice of one of four commercial sizes or for fabrication to the measurement (Fig. 18–28). A 0.045 inch stainless-steel arch wire is made to conform to the shape of the maxillary arch and, after the molar bands are cemented, may be carefully fitted so that it will insert and withdraw quite easily in the mouth. The labial portion of the arch wire should lie as close to the gingival margin as possible without impinging on it. A 12 inch length of 0.055 inch stainless-steel wire is then formed in a paraboloid shape to fit the contours of the face and cheeks at the level of the lips (Fig. 18–29). Thereafter, the labial bow is attached to the arch wire by placing it against the labial surface of the arch wire so that the ends of both the bow and the arch wire are pointed in the same direction.

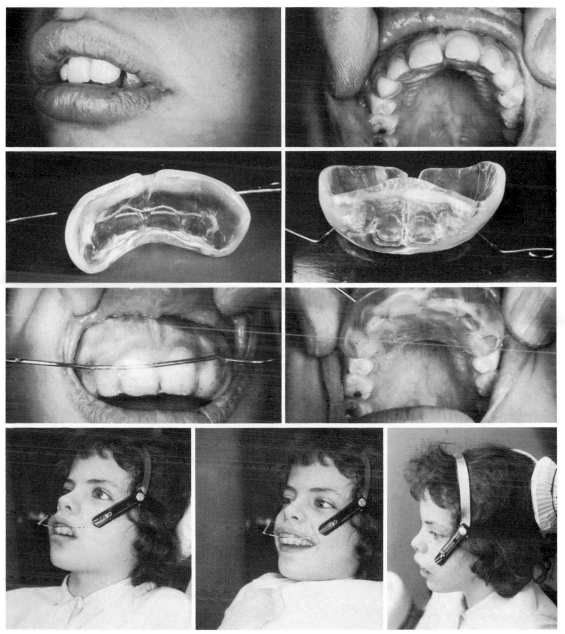

Figure 18–25   Tooth- and tissue-borne elastoplastic, soft acrylic retraction appliance utilizing extraoral force. This type of appliance does not require any fixed attachments and can be used to reduce incisor protrusion and deformation of the premaxillary segment as a result of abnormal perioral muscle function. These appliances are particularly effective in the early mixed dentition period when it is hazardous to place bands on teeth with wide open apices.

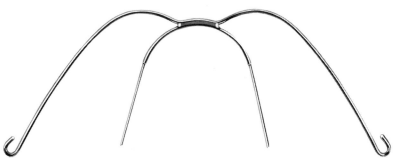

Figure 18–26   Combined extraoral force facial bow and arch wire. (Courtesy Unitek Corp.)

After the midlines of both the bow and arch wire have been matched, a strand of 0.020 inch soft brass ligature wire is wrapped tightly over both wires, extending approximately a quarter of an inch to each side of the midline. If this is done properly, the arch wire and labial bow will look like arcs of concentric circles and will lie fairly flat on the table in the same plane of space (Fig. 18–26). Fluoride flux is applied liberally to the brass wire that has been wrapped around the bow and arch wire, and silver solder is then flowed over the brass wire until a smooth sleeve-like section is obtained. The soldered portion may be polished with pumice-impregnated rubber disks.

The completed assemblage is then carried to the mouth, and the arch wire is inserted into the horizontal molar buccal tubes. Subtle bends are made in the arch wire and labial bow to make sure that the lips close effortlessly over the brass-wire-wrapped and soldered attachment. The labial bow is again checked to make sure that it does not impinge on the corners of the mouth or the cheeks. Hooks are then bent in the ends of the labial bow so that they lie flat against the cheeks, terminating at a point approximately one inch in front of and one inch below the external ear opening.

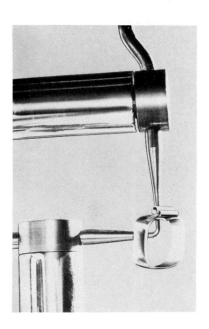

Figure 18–27   Welding of double tube to buccal side of molar band, to receive 0.045 inch diameter inner arch wire. Smaller tube may be used later, if needed, for lighter arch wire and individual banding of selected teeth. Proper positioning of buccal tubes and method of checking is shown in Figures 17–7 and 17–8. (Courtesy Rocky Mountain Dental Products Co.)

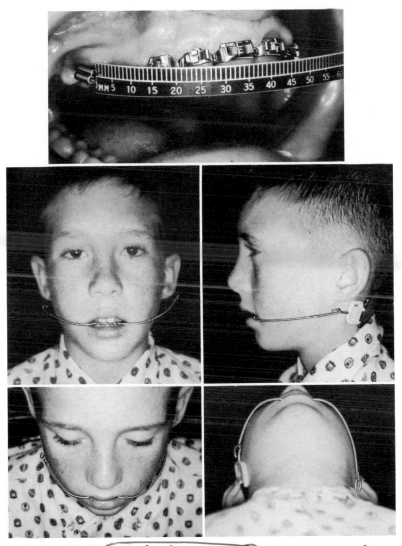

Figure 18–28   (Top) Mayne headgear computer to measure size of inner bow for extraoral arch. Fit of outside arch is shown because this is important both for direction of pull and for comfort to encourage maximum patient wear. (Courtesy W. R. Mayne.)

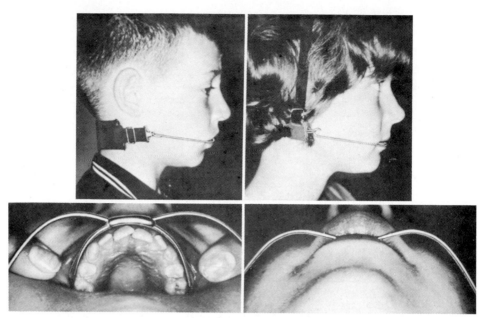

Figure 18–29   The external arm of the headgear arch is motivated by either cervical force (upper left) supplied from an elastic strap, or occipital force, or resistance (upper right) transmitted through an elastic component of the headgear. The fitting of the internal and external bow to the maxillary arch and to the lips is illustrated below. Note that the inner arch stands away from the anterior teeth so that all force is directed against the first permanent molars. (Courtesy W. R. Mayne.)

HEADCAP APPLIANCES

Many types of caps have been designed to serve as a base for the traction on the labial bow.

A number of varieties of headcaps are available from orthodontic supply houses. These are usually made of plastic belting and may be fitted readily and easily (Figs. 18–29, 11–55).

After the face bow and labial bow have been fabricated and the headcap fitted, the arch is inserted into the buccal tubes, and rubber elastics are stretched between the hooks at the end of the facial bow and the hooks on the headcap (Fig. 18–29). If an elastic approximately one centimeter in diameter is used, it should be stretched two to three times for optimal results. If the maxillary incisors are spaced and protruding as a result of abnormal perioral muscle function, and there is only a Class II tendency in the first molar region, with the abnormal perioral muscle activity the primary etiologic factor, it is probably wise to retract the maxillary incisors first. A metal cervical appliance may also be used for this purpose (Fig. 18–30). If the dentist is quite sure that he is dealing with a local problem and has made it clear to the parents that the problem could require further orthodontic treatment later, he may render a valuable service by eliminating deforming muscle patterns and restoring normal function.

INCISOR RETRACTION   To retract the maxillary incisors, the arch or labial bow is allowed to ride freely through the horizontal buccal tubes on the first molar teeth. The elastic traction on the facial bow exerts a force in a lingual direction on the maxillary central and lateral incisors, reducing the arc from canine to canine and closing the spaces. The patient should wear the appliance approximately 12 hours a night, and an hour or two during the day in addition, if possible.

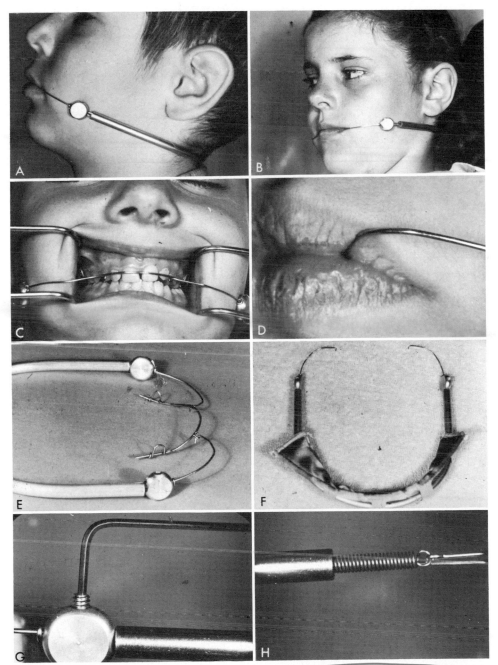

Figure 18–30 Simple extraoral traction, using a cervical aluminum tube with a compressed coil spring inside. Either light (tooth-moving) or heavy orthopedic force may be used with this type of appliance. Tension and adjustment is made with an Allen wrench (G). A pad (F) cushions the neck for added comfort. "J arms" insert around commisure of lip (C and D) to prevent irritation. A .045 inch labial arch with vertical spring loops (see Chap. 17) accepts delivery of extraoral force.

The appliance and the patient's progress should be checked at approximately 3-week intervals by the dentist. He should make sure that the molar bands remain well cemented and that the labial bow is not binding in the molar tubes. The patient is taught how to insert the labial bow and place the occipital cap. He is shown how to attach the elastics between the facial bow and the cap and told that he must use a new elastic on each side every night. Sometimes the cap stretches, reducing the elastic tension. It may be necessary to relocate the elastic hooks to restore optimal force. Sometimes a smaller elastic may be used instead.

Great care must be exercised in the retraction process. The dentist must not encroach on the canine space. If there is an excessive overbite, it may be necessary to use a maxillary bite plate cut away on the lingual side of the maxillary incisors to permit their retraction but with sufficient acrylic to open the bite and allow the posterior teeth to erupt (Fig. 18–31). Most of the overbite problems show an excessive curve of Spee, with overeruption of the mandibular incisors and infraocclusion of the mandibular premolars. Spengeman has designed an appliance he calls the Cosla appliance (curve of Spee leveling appliance), which stimulates eruption of the mandibular premolars. This may be worn in conjunction with extraoral therapy. If this step is successful, further retraction to establish a normal overjet is possible. Because of the danger of excessive lingual inclination of the maxillary incisors, because of the possibility of creating a functional retrusion and a possible temporomandibular joint disturbance and because of the possibility of interfering with the normal eruption of the maxillary canines, the incisors should be retracted only to the point where normal lip function may take place again.

DISTAL MOLAR MOVEMENT   If there is a Class II tendency in the buccal segments, extraoral traction may be employed to move the maxillary first molars distally. Instead of the arch wire being allowed to ride freely through the horizontal buccal tubes on the first molars, it is "stopped." The arch wire is placed in the buccal tubes so that the labial portion of the bow stands away from the labial surface of the maxillary incisors approximately a quarter of an inch. Scratch marks are then made on the arch wire precisely at the mesial end of the horizontal molar tube. Next, the arch wire is removed and small spurs are soldered just mesial to the scratch marks. Two 0.045 inch buccal tubes may be slid on each end of the wire to a point just where the distal end of each tube rests on the scratch mark. These tubes may then be fixed at this point by crimping them sharply or by joining their mesial ends to the arch wire with silver solder. When the arch wire is replaced in the mouth, the spurs or tubes on the wire contact the mesial end of the horizontal molar tubes, preventing the arch wire from sliding distally. The extraoral force is thus directed against the first molar teeth. The same amount of wearing time is required each night as with the retraction of the incisors. If the dentist has been careful in the selection of the proper type of case for this therapy, and has the "blessings and guidance" of his consulting orthodontist, the retraction of the incisors and elimination of the Class II molar relationship should not take more than six months. If it takes longer, he has chosen a case that probably should be handled by the orthodontist himself, or the patient is not cooperating by wearing the headcap the required number of hours each night.[5]

CERVICAL TRACTION APPLIANCES

In many of these muscle perversion problems, where the causation is primarily of a local nature, the protrusion and spacing of the maxillary incisors are

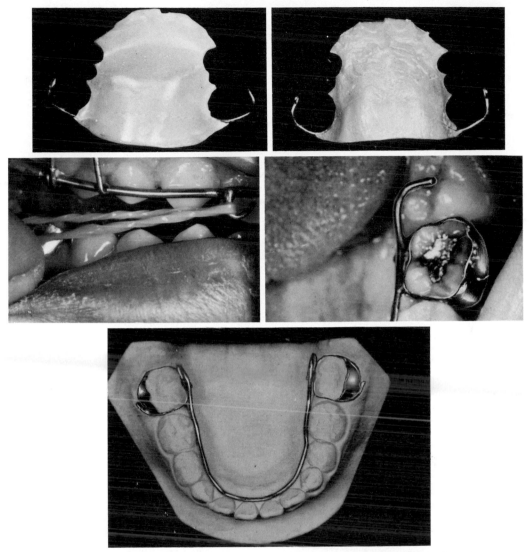

Figure 18–31   Accessory appliances for extraoral traction. Maxillary bite plate (top row) prevents overclosure. Part-time elastic traction to a lower lingual arch (middle and bottom rows) assists in correcting mesiodistal relationship, without dragging lower dental arch forward. If maxillary second molars are slow in erupting and mandibular second molars have already erupted, a finger spring extension to the central fossa will prevent overeruption. Buccal tubes on the lower molars, instead of hooks, may be used as elastic traction hooks.

accompanied by an anterior open bite tendency, or at least a negative overbite situation. The use of cervical traction instead of occipital traction is particularly effective in these cases. Cervical traction may also be used in place of the head-cap appliance just outlined. The direction of pull with a cervical appliance tends to tip the crowns of the maxillary first molar teeth distally more readily than with the occipital assemblage. In the simple Class II tendency problems that are within the sphere of management by the general dentist, however, this tipping may be desired and should not pose too much of a problem over the 4- to 6-month treatment time. Orthopedic force is not necessary, either. (See Chapter 10, *Current Orthodontic Concepts and Techniques.*)

MATERIALS USED

1. Two maxillary first molar bands with 0.045 inch horizontal buccal tubes
2. 0.045 inch stainless-steel arch wire
3. 0.030 inch nichrome or Elgiloy wire for vertical loops at molars and hooks to receive the extraoral appliance
4. Cervical traction appliance (Fig. 18–33)
5. 0.010 inch stainless-steel ligature wire to tie in the arch wire

ARCH WIRE FABRICATION.   The molar bands are made as outlined in Chapter 17. The molar tubes are attached to the buccal surface in the same manner and position as described for the facial bow and occipital assemblage technique.

After the molar bands have been cemented, a 0.045 inch stainless-steel maxillary arch wire is bent to fit the contour of the maxillary arch. As with the labial bow just described, the distal ends of the arch wire should ride freely through the buccal tubes when inserted. Scratch marks are then made on the arch wire with a file at a point 1 cm. mesial to the anterior end of the horizontal buccal tubes. The arch wire is removed and 0.030 inch nichrome or Elgiloy vertical spring loops are soldered to the arch wire (Figs. 17–27, 17–28). The free end of the loop is wrapped around the outside of the arch wire one and a half times so that the end of the wrapped portion is turned toward the gingival tissue and smoothed off.

When the arch wire is replaced, the loop should approximate but not touch the gingival tissue above the second deciduous molar area. With the arch wire fully inserted, the free end of the vertical loop should terminate 2 mm. anterior to

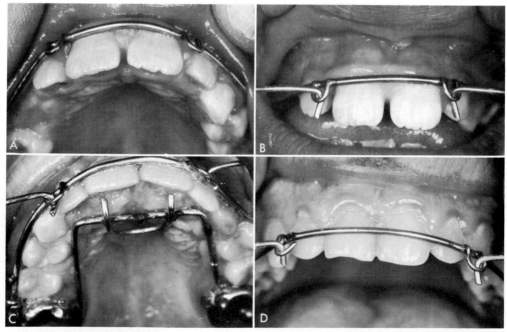

Figure 18–32   A, 0.045 stainless-steel round arch in place with loops soldered on arch to receive extraoral force arms (B, C and D). Appliance may be used in conjunction with a finger habit appliance (C). If part-time elastic traction is required, the extraoral force loop on the arch wire must be open on the mesial side to receive the elastic as well as the extraoral force arms (D).

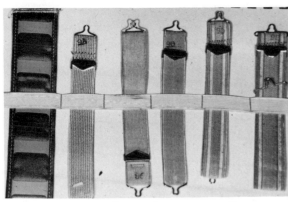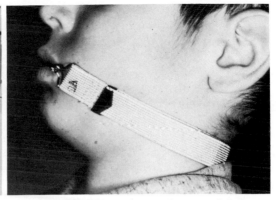

Figure 18–33 Cervical traction appliances come in different thicknesses of elastic and different widths. These elastic straps are placed in the foam rubber pad (left) for comfort, but may be worn alone (right).

the horizontal buccal tubes. Scratch marks are again made with the file on the arch wire, at the right and left lateral-canine embrasures. The arch wire is removed and 0.030 inch nichrome or Elgiloy loops are soldered, with the loop extending downward to receive the extraoral traction arms. The arch wire is then replaced to check the loop positions (Fig. 18–32). These loops should stand away about 2 mm. from the labial surfaces of the lateral incisors to permit the patient to insert and remove the cervical appliance arms.

TYING IN ARCH.   The arch wire is then tied to place with soft stainless-steel ligature wire. The end of the ligature wire is passed through the vertical spring loop and carried distally through the V-shaped notch between the posterior end of the horizontal buccal tubes and the band. The end of the wire is then brought mesially and twisted tightly with the other end of the ligature wire to activate the vertical spring loop. After this procedure is repeated on the opposite side, it is easy to see that there is a constant tension against the labial surfaces of the maxillary incisors as the vertical spring loops attempt to retract the arch wire through the horizontal buccal tubes at the first permanent molars.

The intraoral appliance alone, if allowed to work itself out unaided by extraoral force, would retract the maxillary incisors partly but would move the first molar teeth mesially in the process. This is obviously undesirable, since one of the main objectives is to move the maxillary first permanent molars distally into normal interdigitation with their opposing teeth. An extraoral appliance of the occipital or cervical type is essential (Figs. 18–29, 18–33).

EXTRAORAL ACTIVATION.   If the dentist desires, he may use a metal or plastic tube containing a rubber band that is stretched from each wire arm to provide the necessary tension. Also available are cervical foam rubber padded straps which use elastics to activate the 0.045 inch metal external bow arms that insert into the oral portion of the appliance (Fig. 18–33). Tension with all these appliances should be between 6 and 12 ounces on each side when measured with a tension stress gauge.

Like the headgear previously described, the patient should be instructed to wear his cervical traction unit at least 12 hours out of every 24. Patients are seen at 3-week intervals to maintain the vertical spring loop pressure on the incisors until the spaces are closed and these teeth retracted to the desired position. During this time the extraoral force assists in the retraction process and may actually move the first permanent molars distally.

As soon as the spaces are closed, or after three or four 3-week periods, the distal legs of the vertical spring loops on the arch wire are allowed to contact the mesial ends of the horizontal buccal tubes on the first permanent molars. The arch wire stands away from the maxillary incisors approximately 2 mm. The extraoral force is thus directed primarily against the first permanent molar teeth to correct the Class II relationship. A small amount of expansion is often desirable in the distal ends of the arch wire, since the molars are being moved to a wider part of the mandibular arch. They often show a lingual cross-bite tendency, anyway. At subsequent visits the loops are closed slightly to keep the spaces closed. Appliances are worn for three to six months, depending on tissue response, patient cooperation and growth increments. While restoration of normal perioral muscle function will do much to retain the new positions of the teeth, it is advisable to place a removable Hawley type retainer, to be worn for another three to six months. If treatment response is slower, or more than six months total time is involved, an orthodontic consultation is advisable. In medicine, the specialist frequently continues therapy started by the general practitioner for the benefit of the patient. We would do well to emulate this practice more frequently in dentistry.

MESIAL DRIFT OF MAXILLARY FIRST PERMANENT MOLARS

It was pointed out in Chapter 7 that the premature loss of maxillary second deciduous molars often results in the mesial drift of the first permanent molars. This creates a Class II cuspal relationship and often impacts the erupting second premolars (Fig. 18–34). An extraoral appliance of the type just described is an effective means of moving these first permanent molars distally into normal positions, creating enough space for the eruption of the second premolar teeth. It is imperative that the dentist make sure that the lack of space for eruption of the second premolars is a manifestation of premature loss of second deciduous molars and resultant mesial drift of the first permanent molars. If the arch length deficiency is merely a symptom of a broad and complex orthodontic problem, extraoral force may only aggravate what might well be a full orthodontic appliance situation, requiring the removal of teeth during treatment. As in all these limited corrective orthodontic problems, the dentist should seek competent orthodontic counsel if there is the slightest doubt.[7] For a more detailed dis-

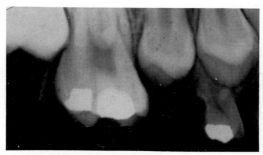
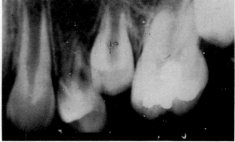

Figure 18–34   Types of problems in which a short period of extraoral force will tip first permanent molars distally to permit impacted second premolars to erupt. One must be sure this arch length deficiency is a local premature loss situation, not a symptom of a broader malocclusion.

cussion of extraoral force and its orthopedic application, see Chapter 10, *Current Orthodontic Concepts and Techniques*, by the author.[9]

THERAPEUTIC PROCEDURES

If the headgear with the labial face-bow combination is used, a spur or tube stop is placed on the arch wire portion so that when the labial bow is inserted into the horizontal buccal tubes the anterior portion stands away from the labial surfaces of the maxillary incisor teeth. This serves to direct the full extraoral force against the maxillary first permanent molars.[4] A small amount of expansion is placed in the labial bow because as molars move distally, they should move a trifle laterally, since the dental arch diverges posteriorly. If the cervical setup is

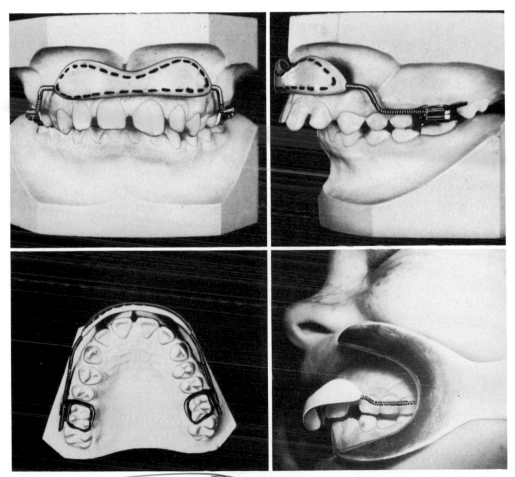

Figure 18–35. Denholz appliance, which uses muscle anchorage to distally drive first permanent molars. Round buccal tubes on first permanent molar bands (or full metal crowns) receive 0.036 or 0.040 inch diameter arch wire. Wire assemblage consists of a vestibular acrylic labial screen and open coil spring segments that fit over the arch. When the arch is inserted by the patient into the tubes, the labial screen stands well away from the anterior teeth. The coil springs are compressed as the lip resists the stretching effect, exerting a distal thrust on the molar teeth. The patient's exercises, one to two hours a day, forcibly closing the lips over the labial screen, will accelerate treatment response. (Courtesy Rocky Mountain Dental Products Co.)

used, the arch wire remains in the mouth all the time, and the vertical spring loops are opened up against the mesial ends of the horizontal buccal tubes on the first molars. This serves to move the arch wire 2 to 3 mm. away from the labial surfaces of the maxillary incisors. As with the headgear, extraoral traction is then directed primarily against the maxillary first permanent molars. After the desired position has been achieved for the first permanent molars, the patient may either use the extraoral appliance two to three nights a week as a retaining mechanism or the operator may choose to place the removable Hawley type retainer. Where the eruption of the second premolars is not expected for a year and a half or two years, fixed space maintainers or a lingual holding arch may be placed to preserve the necessary space. (See Chap. 13, Fabrication.) Where there is mesial drift of the maxillary first permanent molars, and the degree of severity is moderate, so-called muscle anchorage may be used, as shown in Figure 18–35. The Denholz appliance consists of molar bands with horizontal round buccal tubes, a base arch wire of 0.036 or 0.040 inch steel to fit the buccal tubes and a labial ves-

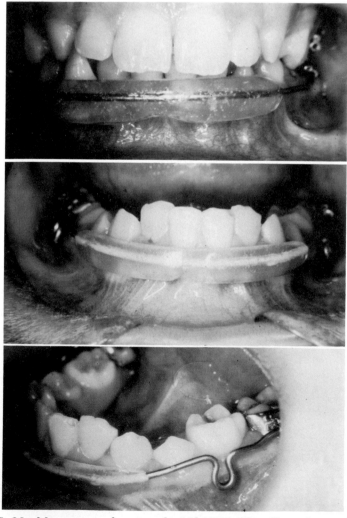

Figure 18–36 Mayne muscle control appliance. This "lip plumper" utilizes lip pressure to exert distal force on molars and to allow tongue to position lower incisors labially, reducing excessive overjet. (Courtesy W. R. Mayne.)

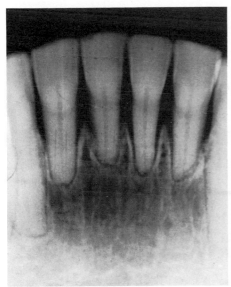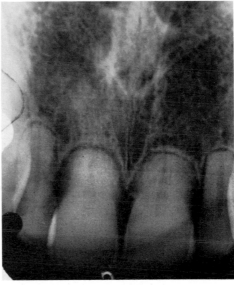

Figure 18–37   The result of inept orthodontic appliance manipulation by a dentist completely unfamiliar with the basic concepts of orthodontic therapy and case selection. The root resorption illustrated here is of a degree not usually seen, but can occur with protracted periods of improperly executed therapy, and with improperly designed appliances, fixed or removable.

tibular screen. Coil spring sections are added to the arch wire so that when the wire-labial screen assembly is inserted into the tubes, the screen stands away from the anterior teeth (Fig. 18–35). The elasticity of the maxillary lip, the resistance to stretching and actual prescribed lip exercises for a definite period each day exert a distal driving force on the maxillary first molar teeth. The wire and coil spring assemblage is usually worn only at home and during the night, but it may be tied in place and worn at all times, if desired. The coil spring must be reactivated occasionally or may be replaced. The mesial end of the spring is attached to the acrylic labial screen, so that it is not lost through patient manipulation.

This last chapter was incorporated in the text with some trepidation. The concern arises from the fact that some of the dentists employing these limited fixed appliance corrective procedures may not heed the warnings given repeatedly about undertaking the correction of orthodontic problems beyond the scope of training and experience of the individual operator. Every appliance and technique described in this chapter has been handled by dental students, and the results obtained have been gratifying. *But all therapy has been under the guidance of trained orthodontists.* That is why the plea is made again that the general practitioner should obtain orthodontic guidance and advice in the selection of cases to be treated and in the actual therapy. If these admonitions are ignored, the dentist who dabbles in orthodontics may get into serious trouble, as Figure 18–36 shows. If they are obeyed, the dentist will experience the tremendous satisfaction of broadening his horizons of professional service by helping to guide and develop the child's best facial and dental pattern, removing any roadblocks that occur on the road to normal occlusion, and maintaining optimum integrity of the dentition throughout the patient's life. These are the rewards of judicious use of preventive, interceptive and limited corrective orthodontic precepts and procedures.[6]

REFERENCES

1. Angle, E. H.: New system of regulation and retention. D. Register, 41:597–603, 1887.
2. Goldstein, M. C.: Orthodontics in crown and bridge and periodontal therapy. D. Clin. North America, July, 1964, pp. 449–459.
3. Wisth, P. J.: The role of zinc phosphate cement in enamel surface changes on banded teeth. Angle Orthodont., 40:329–333, 1970.
4. Miura, F., Nakagawa, K., and Masuhara, E.: New direct bonding system for plastic brackets. Am. J. Orthodont., 59:350–361, 1971.
5. Weber, F. N.: Ortho-rehabilitative procedures. D. Clin. North America, July, 1959, pp. 419–434.
6. Gianelly, A. A., and Goldman, H. M.: Biologic Basis of Orthodontics. Philadelphia, Lea & Febiger, 1971.
7. Gottlieb, E. L.: An aid in establishing and maintaining space of missing upper anterior teeth during orthodontic treatment. Am. J. Orthodont., 52:27–33, 1966.
8. Reid, P. V.: Let's take another look at our problem cases. Am. J. Orthodont., 52:266–282, 1966.
9. Graber, T. M. *in* Graber, T. M. (ed.): Current Orthodontic Concepts and Techniques. Philadelphia, W. B. Saunders Co., 1969.
10. Norton, L. A., and Proffit, W. R.: Molar uprighting as an adjunct to fixed prostheses. J.A.D.A., 76:312–315, 1968.
11. Norton, L. A., and Parker, W. T.: Management of repositioned teeth in preparation for fixed partial dentures, J.A.D.A., 81:916–922, 1970.
12. Brandt, S.: Surgical orthodontics. J. Clin. Orth., 6:196–202, 1972.

APPENDIX

GUIDED READING LIST

The following list of references has been classified into subjects directly and indirectly concerned with orthodontics. After each heading are listed the chapters of this book to which the supplemental reading references pertain. Every effort has been made to select only those books and articles that are relevant and are likely to prove of value to the reader.

1. Histology and embryology (Chaps. 2, 10)
2. Anthropology, evolution and genetics (Chaps. 2, 4, 6, 7)
3. Muscles and physiology of the stomatognathic system (Chaps. 3, 6, 9, 13, 14)
4. Growth and development (Chaps. 2, 3, 4, 6, 11, 15, 18)
5. Habits (Chaps. 3, 6, 13, 14, 16)
6. Temporomandibular joint (Chaps. 2, 3, 4, 9, 16)
7. Cleft palate (Chaps. 2, 6)
8. Cephalometrics (Chaps. 2, 4, 5, 6, 8, 11, 15, 18)
9. Anatomy and occlusion of teeth (Chaps. 2, 3, 4, 5, 6, 7, 8, 9, 15)
10. Tooth measurements (Chaps. 2, 4, 5, 7, 8, 13, 15)
11. Etiology, case analysis and diagnosis (Chaps. 4, 5, 6, 7, 8, 11, 13, 14, 15, 16, 17, 18)
12. The problem of extraction in orthodontics (Chaps. 7, 8, 9, 11, 15)
13. Metallurgy and materia technica (Chaps. 11, 13, 14, 16, 17, 18)
14. Orthodontic therapy (Chaps. 1, 10, 11, 12, 13, 14, 15, 16, 17, 18)
15. Extraoral force and dentofacial orthopedics (Chaps. 11, 18)
16. Retention and post-treatment adjustment (Chaps. 10, 11, 13, 14, 16, 17, 18)
17. Iatrogenic effects (Chaps. 11, 12, 13, 14, 15, 16, 17, 18)
18. Equilibration (Chaps. 11, 12, 14, 17)
19. Patient motivation and management (Chaps. 8, 9, 12, 13, 14, 15, 16)
20. Orthodontic history (Chaps. 1, 11)
21. Surgical orthodontics (Chaps. 5, 11, 15)
22. Statistics (Chaps. 2, 5, 8)
23. Miscellaneous (all chapters)
24. Other textbooks in orthodontics (all chapters)

1. HISTOLOGY AND EMBRYOLOGY

Ackerman, J. L., and Cohen, M. I.: The effects of quantified pressures on bone. Am. J. Orthodont., 52:34–46, 1966.

Anderson, D. J.: Tooth movement in experimental malocclusion. Arch. Oral Biol., 7:7–15, 1962.

Anstendig, H. S., and Kronman, J. H.: A histologic study of pulpal reaction to orthodontic tooth movement in dogs. Angle Orthodont., 42:50–55, 1972.

Atherton, J. D.: The gingival response to orthodontic tooth movement. Am. J. Orthodont., 58:179, 1970.

Avery, J. L., and Devine, R. K.: The development of ossification centers in the face and palate of normal and cleft palate human embryos. Cleft Palate Bull., 9:25–26, 1959.

Bassett, C. A.: Generation of electric potentials by bone in response to mechanical stress. Science, 137:1063–1064, 1962.

Bassett, C. A.: Electrical effects in bone. Sci. Amer., 215:18, 1965.

Bassett, C. A.: Biologic significance of piezoelectricity. Calcif. Tiss. Res., 1:252–272, 1968.

Baumrind, S.: A reconsideration of the propriety of the "pressure-tension" hypothesis. Am. J. Orthodont., 55:12–21, 1969.

Baumrind, S.: Late changes in cell replication and protein synthesis in the periodontal ligament incident to tooth movement. Am. J. Orthodont., 57:109, 1970.

Boese, L. R.: Increased stability of orthodontically rotated teeth following gingivectomy in Macaca nemestrina. Am. J. Orthodont., 56:273, 1969; Am. J. Orthodont., 55:527, 1969.

Brain, W. E.: The effect of surgical transection of free gingival fibers on the regression of orthodontically rotated teeth in the dog. Am. J. Orthodont., 55:50, 1969.

Breitner, C.: Bone changes resulting from experimental orthodontic treatment. Am. J. Orthodont. & Oral Surg., 26:521–547, 1940.

Burket, L. W.: The effects of orthodontic treatment of the soft periodontal tissues. Am. J. Orthodont., 49:660–671, 1963.

Butler, T.: Comparative histologic study of heavy intermittent and light continuous forces. Am. J. Orthodont., 55:304, 1969.

Carollo, D. A., Hoffman, R. L., and Brodie, A. G.: Histology and function of the dental gubernacular cord. Angle Orthodont., 41:300–307, 1971.

Christiansen, R. L., and Burstone, C. J.: Centers of rotation within the periodontal space. Am. J. Orthodont., 55:353, 1969.

DeAngelis, V.: Observations on the response of alveolar bone to orthodontic force. Am. J. Orthodont., 58:284, 1970.

DeShields, R. W.: A study of root resorption in treated class II, division I malocclusions. Angle Orthodont., 39:231, 1969.

Edwards, J. G.: A study of the periodontium during orthodontic rotation of teeth. Am. J. Orthodont., 54:441, 1968.

Eschler, J.: Reaction of the periodontal membrane to the different orthodontic forces. Europ. Orthodont. Soc. Tr., 39:185–201, 1963.

Ford, D. R.: A histologic study of the changes in tissues of the periodontium of the Rhesus monkey with the application of torque force in the third stage of Begg technique. Am. J. Orthodont., 57:193, 1970.

Fullmer, H. M.: The oxytalan fiber. J. Histochem., 6:425, 1958.

Gianelly, A.: The use of parathyroid hormone to assist orthodontic tooth movement. Am. J. Orthodont., 55:305, 1969.

Gillooly, C. J.: Electric potentials recorded from mandibular alveolar bone as a result of forces applied to the tooth. Am. J. Orthodont., 54:649–654, 1968.

Gottlieb, B.: Histologic consideration of the supporting tissues of the teeth. J.A.D.A., 30:1872, 1943.

Gowgiel, J. M.: Observations on the phenomenon of tooth eruption. J. Dent. Res., 46:1325, 1967.

Greear, M. C.: A histologic evaluation of the effects of controlled movement of the maxillary incisor teeth of albino rats receiving therapeutic dosages of proteolytic enzyme. Am. J. Orthodont., 57:91–92, 1970.

Gryson, J. A.: Changes in the periodontal ligament incident to orthodontic therapy. Periodont. Abstr., 13:14–21, 1965.

Hotz, B.: Force determination and control in orthodontics. J. Dent. Ass. S. Africa, 19: 370–373, 1964.

Huettner, R. J.: Experimental histologic study of the effects of orthodontic movement of the gingiva and periodontal membrane in the Macaca rhesus monkey. Abstract Am. J. Orthodont., 46:929, 1960.

Hureau, G. F.: Histological contribution to the study of failures in orthodontic treatment. Orthodont. Franç., 34:381–382, (Fr.).

Iyer, V. S.: Reaction of gingiva to orthodontic force: a clinical study. J. Periodont., 33:26–28, 1962.

Kaplan, H., Aisenberg, M. S., and Erickson, B. E.: Orthodontics and transeptal fibers. Histological interpretation of repair phenomena following the removal of first premolars with retraction of the anterior segment. Am. J. Orthodont. & Oral Surg., 31:1–20, 1945.

Kronman, J. H.: Experimental tooth movement. Angle Orthodont., 41:125, 1971.

Lee, B. W.: Relationship between tooth-movement rate and estimated pressure applied. J. Dent. Res., 44:1053, 1965.

Martuccino, J. V.: An investigation of the deposition of alveolar bone in the orthodontic tipping of teeth in monkeys. Am. J. Orthodont., 55:198, 1969.

McLaughlin, K. D.: Quantitative determination of root resorption during orthodontic treatment. Am. J. Orthodont., 50:143, 1964 (Abstract).

Miller, S.: Rotational axes of human incisor teeth. Am. J. Orthodont., 55:307, 1060.

Murphey, W. H.: Oxytetracycline microfluorescent comparison of orthodontic retraction into recent and healed extraction sites. Am. J. Orthodont., 58:215, 1970.

Oppenheim, A.: Human tissue response to orthodontic intervention. Am. J. Orthodont. & Oral Surg., 28:263, 1942.

Parker, G. R.: Transseptal fibers and relapse following bodily retraction of teeth: A histologic study. Am. J. Orthodont., 61:331–344, 1972.

Parker, W. S., Frisbie, H. E., and Grant, T. S.: The experimental production of dental ankylosis. Angle Orthodont., 34:103–107, 1964.

Reitan, K.: Behavior of Malassez' epithelial rests during orthodontic tooth movement. Acta Odont. Scandinav., 19:443–468, 1961.

Reitan, K.: Effects of force magnitude and direction of tooth movement on different alveolar bone types. Angle Orthodont., 34:244–255, 1964.

Reitan, K.: Influence of variation in bone type and character on tooth movement. Europ. Orthodont. Soc. Tr., 39:137–154, 1963.

Reitan, K.: The initial tissue reaction incident to orthodontic tooth movement. Acta Odont. Scandinav., supp. 6, 1951.

Reitan, K.: Some factors determining the evaluation of forces in orthodontics. Am. J. Orthodont., 43:32–45, 1957.

Reitan, K.: Tissue behavior during orthodontic tooth movement. Am. J. Orthodont., 46:881–900, 1960.

Reitan, K.: Tissue changes following rotation of teeth in the dog. Angle Orthodont., 10:140–147, 1940.

Reitan, K.: Tissue rearrangement during retention of orthodontically rotated teeth. Angle Orthodont., 29:105–113, 1959.

Sandstedt, C.: Einige Beitrage zue Theoriz der Zahnregulierung. Nord. Tandl. Tidskr., 5:236, 1904; 6:141, 1904.

Schwarz, A.: Tissue changes incident to tooth movement. Int. J. Orthodont., 18:331, 1932.

Sicher, H.: Changing concepts of the supporting dental structures. Oral Surg., Oral Med., & Oral Pathol., 12:31–35, 1959.

Sicher, H.: Periodontal ligament. Am. Inst. Oral Biol. Tr., pp. 37–38, 1963.

Sleichter, C. G.: A clinical assessment of light and heavy forces in the closure of extraction spaces. Angle Orthodont., 41:66, 1971.

Stuteville, O. H.: A summary review of tissue changes incident to tooth movement. Angle Orthodont., 8:1–19, 1938.

Utley, K.: Activity of alveolar bone incident to orthodontic tooth movement as studied by oxytetracycline-induced fluorescence. Am. J. Orthodont., 54:167, 1968.

Weinmann, J. P., and Sicher, H.: Bone and Bones, 2nd ed. St. Louis, C. V. Mosby Co., 1955.

Yew, P. K. J., and Shaw, J. H.: Studies of the skull sutures of the rhesus monkey by comparison of the topographic sampling technique autoradiography and vital staining. Arch. Oral Biol., 8:349–362, 1963.

2. ANTHROPOLOGY, EVOLUTION AND GENETICS

Altemus, L. A.: Comparative integumental relationships. Angle Orthodont., 33:217–221, 1963.

Asbell, M. B.: A study of family line transmission of dental occlusion. Am. J. Orthodont., 43:265–285, 1957.

Björk, A., and Björk, L.: Artificial deformation and cranio-facial asymmetry in ancient Peruvians. J. Dent. Res., 43:353–362, 1964.

Dahl, E.: Craniofacial structures in a skull with bilateral cleft lip and palate. Tandlaegebladet, 75:1170–1181, 1971.

Dahlberg, A. A.: Dental Morphology and Evolution. Chicago, University of Chicago Press, 1971.

Garn, S. M., Lewis, A. B., and Vicinus, J. H.: The inheritance of symphyseal size during growth. Angle Orthodont., 33:222–231, 1963.

Gregory, W. K.: The evolution of some orthodontic systems in nature. Am. J. Orthodont., 34:215–234, 1948.

Hausser, E.: (Variability of chin form in the anatomically correct dentition.) Fortschr. Kieferorthop., 25:192–202, 1964 (Ger.).

Hooton, E. A.: Evolution and devolution of the human face. Am. J. Orthodont. & Oral Surg., 32:657–672, 1946.

Horowitz, S. L., Osborne, R. H., and DeGearge, F. V.: Hereditary factors in tooth dimensions, a study of the anterior teeth of twins. Angle Orthodont., 28:87–93, 1958.

Lavelle, C. L. B.: Secular trends in different racial groups. Angle Orthodont., 42:19–25, 1972.

Lavelle, C. L. B., Foster, T. D., and Flinn, R. M.: Dental arches in various ethnic groups, Angle Orthodont., 41:293–299, 1971.

Lundström, A.: The significance of genetic and non-genetic factors in the profile of the facial skeleton. Am. J. Orthodont., 41:910–916, 1955.

Montague, M. F. A.: An Introduction to Physical Anthropology. 3rd ed. Springfield, Ill., Charles C Thomas, 1960.

Shull, A. F.: Heredity. New York, McGraw-Hill Book Co., 1926.

Stein, K. F., Kelley, T. J., and Wood, E.: Influence of heredity in the etiology of malocclusion. Am. J. Orthodont., 42:125–141, 1956.

Stockard, C. R., Section III with A. L. Johnson: The Genetic and Endocrine Basis for Differences in Form and Behavior. Philadelphia, Wistar Institute, 1941.

Stoddard, S. E.: Inheritance of malocclusion. J. Heredity, 38:117–119, 1947.

Wern, G. H.: Comparative radiographic cephalometric study of the mandibular posterior border and maxillary incisor inclination. Texas Dent. J., 81:4–18, 1963.

3.   MUSCLES AND PHYSIOLOGY OF THE STOMATOGNATHIC SYSTEM

Abrams, I. N.: Oral muscle pressures. Angle Orthodont., 33:83–104, 1963.

Abrams, I. N.: Perioral musculature in relation to basal bone and dental arch form. Am. J. Orthodont., 48:633, 1962 (Abstract).

Ahlgren, J.: The silent period in the EMG of the jaw muscles during mastication and its relationship to tooth contact. Acta Odont. Scand., 27:219–227, 1969.

Ahlgren, J., and Owall. B.: Muscular activity and chewing force: A polygraphic study of human mandibular movement. Arch. Oral Biol., 15:271–280, 1970.

Amatulli, G., Nacci, F., and Silla, M.: (Otorhinolaryngological observations of 482 children in the course of orthodontic treatment. An instrument for measuring nasal output. Scope and results of the research.) Rass. Int. Stomat. Prat., 14:165–171, 1963 (It.).

Anderson, W. S.: The relationship of the tongue-thrust syndrome to maturation and other factors. Am. J. Orthodont., 49:264–275, 1963.

Anderson, D. J., and Picton, D. C. A.: Masticatory stress in normal and modified occlusion. J. Dent. Res., 37:312–317, 1958.

Barrett, M. J.: Functioning occlusion. Ann. Aust. Coll. Dent. Surg., 2:68–80, 1969.

Blanton, P., et al.: Electromyographic analysis of the buccinator muscle. J. Dent. Res., 49:389–394, 1970.

Bloomer, H. H.: Speech defects in relation to orthodontics. Am. J. Orthodont., 49:920–929, 1963.

Bosma, J. F.: Maturation of function of the oral and pharyngeal region. Am. J. Orthodont., 49:94–104, 1963.

Brauer, J. S., and Holt, T. V.: Tongue thrust classification. Angle Orthodont., 35:106–112, 1965.

Brodie, A. G.: The apical base: zone of interaction between the intestinal and skeletal systems. Angle Orthodont., 36:136–151, 1966.

Brodie, A. G.: Muscular factors in the diagnosis and treatment of malocclusions. Angle Orthodont., 23:71–77, 1953.

Christensen, J.: Effect of occlusion-raising procedures on the chewing system. Dent. Pract., 20:233–238, 1970.

Cleall, J. F.: Deglutition: a study of form and function. Am. J. Orthodont., 51:566–594, 1965.

Cohen, J.: Highlights of dental electromyographic research over the past fifteen years. Univ. Mich. Sch. Dent. Alum. Bull., 65:35, 37–48, 1963.

Di Salvo, N. A.: Neuromuscular mechanisms involved in mandibular movement and posture. Am. J. Orthodont., 47:330–342, 1961.

Elcan, P. D.: Abnormal deglutition: diagnosis and treatment. J. Dent. Child., 30:256–259, 1963.

Eschler, J.: Mandibulo-motoric coordinated functions and tooth position as a cause for distocclusion of the mandible. Europ. Orthodont. Soc. Tr., 38:220–228, 1962.

Frankl, R.: (Atmospheric pressure, respiration and the soft orofacial tissues.) Deutsch. Zahn-, Mund-Kieferheilk., 43:367–374, 1964 (Ger.).

Franks, A. S. T.: Electromyography relative to the stomatognathic system: a review. D. Practitioner, 8:32–37, 1957.

Fried, K. H.: Palate-tongue relativity. Angle Orthodont., 41:308–323, 1971.

Fuchs, R.: Relationship between the force of masticatory muscles and the electromyogram. Deutsch. Zahn. Z., 24:863–870, 1969.

Garnick, J., and Ramfjord, S. P.: Rest position. J. Prosth. Dent., 12:895–911, 1962.

Garrett, F. A., Angelone, L., and Allen, W. I.: The effect of bite opening, bite pressure, and malocclusion on the electrical response of the masseter muscle. Am. J. Orthodont., 50:435–444, 1964.

Graber, T. M.: Physiological principles in dentistry. Washington Univ. D. J., 23:35–43, 1957.

Graber, T. M.: The "three M's": muscles, malformation, and malocclusion. Am. J. Orthodont., 49:418–450, 1963.

Graber, T. M., Bzoch, K. R., and Aoba, T.: A functional study of the palatal and pharyngeal structures. Angle Orthodont., 29:30–40, 1959.

Griffin, C. J., and Munro, R. R.: Electromyography of the masseter and anterior temporalis muscles in patients with temporomandibular dysfunction. Arch. Oral Biol., 16:929–941, 1971.

Hackworth, H. B.: Lingual articulatory functions in tongue thrust. Angle Orthodont., 35:241–243, 1965.

Harrington, R., and Breinholt, V.: The relation of oral-mechanism malfunction to dental and speech development. Am. J. Orthodont., 49:84–93, 1963.

Jacobs, R. M.: Effects of altered anterior occlusal relationship on perioral muscle forces. Angle Orthodont., 37:144–146, 1967.

Jacobs, R. M.: Treatment objectives and case retention: Cybernetic and myometric considerations. Am. J. Orthodont., 58:552–564, 1970.

Jarabak, J. R.: Adaptability of the temporal and masseter muscles; an electro-myographic study. Angle Orthodont., 24:193–213, 1954.

Koski, F.: Axis of the opening movement of the mandible. J. Prosth. Dent., 12:888–894, 1962.

Kraft, E.: (Physiology and electromyography of the masticatory muscles and their importance in the etiology and therapy of dysgnathism.) Fortschr. Kieferorthop., 25:56–68, 1964 (Ger.).

Kungl, U. S.: Some remarks on the background to certain proprioceptive muscle reflexes with special regard to their occurrence in the jaw muscles. Acta Odont. Scandinav., 18:331–346, 1960.

Kydd, W. L., Akamine, J. S., Mendel, R. A., and Kraus, B. S.: Tongue and lip forces exerted during deglutition in subjects with and without an anterior open bite. J. Dent. Res., 42:858–866, 1963.

Kydd, W. L., and Neff, C. W.: Frequency of deglutition of tongue thrusters compared to a sample population of normal swallowers. J. Dent. Res., 43:363–369, 1964.

Lipke, D., and Posselt, U.: Functional anatomy of the temporomandibular joint. J. West. Soc. Periodont., 8:48–58, 1960.

Lysell, L.: Qualitative and quantitative determination of attrition and the ensuing tooth migration. Acta Odont. Scandinav., 16:267–292, 1958.

Massengill, R., Robinson, M., and Quinn, G.: Cinefluorographic analysis of tongue thrusting. Am. J. Orthodont., 61:402–406, 1972.

Matthews, B., and Yenn, R.: A silent period in the masseter electromyogram following tooth contact in subjects wearing full dentures. Arch. Oral Biol., 15:531–535, 1970.

Moller, E.: Clinical electromyography in dentistry. Int. Dent. J., 19:250–266, 1969.

Moyers, R. E.: Role of musculature in malocclusion. Europ. Orthodont. Soc. Tr., 37:40–59, 1961.

Moyers, R. E.: Tongue problems and malocclusion. D. Clin. North Amer., July, 1964, pp. 529–539.

Munro, R. R., and Griffin, C. J.: Electromyography of the jaw jerk recorded from the masseter and the anterior temporalis muscles in man. Arch. Oral Biol., 16:59–69, 1971.

Powell, R. N.: Tooth contact during sleep; association with other events. J. Dent. Res., 44:959–967, 1965.

Proffit, W., Kydd, W. L., Wilskie, H. H., and Taylor, D. T.: Intraoral pressures in a young adult group. J. Dent. Res., 43:555–562, 1964.

Ramfjord, S. P.: Bruxism, a clinical and electromyographic study. J.A.D.A., 62:21–44, 1961.

Rogers, J. H.: Swallowing patterns of a normal-population sample compared to those of patients from an orthodontic practice. Am. J. Orthodont., 47:674–689, 1961.

Rosenblum, R. E.: Orofacial muscle activity during deglutition as revealed by physiographic cinematography. Angle Orthodont., 33:162–177, 1963.

Solow, B., and Tallgren, A.: Postural changes in craniocervical relationships. Tandlaegebladet, 75:1247–1257, 1971.

Storey, A. T.: Physiology of changing vertical dimension. J. Prosth. Dent., 12:912–921, 1962.

Straub, W. J.: Malfunction of the tongue. Part I. The abnormal swallowing habit: its cause, effects, and results in relation to orthodontic treatment and speech therapy. Am. J. Orthodont., 46:404–424, 1960.

Straub, W. J.: Malfunction of the tongue. Part III. Am. J. Orthodont., 48:486–504, 1962.

Subtelny, J. Daniel, and Subtelny, Joanne D.: Malocclusion, speech, and deglutition. Am. J. Orthodont., 48:685–697, 1962.

Swindler, D. R., and Sassouni, V.: Open bite and thumb sucking in rhesus monkeys. Angle Orthodont., 32:27–37, 1962.

Tulley, W. J.: Adverse muscle forces—their diagnostic significance. Am. J. Orthodont., 42:801–814, 1946.

Walker, D. G.: The tooth, the bone, and the muscle. Brit. Soc. Study Orthodont. Tr., p. 127–130 disc. 130–131, 1961.

Weinstein, S., et al.: On an equilibrium theory of tooth position. Angle Orthodont., 33:1–26, 1963.

Wildman, A. J., Fletcher, S. G., and Cox, B.: Patterns of deglutition. Angle Orthodont., 34:271–291, 1964.

Winders, R. V.: Forces exerted on the dentition by the perioral and lingual musculature during swallowing. Angle Orthodont., 28:226–235, 1958.

Winders, R. V.: Recent findings in myometric research. Angle Orthodont., 32:38–43, 1962.

Yip, A. S. G., and Cleall, J. F.: Cinefluorographic study of velopharyngeal function before and after removal of tonsils and adenoids. Angle Orthodont., 41:251–263, 1971.

4. GROWTH AND DEVELOPMENT

Adams, C. P.: A study of individual dental and facial growth from five to fifteen years. Tandlaegebladet, 75:1235–1246, 1971.

Arita, M., Iwasawa, T., Ono, H., Numata, K., and Seki, O.: Chronological observation of deep overbite patients in their deciduous teeth period. J. Nihon Univ. Sch. Dent., 5:89–98, 1962.

Backlund, E.: (Upper median diastema, frequency and etiology. A longitudinal investigation on 300 children, aged between 9 and 12 years.) Svensk Tandläk. T., 57:273–291, 1964 (Sw.).

Balbach, D. R.: The cephalometric relationship between the morphology of the mandible and its future occlusal position, Angle Orthodont., 39:29–41, 1969.

Bambha, J. K., and Van Natta, P.: Longitudinal study of facial growth in relation to skeletal maturation during adolescence. Am. J. Orthodont., 49:481–493, 1963.

Barrett, M. J., and Brown, T.: A computer based system of dental and cranio-facial measurements and analysis, Aust. Dent. J., 13:207–213, 1963.

Baum, A. T.: Age and sex differences in the dentofacial changes following orthodontic treatment, and their significance in treatment planning. Am. J. Orthodont., 47:355–369, 1961.

Björk, A.: Cranial base development. Am. J. Orthodont., 41:198–225, 1955.

Björk, A.: Variability and age changes in overjet and overbite. Am. J. Orthodont., 39:779–801, 1953.

Björk, A., and Helm, S.: Prediction of age at maximum puberal growth in body height. Angle Orthodont., 37:134–143, 1967.

Broadbent, B. H.: Ontogenetic development of occlusion. Angle Orthodont., 11:223–241, 1941.

Broadbent, B. H.: Ontogenetic development of occlusion in Development of Occlusion. Philadelphia, University of Pennsylvania Press, 1941, pp. 31–48.

Brodie, A. G.: On the growth pattern of the human head from the third month to the eighth year of life. Am. J. Anat., 68:209–262, 1941.

Brown, T., Barrett, M. J., and Grave, K. C.: Facial growth and skeletal maturation at adolescence. Tandlaegebladet, 75:1211–1222, 1971.

Burstone, C. J.: Process of maturation and growth prediction. Am. J. Orthodont., 49: 907–919, 1963.

Cessac, N.: The growth of the dental arches and development of occlusion in twins. Pedodont. Franc., 1:52–60, 1967.

Cheraskin, E., and Ringsdorf, W. M.: Biology of the orthodontic patient: Relationship of chronologic and dental age in terms of vitamin C state. Angle Orthodont., 42:44–49, 1972.

Coben, S. E.: Growth and Class II treatment. Am. J. Orthodont., 52:5–26, 1966.

Cutler, B. S., Hassig, F. H., and Turpin, D. L.: Dentofacial changes produced during and after use of a modified Milwaukee brace on Macaca mulatta. Am. J. Orthodont., 61:115–137, 1972.

Enlow, D. H.: A study of the post-natal growth and remodeling of bone. Am. J. Anat., 11:79–102, 1962.

Enlow, D. H.: A morphogenetic analysis of facial growth. Am. J. Orthodont., 52:283–299, 1966.

Enlow, D. H.: Principles of Bone Remodeling. Springfield, Charles C Thomas, 1963.

Enlow, D. H., and Bang, S.: Growth and remodeling of the human maxilla. Am. J. Orthodont., 51:446–464, 1965.

Enlow, D. H., and Harris, D. B.: A study of postnatal growth of the human mandible. Am. J. Orthodont., 50:25–50, 1964.

Enlow, D. H., Kuroda, T., and Lewis, A. B.: Intrinsic craniofacial compensations. Angle Orthodont., 41:271–285, 1971.

Ford, E. H. R.: Cranial base—growth of the human. Am. J. Orthodont., 44:498–506, 1958.

Graber, T. M.: Cranio-facial and dentitional development. In Falkner, F. (Ed.), Human Development. Philadelphia, W. B. Saunders, 1966.

Haataja, J.: Cephalic, facial and dental growth in Finnish children. A cross-sectional study. Suom. Hammaslääk. Toim. (Suppl.), 59:11–114, 1963.

Harris, J. E.: Cephalometric analysis of mandibular growth rate. Am. J. Orthodont., 48:161–174, 1962.

Harris, J. E.: Cranio-facial growth and malocclusion. Trans. Europ. Orth. Soc., pp. 1–17, 1965.

Harvold, E. P., Chierici, G., and Vargervik, K.: Experiments in the development of dental malocclusion. Am. J. Orthodont., 61:38–44, 1972.

Hellman, M.: The face in its developmental career. D. Cosmos, 77:777–787, 1935.

Helm, S., Siersbaek-Nielsen, S., Skieller, V., and Björk, A.: Skeletal maturation of the hand in relation to maximum puberal growth in body height. Tandlaegebladet, 75:1223–1234, 1971.

Hirschfeld, W.: Time series and exponential smoothing methods applied to the analysis and prediction of growth. Growth, 34:129–143, 1970.

Hirschfeld, W. J., and Moyers, R. E.: Prediction of craniofacial growth: The state of the art. Am. J. Orthodont., 60:435–444, 1971.

Hopkin, G. B.: Development of a malocclusion. A serial study from 8 weeks to 9½ years of age. Brit. Soc. Study Orthodont. Tr., pp. 94–99, 1958.

Johnston, L.: A statistical evaluation of cephalometric prediction. Angle Orthodont., 38:284–304, 1968.

Koski, K., Haataja, J., and Lappalainen, M.: Skeletal development of hand and wrist in Finnish children. Am. J. Phys. Anthrop., 19:379–382, 1961.

Koski, K., Laaksonen, A. L., and Luostarinen, E.: Fate of foetal human bone xenografts in rats. Nature, 193:1092–1093, 1962.

Koski, K., Laaksonen, A. L., and Luostarinen, E.: Heterologous human foetal bone transplants. Ann. Med. Exp. Fenn., 40:318–325, 1962.

Krogman, W. M.: Problems in growth and development of interest to the dentist. D. Clin. North America, July 1958, pp. 497–514.

Krogman, W. M.: The meaningful interpretation of growth and growth data by the clinician. Am. J. Orthodont., 44:411–432, 1958.

Krogman, W. M., and Chung, D. B.: The cranio-facial skeleton at the age of one month. Angle Orthodont., 35:305–310, 1965.

Latham, R. A.: The sella point and postnatal growth of the human cranial base. Am. J. Orthodont., 61:156–162, 1972.

Lebret, L.: Growth changes of the palate. J. Dent. Res., 41:1391–1404, 1962.

Lebret, L. M. L.: (The human palate—its growth. Migration of posterior teeth. Expansion due to two different methods of orthodontic treatment.) Rev. Franç. Odontostomat., 11:1199–1222, 1964 (Fr.).

Maj, G., and Luzi, C.: Longitudinal study of mandibular growth between nine and thirteen years as a basis for an attempt of its prediction. Angle Orthodont., 34:220–230, 1964.

Marschner, J. F., and Harris, J. E.: Mandibular growth and Class II treatment. Angle Orthodont., 36:89–95, 1966.

Melsen, B.: The postnatal growth of the cranial base in macaca rhesus analyzed by the implant method. Tandlaegebladet, 75:1320–1329, 1971.

Merow, W. W.: Cephalometric statistical appraisal of dentofacial growth. Angle Orthodont., 32:205–213, 1962.

Moore, A. W.: Observations on facial growth and its clinical significance. Am. J. Orthodont., 45:399–423, 1959.

Moorrees, C. F. A., Grøn, A. M., Lebret, L. M. L., Yen, P. K. J., and Frohlich, F. J.: Growth studies of the dentition; a review. Am. J. Orthodont., 55:600–616, 1969.

Moss, M. L.: Functional analysis of human mandibular growth. J. Prosth. Dent., 10:1149–1159, 1960.

Moss, M. L.: Vertical growth of the human face. Am. J. Orthodont., 50:359–376, 1964.

Moss, M. L., and Greenberg, S. N.: Postnatal growth of the human skull base. Angle Orthodont., 25:77–84, 1955.

Nakamura, S., Savara, B., and Thomas, D. R.: Norms of size and annual increments of the sphenoid bone from four to sixteen years. Angle Orthodont., 42:35–43, 1972.

Parker, J. II.: Unpredictable growth pattern in orthodontics. J. California D. A., 40:199–223, 250, 1964.

Paulsen, H. U.: Changes in sagittal molar occlusion during growth. Tandlaegebladet, 75:1258–1267, 1971.

Powell, T. V., and Brodie, A. G.: Closure of the spheno-occipital synchondrosis. Anat. Rec., 147:1, 15–24, 1963.

Richardson, E. R., and Brodie, A. G.: Longitudinal study of growth of maxillary width. Angle Orthodont., 34:1–15, 1964.

Ricketts, R. M.: II. Growth, treatment, and clinical significance. Am. J. Orthodont., 50:728–750, 1964.

Rosenstein, S. W.: A longitudinal study of anteroposterior growth of the mandibular symphysis. Angle Orthodont., 34:155–167, 1964.

Sarnat, B. G.: Postnatal growth of the upper face: some experimental considerations. Angle Orthodont., 33:139–161, 1963.

Schudy, F. F.: Vertical growth versus anteroposterior growth as related to function and treatment. Angle Orthodont., 34:75–93, 1964.

Scott, J. H.: Analysis of facial growth from fetal life to adulthood. Angle Orthodont., 33:110–113, 1963.

Scott, J. H.: Cephalometric growth studies. Int. Dent. J., 13:355–371, 1963.

Scott, J. H.: Craniofacial regions. A contribution to the study of facial growth. D. Pract., 5:208–214, 1955.

Scott, J. H.: Facial growth—the analysis of, II. The horizontal and vertical dimensions. Am. J. Orthodont., 44:507–512, 1958.

Scott, J. H.: Facial growth—the analysis of, II. The horizontal and vertical dimensions. Am. J. Orthodont., 44:585–589, 1958.

Scott, J. H.: Growth at facial sutures. Am. J. Orthodont., 42:381–387, 1956.

Scott, J. H.: Growth in width of the facial skeleton. Am. J. Orthodont., 43:366–371, 1957.

Scott, J. H.: The analysis of facial growth from fetal life to adulthood. Angle Orthodont., 33:110–113, 1963.

Sillman, J. H.: Dimensional changes of the dental arches: longitudinal study from birth to 25 years. Am. J. Orthodont., 50:824–842, 1964.

Skieller, V.: Growth stimulation of the upper face in a case of mesial occlusion analyzed by the implant method. Tandlaegebladet, 75:1296–1306, 1971.

van der Linden, F. P. G. M.: Growth in its application to orthodontic therapy. Studieweek, 1965.

Walker, D. G.: A calendar of facial growth. Brit. J. Plast. Surg., 17:424–429, 1964.

Wieslander, L.: Effect of orthodontic treatment on the concurrent development of the craniofacial complex. Am. J. Orthodont., 49:15–27; correction 389, 1963.

5. HABITS

Bockland, E.: Facial growth and the significance of oral habits, mouth breathing, and soft tissues in malocclusion. Am. J. Orthodont., 50:867–875, 1964.

Bowden, B. D.: A longitudinal study of the effects of digit- and dummy-sucking. Am. J. Orthodont., 52:887–901, 1966.

Büttner, M.: Does thumbsucking cause and increase in the incidence of cases with mandibular retroposition? Sweisz. Monatschr. Zahnheilk., 80:32–36, 1970.

Davidson, D. O.: Thumbsucking, Habit or Symptom. J. Dent. Child., 34:252–259, 1967.

Dowling, D.: Influence of musculature & correlation with electromyography. N.U.D.S., 1972. Thesis.

Fisher, H.: Finger, tongue and lip habits in children. Dent. Surv., 45:35–37, 1969.

Fleege, F. J.: Oral habits. Dent. Soc., 43:299–300, 1967.

Freud, S.: Three contributions to the theory of sex, In Brill, A. A., The Basic Writings of Sigmund Freud. New York, Random House, 1938.

Frybarger, R. E.: Tongue thrust, glossopharyngeal syndrome in a quandary. J. Miss. Dent. Assoc., 24:27–31, 1968.

Garliner, D.: Effects of unrecognized abnormal swallowing. J. Canad. Dent. Assoc., 34:301–304, 1968.

Gausman, R. D.: Psychological and dental aspects of thumbsucking. Chron. Omaha Dent. Soc., 33:185, 1970.

Gensior, A. M.: The tongue and Class III. Am. J. Orthodont., 57:256–261, 1970.

Goldstein, I., and Dragon, A.: Case Report: Buccal thumb sucking. Dental Survey, pp. 24–25, February 1970.

Good, S.: Mouth habits—mouth breathing. J. India Dent. Assoc., 38:132–135, 1966.

Graber, T. M.: Thumb and finger sucking, Am. J. Orthodont., 45:258, 1959.

Graf, H.: Bruxism. Dent. Clin. N. Amer., 13:687–724, 1969.

Hanson, M. L., Barnard, L. W., and Case, J. L.: Tongue thrust in preschool children. Am. J. Orthodont., 56:60–69, 1969.

Hanson, M. L., Barnard, L. W., and Case, J. L.: Tongue thrust in pre-school children. II. Dental Occlusal Patterns. Am. J. Orthodont., 57:15–22, 1970.

Haryett, R. D., Hanson, F. C., and Davidson, P. O.: Chronic thumb sucking: A second report on treatment and its psychological effects. Am J. Orthodont., 57:164–178, 1970.

Haryett, R. D., Hanson, F. C., Davidson, P. O., and Sandilands, M. L.: Chronic thumb sucking: The psychologic effects and the relative effectiveness of various methods of treatment. Am. J. Orthodont., 53:569–585, 1967.

Haryett, R. D., Sandilands, M. L., and Davidson, P. O.: Relative effectiveness of various methods of arresting thumbsucking. Canad. Dent. Ass., 34:5–10, 1968.

Hawking, A. C.: Mouth breathing & its relations to malocclusion and facial abnormalities. New Mexico Dent. J., 20:18–21, 1969.

Holt, J. K.: An unusual finger sucking habit. Dent. Prac., 21:238, 1971.

Jacobson, A.: Thumbsucking: A psychological and dental understanding of the problem. Int. J. Orthodont., 1:5–16, 1963.

Jarabak, J. R.: Controlling malocclusion due to sucking habits. Dent. Clin. N. Amer., p. 369, 1959.

Kapoor, D. N.: Effects of deleterious habits on dentofacial complex. Indian. J. Pediat., 37:102–104, 1970.

Klein, E. T.: Thumb sucking. J. Colorado Dent. Ass., 45:1–6, 1967.

Klein, E. T.: Thumbsucking habit, meaningful or empty. Am. J. Orthodont., 59:283–289, 1971.

Kortsch, W. E.: The tongue and its implications in Class II malocclusions. J. Wisconsin Dent. Soc., 41:261, 1965.

Linder-Aronson, S.: A comparison between nose breathers with respect to occlusion and facial dimensions. Odont. Rev., 11:341, 1960.

Littman, J. Y.: Practical approach to torque thrust problems. J. Pract. Orthodont., 2:138, 1968.

Malouf, L.: Thumbsucking Habits. J. S. Calif. Dent. Hyg. Ass., 12:23–30, 1969.

Maschka, P.: Thumbsdown on thumb-sucking. Chron. Omaha Dent. Soc., 33:240–242, 1970.

Massler, M · Oral habits, origin, evolution and current concepts in management. Alpha Omegan, 56:127, 1963.

Miller, H.: Treatment planning for disharmonies caused by noxious habits. J.A.D.A., 79:301–367, 1969.

Moore, R. L.: Oral habits, good and bad. Bull. Phil. Dent. Soc., 31:6–9, 1965.

Moyers, R. E.: Tongue problems and malocclusion. Dent. Clin. N. Amer., p. 529, July, 1964.

Murray, A. B.: The association of incisor protrusion with digit and allergic nasal itching. J. Allergy, 44:239–247, 1969.

Norton, L. A.: Management of digital sucking and tongue thrust in children. Dent. Clin. N. Amer., 363–382, July, 1968.

Picard, P. J.: Bottle feeding as preventive orthodontics. J. Calif. D. S. & Nevada D. S., 35:90–95, 1959.

Popovich, F.: Preventive and interceptive orthodontics. J. Canad. D. A., 28:95–106, 1962.

Popovich, F.: Prevalence of sucking habits and relation to malocclusion. Oral Health, 57:498–499, 1967.

Rasmus, R. L., and Jacobs, R. M.: Mouth breathing and malocclusion. Quantitative technic for measurement of oral and nasal flow velocities. Angle Orthodont., 39: 296–299, 1969.

Rosenberg, J. L.: A gestalt approach to thumb sucking. Arizona Dent. J., 17:10–13, 1971.

Saxene, O. P.: Thumbsucking. J. Indiana Dent. Ass., 39:81–85, 1967.

Siegel, L. R.: Snuff, a causative factor in overbite. Penn. Dent. J., 36:298–300, 1969.

Straub, W. J.: Malfunction of the tongue. I. Am. J. Orthodont., 46:404–424, 1960, II. Am. J. Orthodont., 47:596–617, 1961, III. Am. J. Orthodont., 48:486–503, 1962.

Tewari, A.: Abnormal oral habits and malocclusion. J. Indiana Dent. Ass., 42:81–84, 1970.

Vasilev, P.: Open occlusion due to parafunction of tongue. Stomato, 50:141–144, 1968.

Washbon, R. E.: Thumb sucking: A review and an analysis of a method of treatment. M. S. Thesis, U of Washington, Seattle, 1956.

Weiss, C. E.: Orofacial musculature imbalance and associated symptoms. Brit. J. Disord. Commun., 4:140–145, 1969.

Whitman, C. L.: Correction of oral habits. Dent. Clin. N. Amer., p. 541, 1969.

6. TEMPOROMANDIBULAR JOINT

Agerberg, G., Carlsson, G., and Hasslar, O.: Vascularization of the Temporomandibular Disk. Odont. T., 77:451–460, 1969. Goteborg.

Baume, L. J., and Derichsweiler, H.: Is the condylar growth center responsive to orthodontic therapy? An experimental study in Macaca mulatta. Oral Surg., 14:347–362, 1961.

Choukas, N. C., and Sicher, H.: The structure of the temporomandibular joint. Oral Surg., 13:1203–1213, 1960.

Corbett, N. E.: DeVincenzo, J. P., Huffer, R. A., and Shryock, E. F.: The relation of the condylar path to the articular eminence in mandibular protrusion. Angle Orthodont., 41:286–292, 1971.

Costen, J.: A syndrome of ear and sinus symptoms dependent upon disturbed function of the temporomandibular joint. Ann. Otol., 43:1–15, 1934.

Droel, R., and Isaacson, R. J.: Some relationships between the glenoid fossa position and various skeletal discrepancies. Am. J. Orthodont., 61:64–78, 1972.

Furstman, L.: The early development of the human temporomandibular joint. Am. J. Orthodont., 49:672–682, 1963.

Furstman, L.: The effect of the loss of occlusion upon the mandibular joint. Am. J. Orthodont., 51:245–261, 1965.

Graber, T. M.: Overbite—the dentist's challenge. J.A.D.A., 79:1135–1145, 1969.

Griffin, C. J., and Munro, R. R.: Electromyography of the masseter and anterior temporalis muscles in patients with temporomandibular dysfunction. Arch. Oral Biol., 16:929–941, 1971.

Hjortsjo, C.: Studies on the Mechanics of the Temporomandibular Joint. Lund, Sweden, C.W.K. Gleerup, 1955.

Kawamura, Y., Mayima, T., and Kato, I.: Physiologic role of deep mechanoreceptor in temporomandibular joint capsule. The J. Osaka Univ. Dent. Sch., 7:63–76, 1967.

Keller, J., and Moffett, B. C.: Nerve endings in the temporomandibular joint of the rhesus macaque. Anat. Rec., 160:587–594, 1968.

Klineberg, I.: Structure and function of temporomandibular joint innervation. Ann. Roy. Coll. Surg. Eng., 49:268–288, 1971.

Perry, H. T., Jr.: An electromyographic study of the temporal and masseter muscles of individuals with excellent occlusion and Angle Class II, Division 1 malocclusions. Angle Orthodont., 25:49–58, 1955.

Perry, H. T., Jr.: Implications of myographic research. Angle Orthodont., 25:178–188, 1955.

Perry, H. T., Jr.: Muscle changes associated with temporomandibular joint dysfunction. J.A.D.A., 54:644–653, 1957.

Perry, H. T., Jr.: Static and dynamic orthodontics. Am. J. Orthodont., 48:900–910, 1962.

Perry, H. T., Jr.: The physiology of mandibular displacement. Angle Orthodont., 30:51–60, 1960.

Posselt, U.: Range of movement of the mandible. J.A.D.A., 56:10–13, 1958.

Sarnat, B. G. (ed.): The Temporomandibular Joint. Springfield, Ill., Charles C Thomas, 1963.

Schmid, F.: On the nerve distribution of the temporomandibular joint capsule. Oral Surg., 28:63–65, 1969.

Schweitzer, J. M.: Masticatory function in man. Mandibular repositioning. J. Prosth. Dent., 21:262–291, 1962.

Sicher, H.: Temporomandibular articulation in mandibular overclosure. J.A.D.A., 36:131–139, 1948.

Storey, A. T.: Sensory functions of the temporomandibular joint. J. Canad. Dent. Ass., 34:294–300, 1968.

Thilander, B.: Innervation of the temporo-mandibular joint capsule in man. Trans. Roy. Sch. Dent., 7:1961. Stockholm.

7. CLEFT PALATE

Braver, R. O.: Observations and measurements of nonoperative setback of premaxilla in double cleft patients. Plast. Reconstr. Surg., 35:148–159, 1965.

Coccaro, P. J., Subtelny, J. D., and Pruzansky, S.: Growth of soft palate in cleft palate children. Plast. Reconstr. Surg., 30:1, 43–55, 1962.

Cooper, H. K.: Recent trends in the management of the individual with oral-facial and speech handicaps. Am. J. Orthodont., 49:683–700, 1963.

Cooper, H. K., Long, R. E., Cooper, J. A., Mazaheri, M., and Millard, R. T.: Psychological, orthodontic, and prosthetic approaches in rehabilitation of the cleft palate patient. D. Clin. North America, July, 1960, pp. 381–393.

Crocker, D.: Some implications of superstitions and folk beliefs for counseling parents of children with cleft lip and cleft palate. Cleft Palate J., 7:87, 1970.

Cronin, T. D.: Advances in over-all management of cleft palate. Southern M. J., 58:358–363, 1965.

Dahl, E.: Craniofacial structures in a skull with bilateral cleft lip and palate. Tandlaegebladet, 75:1170–1181, 1971, Kobenhavn.

Fraser, F. C.: Cleft lip and cleft palate. Science, 158:1603, 1967.

Fraser, F. C.: Etiology of cleft lip and palate. Amer. J. Hum. Genet., 22:125, 1970.

Grabb, W. C., Rosenstein, S. W., and Bzoch, K. R.: Cleft Lip and Palate. Little, Brown, Boston, 1971.

Graber, T. M.: A cephalometric analysis of the developmental pattern and facial morphology in cleft palate. Angle Orthodont., 19:91–100, 1949.

Graber, T. M.: A study of craniofacial growth and development in the cleft palate child from birth to six years of age in Hotz, R. (ed.): Early Treatment of Cleft Lip and Palate. Berne, Hans Huber, 1964.

Graber, T. M.: A study of the congenital cleft palate deformity. Ph.D. Thesis, Northwestern University Medical School, Department of Anatomy, 1950.

Graber, T. M.: An appraisal of the developmental deformities in cleft palate and cleft lip individuals. Quart. Bul. Northwest. Univ. Med. Sch., 23:153–169, 1949.

Graber, T. M.: Changing philosophies in cleft palate management. J. Pediat., 37:400–415, 1950.

Graber, T. M.: Cleft palate and harelip. Washington University D. J., 6:76–83, 1940.

Graber, T. M.: Craniofacial morphology in cleft palate and cleft lip deformities. Surg., Gynecol., & Obstet., 88:359–369, 1949.

Graber, T. M.: Craniofacial morphology of cleft lip and cleft palate. Yearbook of Dentistry, 1949, pp. 272–274.

Graber, T. M.: Oral and nasal structures in cleft palate speech. J.A.D.A., 53:693–707, 1956.

Graber, T. M.: Orthodontics for the cleft lip and cleft palate patient. Fortnightly Rev. Chicago D. Soc., 18:9–12, 1949.

Graber, T. M.: The congenital cleft palate deformity. J.A.D.A., 48:375–395, 1954.

Hagerty, R. F., Andrews, E. B., Hill, M. J., Calcote, C. E., Karesh, S. H., Lifschiz, J. M., and Swindler, D. R.: Dental arch collapse in cleft palate. Angle Orthodont., 34:25–36, 1964.

Hagerty, R. F., Andrews, E. B., Hill, M. J., Mendleson, B. P., Karesh, S. H., Lifschiz, J. M., and Swindler, D. R.: Prevention of dental arch collapse. Angle Orthodont., 34:53–57, 1964.

Harvold, E.: A Roentgen Study of the Postnatal morphogenesis of the Facial Skeleton in Cleft Palate. Oslo, Norway, A. W. Broeggers Boktrykkeri, 1954.

Johnston, M. C.: Orthodontic treatment for the cleft palate patient. Am. J. Orthodont., 44:750–763, 1958.

Kraus, B.: Cleft palate research. Cleft Palate J., 7:23, 1970.

Krogman, W. M.: The relation of growth to the cleft palate problem. D. Clin. North America, July, 1960, pp. 373–380.

Mestre, J. C., DeJesus, J., and Subtelny, J. D.: Unoperated oral clefts at maturation. Angle Orthodont., 30:78–85, 1960.

Olin, W. H.: Dental anomalies in cleft lip and palate patients. Angle Orthodont., 34:119–123, 1964.

Pruzansky, S.: Description, classification and analysis of unoperated clefts of the lip and palate. Am. J. Orthodont., 39:590–611, 1953.

Pruzansky, S.: Development of the deciduous occlusion in complete unilateral cleft lip and palate. J. Dent. Res., 43:821 (suppl.) 1964 (Abstract).

Pruzansky, S.: The growth of the premaxillary-vomerine complex in complete bilateral cleft lip and palate. Tandlaegebladet, 75:1157–1169, 1971.

Pruzansky, S.: Factors determining arch form in clefts of the lip and palate. Am. J. Orthodont., 41:827–851, 1955.

Pruzansky, S., and Aduss, H.: Arch form and the deciduous occlusion in complete unilateral clefts. Cleft Palate J., 1:411–418, 1964.

Rosenstein, S. W.: Early orthodontic procedures for cleft lip and palate individuals. Angle Orthodont., 33:127–134, 1963.

Rosenstein, S. W., Jacobson, B. W., Monroe, C., Griffith, B. H., and McKinney, P.: A series of cleft lip and palate children five years after undergoing orthopedic and bone grafting procedures. Angle Orthodont., 42:1–8, 1972.

Skoog, T.: Management of bilateral cleft of primary palate II. Bone grafting. Plast. Reconstr. Surg., 35:140–147, 1965.

Walker, B. C.: "Induction of cleft palate in rats with anti-inflammatory drugs. Teratology, 4:39–42, 1971.

8.   CEPHALOMETRICS AND LAMINAGRAPHY

Altemus, L. A.: A comparison of cephalofacial relationships. Angle Orthodont., 30:223–240, 1960.

Arita, M., and Iwagaki, H.: Studies on the serial observations of the dentofacial region in Japanese children. J. Nihon Univ. Sch. Dent., 1963.

Bennett, G. C., and Kronman, J. H.: A cephalometric study of mandibular development and its relationship to the mandibular and occlusal planes. Angle Orthodont., 40:119–128, 1970.

Berger, H.: Problems and promises of basilar view cephalograms. Angle Orthodont., 31:237–245, 1961.

Björk, A.: Prediction of mandibular growth rotation. Am. J. Orthodont., 55:585–599, 1969.

Björk, A.: The Face in Profile. Lund, Sweden, Svensk Tandläkare Tidskr., supp., 1947.

Björk, A.: The nature of facial prognathism and its relations to normal occlusion of the teeth. Am. J. Orthodont., 37:106–124, 1951.

Brader, A. C.: The application of the principles of cephalometric laminagraphy to studies of the frontal planes of the human skull. Am. J. Orthodont., 35:249–268, 1949.

Broadbent, B. H.: A new x-ray technique and its application to orthodontia. Angle Orthodont., 1:45–66, 1931.

Brodie, A. G., Downs, W. B., Goldstein, A., and Myer, E.: Cephalometric appraisal of orthodontic results: a preliminary report. Angle Orthodont., 8:261–265, 1938.

Brown, T., and Barrett, M. J.: A roentgenographic study of facial morphology in a tribe of Central Australian aborigines. Am. J. Phys. Anthrop., 22:33–42, 1964.

Chan, G. K. H.: A cephalometric appraisal of the Chinese (Cantonese). Am. J. Orthodont., 61:279–285, 1972.

Coben, S. E.: The integration of facial skeletal variants. Am. J. Orthodont., 41:407–434, 1955.

Downs, W. B.: Analysis of the dento-facial profile. Angle Orthodont., 26:191–212, 1956.

Downs, W. B.: Variations in facial relationships: their significance in treatment and prognosis. Am. J. Orthodont., 34:812–840; also Angle Orthodont., 19:145–155, 1949.

Dreyer, C. J., and Joffe, B. M.: A concept of cephalometric interpretation. Angle Orthodont., 33:123–126, 1963.

Fine, H., Barrer, H., and Spengeman, W.: Cephalometrics. J. Pract. Orth., 3:475–478, 1969.

Fletcher, G. G. T.: Cephalometric appraisal of the development of malocclusion. Brit. Soc. Study Orthodont. Tr., p. 124–153 disc. 153–154, 1963.

Goldson, L.: (Importance of premature loss of deciduous teeth with special regard to the effect on overjet and overbite—a cephalometric study.) Svensk Tandläk. T., 56:63–75, 1963 (Sw.).

Graber, T. M.: A critical review of clinical cephalometric radiography. Am. J. Orthodont., 40:1–26, 1954.

Graber, T. M.: Implementation of the roentgenographic cephalometric technique. Am. J. Orthodont., 44:906–932, 1958.

Graber, T. M.: New horizons in case analysis; clinical cephalometrics. Am. J. Orthodont., 38:603–624, 1952.

Graber, T. M.: Panoramic radiography in dentistry. Canad. Dent. Assoc., J., 31:158–173, 1965.

Graber, T. M.: Problems and limitations of cephalometric analysis in orthodontics. J.A.D.A., 53:439–454, 1956.

Harris, J. E.: A cephalometric analysis of mandibular growth rate. Am. J. Orthodont., 48:161–175, 1962.

Harris, J. E., Johnston, L., and Moyers, R. E.: A cephalometric template: Its construction and clinical significance. Am. J. Orthodont., 49:249–263, 1963.

Hasund, A.: Position of the mandibular incisors in relation to orthodontic treatment. Inform. Orthodont. Kieferorthop., 1:22–36, 1969.

Hitchcock, H. P.: A cephalometric supplement. Am. J. Orthodont., 57:47–54, 1970.

Hixon, E. H.: Cephalometrics and longitudinal research. Am. J. Orthodont., 46:36–42, 1960.

Hixon, E. H.: The norm concept and cephalometrics. Am. J. Orthodont., 42:898–906, 1958.

Koski, K.: Growth changes in the relationships between some basicranial planes and the palatal plane. Suom. Hammaslääk. Toim., 57:15–26, 1961.

Maj, G., and Luzi, C.: The role of cephalometrics in the diagnosis and prognosis of malocclusions. Am. J. Orthodont., 48:911–923, 1962.

Marschner, J. F., and Harris, J. E.: Mandibular growth and class II treatment. Angle Orthodont., 36:89–93, 1966.

McDowell, C. S.: A reappraisal of cephalometrics. J. Clin. Orthodont., 4:82–92, 134–145, 1970.

Merow, W. W.: A cephalometric statistical appraisal of dentofacial growth. Angle Orthodont., 32:205–213, 1962.

Miura, F., Inoue, N., and Suzuki, K.: Cephalometric standards for Japanese according to the Steiner analysis. Am. J. Orthodont., 51:288–295, 1965.

Moorrees, C. F. A., and Lebret, L.: The mesh diagram and cephalometrics. Angle Orthodont., 32:214–231, 1962.

Olsson, A., and Posselt, U.: Relationship of various skull reference lines. J. Prosth. Dent., 11:1045–1049, 1961.

Paulson, R. C.: The significance of cephalometric pattern variations. Angle Orthodont., 34:115–118, 1964.

Ricketts, R. M.: Analysis—the interim. Angle Orthodont., 40:129–137, 1970.

Ricketts, R. M., Bench, R. W., Hilgers, J. J., and Schulhof, R.: An overview of computerized cephalometrics. Am. J. Orthodont., 61:1–28, 1972.

Schwarz, A. M.: Practical evaluation of the head x-ray. Europ. Orthodont. Soc. Tr., 37:497–505, 1961.

Steiner, C. C.: Use of cephalometrics as an aid to planning and assessing orthodontic treatment. Report of a case. Am. J. Orthodont., 46:721–735, 1960.

Subtelny, J. D.: Cephalometric diagnosis, growth and treatment: something old, something new? Am. J. Orthodont., 57:262–286, 1970.

Susami, R.: A cephalometric evaluation of dentofacial growth in mandibular protrusion subjects. J. Osaka Univ. Dent. Sch., 9:25–35, 1969.

Tweed, C. H.: The diagnostic facial triangle in the control of treatment objectives. Am. J. Orthodont., 55:651–667, 1969.

Updegrave, W. J.: Radiographic technique for the temporomandibular articulation. Angle Orthodont., 21:181–193, 1951; also Am. J. Orthodont., 39:495–504, 1953.

Updegrave, W. J.: Roentgenology in orthodontics. Am. J. Orthodont., 48:841–847, 1962.

Walker, G. F., Kowalski, C. J.: The distribution of the ANB angle in "normal" individuals. Angle Orthodont., 41:332–335, 1971.

Wei, S. H. Y.: Craniofacial width dimensions. Angle Orthodont., 40:141–147, 1970.

9.   ANATOMY AND OCCLUSION OF TEETH

Adams, C. P.: Investigation into the relation between face width and upper dental arch width in five year old children. Europ. Orthodont. Soc. Tr., 39:265–278 disc. 279–280, 1963.

Adler, P.: Effect of some environmental factors on the sequence of permanent tooth eruption. J. Dent. Res., 42:605–616, 1963.

Altemus, L. A.: Relationships of tooth material and supporting bone. D. Progress, 1:36–41, 1960.

Arita, M., Iwasawa, T., and Namura, S.: Relationship between the curves of Spee in persons with normal occlusion and the occlusal plane (abstract). J. Nihon Univ. Sch. Dent., 6:25–28, 1964.

Backlund, E.: Tooth form and overbite. Europe. Orthodont. Soc. Tr., 36:97–103 disc. 103–104, 1960.

Baume, L. J.: Developmental and diagnostic aspects of the primary dentition. Internat. D. J., 9:349–366, 1959.

Beazley, W. W.: Assessment of mandibular arch length discrepancy utilizing an individualized arch form. Angle Orthodont., 41:45–54, 1971.

Beresford, J. S.: Tooth size and class distinction. Dent. Pract., 20:113–120, 1969.

Beyron, H.: Optimal occlusion. D. Clin. North America, July, 1969.

Bolton, W. A.: Disharmony in tooth size and its relation to the analysis and treatment of malocclusion. Angle Orthodont., 28:113–130, 1958.

Broekman, R. W.: (Unreliability of the indices for the shape of the dental arch.) Schweiz. Mschr. Zahnheilk., 74:238–251, 1964 (Ger.).

Cleall, J. F., and Chebib, F. S.: Coordinate analysis applied to orthodontic studies. Angle Orthodont., 41:214–218, 1971.

Clinch, L. M.: Longitudinal study of the mesiodistal crown diameters of the deciduous teeth and their permanent successors. Europ. Orthodont. Soc. Tr., 39:202–215, 1963.

Dyer, E.: Dental articulation and occlusion. J. Prosth. Dent., 17:238–245, 1967.

Friel, E. S.: The development of ideal occlusion of the gum pads and the teeth. Am. J. Orthodont., 40:196–227, 1954.

Garn, S. M., and Lewis, A. B.: The relationship between third molar agenesis and reduction in tooth number. Angle Orthodont., 32:14–18, 1962.

Garn, S. M., Lewis, A. B., and Kerewsky, R. S.: Sex differences in tooth size. J. Dent. Res., 43:306, 1964.

Gellin, M. E.: A method of predicting the initial eruptive pattern of the mandibular permanent anterior teeth by radiographic analysis. J. Dent. Child., 28:138–149, 1961.

Graber, T. M.: The fundamentals of occlusion. J.A.D.A., 48:177–187, 1954.

Grewe, J. M.: Intercanine width variability in American Indian children. Angle Orthodont., 40:353–358, 1970.

Guichet, N. F.: Applied gnathology, why and how. D. Clin. North America, July, 1969.

Halpert, L. F.: A clinical discussion of occlusion. J. Maryland State Dent. Assn., 34: 197–202, 1968.

Hasund, A., and Sivertsen, R.: Dental arch space and facial type. Angle Orthodont., 41:140–145, 1971.

Hellman, M.: Factors Influencing Occlusion in Development of Occlusion. Philadelphia, University of Pennsylvania Press, 1941.

Hopkins, J. B., and Murphy, J.: Variations in good occlusions. Angle Orthodont., 41:55–65, 1971.

Horowitz, H. S., Cohen, L. K., and Doyle, J.: Occlusal relations in children in an optimally fluoridated community: IV. Clinical and social-psychological findings. Angle Orthodont., 41:189–201, 1971.

Howes, A. E.: Arch width in the premolar region—still the major problem in orthodontics. Am. J. Orthodont., 43:5–31, 1957.

Howes, A. E.: Case analysis and treatment planning based upon the relationship of the tooth material to its supporting bone. Am. J. Orthodont. & Oral Surg., 33:499–533 (correction p. 690), 1947.

Kepron, D.: Experience with modern occlusal concepts, D. Clin. North America, July, 1971.

Knott, V. B., and Meredith, H. V.: Statistics on eruption of the permanent dentition from serial data for North American white children. Angle Orthodont., 36:68–79, 1966.

Lundström, A. F.: Malocclusion of the teeth regarded as a problem in connection with the apical base. Internat. J. Orthodont. & Oral Surg., 11:591–602; 724–731; 793–812; 933–941; 1022–1042; 1109–1133, 1925.

Lundström, A.: Asymmetries in the number and size of the teeth and their aetiological significance. Europ. Orthodont. Soc. Tr., 36:167–185, 1960.

Lysell, L., Magnusson, B., and Thilander, B.: Time and order of eruption of the primary teeth. Odont. Rev., 13:217–234, 1962.

Moorrees, C. F. A.: The Dentition of the Growing Child. Cambridge, Harvard University Press, 1959.

Moorrees, C. F. A., Fanning, E. A., and Hunt, E. E., Jr.: Formation and resorption of three deciduous teeth in children. Am. J. Phys. Anthrop., 21:99–108, 1963.

Moyers, R. E., and Lo, R.: Sequence of eruption of the permanent dentition. Am. J. Orthodont., 39:460, 1953.

Ohnishi, K.: Relationship between apical base and incisal inclination in school children. J. Jap. Orthodont. Soc., 28:12–32, 1969.

Perry, H. T.: Principles of occlusion applied to modern orthodontics. D. Clin. North America, July, 1969.

Ramfjord, S. P., and Ash, M. M.: Occlusion, 2nd Ed. Philadelphia, W. B. Saunders Co., 1971.

Ricketts, R. M.: Occlusion. J. Prosth. Dent. 21:39–60, 1969.

Riedel, R. A.: Maxillo-cranial relations—the relation of maxillary structures to cranium in malocclusion and in normal occlusion. Angle Orthodont., 22:142–145, 1952.

Roth, R.: Gnathological principles and the orthodontically treated case. Bull. Pacif. Coast Soc. Orthodont., 44:20–27, 1969.

Sanin, C., Savara, B. S.: The development of an excellent occlusion. Am. J. Orthodont., 61:345–352, 1972.

Schuyler, C.: Freedom in centric. D. Clin. North America, July, 1969.

Siersbaek-Nielsen, S.: Rate of eruption of central incisors at puberty; an implant study on eight boys. Tandlaegebladet, 75:1288–1295, 1971.

Stahl, S. S.: The role of occlusion in the etiology and therapy of periodontal disease. Angle Orthodont., 40:347–352, 1970.

Stramrud, L.: Incisor-molar relations of the maxilla. Angle Orthodont., 34:168–173, 1964.

10. TOOTH MEASUREMENTS

Baldridge, D. N.: Leveling the curve of Spee: its effect on mandibular arch length. J. Pract. Orthodont., 3:26–41, 1969.

Ballard, M. C., and Wylie, W. L.: Mixed dentition case analysis—estimating size of unerupted teeth. Am. J. Orthodont., 33:754–759, 1947.

Bolton, W. A.: The clinical application of a tooth-size analysis. Am. J. Orthodont., 48: 504–529, 1962.

Carey, C. W.: Linear arch dimensions and tooth size. Am. J. Orthodont., 35:762–775, 1949.

Carlsen, D. B., and Meredith, H. V.: Biologic variation in selected relationships of opposing posterior teeth. Angle Orthodont., 30:162–173, 1960.

Currier, J. H.: A computerized geometric analysis of the human dental arch. Am. J. Orthodont., 56:164–179, 1969.

Dragiff, D. A.: Occlusion of the buccal segments as influenced by disharmony of the buccal teeth. J. Pract. Orthodont., 3:85–91, 1969.

Foresman, R. R.: The maxillary first permanent molar as a causative factor in arch length deficiency. Angle Orthodont., 34:174–180, 1964.

Goldsman, S.: An aid in predicting the fate of crowded teeth. W. Virginia Dent. J., 39:4–5, 1965.

Hasund, A., and Ulstein, G.: The position of the incisors in relation to the lines NA and NB in different facial types. Am. J. Orthodont., 57:1–14, 1970.

Huckaba, G. W.: Arch size analysis and tooth size prediction. D. Clin. North America, July, 1964, pp. 431–440.

Iyer, V. S., and Desai, D. M.: Acceptable deviations in normal dentitions. Angle Orthodont., 33:253–257, 1963.

Kato, S., Kubota, K., Hashimoto, T. Wada, K., Araki, S., and Lee, S. F.: Study on the relative positions of teeth and the average form of dental arches. J. Nihon Univ. Sch. Dent., 6:111–121, September, 1964.

Knott, V. B.: Size and form of the dental arches in children with good occlusion studied longitudinally from age 9 years to late adolescence. Am. J. Orthodont., 48:938–940, 1962.

Lavelle, C. L. B.: Maxillary and mandibular tooth size in different racial groups and in different occlusal categories. Am. J. Orthodont., 61:29–37, 1972.

Lebret, L.: Physiologic tooth migration. J. Dent. Res., 43:610–618, 1964.

Lundström, A.: Intermaxillary tooth width ratio and tooth alignment and occlusion. Acta Odont. Scandinav., 12:265–292, 1954.

Lundström, A.: Variations of tooth size in the etiology of malocclusion. Am. J. Orthodont., 41:872–876, 1955.

Mills, L. F.: Arch width, arch length, and tooth size in young adult males. Angle Orthodont., 34:124–129, 1964.

Mills, L. F., and Hamilton, P. M.: Epidemiological studies of malalignment, a method for computing dental arch circumference. Angle Orthodont., 35:244–248, 1965.

Moorrees, C. F. A., and Chadha, J. M.: Available space for the incisors during dental development—a growth study based on physiologic age. Angle Orthodont., 35:12–22, 1965.

Peck, H., and Peck, S.: An index for assessing tooth shape deviations as applied to mandibular incisors. Am. J. Orthodont., 61:384–401, 1972.

Sanin, C., and Savara, B. S.: An analysis of permanent mesiodistal crown size. Am. J. Orthodont., 59:488–500, 1971.

Solow, B.: The association between spacing of the incisors temporary and permanent dentitions of the same individuals. Acta Odont. Scand., 17:511–527, 1959.

Smith, B., and Bernard, W. V.: The mixed dentition analysis; a prediction of tooth size and arch length relationship. J. Dent. Child., 31:114–119, 1964.

Stifter, J.: A Study of Pont's, Howes', Rees', Neff's and Bolton's analyses on Class I adult dentitions. Angle Orthodont., 28:215–225, 1958.

11. ETIOLOGY, CASE ANALYSIS AND DIAGNOSIS

Ackerman, J. L., and Proffit, W. R.: The characteristics of malocclusion: a modern approach to classification and diagnosis. Am. J. Orthodont., 56:443–454, 1969.

Biederman, W.: The ankylosed tooth. D. Clin. North America, July, 1964, pp. 493–508.

Biggerstaff, R. H.: Computerized diagnostic set-ups and simulations. Angle Orthodont., 40:28–36, 1970.

Biggerstaff, R. H., and Wells, J. A.: Computerized analysis of occlusion in the postcanine dentition. Am. J. Orthodont., 61:245–254, 1972.

Bowden, B. D.: A clinical assessment of mixed dentition crowding. Aust. Dent. J., 14:90–98, 1969.

Bowles, R. M.: Evaluation of tooth size relationships in various intradental and interdental arch segments. Am. J. Orthodont., 57:415–421, 1970.

Burstone, C. J.: Distinguishing developing malocclusion from normal occlusion. D. Clin. North America, July, 1964, pp. 479–491.

Cohen, M. I.: Recognition of developing malocclusion. D. Clin. North America, 299–311, July, 1959.

Cross, S.: Endocrines: their relation to orthodontic diagnosis and treatment planning. Am. J. Orthodont., 34:418–440, 1948.

Dreyer, C. J., and Joffe, B. M.: Concept of cephalometric interpretation. Angle Orthodont., 33:123–126, 1963.

Fleming, H. B.: An investigation of the vertical overbite during the eruption of the permanent dentition. Angle Orthodont., 31:53–62, 1961.

Graber, T. M.: Appliances at the crossroads. Am. J. Orthodont., 42:683–701, 1956.

Graber, T. M.: Extrinsic factors. Am. J. Orthodont., 44:26–45, 1958.

Graber, T. M.: The finger sucking habit and associated problems. J. Dent. Child., 25:145–151, 1958.

Graber, T. M.: The role of upper second molar extraction in orthodontic treatment. Am. J. Orthodont., 41:354–361, 1955.

Graber, T. M.: Thumb and finger-sucking. Am. J. Orthodont., 45:258–264, 1959.

Grewe, J. M., and Hagan, D. V.: Malocclusion indices: a comparative evaluation. Am. J. Orthodont., 61:286–294, 1972.

Grossman, W. J., et al.: Electromyography as an aid in diagnosis and treatment analysis. Am. J. Orthodont., 47:481–497, 1961.

Hahn, G. W.: Treatment planning and therapy in the mixed dentition. Am. J. Orthodont., 49:563–567, 1963.

Harvold, E.: Some biologic aspects of orthodontic treatment in the transitional dentition. Am. J. Orthodont., 49:1–14, 1963.

Harvold, E. P., and Poyton, H. G.: Syndrome of dual bite associated with open bite. J. Canad. Dent. Assoc., 28:617–626, 1962.

Hitchcock, H. P.: A cephalometric supplement. Am. J. Orthodont., 57:47–54, 1970.

Hixon, E. H., and Oldfather, R. E.: Estimation of the sizes of unerupted cuspid and bicuspid teeth. Angle Orthodont., 28:236–240, 1958.

Kuftinec, M. M., and Glass, R. L.: Stability of the IMPA with reference to the Begg method. Angle Orthodont., 41:264–270, 1971.

Leighton, B. C.: Problems of orthodontic consultation. Brit. D. J., 116:234–238, 1964.

Lischer, B. E.: Etiology of dental anomalies. Internat. J. Orthodont. & Dent. Children, 21:9–19, 1935.

Logan, W. R.: Effect of the Milwaukee brace on the developing dentition. Brit. Soc. Study Orthodont. Tr., p. 1–8 disc. 8, 1962.

Lundström, A.: The significance of early loss of deciduous teeth in the etiology of malocclusion. Am. J. Orthodont., 41:819–826, 1955.

Mattila, K.: Prognathism of the upper jaw between the ages of four and nineteen. Odont. T., 77:88–95, 1969.

Mayne, W. R.: A concept, a diagnosis and a discipline. D. Clin. North America, July, 1959, pp. 281–288.

McCartney, T. P. G.: Arch measurements in orthodontic planning. Dent. Pract., 14:14–16, 1963.

Moorrees, C. F. A., Fanning, E. A., Grøn, A., and Lebret, L.: Timing of orthodontic treatment in relation to tooth formation. Europ. Orthodont. Soc. Tr., 38:87–101, 1962.

Mossmann, W. H.: Diagnosis and prevention of some malocclusions. D. Clin. North America, March, 1962, pp. 99–108.

Moyers, R. E., Harvold, E., Jenkins, H., Shultis, K., and Crouch, J. T.: Intraoral factors affecting case assessment. Am. J. Orthodont., 40:341–349, 1954.

Nance, H. N.: The limitations of orthodontic diagnosis and treatment. I. The mixed dentition. II. Diagnosis and treatment in the permanent dentition. Am. J. Orthodont. & Oral Surg., 33:177–223 (Part I); 253–301 (Part II), 1947.

Park, A. W.: Measurement and the oral biologist. Angle Orthodont., 40:138–140, 1970.

Priewe, D. E.: Evaulation of cephalometric analysis and extraction formulas for orthodontic treatment planning. Am. J. Orthodont., 48:414–435, 1962.

Reading, J. F.: Guide to orthodontic diagnosis and treatment planning. Aust. Dent. J., 5:349–355, 1960.

Riedel, R. A.: An analysis of dentofacial relationships. Am. J. Orthodont., 43:103–119, 1957.

Riedel, R. A.: Diagnosis and treatment planning in orthodontics. D. Clin. North America, March, 1963, pp. 175–187.

Riedel, R. A.: Esthetics and its relation to orthodontic therapy. Angle Orthodont., 20:168–178, 1950.

Rosenstein, S.: Interceptive orthodontics. Northwest Dent., 40:277–283, 293, 1961.

Savara, B. S.: The role of computers in dentofacial research and the development of diagnostic aids. Am. J. Orthodont., 61:231–244, 1972.

Schudy, F. F.: Vertical growth versus anteroposterior growth as related to function and treatment. Angle Orthodont., 34:75–93, 1964.

Subtelny, J. D., and Sakuda, M.: Open-bite: diagnosis and treatment. Am. J. Orthodont., 50:337–358, 1964.

Swain, B. F.: Case analysis and treatment planning in Class II, Division 1 cases. Angle Orthodont., 22:187–204, 1952.

Tweed, C. H.: Frankfort-mandibular incisor angle (FMIA) in orthodontic diagnosis, treatment planning and prognosis. Angle Orthodont., 24:121–169, 1954.

Walker, G. F.: A new approach to the analysis of craniofacial morphology and growth. Am. J. Orthodont., 61:221–230, 1972.

Weber, F. N.: Supernumerary teeth. D. Clin. North America, July, 1964, pp. 509–517.

Wei, S. H. Y.: Craniofacial width dimensions. Angle Orthodont., 40:141–147, 1970.

Wylie, W. L., and Johnson, E. L.: Rapid evaluation of facial dysplasia in the vertical plane. Angle Orthodont., 22:165–182, 1952.

12.   THE PROBLEM OF EXTRACTION IN ORTHODONTICS

Barrer, H. G.: Treatment timing of borderline cases. J. Clin. Orthodont., 5:191–199, 1971.

Barron, J. M.: Oral surgery in preventive orthodontics. D. Clin. North America, July, 1964, pp. 461–478.

Buchin, I. D.: Borderline extraction cases, Part One. J. Clin. Orthodont., 5:376–389, 1971. Part Two, 5:421–434, 1971. Part Three, 5:481–491, 1971.

Chipman, M. R.: Second and third molars: their role in orthodontic therapy. Am. J. Orthodont., 47:498–520, 1961.

Dewel, B. F.: A question of terminology. Am. J. Orthodont., 58:78–79, 1970.

Dewel, B. F.: Precautions in serial extraction. Am. J. Orthodont., 60:615–618, 1971.

Dewel, B. F.: Prerequisites in serial extraction. Am. J. Orthodont., 55:633–639, 1969.

Dewel, B. F.: Serial extraction—its limitations and contraindications. Arizona Dent. J., 14:14–30, Sept. 15, 1968.

Dewel, B. F.: Serial extraction: procedures and limitations. Am. J. Orthodont., 43:685–687, 1957.

Fogel, M. S.: Borderline malocclusions, differential diagnosis. Part One, J. Clin. Orthodont., 5:248–259, 1971. Part Two, 5:305–320, 1971.

Graber, T. M. (Ed.): Current Orthodontic Concepts and Techniques. Philadelphia, W. B. Saunders Co., 1969.

Graber, T. M.: Extraction in orthodontics. J. Colorado Dent. Assoc., 53:17–18, 1965.

Graber, T. M.: Maxillary second molar extraction in Class II cases. Am. J. Orthodont., 56:331–353, 1969.

Graber, T. M.: Serial extraction: a continuous diagnostic and decisional process. Am. J. Orthodont., 60:541–575, 1971.

Graber, T. M.: The role of upper second molar extraction in orthodontics. Am. J. Orthodont., 41:354–361, 1955.

Granerus, R.: Some clinical aspects on the problems of impacted upper canines. Europ. Orthodont. Soc. Tr., 37:399–408, 1961.

Heath, J.: Dangers and pitfalls of serial extraction. Europ. Orthodont. Soc. Tr., 37:60–72, 1961.

Hinrichsen, C. F. L.: Serial extraction in mixed dentition orthodontics. Aust. Dent. J., 6:201–209, 1961.

Hitchcock, H. P.: Basis for a modified treatment plan in extraction cases. Alabama J. Med. Sci., 1:123–133, 1964.

Hotz, R.: Active supervision of the eruption of the teeth by extraction. Trans. Europ. Orthodont. Soc., 1947–48, p. 34.

Hotz, R. F.: Guidance of eruption versus serial extraction. Am. J. Orthodont., 58:1–20, 1970.

Jacobs, J.: Cephalometric and clinical evaluation of the Class I discrepancy cases treated by serial extraction procedures. Am. J. Orthodont., 48:631, 1962.

Joondeph, D. D.: Congenitally absent second premolars; an interceptive approach. Am. J. Orthodont., 59:50–55, 1971.

Keedy, R. L.: Indications and Contraindications for extraction procedures. Angle Orthodont., 26:243–349, 1956.

Kessel, S. P.: The rationale of maxillary premolar extraction only in Class II therapy. Am. J. Orthodont., 49:276–293, 1963.

Kjellgren, B.: Serial extraction as a corrective procedure in dental orthopedic therapy. Acta Odont. Scandinav., 8:17–43, 1948; abst., Am. J. Orthodont., 35:471–476, 1949.

Lloyd, Z. B.: Serial extraction as a treatment procedure. Am. J. Orthodont., 42:728–739, 1956.

Mathews, J. R.: Translational movement of first deciduous molars into second molar positions. Am. J. Orthodont., 55:276–285, 1969.

Mayne, W. R.: In Graber, T. H. (Ed.): Current Orthodontic Concepts and Techniques. Philadelphia, W. B. Saunders Co., 1969.

Mayne, W. R.: Serial Extraction—orthodontics at the crossroads. D. Clin. North America, July, 1968.

Moorrees, C. L.: Considerations of dental development in serial extraction. Angle Orthodont., 33:44, 1963.

Nakai, T. T.: The influence of serial extraction procedures on the soft tissues: profiles in Class II, division 1 malocclusions; A Cephalometric Study. Am. J. Orthodont., 54:154, 1968.

Proffit, W. R.: Space maintenance, serial extraction and the general practitioner. J.A.D.A., 74:411–419, 1967.

Ringenberg, Q. M.: Serial extraction: Stop, look, and be certain. Am. J. Orthodont., 50:327–336, 1964.

Ringenberg, O. W.: Influence of serial extraction and development of maxilla and mandible. Am. J. Orthodont., 53:19, 1967.

Schwab, D. T.: The borderline patient and tooth removal. Am. J. Orthodont., 59:126–145, 1971.

Steadman, S. R.: Discussion of "An analysis of second premolar extraction procedures." Angle Orthodont., 34:301–302, 1964.

Swain, B. F.: Borderline extractions cases, guidelines for treatment. J. Clin. Orthodont., 5:539–565, 1971.

Taylor, R. F.: Controlled serial extraction. Am. J. Orthodont., 60:576–599, 1971.

Thilander, B., Jakobsson, S. O., and Skagius, S.: Orthodontic sequelae of extraction of permanent first molars. Odont. T., 71:380–412, 1963.

Tweed, C. H.: Indications for the extraction of teeth in orthodontic procedures. Am. J. Orthodont., 30:405–428, 1944.

Tweed, C. H.: Pre-orthodontic guidance procedures: classification of growth trends; treatment timing, Vistas in Orthodont., Phila., 359–389, 1962.

Tweed, C. H.: Treatment planning and therapy in the mixed dentition. Am. J. Orthodont., 49:881, 1963.

Wilkenson, L. C.: Some things to keep in mind when treating a four bicuspid extraction case. Angle Orthodont., 22:47–52, 1952.

13. METALLURGY AND MATERIA TECHNICA

Andreasen, G. F., and Quenada, F. R.: Evaluation of friction forces in the .022 × .028 edgewise bracket in vitro. J. Biomechanics, 3:151–160, 1970.

Bien, S. M., and Ayers, H. D., Jr.: Solder joints on rustless alloys. J.A.D.A., 58:74–80, 1959.

Billberg, B.: Mechanical properties of stainless steel wire used in orthodontic practice. Svensk. Tandläk. Tidskr., 55:197–210, 405–429, 1962.

Bradel, S. E.: One hundred years of development in metallurgy and its relation to orthodontia. J.A.D.A., 21:1018, 1934.

Cameron, J. C., et al.: Some properties of dental cements of specific importance in the cementation of orthodontic bands. Angle Orthodont., 33:233–245, 1963.

Cutler, R.: A new preparation of British stainless steel. Dent. Record, 52:178, 1932.

Delgado, V. P., and Anderson, J. N.: Tensile and blending properties of stainless steel orthodontic wires. Brit. Dent. J., 114:401–406, 1963.

Denver, P. I.: Heat Treatment of Orthodontic Steel Wire. Masters' thesis. University of Indiana Dental School, Indianapolis, Ind., 1958.

Friel, S.: The practical application of stainless steel in the construction of fixed orthodontic appliances, Int. J. Orthodont., 20:972, 1934.

Funk, A. C.: The heat treatment of stainless steel. Angle Orthodont., 21:129–138, 1951.

Futterman, N. J.: Electrolytic stainless steel polisher. Am. J. Orthodont., 28:652, 1942.

Gardner, J. H.: Some aspects of soldering stainless steel. Dent. Pract., 20:65–76, 1969.

Gaston, N.: Chrome alloy in orthodontics. Am. J. Orthodont., 37:779, 1951.

Griffin, J. N.: The use of chrome alloy in edgewise technique. Am. J. Orthodont., 40:450, 1954.

Heideborn, M. O.: Disadvantages of orthodontic bands and first experiments with a new plastic bracket for direct attachment. Zahnarztl. Welt., 78:933–938, 1969.

Hillam, H. G.: Relationship of structure to physical properties of soldered cobalt chromium orthodontic wires. Masters' thesis. Northwestern University Dental School, Chicago, Ill., 1966.

Howe, G. L.: Mechanical properties and stress relief of stainless steel orthodontic wire. Angle Orthodont., 38:244–249, 1968.

Kemler, E. A.: A study of the effect of low temperature heat treatment on the physical properties of orthodontic wire. Thesis. Northwestern University, Chicago, Ill., 1955.

Kohl, R. W.: Metallurgy in orthodontics. Angle Orthodont., 34:37–42, 1964.

Mutchler, R. W.: The effect of heat treatment on the mechanical properties of orthodontic cobalt-chromium steel wires as compared with chromium nickel wire. Master's Thesis, Northwestern University Dental School, Chicago, Ill., 1959.

Newman, G. V.: Adhesion and orthodontic plastic attachments. Am. J. Orthodont., 56:573–588, 1969.

Newman, G. V.: Biophysical properties of orthodontic rubber elastics. J. New Jersey Dent. Soc., 35:95–103, 1963.

Newman, G. V.: Bonding plastic orthodontic attachments. J. Pract. Orthodont., 3:231–238, 1969.

Newman, G. V.: Clinical treatment with bonded plastic attachments. Am. J. Orthodont., 60:600–610, 1971.

Newman, G. V.: Bonding plastic orthodontic attachments to tooth enamel. J. New Jersey Dent. Soc., 35:346–358, 1964.

Ohkawa, T.: A study of the heat-treatment hardening of cobalt base alloy wires for use in orthodontics. Shikwa Gaku, 69:59–87, 1969.

Parker, J. H.: Improved soldering technic. Angle Orthodont., 30:95–98, 1960.

Paskow, H.: Resins for use in making orthodontic appliances. (A letter to the editor.) Am. J. Orthodont., 50:203–204, 1964.

Pullen, H. A.: Seamless incisor bands in orthodontics. Am. Soc. Orthodont. Proceedings, 31:281, 1930.

Richman, G. Y.: Practical metallurgy for the orthodontist. Am. J. Orthodont., 42:573–587, 1956.

Sarantos, S. R.: Cementation of orthodontic bands. J. New Jersey Dent. Soc., 36:62–68, 1964.

Schmidt, D. A.: Stainless steel crowns and the child patient. D. Digest, 67:299, 1961.

Siersma, G. H.: The use of chrome alloy. Am. J. Orthodont., 26:875, 1940.

Vassar, R. J.: A metallographic study of the welded bond between two pieces of stainless steel band material. Master's Thesis, Northwestern University Dental School, Chicago, Ill., 1957.

Wilkinson, J. V.: Effect of high temperatures on stainless steel orthodontic arch wire. Aust. Dent. J., 5:264–268, 1960.

Wilkinson, J. V.: Soldering stainless steel. Angle Orthodont., 33:284–289, 1963.

Yost, H.: Practicality of chrome-nickel alloys for orthodontic use. J.A.D.A., 23:798, 1936.

14.   ORTHODONTIC THERAPY

Ackerman, J. L., and Proffit, W. R.: Treatment response as an aid in diagnosis and treatment planning. Am. J. Orthodont., 57:490–496, 1970.

Ahlgren, J.: Response to activator therapy. Dent. Abstr., 6:488–489, 1961.

Andreasen, G. F., and Brady, P. R.: A use hypothesis for 55 nitinol wire for orthodontics. Angle Orthodont., 42:172–177, 1972.

Armstrong, C. J.: Clinical evaluation of the chin cup. Aust. Dent. J., 8:492–499, 1963.

Atherton, J. D., and Wynne, T. H. M.: Long-term assessment of the facial pattern in children who had received orthodontic treatment. D. Pract., 14:317–322, 1964.

Baker, R. W., Guay, A. H., and Peterson, H. W.: Current concepts of anchorage management. Angle Orthodont., 42:129–138, 1972.

Barrer, H. G.: Non-extraction treatment with the Begg technique. Am. J. Orthodont., 56:365–378, 1969.

Barrer, H. G., Buchin, I. D., Fogel, M. S., Swain, B. S., and Ackerman, J. L.: Borderline extraction cases. J. Clin. Orthodont., 5:658–669, 1971.

Begg, P. R.: Choice of bracket for the light wire technique. Begg J. Orthodont. Theory & Treat., 1:11–18, 1962.

Begg, P. R.: Light arch wire technique employing the principle of differential force. Am. J. Orthodont., 47:30–48, 1961.

Begg, P. R., and Kesling, P. C.: Begg Orthodontic Theory and Technique, 2nd edition. Philadelphia, W. B. Saunders Co., 1971.

Bernstein, L.: Root torque with Warren springs. J. Clin. Orthodont., 5:167–169, 1971.

Bishara, S. E.: Management of diastemas in orthodontics. Am. J. Orthodont., 61:55–63, 1972.

Blodgett, G. B., and Andreason, G. F.: Comparison of applying two methods of lingual root torque to Maxim incisors. Angle Orthodont., 38:216, 1968.

Broussard, G. J., Broussard, C. J., Buck, H. R., and Shia, G. J.: Clinical applications of the Broussard auxiliary edgewise bracket. Am. J. Orthodont., 50:881–899, 1964.

Broussard, J. E.: Vertical dimension changes in 8-tooth extraction cases. Master's thesis, University of Tennessee, 1969.

Burstone, C. J.: Rationale of the segmented arch. Am. J. Orthodont., 48:805–822, 1962.

Burstone, C. J.: The mechanics of the segmented arch technique. Angle Orthodont., 36:99–120, 1966.

Burstone, C. J., Baldwin, J. J., and Lawless, D. T.: Application of continuous forces to orthodontics. Angle Orthodont., 31:1–14, 1961.

Carr, M. K., and Blafer, J. L.: Segmented arch technique. J. Clin. Orthodont., 5:501–509, 1971.

Chaconas, S. J.: Removable orthodontic appliances. J. Clin. Orthodont., 5:363–375, 1971.

Chavoor, A. G.: Adult orthodontics Class II, Division 1. Europ. Orthodont. Soc., 44:257–268, 1968.

Cheney, E. A.: Indications and methods for the interception of functional crossbites and inlockings. D. Clin. North America, July, 1959, pp. 385–402.

Cohen, M. I.: Mandibular prognathism. Am. J. Orthodont., 51:368–379, 1965.

Denholtz, M.: Effective procedure to help guide the developing dentition into proper occlusion. J. Dent. Child., 31:192–197, 1964.

Dipaolo, R. J., and Boruchov, M. J.: Thought on stripping of anterior teeth. J. Clin. Orthodont., 5:510–511, 1971.

Fastlicht, J.: More about the Universal Appliance. J. Clin. Orthodont., 5:72–81, 1971.

Freeman, R. S.: Are Class II elastics necessary? Am. J. Orthodont., 49:365–385, 1963.

Graber, T. M.: The edgewise appliance in routine practice. Am. J. Orthodont., 46:1–23, 1960.

Graber, T. M. (Ed.): Current Orthodontic Concepts and Techniques, 2 vols. Philadelphia. W. B. Saunders Co., 1969.

Grossmann, W., and Moss, J. P.: Role of functional jaw orthopaedics in orthodontics. D. Pract., 14:405–412, 1964.

Haack, D. C.: Science of mechanics and its importance to analysis and research in the field of orthodontics. Am. J. Orthodont., 49:330–344, 1963.

Harvold, E.: Some biologic aspects of orthodontic treatment in the transitional dentition. Am. J. Orthodont., 49:1–14, 1963.

Hixon, E. H., Atikian H., Callow, G. E., McDonald, H. W., and Tracy, R. J.: Optimal force, differential force, and anchorage. Am. J. Orthodont., 55:437–457, 1969.

Isaacson, R. J., and Ingram, A. H., II: Forces present during treatment. Angle Orthodont., 34:261–270, 1964.

Isaacson, R. J., and Murphy, T. D.: Some effects of rapid maxillary expansion in cleft lip and palate patients. Angle Orthodont., 34:143–154, 1964.

Isaacson, R. J., Wood, J. L., and Ingram, A. H.: Forces produced by rapid maxillary expansion: I. Design of force measuring system. Angle Orthodont., 34:256–260, 1964.

Levitt, H. L.: Adult orthodontics. J. Clin. Orthodont., 5:130–146, 1971.

Lewis, P. D.: Canine retraction. Am. J. Orthodont., 57:543–560, 1970.

Mathews, J. R.: Clinical management and supportive rationale in early orthodontic therapy. Angle Orthodont., 31:35–52, 1961.

McDowell, C. S.: Static anchorage in the Begg technique. Angle Orthodont., 39:162–170, 1969.

Mehta, J. D., and Barnett, E. M.: How to avoid problems in minor orthodontic procedures. New York. J. Dent., 36:24–28, 1970.

Miller, B. H.: Adult orthodontics. J. Dent. Ass. S. Africa., 24:81–91, 1969.

Muchnic, H. V.: Retention or continuing treatment. Am. J. Orthodont., 57:23–34, 1970.

Nahoum, H. I.: Torque: a round wire technique. Angle Orthodont., 32:242–251, 1962.

Nance, H. N.: The limitations of orthodontic treatment. Am. J. Orthodont. & Oral Surg., 33:177–223, 253–301, 1947.

Nasby, J. A., Isaacson, R. J., Worms, F. W., and Speidel, T. M.: Orthodontic extractions and the facial skeletal pattern. Angle Orthodont., 42:116–122, 1972.

Parker, W. S.: Mechanical principles and orthodontic appliances. Angle Orthodont., 30:241–247, 1960.

Poulton, D. R.: A three-year study of Class II malocclusions with and without headgear therapy. Angle Orthodont., 34:181–192, 1964.

Prescott, G. O.: Adult orthodontics. J. Rhode Isl. Dent. Ass., 2:9–10, 1969.

Rauch, E. D.: Torque and its application to orthodontics. Am. J. Orthodont., 45:817–830, 1959.

Rocke, R. A.: Management of overbite within the vertical dimension. Begg J. Orthodont. Theory Treat., 3:9–18, 1964.

Ruff, R. M.: Orthodontic treatment in the mixed dentition. Am. J. Orthodont., 57:502–518, 1970.

Seide, L. J.: Adult orthodontics. J. Prosth. Dent., 24:83–93, 1970.

Sims, M. R.: Begg philosophy and fundamental principles. Am. J. Orthodont., 50:15–24, 1964.

Sims, M. R.: Loop systems—a contemporary reassessment. Am. J. Orthodont., 61:270–278, 1972.

Spurrier, H. S.: Edgewise treatment of the Class II, Division 1 malocclusion. J. Pract. Orthodont., 3:362–369, 1969.

Stockfish, H.: Experience in active and functional plate treatment and the utilization of kinetic muscle energy in jaw-orthopedic methods. Int. J. Orthodont., 2:24–32, 1964 (Reprint).

Swain, B. F.: Guidelines for early treatment, headgear treatment, serial extraction without immediate treatment, non-extraction trial, and one-arch extraction treatment. J. Clin. Orthodont., 5:538–565, 1971.

Thilander, B.: Treatment of Angle Class III malocclusion with chin-cap. Europ. Orthodont. Soc. Tr., 39:384–397 disc. 398, 1963.

Thörne, N. A. H.: Expansion of maxilla. Spreading the midpalatal suture; measuring the widening of the apical base and the nasal cavity on serial roentgenograms. Am. J. Orthodont., 46:626, 1960 (Abstract).

Tweed, C. H.: Treatment planning and therapy in the mixed dentition. Am. J. Orthodont., 49:881–906, 1963.

Weber, F. N.: Corrective measures during the mixed dentition. Am. J. Orthodont., 43:639–660, 1957.

Weber, F. N.: Orthorehabilitative procedures. D. Clin. North America, July, 1959, pp. 419–434.

Weinstein, S., Haack, D. C., Morris, L. Y., Snyder, B. B., and Attaway, H. E.: On an equilibrium theory of tooth position. Angle Orthodont., 33:1–26, 1963.

Zimring, J. F., and Isaacson, R. J.: Forces produced by rapid maxillary expansion. Angle Orthodont., 35:178–186, 1965.

15.   EXTRAORAL FORCE AND ORTHOPEDICS

Baalack, I. B.: Occipital anchorage for distal movement of the maxillary first molars. Acta Odont. Scand., 24:307–321, 1966.

Dewel, B. F.: Class II treatment in the mixed dentition with the edgewise appliance and extraoral traction. E.O.S. Proceed., 307–319, 1968.

Gould, I. E.: Mechanical principles in extra-oral anchorage. Am. J. Orthodont., 43:319–333, 1957.

Graber, T. M.: A cephalometric appraisal of the result of cervical gear therapy. Am. J. Orthodont., 40:60, 1954.

Graber, T. M.: Current Orthodontic Concepts and Techniques, Chapter 10. W. B. Saunders Co., Philadelphia, 1969.

Graber, T. M.: Extra-oral force—facts and fallacies. Am. J. Orthodont., 41:490–505, 1955.

Graber, T. M., Chung, D. D. B., and Aoba, J. T.: Dentofacial orthopedics versus orthodontics. Aust. J. Orth., 1:84–105, 1968.

Graber, T. M., Chung, D. D. B., and Aoba, J. T.: Dentofacial orthopedics versus orthodontics. J.A.D.A., 75:1145–1166, 1967.

Graber, T. M., Moyers, R. E., Woodside, D. G., and Kaplan, H.: Extraoral force. J. Clin. Orthodont., 4:554–577, 618–641, 1970.

Greenspan, R. A.: Reference charts for controlled extraoral force application to maxillary molars. Am. J. Orthodont., 58:486–491, 1970.

Gregorak, W.: Eruption path of permanent maxillary molars in Class II, Division 1 malocclusion using headgear. Am. J. Orthodont., 48:367–381, 1962.

Henry, R. G.: Cervical anchorage and the upper first permanent molar. Aust. Dent. J., 6:260–268, 1961.

Klein, P. L.: An evaluation of cervical traction on the maxilla and the upper first permanent molars. Angle Orthodont., 27:61–68, 1957.

Kloeffler, G. D.: A report on maxillary orthopedics in cleft palate treatment. J. Prosth. Dent., 23:227–231, 1970.

Kloehn, S. J.: Analysis and treatment in mixed dentitions, a new approach. Am. J. Orthodont., 39:161–186, 1953.

Kuhn, R. J.: Control of anterior vertical dimension and proper selection of extra-oral anchorage. Angle Orthodont., 38:340–349, 1968.

Merrifield, L., Cross, J. J.: Directional forces. Am. J. Orthodont., 57:435–464, 1970.

Pfeiffer, J. P., and Grobety, D.: Simultaneous use of cervical appliance and activator: An orthodontic approach to fixed appliance therapy. Am. J. Orthodont., 61:353–373, 1972.

Poulton, D. R.: Changes in Class II malocclusions with and without occipital headgear therapy. Angle Orthodont., 29:232–250, 1959.

Poulton, D. R.: The influence of extraoral traction. Am. J. Orthodont., 53:8–18, 1967.

Poulton, D. R.: Three-year survey of Class II malocclusions with and without headgear therapy. Angle Orthodont., 34:181–193, 1964.

Rosenstein, S. W.: A new concept in the early orthopedic treatment of cleft lip and palate. Am. J. Orthodont., 55:765–775, 1969.

Seward, S.: Extra-oral anchorage. Aust. Dent. J., 9:419–425, 1964.

16.   RETENTION AND POST-TREATMENT ADJUSTMENT

Atherton, J. D., and Wynne, T. H. M.: Long-term assessment of the facial pattern in children who had received orthodontic treatment. D. Pract., 14:317–322, 1964.

Bates, D. E.: The removeable cast orthodontic retainer. Int. J. Orthodont., 8:106–112, 1970.

Baum, A. T., and Marshall, P. D.: Esthetic removal fixed retention. Angle Orthodont., 42:103–106, 1972.

Boese, L. R.: Increased stability of orthodontically rotated teeth following gingivectomy in Macaca nemestrina. Am. J. Orthodont., 56:273–290, 1969.

Broekman, R. W.: (Relapses in orthodontic treatment.) Nederl. T. Tandheelk., 69:278–290, 1962 (Dut.).

Chateau, M., and Démogé, P. H.: Evaluation of long term results of orthodontic therapy. Int. Dent. J., 11:29–46, 1961.

Cousins, A. J. P., Brown, W. A. B., and Harkness, E. M.: An investigation into the effect of the maxillary biteplate on the height of the lower incisor teeth. Dent. Pract., 20:107–121, 1969.

Dwight, O. D.: Simplified retaining and debanding procedures. Angle Orthodont., 39:230–238, 1969.

Edwards, J. G.: The prevention of relapse in extraction cases. Am. J. Orthodont., 60:128–141, 1971.

Galen, R.: Retention can be less of a problem. J. Clin. Orthodont., 6:102–106, 1972.

Holden, T. M.: Effects of the tooth positioner on the oral mechanism following orthodontic treatment. Am. J. Orthodont., 48:630, 1962 (Abstract).

Hopkins, S. C.: Inadequacy of mandibular anchorage—five years later. Am. J. Orthodont., 46:440–455, 1960.

Huggins, D. G.: Functional retention. Brit. Soc. Study Orthodont. Tr., pp. 77–80, 1963.

Huggins, D. G., et al.: Cephalometric investigation of stability of upper incisors following their retraction. Am. J. Orthodont., 50:852–856, 1964.

Jacobs, R. M.: Treatment objectives and case retention: cybernetics and "Myometric" Considerations. Am. J. Orthodont., 58:552–564, 1970.

Khouw, F. E.: Band space closure and retention. J. Pract. Orthodont., 3:424–425, 1969.

Korkhaus, G. (moderator), et al.: Post-treatment appraisal of orthodontic results. Round table discussion. Europ. Orthodont. Soc. Tr., 37:73–97, 1961.

Kraut, A.: Tooth changes three to nine years out of retention. Bul. Monmouth Co. D. Soc., Vol. 16, November, 1962.

Levitt, H.: High labial retainer. J. Clin. Orthodont., 6:35–39, 1972.

Lombardi, A.: Mandibular incisor crowding in completed cases. Am. J. Orthodont., 61:374–383, 1972.

Muchnic, H. V.: Retention or continuing treatment. Am. J. Orthodont., 57:23–35, 1970.

Nielsen, I. L.: Transsection of supra-alveolar fibers on orthodontically rotated teeth in monkeys. Tandlaegebladet, 75:1330–1340, 1971.

Reitan, K.: Biomechanical principles and reactions. In Graber, T. M. (Ed.): Current Orthodontic Concepts and Techniques, pp. 56–160, Philadelphia, W. B. Saunders Co., 1969.

Reitan, K.: Clinical and histologic observations on tooth movement during and after orthodontic treatment. Am. J. Orthodont., 53:721–745, 1967.

Reitan, K.: Experiments on rotation of teeth and their subsequent retention. Europ. Orthodont. Soc. Trans., 34:124–140, 1958.

Reitan, K.: Tissue rearrangement during retention of orthodontically rotated teeth. Angle Orthodont., 29:105–113, 1959.

Riedel, R. A.: A review of the retention problem. Angle Orthodont., 30:179–199, 1960.

Riedel, R. A.: Retention. In Graber, T. M. (Ed.): Current Orthodontic Concepts and Techniques. Philadelphia, W. B. Saunders Co., 1969.

Rosenstein, S. W., and Jacobson, B. N.: Retention: An Equal Partner. Am. J. Orthodont., 59:323–332, 1971.

Steadman, S. R.: A philosophy and practice of orthodontic retention. Angle Orthodont., 37:175–185, 1967.

Steadman, S. R.: Changes of intermolar and intercuspid distances following orthodontic treatment. Angle Orthodont., 31:207–215, 1961.

Theuveny, F.: Retention with a fixed bandless archwire. J. Clin. Orthodont., 5:392–393, 1971.

Tulley, W. J.: Long-term orthodontic results. Brit. Soc. Study Orthodont. Tr., pp. 73–80 disc. 81–82, 1961.

Weiss, H., and Gurman, M.: The tooth aligner. J. Clin. Orthodont., 5:655–657, 1971.

17. IATROGENIC EFFECTS

Adams, R. J.: The effects of fixed orthodontic appliances on the cariogenicity, quantity, and microscopic morphology of oral lactobacilli. J. Oral Med., 22:88–98, 1967.

Balenseifen, J. W., and Madonia, J. V.: Study of dental plaque in orthodontic patients. J. Dent. Res., 49:320–324, 1970.

Becks, H.: Orthodontic prognosis: evaluation of routine dentomedical examinations to determine "good and poor risks." Am. J. Orthodont., 25:610–624, 1939.

Becks, H.: Root resorptions and their relation to pathologic bone formation, Part II. Am. J. Orthodont., 28:513–526, 1942.

Bloom, R. H., and Brown, L. R.: A study of the effects of orthodontic appliances on the oral microbial flora. Oral Surg., 17:658–667, 1964.

Bogucki, Z.: A comparison of apical root resorptions incident to Begg and edgewise orthodontic therapy. Master's Thesis, Department of Orthodontics, College of Dentistry, Fairleigh Dickinson University, Teaneck, New Jersey, 1966.

Carpol, H.: A qualitative roentgenographic evaluation of root lengths in hypothyroid patients. Am. J. Orthodont., 47:588–589, 1961.

Carr, W. K.: Simultaneous mass retraction of maxillary anteriors with lingual root torque. J. Clin. Orthodont., 5:200–204, 1971.

DeShields, R. W.: A study of root resorption in treated Class II, Division 1 malocclusions. Angle Orthodont., 39:231–245, 1969.

Docking, A. R., Newbury, C. R., Donnison, J. A., and Storey, E.: The effect of orthodontic cements on tooth enamel. Dent. Rec., 72:243–256, 1952.

Dougherty, H. L.: The effect of mechanical forces upon the mandibular buccal segments during orthodontic treatment. Am. J. Orthodont., 54:29–49, 83–103, 1968.

Furstman, L., and Bernick, S.: Clinical considerations of the periodontium. Am. J. Orthodont., 61:138–155, 1972.

Gaudet, E. L.: Tissue changes in the monkey following root torque with the Begg technique. Am. J. Orthodont., 58:164–178, 1970.

Graber, T. M.: Post-treatment postmortems. Am. J. Orthodont., 52:331–352, 1966.

Gross, D. J.: The solubility of enamel as affected by cement under orthodontic bands. New York Dent. Soc. J., 17:201–206, 1951.

Haryett, R. D.: Study of traumatic tooth movement. Am. J. Orthodont., 48:627, 1962 (Abstract).

Hemley, S.: The etiology of root resorption of vital permanent teeth. Bull. Dent. Soc. N.Y., 5:7–19, Jan. 1938.

Hemley, S.: The incidence of root resorption of vital permanent teeth. J. Dent. Res., 20:133–141, 1941.

Henry, J. L., and Weinmann, J. P.: The pattern of resorption and repair of human cementum. J.A.D.A., 42:270–290, 1951.

Houston, W. J. B., and Miller, M. W.: Cements for orthodontic use. Dent. Practit., 19:104–109, 1968.

Ketcham, A. H.: A radiographic study of orthodontic tooth movement: a preliminary report. J.A.D.A., 42:1577–1598, 1927.

Ketcham, A. H.: A progress report of an investigation of apical root resorption of vital permanent teeth. Int. J. Orthodont., 15:310–328, 1929.

Lefkowitz, W.: Histological evidence of the harmful effect of cement under orthodontic bands. J. Dent. Res., 19:47–55, 1940.

Marshall, J. J.: Studies on apical absorption of permanent teeth, Part I. Int. J. Orthodont., 16:1–19, 1930.

Marshall, J. A.: Studies on apical absorption of permanent teeth, Part II. Int. J. Orthodont., 16:1035–1049, 1930.

Marshall, J. A.: The classification, etiology, diagnosis, prognosis, and treatment of radicular resorption of teeth. Int. J. Orthodont., 20:731–745, 1934.

Massler, M.: Root resorption in human permanent teeth. Am. J. Orthodont., 40:619–633, 1954.

McLaughlin, K. D.: Quantitative determination of root resorption during orthodontic treatment. Am. J. Orthodont., 50:143–150, 1964.

Muhler, J. C.: Dental Caries – Orthodontic Appliances – SnF_2. J. Dent. Child., 37:218–221, 1970.

Nabers, C. L.: Open contacts caused by night guard appliance. Case report. J. Periodont., 34:436–437, 1963.

Oppenheim, A.: Biologic orthodontic therapy and reality. Angle Orthodont., 6:5–38; 6:69–116, 1936.

Oppenheim, A.: Human response to orthodontic intervention of short and long duration. Am. J. Orthodont., 28:263–301, 1942.

Orban, R.: Biological problems in orthodontics. J.A.D.A., 23:1870, 1936.

Phillips, J. R.: Apical root resorption under orthodontic therapy. Angle Orthodont., 25:1–22, 1955.

Rudolph, C. E.: A comparative study in root resorption in permanent teeth. J.A.D.A., 23:822–826, 1936.

Rudolph, C. E.: An evaluation of root resorption occurring during orthodontic treatment. J. Dent. Res., 19:367–371, 1940.

Sakamaki, S. T., and Bahn, A. N.: Effect of orthodontic banding on localized oral lacto-bacilli. J. Dent. Res., 47:275–279, 1968.

Schluger, S.: The periodontist and the postorthodontic patient. D. Clin. North America, July, 1968, pp. 525–527.

Schwarz, A. M.: Tissue changes incident to orthodontic tooth movement. Int. J. Orthodont., 18:331–352, 1932.

Smith, R. S.: A radiographic evaluation of apical root resorption during orthodontic treatment. (Master's Thesis.) Northwestern University Dental School, Chicago, 1964.

Soltis, J. E., Makfoor, P. R., and Bowman, D. C.: Changes in ability of patients to differentiate intensity of forces applied to maxillary central incisors. J. Dent. Res., 50:590, 1971.

Steadman, S. R.: Resume of the literature on root resorption. Angle Orthodont., 12:28–38, 1942.

Thompson, H. E.: Orthodontic relapses analyzed in a study of connective tissue fibers. Am. J. Orthodont., 45:93–109, 1959.

Tirk, T. M.: Limitations in orthodontic treatment. Angle Orthodont., 35:165–177, 1965.

Zachrisson, S., and Zachrisson, B. U.: Gingival condition associated with orthodontic treatment. Angle Orthodont., 42:26–34, 1972.

Ziegler, J. T.: The comparative merits of cementing orthodontic bands on non-dehydrated and air-dried teeth. Am. J. Orthodont., 45:869–870, 1959.

18. EQUILIBRATION

Blume, D. G.: A study of occlusal equilibration as it relates to orthodontics. Am. J. Orthodont., 44:575–584, 1958.

Heide, M., and Thorpe, C. W.: The necessity for postorthodontic precision grinding for balanced occlusion. Angle Orthodont., 35:113–120, 1965.

Heimlich, A. C.: Occlusal equilibration in relation to orthodontic treatment. D. Clin. North America, November, 1960, pp. 807–813.

Posselt, U.: Occlusal rehabilitation. D. Pract., 9:255–259, 1959.

Ratcliff, P. A.: Relationship of periodontics and orthodontics with special reference to the periodontal problems created and helped by orthodontics. Bul. Pacific Coast Soc. Orthodont., 36:11–13, 1961 (Abstract).

Sved, A.: Occlusal equilibration in relation to orthodontic treatment. Equilibration as a postretention measure. D. Clin. North America, November, 1960, pp. 815–820.

19. PATIENT MOTIVATION AND MANAGEMENT

Allan, T. K., and Hodgson, E. W.: The use of personality measurements as a determinant of patient cooperation in an orthodontic practice. Am. J. Orthodont., 54:433–440, 1968.

Ando, Y.: Psychological responses of patients in orthodontic treatment. Am. J. Orthodont., 48:712–713, 1962 (Abstract).

Ash, A. S.: Psychosomatic considerations in orthodontics. Am. J. Orthodont., 36:292–300, 1950.

Astrachan, A.: Influence of emotional factors on orthodontic patients. Rev. Port. Estomat., 9:105–115, 1969.

Baldwin, D. C., Barnes, M. L., et al.: Social and cultural variables in the decision for orthodontic treatment. J. Dent. Res., 77:309–314, 1967.

Broekman, R. W.: The cooperation of patients in orthodontic treatment. Nederl. Tandheelk., 74:355–361, 1967.

Burns, M. H.: Personality rating scale for orthodontic patients. (Master's Thesis.) University of Tennessee, 1968.

Feldstein, L.: Problems of orthodontists in treating adolescents. Am. J. Orthodont., 45:131–140, 1959.

Fränkl, R.: (Handling of orthodontic appliances and the psychological preparation of patients.) Deutsch. Stomat., 14:287–300, 1964 (Ger.).

Gajda, Z.: The patient undergoing orthodontic treatment. Czas. Stomat., 23:141–156, 1970.

Gardner, J. H.: Crooked teeth: their prevention and cure. Dist. Nurs., 84:6–14, 1969.

Graber, T. M.: Patient motivation. J. Clin. Orthodont., 5:670–687, 1971.

Harris, J. G.: Some psychological differences between children with well-aligned incisors and those with spaced protrusive incisors as revealed by the "Blacky" projective test. Am. J. Orthodont., 48:625, 1962 (Abstract).

Hennis, I.: (Psychological considerations in orthodontic treatment.) Zahnärztl. Welt, 65:801–806, 1964 (Ger.).

Jarabak, J. R.: Patient motivation, discussion. J. Clin. Orthodont., 5:688–691, 1971.

Jenks, L.: How the dentist's behavior can influence the child's behavior. J. Dent. Child., 31:358–366, 1964.

Kreit, L. W., Burstone, C., and Delman, L.: Patient cooperation and orthodontic treatment. J. Am. Coll. Dent., 35:327–332, 1968.

Lewit, D. W., and Virolainen, K. M.: Conformity and independence in adolescents' motivation for orthodontic treatment. Child Develop., 39:1189–1200, 1968.

Lustman, S. L.: Emotional problems of children as they relate to orthodontics. Am. J. Orthodont., 46:358–362, 1960.

MacGregor, F. C.: Some psycho-social problems associated with facial deformities. Amer. Sociol. Rev., 16:629–638, 1951.

Maj, G., Grilli, S., and Belletti, M. F.: Psychological appraisal of children facing orthodontic treatment. Am. J. Orthodont., 53:849–857, 1967.

Mattingly, J. B.: An evaluation of patient attitude and cooperation. (Master's Thesis.) Northwestern University, Chicago, 1971.

Mueller, G., and Kloeters, R.: The professional psychologist as an assistant in the orthodontic clinic. Fortschr. Kieferorthop., 28:24–80, 1967.

Okun, J. H.: Increasing patient cooperation. J. Clin. Orthodont., 5:50–51, 1971.

Reitan, K.: Orthodontic treatment of patients with psychogenic, muscular and articulation disturbances. Tandlaegebladet, 75:1182–1197, 1971.

Sheldon. G. H.: Psychological factors in the etiology of malocclusion. New York Dent. J., 35:277–284, 1969.

Stricker, G.: Psychological issues pertaining to malocclusion. Am. J. Orthodont., 58:276–283, 1970.

20.   ORTHODONTIC HISTORY

Allen, W. I.: Historical aspects of roentgenographic cephalometry. Am. J. Orthodont., 49:451–459, 1963.

Anderson, G. M.: Years of change. Am. J. Orthodont., 50:521–527, 1964.

Angle, E. H.: Orthodontia as a specialty. Dental Cosmos, 44:905–910, 1902.

Baker, C. R.: Early orthodontics in the Chicago area. Am. J. Orthodont., 48:29–33, 1962.

Berg, R., and Johannesen, B.: The present status of orthodontics in Norway. J. Clin. Orthodont., 4:225–227, 1970.

Besombes, A.: Pierre Fauchard, Orthodontist. Rev. Belg. Méd. Dent., 18:839–850, 1963 (Fr.).

Brader, A. C.: Historical review of research findings of growth and development prior to the introduction of roentgenographic cephalometry. Angle Orthodont., 26:1–9, 1956.

Brodie, A. G.: Erratic evolution of orthodontics. Am. J. Orthodont., 47:116–123, 1961.

Case, C. S.: Question of extraction in orthodontia. (1911 debate) Am. J. Orthodont., 50:658–691; disc. 751–768: 843–851 editorial comment 862–865, 1964.

Castro, Frank M.: A historical sketch of orthodontics. Dental Cosmos, 76:130–134, 1931.

Chapman, H.: Orthodontics: fifty years in retrospect. Am. J. Orthodont., 42:421–442, 1956.

Cunat, J. J.: A perspective on orthodontics. Bull. Hist. Dent., 17:37–40, 1969.

Dewel, B. F.: Orthodontics' achievements and responsibilities. Am. J. Orthodont., 54:823–830, 1968.

"Father of Orthodontia." Pacific Dental Gazette, 38:744–745, 1930.

Hahn, G. W.: Edward Hartley Angle (1855–1930). New York J. Dent., 37:116–118, 1967.

Harding, J. F. A.: Orthodontic practice in New Zealand. J. Pract. Orthodont., 3:92–93, 1969.

Lischer, B. E.: Time to Tell: A Comment on Orthodontic Orthodoxy and Other Essays. New York, Vantage Press, 1955.

Neumann, B. Orthodontic therapy. Cesk. Stomat., 69:323–333, 1969.

Noyes, Frederick B.: The teaching of orthodontia as he viewed it. Dental Cosmos, 73:802–808, 1931.

Osburn, R. C.: The breadth of his vision as a specialist. Dental Cosmos, 73:808–821, 1931.

Pollock, H. C.: Extraction debate of 1911 by Case, Dewey, and Cryer. Introduction. Am. J. Orthodont., 50:656–657, 1964.

Pollock, H. C., Sr.: Genesis of specialization. Am. J. Orthodont., 48:21–28, 1962.

Shankland, W. M.: The American Association of Orthodontists: the biography of a specialty organization. St. Louis, American Association of Orthodontists, 1971.

Weinberger, B. W.: Historical resume of the evaluation and growth of orthodontia. J.A.D.A., 21:2001–2021, 1934.

Weinberger, B. W.: Orthodontics, an Historical Review of Its Origin and Evolution. St. Louis, C. V. Mosby Co., 1926.

Wylie, W. L.: Orthodontic concepts since Edward H. Angle. Angle Orthodont., 26:59–67, 1956.

21. SURGICAL ORTHODONTICS

Angle, E. H.: Double resection for the treatment of mandibular protrusion. Dental Cosmos, 45:268–274, 1903.

Barton, P. R., and Rayne, J.: The role of alveolar surgery in the treatment of malocclusion. Brit. Dent. J., 126:11–27, 1969.

Bell, W. H.: Surgical-orthodontic correction of adult malocclusions. Angle Orthodont., 23:71–77, 1953.

Bell, W. H.: Alessandra, P. A., and Condit, C. L.: Surgical-orthodontic correction of Class II malocclusion. J. Oral Surg., 26:265–272, 1968.

Brandt, S.: Surgical orthodontics. J. Clin. Orthodont., 6:196–202, 1972.

Byrd, D. L., and Murphey, P. J.: The surgical approach to Class III malocclusions. J.A.D.A., 28:813–818, 1971.

Buchanan, G.: Surgical intervention as an aid to orthodontics. Ann. Aust. Coll. Dent. Surg., 1:70–77, 1967.

Castro, O. O.: Surgical correction of prognathism: angled osteoplasty of the mandibular rami. Brit. J. Plast. Surg., 20:57, 1967.

Charest, A., and Maranda, G.: New method for surgical correction of maxillary protrusion. J. Canad. Dent. Ass., 34:630–635, 1968.

Converse, J. M., and Horowitz, S. L.: The surgical orthodontic approach to the treatment of dentofacial deformities. Am. J. Orthodont., 55:217–243, 1969.

Dingman, R. O., and Dodenhoff, T. G.: Surgical correction of mandibular deformities. *In* Grabb, W. C., Rosenstein, S. W., and Bzoch, K. R. (ed.): Cleft Lip and Palate. Boston, Little, Brown, and Company, 1971, p. 499.

Edwards, J. G.: A surgical procedure to eliminate rotational relapse. Am. J. Orthodont., 57:35–46, 1970.

Ewen, S. J.: Periodontal surgery—an adjunct to orthodontic therapy. J. Periodont., 21:162, 1964.

Graber, T. M.: Team effort—oral surgery and orthodontics. J. Oral Surg., 25:201–224, 1967.

Hamula, W.: Surgical alteration of muscle attachments to enhance esthetics and denture stability. Am. J. Orthodont., 57:327–369, 1970.

Hawkinson, R. T.: Retrognathia correction by means of an arcing osteotomy in the ascending ramus. J. Prosth. Dent., 20:77–86, 1968.

Henry, T. C., and Wreakes, G.: The surgical positioning of labial segments in the treatment of malocclusion. Dent. Pract., 18:329–341, 1968.

Hinds, E. C., Galbreath, J. C., and Sills, A. H.: Selection of procedure in the management of jaw deformities. Plast. Reconstr. Surg., 29:176–185, 1962.

Hinds, E. C., Broussard, G. J., and Norris, C. W.: The team approach in the correction of maxillary protrusion. J.A.D.A., 73:1337–1341, 1966.

Hovell, J. H.: Orthodontic considerations in the surgical correction of mandibular prognathism. Europ. Orthodont. Soc. Tr., 37:205–215, 1961.

Laskin, D. M., and Peskin, S.: Surgical aids in orthodontics. D. Clin. North America, July, 1968, pp. 509–524.

MacIntosh, R. B.: Orthodontic surgery; comments on diagnostic modalities. J. Oral Surg., 28:249–259, 1970.

MacIntosh, R. B.: The surgical approach to Class II, Division 1 Malocclusion. J.A.D.A., 28:796–804, 1971.

Moss, J. P.: The transplantation of maxillary canines. J. Clin. Orthodont., 4:77–81, 1970.

Mills, P. B.: The orthodontist's role in surgical correction of dentofacial deformities. Am. J. Orthodont., 56:266–272, 1969.

Murphey, P. J., and Walker, R. V.: Correction of maxillary protrusion by ostectomy and orthodontic therapy. J. Oral Surg., 21:275–290, 1963.

Murphey, P. J., and Walker, R. V.: Orthodontic and surgical procedures for correction of severe oral and facial malformation. J.A.D.A., 79:1431–1440, 1969.

Nordenram, A.: Vertical subcondylar osteotomy in the treatment of mandibular protrusion. Norske Tanlaeg. Tid., 78:394–407, 1968.

Obwegeser, H. L.: Surgical correction of maxillary deformities. *In* Grabb, W. C., Rosenstein, S. W., and Bzoch, K. R. (ed.): Cleft Lip and Palate. Boston, Little, Brown, and Co., 1971, p. 515.

Peskin, S., and Graber, T. M.: Surgical positioning of teeth. J.A.D.A., 80:1320–1326, 1970.

Peterson, L. W., and Wilson, A. E.: Surgical adjuncts to orthodontic treatment. D. Clin. North America, July, 1964, pp. 371–382.

Proffit, W. R., and White, R. P.: Treatment of severe malocclusions by correlated surgical-orthodontic procedures. Angle Orthodont., 40:1–10, 1970.

Revell, J. H.: Surgical orthodontics. New methods to stimulate and direct eruption. Int. J. Orthodont., 2:5–20, 1964.

Robinson, M.: Open vertical osteotomies of the rami for correction of mandibular deformities. Am. J. Orthodont., 46:425–432, 1960.

Robinson, M., and Dougherty, H. L.: Mandibulofacial dysostosis—report of surgical orthodontic occlusion treatment of a case. J. S. Calif. Dent. Ass., 37:457–460, 1969.

Robinson, M., and Dougherty, H. L.: Prognathism questions in the surgical-orthodontic team. Am. J. Orthodont., 47:531–533, 1961.

Robinson, M., and Stoughton, D.: Surgical-orthodontic treatment of a case of hemifacial microsomia. Am. J. Orthodont., 57:287–292, 1970.

Salzmann, J. A.: An appraisal of surgical orthodontics. Am. J. Orthodont., 61:105–114, 1972.

Straith, R. E., and Lawson, J. M.: Surgical orthodontia: a new horizon for plastic surgery. Plast. Reconstr. Surg., 39:366–372, 1967.

Williamson, J. J.: Surgical positioning of maxillary canines. Report of a case. Oral Surg., 17:289–295, 1964.

Zadok, B.: Minor surgery in the maxilla preceding orthodontic treatment of the jaws. Sweisz. Monatschr. Zahnheilk., 78:426–430, 1968.

22. STATISTICS

Armitage, S.: Statistical Methods in Medical Research. New York, John Wiley & Sons, 1971.

Bliss, C. I.: Statistics in Biology: Statistical Methods for Research in the Natural Sciences. New York, McGraw-Hill, 1967.

Dixon, W. J., and Massey, F. J.: Introduction to Statistical Analysis. 3rd ed. New York, McGraw-Hill, 1968.

Fisher, R. A.: Statistical methods for research workers. 13th ed. New York, Hafner, 1967.

Garn, S. M.: Statistics: a review. Angle Orthodont., 28:149–165, 1958.

Hill, A. B.: Principles of Medical Statistics. 7th ed. New York, Oxford University Press, 1961.

Hodges, J. L., and Lehman, E. L.: Basic Concepts of Probability and Statistics. San Francisco, Holden-Day, 1964.

Mosteller, F., Rourke, R. E. K., and Thomas, G. B.: Probability, a First Course. 2nd ed. Reading, Addison-Wesley, 1970.

Romington, R. D., and Schork, M. A.: Statistics with Applications to the Biological and Health Sciences. Englewood Cliffs, N.J. Prentice-Hall, 1970.

Snedecor, G. W., and Cochran, W. G.: Statistical Methods. 6th ed. Ames, Iowa, Iowa State University Press, 1967.

Tanur, J., et al.: Statistics; A Guide to the Unknown. San Francisco, Holden-Day, 1972.

Thurow, R. C.: Statistics — lighthouse or Lorelei? Angle Orthodont., 28:61–78, 1958.

23. MISCELLANEOUS

Adler, T., Conark, S. C., Cote, E. F., Fields, R. S. Fine, H. S., Gurin, L. R., and Thomas, A. I.: Owning, planning, equipping an orthodontic office. J. Clin. Orthodont., 6: 221–230, 1972.

Andreasen, G. F.: Selection of the square and rectangular wires in clinical practice. Angle Orthodont., 42:81–84, 1972.

Ash, M. M., Jr.: Occlusion as taught at the University of Michigan. J. Dent. Educ., 33:83–88, 1969.

Bernstein, M.: Orthodontics in periodontal and prosthetic therapy. J. Periodont., 40: 577–587, 1969.

Blount, W. P.: Early recognition and prompt evaluation of spinal deformity. Wisc. Med. J., 68:245–249, 1967.

Brouwer, H., and Van Hillegondsberg, A. J.: Standardized intraoral photography. J. Pract. Orthodont., 3:239–246, 1969.

Campbell, M. E. A.: Post-treatment loss of teeth in a group of orthodontic patients. Brit. Dent. J., 127:469–471, 1969.

Chavoor, A. G.: Relation of the general practitioner of dentistry and the orthodontist. J.A.D.A., 63:632–635, 1961.

Dewel, B. F.: Two decades: one past, one future. Am. J. Orthodont., 57:79–83, 1970.

Foster, H. R.: Malocclusion associated with poliomyelitis. Am. J. Orthodont., 51:595–603, 1965.

Galante, J., et al.: Forces acting in the Milwaukee brace on patients undergoing treatment for idiopathic scoliosis. J. Bone Joint Surg., 52:498–506, 1970.

Gerdin, O.: Supervised bite development from the age of six years. Frequency of disturbances of bite development and need for their treatment. Early diagnosis and early therapy. Svensk. Tandläk. Tid., 62:296–309, 1969.

Graber, T. M.: Auxiliary personnel—pillars of practice procedure. Am. J. Orthodont., 51:412–434, 1965.

Graber, T. M.: Countdown in orthodontic education. J. Dent. Educ., 31:128–137, 1967.

Graber, T. M.: Current concepts of orthodontic treatment in the United States. Aust. Dent. J., 7:355–362, 1962.

Graber, T. M.: Requisites of orthodontic techniques in general practice. J. Tennessee Dent. A., 43:196–204, 1963.

Graber, T. M.: Visual and auditory aids: their role in national and sectional orthodontic meetings. Am. J. Orthodont., 45:528–533, 1959.

Graber, T. M., and Chung, D. B.: Orthodontics in 1969. Am. J. Orthodont., 45:655–681, 1959.

Hannett, H. A.: Undergraduate education. Am. J. Orthodont., 49:507–520, 1963.

Herzog, P. W.: Have you considered the incorporation of your orthodontic practice? Am. J. Orthodont., 56:613–616, 1969.

Hitchcock, H. P.: Malocclusion associated with scoliosis. Angle Orthodont., 39:64–68, 1969.

Horowitz, H. S., Thorburn, B. R., and Summers, C. J.: Occlusal relations in an optimally fluoridated community: I. Clinical methods. Angle Orthodont., 40:59–68, 1970.

Horowitz, H. S., and Doyle, J.: Occlusal relations in children born and reared in an optimally fluoridated community. II. Clinical findings. Angle Orthodont., 40:104–111, 1970.

Howard, C. C.: A preliminary report of infraocclusion of the molars and premolars produced by orthopedic treatment of scoliosis. Int. J. Orthodont., 12:434–437, 1926.

Hull, D. F.: An electromyographic study of the effects of the Milwaukee brace on the temporal and masseter muscles. Am. J. Orthodont., 54:151–152, 1968.

Joondeph, D. R.: Pont's index; a clinical evaluation. Angle Orthodont., 40:112–118, 1970.

Leighton, B. C.: The time factor in orthodontics. Brit. Dent. J., 124:161–166, 1968.

Lindegard, B., Lindegard, L., Carlson, M., and Larsson, S.: Need and demand for orthodontic treatment. Tandlaegebladet, 75:1198–1210, 1971.

Luedtke, G. L.: Management of the dentition of patients under treatment for scoliosis using the Milwaukee brace. Am. J. Orthodont., 57:607–614, 1970.

Mayerson, M.: Group practice—how and why? Angle Orthodont., 41:324–331, 1971.

Millstein, P. L., Kronman, J. H., and Clark, R. E.: Hydroptic measuring system for testing the accuracy of interocclusal recording mediums. J. Dent. Res., 49:462–463, 1970.

Nasby, J. A., Isaacson, R. J., Worms, F. W., and Speidel, T. M.: Orthodontic extractions and the facial skeletal pattern. Angle Orthodont., 42:116–122, 1972.

Pollack, J. J.: The effects of the Milwaukee brace on the dentition and jaws. J. Nat. Med. Ass., 62:27–35, 1970.

Proffit, W. R., et al.: Generalized muscular weakness with severe anterior open bite. Am. J. Orthodont., 54:104–110, 1968.

Rathbone, J. S., and Reynolds, J. M.: The management of transfer cases. Am. J. Orthodont., 56:252–265, 1969.

Reitan, K.: To what extent can orthodontics be a contributory factor in the treatment of periodontic cases? Am. J. Orthodont., 48:934–938, 1962 (Abstract).

Ringqvist, M., and Thilander, B.: The frequency of partial anodontia in orthodontics. Svensk. Tandlak. Tid., 62:535–541, 1969.

Rock, W. P., and Baker, R.: The effect of the Milwaukee brace upon dentofacial growth. Angle Orthodont., 42:96–102, 1972.

Rogers, G. A., and Wagner, M. J.: Protection of stripped enamel surfaces with topical fluoride applications. Am. J. Orthodont., 56:551–559, 1969.

Roth, N. M.: The modified monobloc appliance in scoliosis treatment. Am. J. Orthodont., 55:506–509, 1969.

Rubin, A.: Legal aspects of administrative problems. J. Clin. Orthodont., 6:203–217, 1972.

Shankland, W. M.: The AAO library: A major accomplishment. 61:409–412, 1972.

Stuteville, O. H.: Injuries caused by orthodontic forces and the ultimate result of these injuries. Am. J. Orthodont & Oral Surg., 24:103–118, 1938.

Swain, B. F.: Cooperation between general practitioner and orthodontist. J.A.D.A., 67:405–410, 1963.

Wagers, L. E.: Clean and check. J. Pract. Orthodont., 3:370–374, 1969.

Weber, F. N.: How can we educate more orthodontists? Am. J. Orthodont., 51:58–64, 1965.

Stoller, A. E.: The Universal Appliance. St. Louis, C. V. Mosby Co., 1971.

Thurow, R. C.: Atlas of Orthodontic Principles. St. Louis, C. V. Mosby Co., 1970.

Thurow, R. C.: Edgewise Orthodontics. 3rd edition. St. Louis, C. V. Mosby Co., 1973.

Tweed, C. H.: Clinical Orthodontics. St. Louis, C. V. Mosby Co., 1966.

24.   OTHER TEXTBOOKS IN ORTHODONTICS

Adams, C. P.: The Design and Construction of Removable Orthodontic Appliances. 4th ed. Bristol, John Wright & Sons, 1060.

Anderson, G. M.: Practical Orthodontics. St. Louis, C. V. Mosby Co., 1960.

Angle, E. H.: Malocclusion of the Teeth. 7th ed. Philadelphia, S. S. White Dental Mfg. Co., 1907.

Begg, P. R., and Kesling, P. C.: Begg Orthodontic Theory and Technique. 2nd ed. Philadelphia, W. B. Saunders Co., 1971.

Case, C. S.: Dental Orthopedia. New York, Leo Bruder, 1963.

Dahlberg, A. A.: Dental Morphology and Evolution. Chicago, University of Chicago Press, 1971.

Dickson, G. C.: Orthodontics in General Dental Practice. Rev. ed. London, Pitman Medical Publishing Co., Ltd., 1964.

Fastlicht, J.: The Universal Appliance Technique. Philadelphia, W. B. Saunders Co., 1972.

Fogel, M. S., and Magill, J. M.: The Combination Technique in Orthodontic Practice. Philadelphia, J. B. Lippincott Co., 1972.

Graber, T. M. (ed.): Current Orthodontic Concepts and Techniques. Philadelphia, W. B. Saunders Co., 1969.

Hemley, S.: A Text on Orthodontics. Washington, Coiner Publications, 1971.

Horowitz, S. L., and Hixon, E. H.: The Nature of Orthodontic Diagnosis. St. Louis, C. V. Mosby Co., 1966.

Hotz, R.: Early Treatment of Cleft Lip and Palate. Berne, Hans Huber, 1964.

Hotz, R.: Orthodontics in Everyday Practice. Berne, Hans Huber, 1963.

Hotz, R.: Orthodontie in der taglichen Praxis. Bern, Hans Huber, 1970.

Jarabak, J. R.: Management of an Orthodontic Practice. St. Louis, C. V. Mosby Co., 1965.

Jarabak, J. R.: Technique and Treatment with the Light Wire Appliance. 2nd edition. St. Louis, C. V. Mosby Co., 1973.

Lischer, B. E.: Principles and Methods of Orthodontics. Philadelphia, Lea & Febiger, 1912.

Moyers, R. E.: Handbook of Orthodontics. 3rd edition. Chicago, Yearbook Medical Publishers, 1973.

Lundström, A.: Introduction to Orthodontics. New York, McGraw-Hill, 1961.

Pruzansky, S.: Congenital Anomalies of the Face and Associated Structures. Springfield, Charles C Thomas, 1961.

Riedel, R. A., and Kraus, B. S.: Vistas in Orthodontics. Philadelphia, Lea & Febiger, 1962.

Salzmann, J. A.: Practice of Orthodontics. Philadelphia, J. B. Lippincott Co., 1966.

Sassouni, V., and Forrest, E. J.: Orthodontics in Dental Practice. St. Louis, C. V. Mosby Co., 1971.

Schwarz, A. M., and Gratzinger, M.: Removable Orthodontic Appliances. Philadelphia, W. B. Saunders Co., 1966.

Shepard, E. S.: Technique and Treatment With the Twin Wire Appliance. St. Louis, C. V. Mosby Co., 1961.

Simon, P. W.: Fundamental Principles of Systematic Diagnosis of Dental Anomalies. (Trans. B. E. Lischer) Boston, The Stratford Co., 1926.

Stoller, A. E.: The Universal Appliance. St. Louis, C. V. Mosby Co., 1971.

AUDIO-VISUAL MATERIALS IN ORTHODONTICS AND ASSOCIATED DENTAL FIELDS

Programmed teaching, computer-assisted instruction and the programmed individual presentation system are now an academic way of life. All make heavy use of relevant audio-visual aids. Whether these are under control of the student, instructor or both, audio-visual sequences provide information and stimulate learning in a manner not possible with conventional lecture techniques.

A large number of films and sequences are now available from dental schools, professional societies and commercial sources. Those interested in obtaining these teaching (and learning) aids should write to the Bureau of Audio-Visual Service, American Dental Association, 211 East Chicago, Chicago, Illinois 60611. A complete film and slide catalogue of selections currently available from the A.D.A. Library will be sent on request. Many of these may either be rented or purchased for a nominal sum.

The American Association of Orthodontists, 7477 Delmar, St. Louis, Missouri 63130, has developed the most comprehensive specialty audio-visual service available anywhere. Automated slide-tape sequences and movies on a large variety of orthodontic subjects, by outstanding authorities, are available for rental. Some may be purchased by educational institutions merely for the cost of duplication and processing. Information may be obtained from the A.A.O. by writing to the Executive Director.

In 1972, a new continuing education program was introduced by the American Association of Orthodontists, providing a series of sequences, obtainable on a two-year subscription basis. Each month a program is being sent, including a filmstrip, audio cassette and program guide. A biographical sketch of the author and a bibliography is included, when applicable. Selected audio-visual equipment is distributed with the subscription, along with custom-designed cassette/filmstrip binders, which all become the property of the subscriber. Information on this continuing education program may be obtained from the American Association of Orthodontists, or from Communico, Inc., Educational Systems Division, 1315 North Highway Drive, Fenton, Missouri 63026.

AUTHOR
REFERENCE INDEX

SUBJECT INDEX

Page numbers given in *italic* type refer to illustrations.

A

ACCIDENTS, and malocclusion, 328, 485, *485*
  as cause of missing teeth, 348, *355–356*
Acromegaly, and malocclusion, 288, *291*
  effects on mandible, 132, *132*
Age, as factor in tooth movement, 516–518, *517*
All or none law, and muscle physiology, 137
Alveolar bone. See *Bone.*
Anchorage, Baker, 531, *532*
  extraoral, *520*, 522
  intermaxillary, *520*, 522
  intramaxillary, *520*, 522
  intraoral, *520*, 521
  multiple, *520*, 522
  reciprocal, *520*, 521
  stationary, 519, *520*
  types of, 519–522, *520*
Angle, E. H., career of, 3
  classification of occlusion, 227, 228
  edgewise appliance of, 534, *535*

Angle, E. H. *(Continued)*
  pin and tube appliance of, 530, *531*
  ribbon arch appliance of, 530, *531*
  theories of occlusion, 183, *183*
Ankylosis, in child patient, 390–393, *391*
Anodontia, 348, *348*
Apical base. See *Base.*
Appliance(s), habit control, in cheek biting, 699, *699–702*
  in finger sucking, 679–686, *682–685*, 687
  in lip biting and sucking, 693–699, *695–698*
  in tongue thrust, 688–693, *689–692*
  removable, 699–703, *699–702*
 orthodontic, 528–608
  Baker anchorage for, 531, *532*
  cervical traction, 884–888, *886–887*
  chincap, *706*
  development of, 528–541, *529–533, 535–542*
  differential light force, development of, 538, *539–542*